MYOCARDITIS

From Bench to Bedside

MYOCARDITIS

From Bench to Bedside

EDITED BY

Leslie T. Cooper, Jr., MD

Consultant, Division of Cardiovascular Diseases
and Internal Medicine, Mayo Clinic;
Assistant Professor of Medicine, Mayo Medical School;
Rochester, Minnesota

HUMANA PRESS
TOTOWA, NEW JERSEY

Cover design by Kathryn K. Shepel.

This publication is printed on acid-free paper. ∞
ANSI Z39.48-1984 (American National Standards Institute)
Permanence of Paper for Printed Library Materials.

Printed in the United States of America. 10 9 8 7 6 5 4 3 2 1

Library of Congress Cataloging-in-Publication Data

Myocarditis: from bench to bedside / edited by Leslie T. Cooper, Jr.
     p. ; cm.
   Includes bibliographical references and index.
   ISBN 1-58829-112-X/03 (alk. paper)
   1. Myocarditis.   I. Cooper, Leslie T.
   [DNLM: 1. Myocarditis. 2. Cardiomyopathy, Congestive. WG 280 M99758 2002]
   RC685.M92 M64 2002
   616.1'24--dc21   2002069097

Preface

Many readers may recall a family member, friend, or acquaintance who died suddenly with no history of heart disease or who acutely developed heart failure of unknown cause. These are common clinical presentations of patients who have acute myocarditis. Myocarditis, often related to a viral infection, contributes substantially to dilated cardiomyopathy and the burden of heart failure worldwide. In the 8 years since the last monograph on myocarditis was published, knowledge of viral-induced myocardial injury, autoimmune pathways in the heart, and the clinical treatment of myocarditis has advanced significantly. New cardiotropic viruses have been described. The causal mechanisms between acute viral infection and dilated cardiomyopathy have been elucidated in great detail. It is timely to draw together in one volume the threads of research on viral myocarditis, autoimmune myocardial injury, and clinical advances in myocarditis for the benefit of the practicing physician and the specialized researcher. This book is written equally for the clinician confronted with suspected myocarditis and the specialized investigator. It seeks to give each a framework and greater context for study.

This is the first volume that attempts to cover the entire spectrum of myocarditis from basic research to bedside medicine. The first chapter provides an introduction to experimental myocarditis. Dr. Charles Gauntt is an authority in the field of virology who is well equipped to provide such an overview. The members of Dr. Steven Tracy's premier enteroviral research laboratory contributed the second chapter on viral life cycle and the earliest events in the molecular pathogenesis of experimental coxsackie and adenoviral myocarditis.

Chapters 3 through 6 address the immune reaction that results in postviral myocarditis. The multifaceted immune response is described by several closely related topics. Dr. Sally Huber begins the discussion with a chapter on the cellular immune response, followed by Dr. Bernhard Maisch's chapter on the humoral immune response. These chapters emphasize the central role of Th1 and Th2 lymphocytes in postviral autoimmune myocarditis. In Chapter 5, Dr. Akira Matsumori, discusses the beneficial and detrimental roles of cytokines in postviral myocarditis. The terrific expansion of knowledge of nitric oxide biology justified a separate chapter by Drs. Joshua Hare and Charles Lowenstein on the roles of nitric oxide in viral infection and postviral heart disease.

The next 4 chapters cover translational research and seek to bridge basic biologic investigations and the clinical disorders. Dr. Bruce McManus and his laboratory colleagues cover extensive experimental data on the role of programmed cell death, apoptosis, in viral myocarditis in Chapter 7. Dr. Makoto Kodama describes experimental autoimmune (versus postviral) giant cell and lymphocytic myocarditis in rat and mouse models in Chapter 8. The role of the adrenergic system in experimental and human dilated cardiomyopathy and the implications for treatment of human disease are described next. This section concludes with a chapter on the latest available data on enteroviral proteases and cardiomyopathy from Dr. Kirk Knowlton's laboratory.

The diagnosis, prognosis, and treatment of nonspecific and specific myocarditides are covered in Chapters 11 through 24. The strengths and limitations of noninvasive tests, including serologic biomarkers, measures of apoptosis, nuclear imaging, and echocardiography, are covered in detail. The technique and interpretation of endomyocardial biopsy are placed at the center of this section. Separate chapters are devoted to major idiopathic clinical entities, including cardiac sarcoidosis, giant cell myocarditis, and the eosinophilic myocarditides. Specific infectious diseases that affect the heart include Chagas disease, rheumatic fever, and human immunodeficiency virus-related cardiomyopathy. The book concludes with state-of-the-art chapters on myocarditis in children and peripartum cardiomyopathy.

A second objective of this book is to foster exchange of new ideas between basic and clinical investigators through a collation of parallel, related research. Leaders in experimental myocarditis can read of their clinical colleagues' latest progress and opinions and vice versa. I hope this book forms a platform for new research collaborations to grow. I am heartened that students of the clinical and basic sciences can glimpse in these chapters the excitement of participation in a decades-long, worldwide, multidisciplinary effort and sense the satisfaction of many investigators.

I thank all of my colleagues who have generously contributed to this work, in particular, Dr. Kirk U. Knowlton for his counsel and encouragement early on, for without him this project would not have started; Dr. Joseph G. Murphy, whose experience I sought on many occasions and who heard my frustrations and shared in the pleasure of the final proof; Dr. Carol L. Kornblith (editor), who read every word at least four times and patiently heard and taught me; and the production staff, including Kathryn K. Shepel (art director), Roberta J. Schwartz (production editor), Virginia A. Dunt (editorial assistant), and John P. Hedlund (proofreader). I thank my dear wife, Jane, without whose support and encouragement (and ruthless editing) this project could not have happened.

Leslie T. Cooper, Jr., MD

Dedication

This book is dedicated to my mentors.

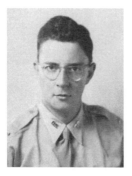

John Joyce Saÿen, MD

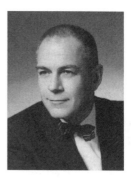

John J. Joyce III, MD

Contents

Contributors

Yoshifusa Aizawa, MD, The First Department of Internal Medicine, Niigata University School of Medicine, Niigata, Japan

Kristen A. Atkins, MD, Clinical Instructor in Surgical Pathology, Department of Pathology, Stanford University Medical Center, Stanford, California; Presently, Assistant Professor of Pathology, Medical College of Virginia, Richmond, Virginia

Cornel Badorff, MD, Department of Medicine, Goethe-University, Frankfurt, Germany

Ragavendra Baliga, MD, Clinical Assistant Professor of Medicine, University of Michigan, Ann Arbor, Michigan

Gerald J. Berry, MD, Associate Professor of Pathology, Director of Cardiac Pathology, Stanford University Medical Center, Stanford, California

Neil E. Bowles, PhD, Department of Pediatrics (Cardiology), Baylor College of Medicine, Houston, Texas

Steven D. Carson, PhD, Department of Pathology and Microbiology, University of Nebraska Medical Center, Omaha, Nebraska

Chris Carthy, BSc, Department of Pathology and Laboratory Medicine, University of British Columbia (UBC)-St. Paul's Hospital, Providence Health Care, Vancouver, British Columbia, Canada

Y. Chandrashekhar, MD, Associate Professor of Medicine, Division of Cardiology, University of Minnesota School of Medicine, Minneapolis, Minnesota

Nora M. Chapman, PhD, Department of Pathology and Microbiology, University of Nebraska Medical Center, Omaha, Nebraska

Paul Cheung, BSc, Department of Pathology and Laboratory Medicine, University of British Columbia (UBC)-St. Paul's Hospital, Providence Health Care, Vancouver, British Columbia, Canada

Prem Chopra, MD, Professor of Pathology, Cardiothoracic Center, All India Institute of Medical Sciences, New Delhi, India

Jonathan Choy, BSc, Department of Pathology and Laboratory Medicine, University of British Columbia (UBC)-St. Paul's Hospital, Providence Health Care, Vancouver, British Columbia, Canada

Leslie T. Cooper, Jr., MD, Consultant, Division of Cardiovascular Diseases and Internal Medicine, Mayo Clinic; Assistant Professor of Medicine, Mayo Medical School; Rochester, Minnesota

Darya Dabiri, Department of Pathology and Laboratory Medicine, University of British Columbia (UBC)-St. Paul's Hospital, Providence Health Care, Vancouver, British Columbia, Canada

G. William Dec, MD, Medical Director, Cardiac Transplantation Program, Massachusetts General Hospital, Boston, Massachusetts

Mitra Esfandiarei, MSc, Department of Pathology and Laboratory Medicine, University of British Columbia (UBC)-St. Paul's Hospital, Providence Health Care, Vancouver, British Columbia, Canada

Robert P. Frantz, MD, Consultant, Division of Cardiovascular Diseases and Internal Medicine, Mayo Clinic; Assistant Professor of Medicine, Mayo Medical School; Rochester, Minnesota

Charles J. Gauntt, PhD, Department of Microbiology, The University of Texas Health Science Center at San Antonio, Texas

Gerald J. Gleich, MD, Consultant, Division of Allergic Diseases and Internal Medicine and the Department of Immunology, Mayo Clinic; Professor of Medicine and of Immunology, Mayo Medical School; Rochester, Minnesota

David Granville, PhD, Department of Pathology and Laboratory Medicine, University of British Columbia (UBC)-St. Paul's Hospital, Providence Health Care, Vancouver, British Columbia, Canada

James M. Hagar, MD, Associate Clinical Professor of Medicine, University of California Irvine, School of Medicine, Irvine, California

Joshua M. Hare, MD, Division of Cardiology, Department of Medicine, The Johns Hopkins Medical Institutions, Baltimore, Maryland

Katja Höfling, MD, Department of Pathology and Microbiology, University of Nebraska Medical Center, Omaha, Nebraska

Sally A. Huber, PhD, Professor of Pathology, Department of Pathology, University of Vermont, Burlington, Vermont

Tohru Izumi, MD, The Second Department of Internal Medicine, Kitasato University School of Medicine, Sagamihara, Japan

Allan S. Jaffe, MD, Consultant, Division of Cardiovascular Diseases and Internal Medicine and Department of Laboratory Medicine and Pathology, Mayo Clinic; Professor of Medicine, Mayo Medical School; Rochester, Minnesota

Gail M. Kephart, BS, Research Technologist, Division of Allergic Diseases and Internal Medicine, Mayo Clinic, Rochester, Minnesota

Kyung-Soo Kim, PhD, Department of Pathology and Microbiology, University of Nebraska Medical Center, Omaha, Nebraska

Karin Klingel, MD, Department of Molecular Pathology, University Hospital of Tübingen, Germany

Kirk U. Knowlton, MD, Department of Medicine, University of California, San Diego, California

Makoto Kodama, MD, The First Department of Internal Medicine, Niigata University School of Medicine, Niigata, Japan

Ismail Laher, PhD, Department of Pharmacology and Therapeutics, Faculty of Medicine, University of British Columbia, Vancouver, British Columbia, Canada

Charles J. Lowenstein, MD, Division of Cardiology, Department of Medicine, The Johns Hopkins Medical Institutions, Baltimore, Maryland

Amy Lui, MSc, Department of Pathology and Laboratory Medicine, University of British Columbia (UBC)-St. Paul's Hospital, Providence Health Care, Vancouver, British Columbia, Canada

Honglin Luo, MD, Department of Pathology and Laboratory Medicine, University of British Columbia (UBC)-St. Paul's Hospital, Providence Health Care, Vancouver, British Columbia, Canada

Bernhard Maisch, MD, Director and Professor, Department of Internal Medicine—Cardiology, Philipps University, Marburg, Germany

Ružica Maksimović, MD, PhD, University Institute for Cardiovascular Diseases, Medical Center of Serbia, Belgrade

Jay W. Mason, MD, Jack M. Gill Professor; Chairman, Department of Medicine, University of Kentucky, Lexington, Kentucky

Akira Matsumori, MD, PhD, Department of Cardiovascular Medicine, Kyoto University Graduate School of Medicine, Kyoto, Japan

Bruce M. McManus, MD, PhD, Department of Pathology and Laboratory Medicine, University of British Columbia (UBC)-St. Paul's Hospital, Providence Health Care, Vancouver, British Columbia, Canada

Joseph G. Murphy, MD, Consultant, Division of Cardiovascular Diseases and Internal Medicine, Mayo Clinic; Associate Professor of Medicine, Mayo Medical School; Rochester, Minnesota

Jagat Narula, MD, PhD, Thomas J. Vischer Professor, Department of Medicine, Director, Heart Failure and Transplantation Center, MCP-Hahnemann University School of Medicine, Philadelphia, Pennsylvania

Navneet Narula, MD, Assistant Professor, Department of Pathology, University of Pennsylvania School of Medicine, Philadelphia, Pennsylvania

Yuji Okura, MD, The First Department of Internal Medicine, Niigata University School of Medicine, Niigata, Japan

Lyle J. Olson, MD, Consultant, Division of Cardiovascular Diseases and Internal Medicine, Mayo Clinic; Associate Professor of Medicine, Mayo Medical School; Rochester, Minnesota

Shahbudin H. Rahimtoola, MB, George C. Griffith Professor of Cardiology, Chairman, Griffith Center, Professor of Medicine, Keck School of Medicine at University of Southern California, Los Angeles, California

Arsen D. Ristić, MD, MSc, University Institute for Cardiovascular Diseases, Medical Center of Serbia, Belgrade, and Department of Internal Medicine–Cardiology, Philipps University, Marburg, Germany

Petar M. Seferović, MD, PhD, University Institute for Cardiovascular Diseases, Medical Center of Serbia, Belgrade

Simon Sinn, BSc, Department of Pathology and Laboratory Medicine, University of British Columbia (UBC)-St. Paul's Hospital, Providence Health Care, Vancouver, British Columbia, Canada

Jeffrey A. Towbin, MD, Departments of Pediatrics (Cardiology), Molecular and Human Genetics, and Cardiovascular Sciences, Baylor College of Medicine, Texas Children's Hospital, Houston, Texas

Steven Tracy, PhD, Department of Pathology and Microbiology, University of Nebraska Medical Center, Omaha, Nebraska

Aikun Wang, MD, Department of Pathology and Laboratory Medicine, University of British Columbia (UBC)-St. Paul's Hospital, Providence Health Care, Vancouver, British Columbia, Canada

Kevin Wei, MD, Cardiovascular Division, Faculty of Medicine, University of Virginia, Charlottesville, Virginia

Janet E. Wilson, BSc, MT, Department of Pathology and Laboratory Medicine, University of British Columbia (UBC)-St. Paul's Hospital, Providence Health Care, Vancouver, British Columbia, Canada

Lambert A. Wu, MD, Senior Associate Consultant, Division of Cardiovascular Diseases and Internal Medicine, Mayo Clinic, Rochester, Minnesota

Dingding Xiong, MD, PhD, Department of Medicine, University of California, San Diego, California

Bobby Yanagawa, BSc, Department of Pathology and Laboratory Medicine, University of British Columbia (UBC)-St. Paul's Hospital, Providence Health Care, Vancouver, British Columbia, Canada

Decheng Yang, PhD, Department of Pathology and Laboratory Medicine, University of British Columbia (UBC)-St. Paul's Hospital, Providence Health Care, Vancouver, British Columbia, Canada

Mary Zhang, MSc, Department of Pathology and Laboratory Medicine, University of British Columbia (UBC)-St. Paul's Hospital, Providence Health Care, Vancouver, British Columbia, Canada

Introduction and Historical Perspective on Experimental Myocarditis

Charles J. Gauntt, Ph.D.

INTRODUCTION

MILESTONES IN ANIMAL MODEL STUDIES OF
COXSACKIEVIRUS-INDUCED MYOCARDITIS
 Isolation of the Coxsackieviruses Group B
 Defining Innate Responses to CVB Infections
 Humoral Immune Responses During CVB Infections
 Role(s) of T Lymphocytes in CVB3-Induced Myocarditis
 Identification of Cardiovirulence Determinants in
  the CVB3 Genome
 Persistence of Viral RNA in Heart Tissues of Mice With
  Chronic Myocarditis
 Nutritional Deficiencies and CVB3-Induced Myocarditis

CONCLUSIONS AND PREDICTIONS

INTRODUCTION

During the last half century, funds for research and advances in technology permitted cardiologists, immunologists, infectious disease researchers, pathologists, and virologists to make significant progress in understanding how numerous infectious agents, including bacteria, fungi, and viruses, can induce myocarditis in humans. Although more than 20 common viruses have been associated with myocarditis in humans, serologic evidence indirectly suggested that enteroviruses classified as the coxsackieviruses group B (CVB), particularly serotypes B1-B5, were the major etiologic agents of this inflammatory heart disease.

The majority of studies on the sequence of events and molecular basis of pathogenesis in myocarditis used murine models infected with CVB3. Researchers showed that murine models of CVB3-induced acute or chronic myocarditis could be established, but the outcome depended on the genetic background of the murine strain being challenged with a cardiovirulent CVB3. Studies of murine host responses to a CVB3 infection found that virus-induced interferon and activation of natural killer cells could contribute to defense against induction of myocarditis until antiviral antibodies were produced.

The virus-induced antibody story got complicated with tales of antibodies that cross-reacted with other CVB serotypes or with several normal cellular proteins and proteins on and in normal tissue. Antiviral antibodies can contribute to heart disease. If that outcome was not sufficiently complicated, the T-lymphocyte story evolved into chapters that had subsets of these cells serving as bodyguards to the murine host or contributing to heart disease as vicious thugs might in a street brawl, directly or indirectly via cytokines. Some T-lymphocyte cells favored attacks on normal cardiac tissues instead of cells in the host that were producing virus. The parasites (CVB3 virions or genomes) lysed various cells during their replication or persisted as genomic viral RNA, according to some nightmarish plan. The intracellular presence of CVB3 genomic RNA disrupted various homeostatic heart tissue functions and mimicked, exposed, or released numerous antigens that have been presumed to play a role(s) in further dysfunction or destruction of heart tissues. One antigen, cardiac myosin, induced a similar parallel autoimmune disease with many similarities to CVB3-induced acute or chronic myocarditis, depending on the host strain of mouse involved.

Molecular studies showed that cardiovirulence in the single-stranded RNA genome could be mapped to a region, a gene, or even a single nucleotide. Heretical notions of CVB3 persisting only as RNA genomes, likely in dsRNA form, and not as infectious virus particles or in a cDNA form in heart tissues were proposed from molecular detection studies of human biopsy specimens and confirmed with mouse heart tissues from mice with CVB3-induced chronic myocarditis. Subtle dietary deficiencies significantly exacerbate CVB3-induced cardiopathology. CVB3-challenge of transgenic knock-out and immunodeficient murine strains identified specific proteins or immune system responses that were required for induction of myocarditis.

So what causes the cardiopathology in CVB3-murine models: virus-induced or immune-response processes? Data supporting each hypothesis usually were presented in a 1-sided manner during the past 20 plus years. Today, proponents of each hypothesis still wearily line up for discussions, although the sheer weight of data on both sides suggests each group is right for a given set of experimental conditions, but it is likely that both hypotheses are correct in many CVB3-murine models. Data from CVB3-murine model studies have contributed to changes in the ways in which patients with myocarditis are diagnosed, treated, and given a prognosis about recovery. The complexities of virus-induced processes and the hosts' responses have confirmed many researchers' findings that an answer(s) to 1 piece of the puzzle merely complicates the complete picture. Being scientists, we can only appreciate nature's hidden secrets and eagerly await colleagues' latest discoveries.

MILESTONES IN ANIMAL MODEL STUDIES OF COXSACKIEVIRUS-INDUCED MYOCARDITIS

ISOLATION OF THE COXSACKIEVIRUSES GROUP B

In early 1948, newborn mice were the initial animal model used to isolate previously unknown filterable infectious agents associated with a small outbreak of paralytic disease in children in Coxsackie, New York.[1] Intracranial inoculation of suckling white albino mice with a 20% stool specimen from 2 small children induced paralysis in 3- to 7-day-old mice but not in mice more than 12 days old.[1] The following year, Melnick and coworkers[2] reported the isolation, in infant mice, of 2 additional distinct nonpoliovirus agents from 2 patients with aseptic meningitis and from 2 patients with fever of unknown origin in New Haven, Connecticut. Antisera to Melnick's isolates indicated serologic relatedness among his isolates, but not to Dalldorf's isolates. Gifford and Dalldorf[3] recognized that these new viruses induced 2 different pathologic conditions in the suckling mouse: group A isolates induced a generalized myositis whereas group B isolates induced focal myositis and inflammatory lesions in many viscera, including pancreas, heart, and liver, and in the central nervous system. Use of the infant mouse to isolate the 2 groups of coxsackieviruses was highly significant, because tissue culture methodology for the detection and study of animal viruses was not available to Dalldorf or Melnick and their colleagues during these virus isolations.[4]

Enders et al.[5] published their classic work on use of human embryonic tissue fragments to propagate the Lansing strain of poliovirus the same year that Melnick reported the discovery of the initial coxsackie group B virus (Dalldorf's classification). Kilbourne and Horsfall[6] provided an early demonstration that immunosuppression of the normally resistant adult mouse with cortisone subsequently rendered mice susceptible to replication of coxsackievirus B1 (Conn-5 strain) and death. The number of group B coxsackievirus serotypes was extended slowly to 3 by 1950 through the work by Melnick and colleagues.[4]

The Committee on the Enteroviruses was established in 1957 to bring some order to the classification of viruses within the poliomyelitis, coxsackie A and B, and ECHO groups.[7] This committee reported that there were 3 polioviruses, 19 coxsackie A viruses, 5 coxsackie B viruses, and 19 ECHO viruses.[7] Coxsackievirus B6 was isolated subsequently from stool samples, as were the other 5 serotypes.[4]

In 1962, an International Subcommittee on Virus Nomenclature was established to classify major groups of viruses on the basis of biochemical and biophysical properties.[8] The work of this committee was a major event, because it allowed researchers and clinicians all over the world to compare findings, knowing that they were talking about a given virus. Thus, this virology classification became an international language that broke barriers and led to many friendships and collaborations across national borders. This international body introduced the term "picornavirus" to describe the small (pico)-RNA genome-nonenveloped viruses of human origin that included enteroviruses, rhinoviruses, and unclassified groups. Family status of the Picornaviridae was not achieved until 1973.[9] Genus status for the enteroviruses was accorded in 1976.[10]

Human studies that associated CVB with myocarditis were conducted by various methods.[11-26] Subsequently, several laboratories spent many years identifying cardiovirulent CVB strains and suitable murine strains to study development of myocarditis[27-33] or explored other CVB-animal models of heart disease.[34-37]

The early researchers who initially isolated the CVB serotypes in infant mice also described the pathologic features wrought by these viruses in the major organs, and they noticed that the heart often was involved. These and other pioneering researchers established several facts about the CVB that have contributed to their intensive study in the last 50 plus years. This small group of 6 related viruses: 1) is associated with a wide variety of diseases in humans of all races on all continents;[38] 2) is widely distributed in the environment, with humans being the major natural hosts, although there are a few other natural hosts (eg, swine that become infected by a CVB5 strain);[39] 3) is highly stable in the environment, especially in water;[40,41] 4) induces inapparent infections in the vast majority of humans;[38] 5) induces an array of host responses, particularly immune responses, that may play a role in cardiopathology;[40,42-45] 6) induces infections whose outcome is considerably influenced by age, sex, and nutritional status of the host;[46-50] and 7) depends on the type of nucleotide or small sequence of nucleotides of the virus to determine "fitness" of a CVB strain for induction of particular disease in a murine model.[51,52]

DEFINING INNATE RESPONSES TO CVB INFECTIONS

Murine models have been quite useful in identifying several innate responses against a

CVB3 infection.[53,54] Following an oral[55,56] or the more usual intraperitoneal challenge of adolescent mice with a suitable dose of a cardiovirulent CVB3, a rapid viremia ensues and is maintained for 1 to 3 days.[57] Virus is found in the plasma phase and in association with circulating lymphocytes.[57] Cells involved in the initial replication are likely endothelial cells[44,57] but cells in the spleen, liver, pancreas, and heart also produce nascent virions.[50,58,59] Noncardiovirulent CVB3 strains replicate poorly in murine organs and the level of infectious virus in the viremic phase is generally 100- to 500-fold lower than that found for cardiovirulent strains.[54,57] Whereas earlier work failed to detect replication of a CVB3 in leukocytes,[57] more recent molecular detection studies show that virus replication does occur in B lymphocytes[60,61] and perhaps contributes to immune deviation of Th_0 subsets to Th_1 instead of Th_2 cells.[40] Infection induces production of interferons-β and -γ,[62,63] and administration of interferon-β ± 24 h of virus challenge generally does not reduce CVB3 titers in heart tissues but does reduce the severity of myocarditis.[64]

Natural killer (NK) cells are activated by infection, and most likely by the interferon induced in mice.[63,65] NK cells are detected around 2 days postinoculation and these cells participate in reducing virus titers in the heart, as evidenced by finding significantly higher titers of virus in hearts of mice depleted of NK cells by administration of anti-asialo-GM antiserum.[63] Heart tissues of mice developing focal myocardial lesions contain NK cells at the earliest detection of foci containing leukocytes adjacent to damaged myocytes.[66] Macrophages, helper T cells, and likely fibroblasts are also found in the developing myocarditis lesions.[66] Thus, both interferon and activated NK cells serve as innate first lines of defense against virus replication in the mouse, and both play roles in amelioration of CVB3-induced myocarditis.

Inducible nitric oxide synthase is induced by a CVB3 infection, and inhibitors of inducible nitric oxide synthase increase virus production and mortality in mice, showing that NO is a nonspecific defense against viral infection.[67] Long-term expression of inducible nitric oxide synthase correlates with transition of CVB3-induced acute-to-chronic myocarditis only in a murine strain capable of developing chronic heart disease.[68]

HUMORAL IMMUNE RESPONSES DURING CVB INFECTIONS

Most CVB strains must replicate to some extent in humans, as evidenced by detection of antiviral antibodies in sera of hosts with illnesses or serious diseases such as inflammatory heart disease.[43,44,55,69] Depending on the serotype and socioeconomic level of a person, by age 30 years 18% to 94% of humans have antibodies to at least 1, sometimes 2 or 3, of the CVB serotypes.[70-73] A protective role for antibodies against CVB3-induced myocarditis or death was established early with murine models. Anti-CVB3 neutralizing antibodies could protect newborn mice from CVB3-induced death if administered 24 h before or 2 h postinoculation of CVB3, but not if given 24 h postinoculation.[74-76] Adolescent mice passively administered anti-CVB3 hyperimmune mouse sera at 24 h pre- or post-CVB3 challenge had a reduced number of myocarditis lesions.[77]

The speed with which mice produced antibodies is a major factor in reducing CVB3-induced heart disease. Inbred murine strains capable of responding to a CVB3 infection by day 3 postinoculation exhibited a reduced level of cardiopathology compared with strains that delayed production of antibodies by 1 day or more.[78-81] Comparative studies in female versus male mice showed that females responded quicker and produced more antibodies than males after a CVB3 challenge.[49] The female response to a CVB3 infection is primarily associated with Th_2 cells and production of IgG_1 antibodies; in contrast, males generally respond to a CVB3 infection with production of Th_1 cells and an IgG_{2a} antibody response.[82] Comparative studies between homozygous (nu/nu) nude and euthymic (nu/+) mice showed that antibody alone was insufficient to clear CVB3 and prevent development of myocardial lesions, suggesting that virus-specific T cells were also required.[83] However, several early vaccination studies using murine-CVB3 models found that antibodies produced to a challenge with CVB3 virions or inactivated virus particles were protective against heart disease induced by a cardiovirulent CVB3 (reviewed in reference 43).

Several studies by Maisch and Schultheiss and their colleagues reported that CVB3 infections in humans induced autoreactive antibodies. Patients with myocarditis had serum antibodies to a CVB and autoantibodies to heart tissues.[84-92] About half of the cases of myocarditis and up to one-fifth of the cases of idiopathic dilated cardiomyopathy, a sequela of myocarditis, are associated with the CVB, and 40% to 100% of the latter patients have autoantibodies to heart tissue antigens.[85,87,92-102] Autoantibodies were directed against cardiac myosin, laminin, branched chain keto acid dehydrogenase, adenine nucleotide translocator, calcium channel proteins, β-adrenergic receptor, actin, and fibrillary proteins (reviewed in reference 43). Antibodies to several autoantigens recognized epitopes on purified CVB3 or CVB4 particles.[93,103] Autoantibodies could be detected as deposits on human heart tissues in biopsy specimens, some in combination with complement components.[93]

Mouse models of CVB3-induced myocarditis were studied extensively to confirm and extend the observations that a CVB3 infection stimulated production of autoantibodies.[104] The next question was whether these autoantibodies contributed to cardiopathology. In initial studies, a significant fraction of the autoantibodies were directed against cardiac myosin,[80,105] particularly epitopes found on the H chain of cardiac myosin.[106] Significantly, induction of autoantibodies during a CVB3 infection depended on the genetics of the murine strain under study.[107] Only those few murine strains that developed CVB3-induced acute myocarditis and then chronic heart disease developed heart-specific IgG autoantibodies, whereas murine strains that developed only the acute disease and resolved it produced low titers of IgM autoantibodies.[108] Some IgG autoantibodies bound to mouse heart tissues and, on elution, they reacted in immunoblots with heart tissue antigens of a broad range of molecular sizes,[109] including molecules of the size of branched chain keto acid dehydrogenase and adenine nucleotide translocator.[110] Severity of chronic myocarditis correlated with deposition of anticardiac myosin, anti-branched chain keto acid dehydrogenase, or antisarcolemma antibodies on mouse heart tissues.[110-112] Studies in another CVB3-murine model showed that CVB3 induced autoantibodies reactive with heart tissue antigens, and the timing of this response correlated with development of chronic myocarditis; titers of these antibodies often correlated with severity of myocarditis.[44,113-115]

The autoantibodies were induced in mice given highly purified CVB3 particles, obviating the question of whether the inducing antigens in the virus-challenge inocula were viral antigens or cell lysate contaminants.[116] Conclusive proof of nonviral heart tissue antigens was obtained using murine models of cardiac myosin-induced myocarditis;[43,96,97,110] other heart tissue antigens were also cardiopathologic in mouse models (reviewed in references 40, 45, 98, 103, 117). Autoantibodies induced by a CVB3 infection were nonreactive with the strain of CVB3 used in pediatric-CVB3 models of acute and chronic myocarditis,[118] whereas another cardiovirulent CVB3 strain (CVB3$_m$) used in adolescent mouse models of acute and chronic myocarditis was blocked in binding to myocytes by a monoclonal antibody generated against murine cardiac myosin.[119] This monoclonal antibody also recognized an epitope on adenine nucleotide translocator,[103] an inner mitochondrial membrane protein that shares an epitope with cardiac myosin and the surface calcium channel protein;[120] not surprisingly, this monoclonal antibody could also reduce the extent of myocarditis induced by the CVB3$_m$ strain in mice.[121] Studies with a panel of anti-CVB3 neutralizing monoclonal antibodies generated against a purified cardiovirulent strain found that several monoclonal antibodies recognized epitopes on murine and cardiac myosin, could participate in complement-mediated lysis of normal murine cardiac fibroblasts, and could induce cardiopathologic alterations in heart tissues of several strains of normal mice.[46,116,122-124] Additionally, some of the latter monoclonal antibodies reacted with epitopes on laminin, actin, elastin, and vimentin in enzyme-linked immunosorbent assay.[46] Monoclonal antibodies directed against M protein of group A streptococci neutralized the cardiovirulent CVB3$_m$ strain and recognized epitopes on human and mouse cardiac myosin.[125] One of the anti-streptococcal monoclonal antibodies was used to select an escape mutant of CVB3 that had an altered murine strain host range; the escape mutant induced more severe myocarditis than the parent CVB3 in several congenic strains.[126] Thus, data from the above direct and indirect studies provide evidence that autoantibodies induced during a CVB3 infection of mice can participate in several types of autoimmune reactions that can contribute to cardiopathology.

As noted above, several vaccination trials in mice used candidate CVB3 strains and strain preparations that showed efficacy against a subsequent challenge with a cardiovirulent CVB3.[43,127,128] Several naturally occurring CVB3 isolates were noncardiovirulent and were regarded as potential candidate strains.[53,129] A recent reexamination of several of these strains showed that although they do not infect heart tissues, they do infect the murine pancreas and thus they suggest the possibility of contributing to development of diabetes mellitus type 1.[130] Data from human studies over several years suggested that infection of a person with a CVB serotype induced homotypic antibody production, and if this person was subsequently infected with a different CVB serotype, the anti-CVB antibody response was heterotypic.[43,131] A role for heterotypic anti-CVB antibodies in health and disease has been found using mouse models in which sequential challenges of mice were made with different serotypes of a CVB. In some studies, an antecedent infection with a heterologous CVB serotype reduced cardiopathology induced by a second CVB serotype, whereas in other studies the antecedent heterologous CVB infection either had no effect or exacerbated severity of the disease (reviewed in reference 43). Although a rational explanation is not at hand, these data must be taken into account when testing potential CVB vaccines in the future. At issue is whether having previous antibodies to a shared antigen (eg, the CVB group antigen) results in antibody-enhanced infection via F_c receptors and induction of a new or more serious disease, as occurs in sequential infections involving the dengue viruses.

ROLE(S) OF T LYMPHOCYTES IN CVB3-INDUCED MYOCARDITIS

Inflammatory mononuclear cells, focally associated with degenerating or necrotic myofibers, are a hallmark of coxsackievirus-induced myocarditis in human and murine models of the disease.[44,49,50,59,132-136] The focal myocardial lesions in CVB3-challenged mouse hearts histopathologically resemble lesions found in human hearts with myocarditis.[50,137,138] Earlier data identified the inflammatory cell composition of the focal myocardial lesion, ie, macrophages, T helper (likely Th1) lymphocytes, NK cells, and CD8+-T cells.[66] Subsequent important studies showed that γδ T cells congregate at the lesion site.[40,139,140] These inflammatory cells likely are responding to a virus-induced increase in expression of a 65-kDa heat-shock protein in the stressed myocytes.[141] CVB3 infection of cells within or at the edges of the focal inflammatory lesion has been well documented for both acute and chronic myocarditis,[45,54,142,143] suggesting that the infiltrating inflammatory cells were responding in a protective manner to the infection.

Studies in T-lymphocyte-deficient mice or in mice with severe combined immunodeficiency showed that CVB3 infections result in far greater virus replication in heart tissues and more severe myocarditis than in similar CVB3 infections in related euthymic mice.[43-45,76,83] These data were interpreted to suggest that the leukocytes responding to the virus-induced inflammation must have a protective role. Other studies in CVB3-challenged euthymic mice strongly suggest that, whereas the early inflammatory response could be beneficial to the murine host, the continued presence of inflammatory cells in the lesion most likely contributes to cardiopathology.[44-46,50,97,144] Selective depletion of T cells from mice before challenge with a cardiovirulent CVB3 significantly reduced myocyte necrosis and the inflammatory infiltrate that formed lesions.[145] Subsequent studies by Huber and colleagues[44,45,113-115,139] showed that the outcome depended highly on the murine strain used in each study.

In a classic study, CD8[+] T cells were the major effector cell of cardiac tissue injury in BALB/c mice, whereas CD4[+] T lymphocytes assumed this role in mice of the DBA/2 strain, along with deposition of IgG autoantibodies in heart tissues.[113] Additional studies showed that in BALB/c mice, a CVB3 infection preferentially activated CD4[+] Th$_1$ cells that stimulated, via cytokines, activation of CD8[+] T lymphocytes, whereas in DBA/2 mice, a CVB3 infection activated CD4[+] Th$_2$ cells whose cytokines stimulated B-cell differentiation.[44,45] Early studies also identified 2 subpopulations of cytotoxic T lymphocytes activated in mice by a CVB3 infection; 1 type reacted against virus-infected cells in vitro, whereas the other type reacted against only uninfected syngeneic host target cells in culture.[44,50,114,137] Transfer of only the latter cytotoxic T lymphocytes to uninfected mice induced myocardial pathology, whereas transfer of virus-specific cytotoxic T lymphocytes to uninfected mice caused no cardiopathology.[146]

T-cell epitopes have been identified on the largest of the 3 surface capsid proteins of CVB3 virions, VP1, that through peptide immunization studies can either reduce or exacerbate CVB3-induced myocarditis in mice.[45] A new type of T lymphocyte, the γδ T cell, infiltrated the infected myocardium to produce an immune deviation toward the Th$_1$ inflammatory cell type in heart tissue.[45,139,140] As these findings unfolded, the explanations became more complicated, eg, the major histocompatibility complex was a major factor in determining susceptibility to particular CVB3 strains during induction of myocarditis.[40,45,80,97,111,112,139] It was then found that activated γδ[+] T-cell subpopulations may act through regulation of the major histocompatibility complex class II IE antigen that controls susceptibility to CVB3-induced myocarditis.[147] Also, up-regulation of intercellular adhesion molecule-1 via expression of cytokines, tumor necrosis factor-α and interferon-γ, by Th$_1$ cells further promoted infiltration of T cells and macrophages into CVB3-induced myocardial lesions.[148]

The type and quantity of cytokines induced during a CVB3 infection, whether from infected myocytes or from activated leukocytes in the myocardial lesion, also contributed to the inflammatory milieu in the myocardium and promoted or reduced cardiopathology, depending on the type of cytokine and time of the presence of each relative to development of the myocardial lesion.[64,68,82,148-153] CVB3 infection of human monocytes in culture readily induces tumor necrosis factor-α, interleukin-1β, and interleukin-6,[149] cytokines that can contribute to CVB3-induction or maintenance of myocarditis in mice.[68,150-153] Exogenous administration of several proinflammatory cytokines can significantly increase the susceptibility of mice to development of CVB3-induced myocarditis in several murine models of disease in which the virus is minimally cardiovirulent, a scenario similar to using a cardiovirulent CVB3 strain that induces proinflammatory cytokines.[117]

Knock-out and transgenic mice have provided information on what cells or processes are required for the cardiopathology by CVB3 in murine models of myocarditis. Minimally susceptible C57B1/6J mice become highly susceptible to CVB3-induction of myocarditis when genetically altered to be devoid of CD4[+] and β_2-microglobulin, suggesting that these deletions remove an inhibitory action that was directed against CD8[+] T cells, which could then contribute more to the cardiopathology.[149] Some CD8[+] T lymphocytes can lyse virus-infected cells via a perforin-mediated mechanism; however, perforin knock-out mice exhibit significantly reduced myocarditis and fewer die of infection even though virus clearance is not altered.[154] Mice made genetically mutant (knock-out mice) in macrophage inflammatory protein-1α were resistant to CVB3-induced myocarditis, in contrast to genetically intact animals that were susceptible.[155] Transgenic nonobese diabetic mice expressing interferon-γ in pancreatic β cells do not develop myocarditis in response to a CVB3 challenge, probably because of decreased virus titers in heart tissues.[156] The founder nonobese diabetic mice died quickly in response to the CVB3 challenge.

IDENTIFICATION OF CARDIOVIRULENCE DETERMINANTS IN THE CVB3 GENOME

With the goal of ultimately describing safe efficacious vaccine candidate strains, mice have served as useful hosts in assessing cardiovirulence of CVB3 strains. Candidate mutant and chimeric variants of CVB3 (ie, molecular constructs composed of nucleotide sequences derived from cardiovirulent and noncardiovirulent CVB3 strains) have been tested. Cardiovirulence has been mapped to several different single nucleotides in the 5′-non-translated region,[129,157] to an unknown sequence in the 5′-nontranslated region,[52,158] or to VP2 in the capsid region.[159] Additional genomic sequences that may contribute to cardiovirulence have been described as well as different multicompensatory nucleotide sequences that may be associated with cardiovirulence or attenuation.[51] However, for most naturally occurring or laboratory CVB3 strains that have been molecularly analyzed, cardiovirulence maps to the 5′-nontranslated region.[51]

PERSISTENCE OF VIRAL RNA IN HEART TISSUES OF MICE WITH CHRONIC MYOCARDITIS

Enteroviruses can persist in heart tissues of murine strains, but the majority of studies involved hosts that were either immunosuppressed or immunodeficient.[83,160,161] Immunodeficient mice produced high titers of anti-CVB3 antibodies but could not clear the virus from the heart or other organs,[43,57] perhaps suggesting a protective role for cell-mediated immune reactions in clearance of virions. However, several studies show that enteroviruses can persist only as replicating viral RNA, likely in the more stable double-stranded RNA replication form, in heart tissues (and likely pancreatic tissues also) of certain strains of mice that develop CVB3-induced chronic myocarditis. These data suggest that the genetic background of some murine strains precludes virus clearance.

Initial studies in this area used in situ hybridization analyses of human heart biopsy specimens with cDNA probes to CVB strains that were broadly reactive with enterovirus genomes.[162-168] Subsequent studies using polymerase chain reaction confirmed and extended the sensitivity of the findings—ie, enterovirus RNA does indeed persist in approximately 30% of human heart biopsy specimens from patients with myocarditis and the sequela, cardiomyopathy.[165,169] Patients with positive viral RNA biopsy reports had adverse outcomes (death) far more frequently than those with negative viral RNA biopsy reports.[170]

Studies in human tissues have been confirmed in highly reproducible murine models of CVB3-induced acute and chronic myocarditis.[83,142,143] In general, these and other data (Gauntt, Wood, and Montellano, unpublished data) show that inbred strains of mice that develop only acute but resolved myocarditis in response to a cardiovirulent CVB3 strain infection do not permit persistence of viral RNA in heart tissues, whereas murine strains that develop CVB3-induced chronic myocarditis can harbor CVB3 RNA for at least up to 90 days postinoculation in their heart tissues; noncardiovirulent CVB3 strains do not persist as viral RNA in any murine strains. During persistence, viral RNA is expressed and 1 protease (2A) has many potential lethal effects on cells,[171] such as destruction of the poly A-binding protein, involved in cell mRNA production,[172] and cleavage of dystrophin, a key cytoskeletal protein in myocytes.[173] Detection of enteroviral RNA in heart tissues by polymerase chain reaction is a diagnostically significant finding, because isolation of infectious enterovirus particles from heart tissues is rare.[167,168]

NUTRITIONAL DEFICIENCIES AND CVB3-INDUCED MYOCARDITIS

Murine models of CVB3-induced myocarditis have also been exploited to examine the effects of deficient, nutrient-limited, or excessive nutrition (hypercholesterol) diets on the severity or outcome of an infection. In general, mice on diets with nutrient deprivation or hypercholesteremic, vitamin E-deficient, or selenium-deficient diets develop more severe myocarditis than matched groups on normal healthy diets.[48,174] Recall that most naturally occurring CVB3 strains are not cardiovirulent for susceptible mouse strains.[53,129] An important finding from selenium- and vitamin E-deficient diet studies was that revertant cardiovirulent variants were readily selected from the challenge inocula population of non-cardiovirulent CVB3 viruses, established residence in heart tissues, and induced severe heart disease.[174] Early studies of mice on deficient diets that were forced to exercise reported higher titers of virus in heart tissues and more severe disease, often leading to death (reviewed in references 48 and 174). The latter findings suggested that patients with myocarditis should not engage in any exercise and therefore bed rest has long been part of recovery.

CONCLUSIONS AND PREDICTIONS

The voluminous data on murine models of CVB-, predominantly CVB3-, induced myocarditis show that many factors contribute to recovery from acute myocarditis or the transformation to chronic myocarditis. Chance determines whether a person is infected with a cardiovirulent CVB3 or reacts unfavorably to a noncardiovirulent strain when immunosuppressed or consuming an inadequate diet. Murine models have established that a heart disease outcome depends on the genetic background, sex, and age of the host; nutritional and immunologic status of the host; and innate and immunologic systems responses to the CVB infection. The researcher has the advantage of being able to control most of these variables to design the disease needed for further study.

Decades have been spent searching for diagnostic tests whose results would covary with detection or severity of myocarditis induced in CVB3-murine models. Perhaps a potential method has been found in the use of polymerase chain reaction to monitor enteroviral RNA values in mouse hearts that develop chronic disease and are given various treatments. Quantitative values of viral RNA, cytokine mRNA profiles, or type of T-cell receptor in circulating leukocytes could have diagnostic significance for humans with heart disease due to CVB or even other viruses. With the abundance of myocardial tissues for sampling, the murine models offer the best approach for developing effective therapies, perhaps designing more heart-healthy diets or establishing new approaches to controlling unwanted immune responses in heart tissues. Murine models of CVB3-induced myocarditis have also confirmed and extended patients' data on virus-induced, potentially cardiopathologic, autoimmune responses, findings that can adversely affect development of a safe CVB vaccine.

With the release of dual sets of sequence data on the entire human genome, the future potential for assessing each individual's genome is possible. It seems possible that an individual's data will be useful information about the potential for developing or prognosis for recovery from CVB-induced heart disease. Will we bring a genomic background computer microchip card to the physician for each visit for future predictions about our health? Similar murine genomic information about potentially defective genes could likely be useful in predicting outcomes in murine models of CVB3-induced myocarditis. For example, it was recently shown that mice lacking the sarcoma family kinase LcK (p56[lck]) gene did not develop CVB3-induced myocarditis, whereas CVB3 infection of wild-type founder mice resulted in severe myocarditis.[175] Identification of host genes up-regulated during

CVB3-induced acute and chronic myocarditis in appropriate murine strains will be important information, offering possibilities for therapeutic intervention.[176] We continue to make progress on a heart disease first described more than a hundred years ago.[177]

ACKNOWLEDGMENT

This work was supported by a grant (9950138N) from the American Heart Association.

REFERENCES

1. Dalldorf G, Sickles GM. Unidentified filtrable agent isolated from feces of children with paralysis. Science 1948;108:61-62.
2. Melnick JL, Shaw EW, Curnen EC. Virus isolated from patients diagnosed as non-paralytic poliomyelitis or aseptic meningitis. Proc Soc Exp Biol Med 1949;71:344-349.
3. Gifford R, Dalldorf G. Morbid anatomy of experimental coxsackie virus infection. Am J Pathol 1951;27:1047-1063.
4. Crowell RL, Landau BJ. A short history and introductory background on the coxsackieviruses of group B. Curr Top Microbiol Immunol 1997;223:1-11.
5. Enders JF, Weller TH, Robbins FC. Cultivation of Lansing strain of poliomyelitis virus in cultures of various human embryonic tissues. Science 1949;109:85-87.
6. Kilbourne ED, Horsfall FL Jr. Lethal infection with coxsackie virus of adult mice given cortisone. Proc Soc Exp Biol Med 1951;77:135-138.
7. Committee on the Enteroviruses. The enteroviruses. Am J Public Health 1957;47:1556-1566.
8. Melnick JL, Cockburn WC, Dalldorf G, Gard S, Gear JHS, Hammon WMcD, Kaplan MM, Nagler FP, Oker-Blom N, Rhodes AJ, Sabin AB, Verlinde JD, von Magnus H. Picornavirus group. Virology 1963;19:114-116.
9. Melnick JL. Classification and nomenclature of viruses, 1973. Prog Med Virol 1973;16:337-342.
10. Fenner F. Classification and nomenclature of viruses. Second report of the International Committee on Taxonomy of Viruses. Intervirology 1976;7:1-115.
11. Burch GE, Giles TD. The role of viruses in the production of heart disease. Am J Cardiol 1972;29:231-240.
12. Burch GE, Sun SC, Colcolough HL, Sohal RS, DePasquale NP. Coxsackie B viral myocarditis and valvulitis identified in routine autopsy specimens by immunofluorescent techniques. Am Heart J 1967;74:13-23.
13. Burch GE, Sun SC, Chu KC, Sohal RS, Colcolough HL. Interstitial and coxsackievirus B myocarditis in infants and children. A comparative histologic and immunofluorescent study of 50 autopsied hearts. JAMA 1968;203:1-8.
14. Connolly JH. Myocarditis during coxsackie B5 infection. Br Med J 1961;1:877-878.
15. Gear JH. Coxsackie virus infections of the newborn. Prog Med Virol 1958;1:106-121.
16. Gear JHS, Measroch V. Coxsackievirus infections of the newborn. Prog Med Virol 1973;15:42-62.
17. Grist NR, Bell EJ. Coxsackie viruses and the heart. Am Heart J 1969;77:295-300.

18. Helin M, Savola J, Lapinleimu K. Cardiac manifestations during a Coxsackie B5 epidemic. Br Med J 1968;3:97-99.

19. Hirschman SZ, Hammer GS. Coxsackie virus myopericarditis. A microbiological and clinical review. Am J Cardiol 1974;34:224-232.

20. Hosier DM, Newton WA Jr. Serious coxsackie infection in infants and children. Am J Dis Child 1958;96:251-267.

21. Javett SN, Heymann S, Mundel B, Pepler WJ, Lurie HI, Gear J, Measroch V, Kirsch Z. Myocarditis in the newborn infant: a study of an outbreak associated with coxsackie group B virus infection in a maternity home in Johannesburg. J Pediatr 1956;48:1-22.

22. Kibrick S, Benirschke K. Acute aseptic myocarditis and meningoencephalitis in the newborn child infected with coxsackie virus group B, type 3. N Engl J Med 1956;255:883-889.

23. Lansdown AB. Viral infections and diseases of the heart. Prog Med Virol 1978;24:70-113.

24. Montgomery J, Gear J, Prinsloo FR, Kahn M, Kirsch ZG. Myocarditis of the newborn: an outbreak in a maternity home in Southern Rhodesia associated with coxsackie group-B virus infection. South African Med J 1955;29:608-612.

25. Nouaille J, Gautier M. Viral infections in which cardiovascular manifestations predominate. In: Debré R, Celers J, eds. Clinical virology: the evaluation and management of human viral infections. Philadelphia: WB Saunders Company, 1970:485-496.

26. Van Creveld S, de Jager H. Myocarditis in newborns, caused by coxsackie virus. Clinical and pathological data. Ann Paediatr 1956;187:100-112.

27. Gauntt CJ, Gomez PT, Duffey PS, Grant JA, Trent DW, Witherspoon SM, Paque RE. Characterization and myocarditic capabilities of coxsackievirus B3 variants in selected mouse strains. J Virol 1984;52:598-605.

28. Gauntt CJ, Trousdale MD, LaBadie DR, Paque RE, Nealon T. Properties of coxsackievirus B3 variants which are amyocarditic or myocarditic for mice. J Med Virol 1979;3:207-220.

29. Paque RE, Gauntt CJ, Nealon TJ, Trousdale MD. Assessment of cell-mediated hypersensitivity against coxsackievirus B3 viral-induced myocarditis utilizing hypertonic salt extracts of cardiac tissue. J Immunol 1978;120:1672-1678.

30. Paque RE, Straus DC, Nealon TJ, Gauntt CJ. Fractionation and immunologic assessment of KC1-extracted cardiac antigens in coxsackievirus B3 virus-induced myocarditis. J Immunol 1979;123:358-364.

31. Rabin ER, Hassan SA, Jenson AB, Melnick JL. Coxsackie virus B3 myocarditis in mice. An electron microscopic, immunofluorescent and virus-assay study. Am J Pathol 1964;44:775-797.

32. Reyes MP, Smith FE, Lerner AM. An enterovirus-induced murine model of an acute dilated-type cardiomyopathy. Intervirology 1984;22:146-155.

33. Rytel MW, Kilbourne ED. Differing susceptibility of adolescent and adult mice to non-lethal infection with coxsackievirus B_3. Proc Soc Exp Biol Med 1971;137:443-448.

34. Hoshino T, Kawai C, Tokuda M. Experimental coxsackie B viral myocarditis in cynomolgus monkeys. Jpn Circ J 1983;47:59-66.

35. Horita H, Kitaura Y, Deguchi H, Kotaka M, Kawamura K. Experimental coxsackie B3 virus myocarditis in golden hamsters. II. Evaluation of left ventricular function in intact *in situ* heart 14 months after inoculation. Jpn Circ J 1984;48:1097-1106.

36. Paque RE, Gauntt CJ, Nealon TJ. Assessment of cell-mediated immunity against coxsackievirus B3-induced myocarditis in a primate model (*Papio papio*). Infect Immun 1981;31:470-479.

37. Rhodes AJ, Van Rooyen CE. Textbook of virology: for students and practitioners of medicine and the other health sciences. 5th ed. Baltimore: Williams & Wilkins Company, 1968:129-131.

38. Pallansch MA. Epidemiology of group B coxsackieviruses. In: Bendinelli M, Friedman H, eds. Coxsackieviruses: a general update. New York: Plenum Press, 1988:399-417.

39. Mahy BWJ. Classification and general properties. In: Bendinelli M, Friedman H, eds.

Coxsackieviruses: a general update. New York: Plenum Press, 1988:1-18.

40. Gauntt CJ, Sakkinen P, Rose NR, Huber SA. Picornaviruses: immunopathology and autoimmunity. In: Cunningham MW, Fujinami RS, eds. Effects of microbes on the immune system. Philadelphia: Lippincott Williams & Wilkins, 2000:313-329.

41. Rueckert RR. Picornaviridae: the viruses and their replication. In: Fields BN, Knipe DM, Howley PM, Chanock RM, Melnick JL, Monath TP, Roizman B, Straus SE, eds. Fundamental virology. 3rd ed. Philadelphia: Lippincott-Raven, 1996:477-522.

42. Gauntt CJ. Cellular and humoral immune responses in coxsackievirus myocarditis. In: Kawai C, Abelmann WH, Matsumori A, eds. Pathogenesis of myocarditis and cardiomyopathy: recent experimental and clinical studies. Tokyo: University of Tokyo Press, 1987:49-61.

43. Gauntt CJ. Roles of the humoral response in coxsackievirus B-induced disease. Curr Top Microbiol Immunol 1997;223:259-282.

44. Leslie K, Blay R, Haisch C, Lodge A, Weller A, Huber S. Clinical and experimental aspects of viral myocarditis. Clin Microbiol Rev 1989;2:191-203.

45. Schwimmbeck PL, Huber SA, Schultheiss HP. Roles of T cells in coxsackievirus B-induced disease. Curr Top Microbiol Immunol 1997;223:283-303.

46. Gauntt C, Higdon A, Bowers D, Maull E, Wood J, Crawley R. What lessons can be learned from animal model studies in viral heart disease? Scand J Infect Dis Suppl 1993;88:49-65.

47. Huber SA, Job LP, Auld KR, Woodruff JF. Sex-related differences in the rapid production of cytotoxic spleen cells active against uninfected myofibers during Coxsackievirus B-3 infection. J Immunol 1981;126:1336-1340.

48. Loria RM. Host conditions affecting the course of coxsackievirus infections. In: Bendinelli M, Friedman H, eds. Coxsackieviruses: a general update. New York: Plenum Press, 1988:135-157.

49. Wong CY, Woodruff JJ, Woodruff JF. Generation of cytotoxic T lymphocytes during coxsackievirus B-3 infection. III. Role of sex. J Immunol 1977;119:591-597.

50. Woodruff JF. Viral myocarditis. A review. Am J Pathol 1980;101:425-484.

51. Chapman NM, Ramsingh AI, Tracy S. Genetics of coxsackievirus virulence. Curr Top Microbiol Immunol 1997;223:227-258.

52. Lee C, Maull E, Chapman N, Tracy S, Gauntt C. Genomic regions of coxsackievirus B3 associated with cardiovirulence. J Med Virol 1997;52:341-347.

53. Gauntt CJ. The possible role of viral variants in pathogenesis. In: Bendinelli M, Friedman H, eds. Coxsackieviruses: a general update. New York: Plenum Press, 1988:159-179.

54. Gauntt CJ, Godeny EK, Lutton CW, Arizpe HM, Chapman NM, Tracy SM, Revtyak GE, Valente AJ, Rozek MM. Mechanism(s) of coxsackievirus-induction of acute myocarditis in a mouse model. In: de la Maza LM, Peterson EM, eds. Medical virology VIII. Hillsdale, NJ: Lawrence Erlbaum Associates, 1988:161-182.

55. Reyes MP, Lerner AM. Coxsackievirus myocarditis—with special reference to acute and chronic effects. Prog Cardiovasc Dis 1985;27:373-394.

56. Loria RM, Kibrick S, Broitman SA. Peroral infection with group B coxsackievirus in the newborn mouse: a model for human infection. J Infect Dis 1974;130:225-230.

57. Gauntt CJ, Godeny EK, Lutton CW. Host factors regulating viral clearance. Pathol Immunopathol Res 1988;7:251-265.

58. Abelmann WH. Virus and the heart. Circulation 1971;44:950-956.

59. McManus BM, Cassling RS, Gauntt CJ. Immunologic basis of myocardial injury. Cardiovasc Clin 1986;18:163-184.

60. Anderson DR, Wilson JE, Carthy CM, Yang D, Kandolf R, McManus BM. Direct interactions of coxsackievirus B3 with immune cells in the splenic compartment of mice susceptible or resistant to myocarditis. J Virol 1996;70:4632-4645.

61. Klingel K, Stephan S, Sauter M, Zell R, McManus BM, Bultmann B, Kandolf R. Pathogenesis of murine enterovirus myocarditis: virus dissemination and immune cell targets. J Virol 1996;70:8888-8895.

62. Gauntt CJ, Paque RE, Trousdale MD, Gudvangen RJ, Barr DT, Lipotich GJ, Nealon TJ, Duffey PS. Temperature-sensitive mutant of coxsackievirus B3 establishes resistance in neonatal mice that protects them during adolescence against coxsackievirus B3-induced myocarditis. Infect Immun 1983;39:851-864.

63. Godeny EK, Gauntt CJ. Involvement of natural killer cells in coxsackievirus B3-induced murine myocarditis. J Immunol 1986;137:1695-1702.

64. Lutton CW, Gauntt CJ. Ameliorating effect of IFN-β and anti-IFN-β on coxsackievirus B3-induced myocarditis in mice. J Interferon Res 1985;5:137-146.

65. Godeny EK, Gauntt CJ. Murine natural killer cells limit coxsackievirus B3 replication. J Immunol 1987;139:913-918.

66. Godeny EK, Gauntt CJ. In situ immune autoradiographic identification of cells in heart tissues of mice with coxsackievirus B3-induced myocarditis. Am J Pathol 1987;129:267-276.

67. Lowenstein CJ, Hill SL, Lafond-Walker A, Wu J, Allen G, Landavere M, Rose NR, Herskowitz A. Nitric oxide inhibits viral replication in murine myocarditis. J Clin Invest 1996;97:1837-1843.

68. Freeman GL, Colston JT, Zabalgoitia M, Chandrasekar B. Contractile depression and expression of proinflammatory cytokines and iNOS in viral myocarditis. Am J Physiol 1998;274(1 Pt 2): H249-H258.

69. Martino TA, Liu P, Petric M, Sole MJ. Enteroviral myocarditis and dilated cardiomyopathy: a review of clinical and experimental studies. In: Rotbart HA, ed. Human enterovirus infections. Washington, DC: ASM Press, 1995:291-351.

70. Grist NR, Bell EJ, Assaad F. Enteroviruses in human disease. Prog Med Virol 1978;24:114-157.

71. Kogon A, Spigland I, Frothingham TE, Elveback L, Williams C, Hall CE, Fox JP. The virus watch program: a continuing surveillance of viral infections in metropolitan New York families. VII. Observations on viral excretion, seroimmunity, intrafamilial spread and illness association in coxsackie and echovirus infections. Am J Epidemiol 1969;89:51-61.

72. Lau RC. Coxsackie B virus infections in New Zealand patients with cardiac and non-cardiac diseases. J Med Virol 1983;11:131-137.

73. Roggendorf M. Experience with enzyme-linked immunosorbent assay for the detection of antibodies of the IgM class against coxsackie B viruses. In: Bolte H-D, ed. Viral heart disease. Berlin: Springer-Verlag, 1984:116-123.

74. Cho CT, Feng KK, McCarthy VP, Lenahan MF. Role of antiviral antibodies in resistance against coxsackievirus B3 infection: interaction between preexisting antibodies and an interferon inducer. Infect Immun 1982;37:720-727.

75. Rager-Zisman B, Allison AC. The role of antibody and host cells in the resistance of mice against infection by coxsackie B-3 virus. J Gen Virol 1973;19:329-338.

76. Takada H, Kishimoto C, Hiraoka Y. Therapy with immunoglobulin suppresses myocarditis in a murine coxsackievirus B3 model. Antiviral and anti-inflammatory effects. Circulation 1995;92:1604-1611.

77. Godney EK, Arizpe HM, Gauntt CJ. Characterization of the antibody response in vaccinated mice protected against coxsackievirus B3-induced myocarditis. Viral Immunol 1987-1988;1:305-314.

78. Herskowitz A, Beisel KW, Wolfgram LJ, Rose NR. Coxsackievirus B3 murine myocarditis: wide pathologic spectrum in genetically defined inbred strains. Hum Pathol 1985;16:671-673.

79. Herskowitz A, Wolfgram LJ, Rose NR, Beisel KW. Coxsackievirus B3 murine myocarditis: a pathologic spectrum of myocarditis in genetically defined inbred strains. J Am Coll Cardiol 1987;9:1311-1319.

80. Wolfgram LJ, Beisel KW, Herskowitz A, Rose NR. Variations in the susceptibility to coxsackievirus B3-induced myocarditis among different strains of mice. J Immunol 1986;136:1846-1852.

81. Wolfgram LJ, Rose NR. Coxsackievirus infection as a trigger of cardiac autoimmunity. Immunol Res 1989;8:61-80.

82. Huber SA, Pfaeffle B. Differential Th_1 and Th_2 cell responses in male and female BALB/c mice infected with coxsackievirus group B type 3. J Virol 1994;68:5126-5132.

83. Sato S, Tsutsumi R, Burke A, Carlson G, Porro V, Seko Y, Okumura K, Kawana R, Virmani R. Persistence of replicating coxsackievirus B3 in the athymic murine heart is associated with development of myocarditic lesions. J Gen Virol 1994;75:2911-2924.

84. Maisch B. Cardiocytolysis by sera of patients suffering from acute perimyocarditis. In: Bolte H-D, ed. Viral heart disease. Berlin: Springer-Verlag, 1984:121-130.

85. Maisch B. Diagnostic relevance of humoral and cell-mediated immune reactions in patients with acute myocarditis and congestive cardiomyopathy. In: Chazov EI, Smirnov VN, Oganov RG, eds. Cardiology. London: Plenum, 1984:1327-1338.

86. Maisch B. Immunologic regulator and effector functions in perimyocarditis, postmyocarditic heart muscle disease and dilated cardiomyopathy. Basic Res Cardiol 1986;81 Suppl 1:217-241.

87. Maisch B. Autoreactivity to the cardiac myocyte, connective tissue and the extracellular matrix in heart disease and postcardiac injury. Springer Semin Immunopathol 1989;11:369-395.

88. Maisch B. Myocarditis. Curr Opin Cardiol 1990;5:320-327.

89. Maisch B, Berg PA, Kochsiek K. Clinical significance of immunopathological findings in patients with post-pericardiotomy syndrome. I. Relevance of antibody pattern. Clin Exp Immunol 1979;38:189-197.

90. Maisch B, Berg PA, Kochsiek K. Autoantibodies and serum inhibition factors (SIF) in patients with myocarditis. Klin Wochenschr 1980;58:219-225.

91. Maisch B, Deeg P, Liebau G, Kochsiek K. Diagnostic relevance of humoral and cytotoxic immune reactions in primary and secondary dilated cardiomyopathy. Am J Cardiol 1983;52:1072-1078.

92. Maisch B, Trostel-Soeder R, Stechemesser E, Berg PA, Kochsiek K. Diagnostic relevance of humoral and cell-mediated immune reactions in patients with acute viral myocarditis. Clin Exp Immunol 1982;48:533-545.

93. Maisch B, Bauer E, Cirsi M, Kochsiek K. Cytolytic cross-reactive antibodies directed against the cardiac membrane and viral proteins in coxsackievirus B3 and B4 myocarditis: characterization and pathogenetic relevance. Circulation 1993;87 Suppl 4:49-65.

94. Maisch B, Outzen H, Roth D, Hiby A, Herzum M, Hengstenberg C, Hufnagel G, Schönian U, Kochsiek K. Prognostic determinants in conventionally treated myocarditis and perimyocarditis—focus on antimyolemmal antibodies. Eur Heart J 1991;12 Suppl D:81-87.

95. Neumann DA, Burek CL, Baughman KL, Rose NR, Herskowitz A. Circulating heart-reactive antibodies in patients with myocarditis or cardiomyopathy. J Am Coll Cardiol 1990;16:839-846.

96. Rose NR, Herskowitz A, Neumann DA, Neu N. Autoimmune myocarditis: a paradigm of postinfection autoimmune disease. Immunol Today 1988;9:117-120.

97. Rose NR, Neumann DA, Herskowitz A. Coxsackievirus myocarditis. Adv Intern Med 1992;37:411-429.

98. Schultheiss HP. The significance of autoantibodies against the ADP/ATP carrier for the pathogenesis of myocarditis and dilated cardiomyopathy—clinical and experimental data. Springer Semin Immunopathol 1989;11:15-30.

99. Schultheiss HP, Bolte HD. Immunological analysis of auto-antibodies against the adenine nucleotide translocator in dilated cardiomyopathy. J Mol Cell Cardiol 1985;17:603-617.

100. Schultheiss H-P, Schulze K, Kühl U, Ulrich G, Klingenberg M. The ADP/ATP carrier as a mitochondrial auto-antigen—facts and perspectives. Ann NY Acad Sci 1986;488:44-63.

101. Schulze K, Becker BF, Schultheiss HP. Antibodies to the ADP/ATP carrier, an autoantigen in myocarditis and dilated cardiomyopathy, penetrate into myocardial cells and disturb energy metabolism *in vivo*. Circ Res 1989;64:179-192.

102. Schwimmbeck PL, Schultheiss H-P, Strauer BE. Identification of a main autoimmunogenic epitope of the adenine nucleotide translocator which cross-reacts with coxsackie B3 virus: use in the diagnosis of myocarditis and dilative cardiomyopathy (abstract). Circulation 1989;80 Suppl 2:II-665.

103. Schwimmbeck PL, Schwimmbeck NK, Schultheiss HP, Strauer BE. Mapping of antigenic determinants of the adenine-nucleotide translocator and coxsackie B3 virus with synthetic peptides: use for the diagnosis of viral heart disease. Clin Immunol Immunopathol 1993;68:135-140.

104. Herskowitz A, Traystman MD, Beisel KW. Murine viral myocarditis—new insights into mechanisms of disease. Heart Failure 1986;2:86-91.

105. Wolfgram LJ, Beisel KW, Rose NR. Heart-specific autoantibodies following murine coxsackievirus B3 myocarditis. J Exp Med 1985;161:1112-1121.

106. Alvarez FL, Neu N, Rose NR, Craig SW, Beisel KW. Heart-specific autoantibodies induced by coxsackievirus B3: identification of heart autoantigens. Clin Immunol Immunopathol 1987;43:129-139.

107. Rose NR, Neumann DA, Herskowitz A, Traystman MD, Beisel KW. Genetics of susceptibility to viral myocarditis in mice. Pathol Immunopathol Res 1988;7:266-278.

108. Neu N, Beisel KW, Traystman MD, Rose NR, Craig SW. Autoantibodies specific for the cardiac myosin isoform are found in mice susceptible to coxsackievirus B_3-induced myocarditis. J Immunol 1987;138:2488-2492.

109. Neumann DA, Lane JR, LaFond-Walker A, Allen GS, Wulff SM, Herskowitz A, Rose NR. Heart-specific autoantibodies can be eluted from the hearts of coxsackievirus B3-infected mice. Clin Exp Immunol 1991;86:405-412.

110. Neumann DA, Rose NR, Ansari AA, Herskowitz A. Induction of multiple heart autoantibodies in mice with coxsackievirus B3- and cardiac myosin-induced autoimmune myocarditis. J Immunol 1994;152:343-350.

111. Beisel KW, Rose NR. Relationship of coxsackievirus to cardiac autoimmunity. In: Bendinelli M, Friedman H, eds. Coxsackieviruses: a general update. New York: Plenum Press, 1988:271-292.

112. Traystman MD, Beisel KW. Genetic control of coxsackievirus B3-induced heart-specific autoantibodies associated with chronic myocarditis. Clin Exp Immunol 1991;86:291-298.

113. Huber SA, Lodge PA. Coxsackievirus B-3 myocarditis. Identification of different pathogenic mechanisms in DBA/2 and Balb/c mice. Am J Pathol 1986;122:284-291.

114. Huber SA, Weller A, Herzum M, Lodge PA, Estrin M, Simpson K, Guthrie M. Immunopathogenic mechanisms in experimental picornavirus-induced autoimmunity. Pathol Immunopathol Res 1988;7:279-291.

115. Lodge PA, Herzum M, Olszewski J, Huber SA. Coxsackievirus B-3 myocarditis. Acute and chronic forms of the disease caused by different immunopathogenic mechanisms. Am J Pathol 1987;128:455-463.

116. Gauntt CJ, Lutton CW, Arizpe HM, Higdon AH, Tracy SM. Autoimmune reactions in coxsackievirus B3-induced murine myocarditis. Life Sci Adv 1991;10:23-31.

117. Huber SA, Gauntt CJ, Sakkinen P. Enteroviruses and myocarditis: viral pathogenesis through replication, cytokine induction, and immunopathogenicity. Adv Virus Res 1998;51:35-80.

118. Neu N, Craig SW, Rose NR, Alvarez F, Beisel KW. Coxsackievirus induced myocarditis in mice: cardiac myosin autoantibodies do not cross-react with the virus. Clin Exp Immunol 1987;69:566-574.

119. Weller AH, Simpson K, Herzum M, Van Houten N, Huber SA. Coxsackievirus-B3-induced

myocarditis: virus receptor antibodies modulate myocarditis. J Immunol 1989;143:1843-1850.

120. Ulrich G, Kühl U, Melzner B, Janda I, Schäfer B, Schultheiss H-P. Antibodies against the adenosine di-/triphosphate carrier cross-react with the Ca channel—functional and biochemical data. In: Schultheiss H-P, ed. New concepts in viral heart disease: virology, immunology, and clinical management. Berlin: Springer-Verlag, 1988:225-235.

121. Loudon RP, Moraska AF, Huber SA, Schwimmbeck P, Schultheiss P. An attenuated variant of cox-sackievirus B3 preferentially induces immunoregulatory T cells *in vivo*. J Virol 1991;65:5813-5819.

122. Gauntt CJ, Arizpe HM, Higdon AL, Rozek MM, Crawley R, Cunningham MW. Anti-coxsackievirus B3 neutralizing antibodies with pathological potential. Eur Heart J 1991;12 Suppl D:124-129.

123. Gauntt CJ, Arizpe HM, Higdon AL, Wood HJ, Bowers DF, Rozek MM, Crawley R. Molecular mimicry, anti-coxsackievirus B3 neutralizing monoclonal antibodies, and myocarditis. J Immunol 1995;154:2983-2995.

124. Gauntt CJ, Higdon AL, Arizpe HM, Tamayo MR, Crawley R, Henkel RD, Pereira ME, Tracy SM, Cunningham MW. Epitopes shared between coxsackievirus B3 (CVB3) and normal heart tissue contribute to CVB3-induced murine myocarditis. Clin Immunol Immunopathol 1993;68:129-134.

125. Cunningham MW, Antone SM, Gullizia JM, McManus BM, Fischetti VA, Gauntt CJ. Cytotoxic and viral neutralizing antibodies crossreact with streptococcal M protein, enteroviruses, and human cardiac myosin. Proc Natl Acad Sci U S A 1992;89:1320-1324.

126. Huber SA, Moraska A, Cunningham M. Alterations in major histocompatibility complex associa-tion of myocarditis induced by coxsackievirus B3 mutants selected with monoclonal antibodies to group A streptococci. Proc Natl Acad Sci U S A 1994;91:5543-5547.

127. Fohlman J, Pauksen K, Morein B, Bjare U, Ilbäck N-G, Friman G. High yield production of an inactivated coxsackie B3 adjuvant vaccine with protective effect against experimental myocarditis. Scand J Infect Dis Suppl 1993;88:103-108.

128. Trousdale MD, Paque RE, Nealon T, Gauntt CJ. Assessment of coxsackievirus B3 ts mutants for induction of myocarditis in a murine model. Infect Immun 1979;23:486-495.

129. Gauntt CJ, Pallansch MA. Coxsackievirus B3 clinical isolates and murine myocarditis. Virus Res 1996;41:89-99.

130. Tracy S, Hofling K, Pirruccello S, Lane PH, Reyna SM, Gauntt CJ. Group B coxsackievirus myocarditis and pancreatitis: connection between viral virulence phenotypes in mice. J Med Virol 2000;62:70-81.

131. Beck MA, Chapman NM, McManus BM, Mullican JC, Tracy S. Secondary enterovirus infection in the murine model of myocarditis. Pathologic and immunologic aspects. Am J Pathol 1990;136:669-681.

132. Huber SA, Job LP. Differences in cytolytic T cell response of BALB/c mice infected with myocarditic and non-myocarditic strains of coxsackievirus group B, type 3. Infect Immun 1983;39:1419-1427.

133. Huber SA, Job LP, Woodruff JF. Lysis of infected myofibers by coxsackievirus B-3 immune T lymphocytes. Am J Pathol 1980;98:681-694.

134. Lerner AM. Coxsackievirus myocardiopathy. J Infect Dis 1969;120:496-499.

135. Wong CY, Woodruff JJ, Woodruff JF. Generation of cytotoxic T lymphocytes during coxsackievirus B-3 infection. I. Model and viral specificity. J Immunol 1977;118:1159-1164.

136. Wong CY, Woodruff JJ, Woodruff JF. Generation of cytotoxic T lymphocytes during coxsackievirus tb-3 infection. II. Characterization of effector cells and demonstration of cytotoxicity against viral-infected myofibers. J Immunol 1977;118:1165-1169.

137. Huber SA, Lodge PA. Coxsackievirus B-3 myocarditis in Balb/c mice. Evidence for autoimmunity to myocyte antigens. Am J Pathol 1984;116:21-29.

138. Lerner AM, Wilson FM. Virus myocardiopathy. Prog Med Virol 1973;15:63-91.

139. Huber SA. Coxsackievirus-induced myocarditis is dependent on distinct immunopathogenic responses in different strains of mice. Lab Invest 1997;76:691-701.

140. Huber SA, Mortensen A, Moulton G. Modulation of cytokine expression by CD4⁺ T cells during coxsackievirus B3 infections of BALB/c mice initiated by cells expressing the γδ⁺ T-cell receptor. J Virol 1996;70:3039-3044.

141. Huber SA. Heat-shock protein induction in adriamycin and picornavirus-infected cardiocytes. Lab Invest 1992;67:218-224.

142. Klingel K, Hohenadl C, Canu A, Albrecht M, Seemann M, Mall G, Kandolf R. Ongoing enterovirus-induced myocarditis is associated with persistent heart muscle infection: quantitative analysis of virus replication, tissue damage, and inflammation. Proc Natl Acad Sci U S A 1992;89:314-318.

143. Klingel K, Kandolf R. The role of enterovirus replication in the development of acute and chronic heart muscle disease in different immunocompetent mouse strains. Scand J Infect Dis Suppl 1993;88:79-85.

144. Kishimoto C, Abelmann WH. In vivo significance of T cells in the development of coxsackievirus B3 myocarditis in mice: immature but antigen-specific T cells aggravate cardiac injury. Circ Res 1990;67:589-598.

145. Woodruff JF, Woodruff JJ. Involvement of T lymphocytes in the pathogenesis of coxsackie virus B3 heart disease. J Immunol 1974;113:1726-1734.

146. Guthrie M, Lodge PA, Huber SA. Cardiac injury in myocarditis induced by coxsackievirus group B, type 3 in Balb/c mice is mediated by Lyt2⁺ cytolytic lymphocytes. Cell Immunol 1984;88:558-567.

147. Huber SA, Stone JE, Wagner DH Jr, Kupperman J, Pfeiffer L, David C, O'Brien RL, Davis GS, Newell MK. γδ⁺ T cells regulate major histocompatibility complex class II(IA and IE)-dependent susceptibility to coxsackievirus B3-induced autoimmune myocarditis. J Virol 1999;73:5630-5636.

148. Seko Y, Matsuda H, Kato K, Hashimoto Y, Yagita H, Okumura K, Yazaki Y. Expression of inter-cellular adhesion molecule-1 in murine hearts with acute myocarditis caused by coxsackievirus B3. J Clin Invest 1993;91:1327-1336.

149. Henke A, Mohr C, Sprenger H, Graebner C, Stelzner A, Nain M, Gemsa D. Coxsackievirus B3-induced production of tumor necrosis factor-α, IL-1β, and IL-6 in human monocytes. J Immunol 1992;148:2270-2277.

150. Huber SA, Polgar J, Schultheiss P, Schwimmbeck P. Augmentation of pathogenesis of coxsackievirus B3 infections in mice by exogenous administration of interleukin-1 and interleukin-2. J Virol 1994;68:195-206.

151. Lane JR, Neumann DA, Lafond-Walker A, Herskowitz A, Rose NR. Role of IL-1 and tumor necrosis factor in coxsackie virus-induced autoimmune myocarditis. J Immunol 1993;151:1682-1690.

152. Liu P. The role of cytokines in the pathogenesis of myocarditis. In: Schultheiss H-P, Schwimmbeck P, eds. The role of immune mechanisms in cardiovascular disease. Berlin: Springer-Verlag, 1997:44-56.

153. Neumann DA, Lane JR, Allen GS, Herskowitz A, Rose NR. Viral myocarditis leading to cardio-myopathy: do cytokines contribute to pathogenesis? Clin Immunol Immunopathol 1993;68:181-190.

154. Gebhard JR, Perry CM, Harkins S, Lane T, Mena I, Asensio VC, Campbell IL, Whitton JL. Coxsackievirus B3-induced myocarditis: perforin exacerbates disease, but plays no detectable role in virus clearance. Am J Pathol 1998;153:417-428.

155. Cook DN, Beck MA, Coffman TM, Kirby SL, Sheridan JF, Pragnell IB, Smithies O. Requirement of MIP-1α for an inflammatory response to viral infection. Science 1995;269:1583-1585.

156. Horwitz MS, La Cava A, Fine C, Rodriguez E, Ilic A, Sarvetnick N. Pancreatic expression of inter-

feron-γ protects mice from lethal coxsackievirus B3 infection and subsequent myocarditis. Nat Med 2000;6:693-697.

157. Tu Z, Chapman NM, Hufnagel G, Tracy S, Romero JR, Barry WH, Zhao L, Currey K, Shapiro B. The cardiovirulent phenotype of coxsackievirus B3 is determined at a single site in the genomic 5' nontranslated region. J Virol 1995;69:4607-4618.

158. Dunn JJ, Chapman NM, Tracy S, Romero JR. Genomic determinants of cardiovirulence in coxsackie-virus B3 clinical isolates: localization to the 5' nontranslated region. J Virol 2000;74:4787-4794.

159. Knowlton KU, Jeon ES, Berkley N, Wessely R, Huber S. A mutation in the puff region of VP2 attenuates the myocarditic phenotype of an infectious cDNA of the Woodruff variant of coxsackie-virus B3. J Virol 1996;70:7811-7818.

160. Khatib R, Probert A, Reyes MP, Khatib G, Chason JL. Mouse strain-related variation as a factor in the pathogenesis of coxsackievirus B3 murine myocarditis. J Gen Virol 1987;68:2981-2988.

161. Schnurr DP, Schmidt NJ. Persistent infections. In: Bendinelli M, Friedman H, eds. Coxsackie-viruses: a general update. New York: Plenum Press, 1988:181-201.

162. Baboonian C, Davies MJ, Booth JC, McKenna WJ. Coxsackie B viruses and human heart disease. Curr Top Microbiol Immunol 1997;223:31-52.

163. Bowles NE, Richardson PJ, Olsen EG, Archard LC. Detection of coxsackie-B-virus-specific RNA sequences in myocardial biopsy samples from patients with myocarditis and dilated cardiomyopathy. Lancet 1986;1:1120-1123.

164. Easton AJ, Eglin RP. The detection of coxsackievirus RNA in cardiac tissue by *in situ* hybridization. J Gen Virol 1988;69(Pt 2):285-291.

165. Hilton DA, Variend S, Pringle JH. Demonstration of coxsackie virus RNA in formalin-fixed tissue sections from childhood myocarditis cases by *in situ* hybridization and the polymerase chain reaction. J Pathol 1993;170:45-51.

166. Kandolf R. The impact of recombinant DNA technology on the study of enterovirus heart disease. In: Bendinelli M, Friedman H, eds. Coxsackieviruses: a general update. New York: Plenum Press, 1988:293-318.

167. Tracy S, Chapman NM, McManus BM, Pallansch MA, Beck MA, Carstens J. A molecular and serologic evaluation of enteroviral involvement in human myocarditis. J Mol Cell Cardiol 1990;22:403-414.

168. Tracy S, Wiegand V, McManus B, Gauntt C, Pallansch M, Beck M, Chapman N. Molecular approaches to enteroviral diagnosis in idiopathic cardiomyopathy and myocarditis. J Am Coll Cardiol 1990;15:1688-1694.

169. Jin O, Sole MJ, Butany JW, Chia WK, McLaughlin PR, Liu P, Liew CC. Detection of enterovirus RNA in myocardial biopsies from patients with myocarditis and cardiomyopathy using gene amplification by polymerase chain reaction. Circulation 1990;82:8-16.

170. Why HJ, Meany BT, Richardson PJ, Olsen EG, Bowles NE, Cunningham L, Freeke CA, Archard LC. Clinical and prognostic significance of detection of enteroviral RNA in the myocardium of patients with myocarditis or dilated cardiomyopathy. Circulation 1994;89:2582-2589.

171. Wessely R, Henke A, Zell R, Kandolf R, Knowlton KU. Low-level expression of a mutant coxsackie-viral cDNA induces a myocytopathic effect in culture: an approach to the study of enteroviral persistence in cardiac myocytes. Circulation 1998;98:450-457.

172. Kerekatte V, Keiper BD, Badorff C, Cai A, Knowlton KU, Rhoads RE. Cleavage of poly(A)-binding protein by coxsackievirus 2A protease in vitro and in vivo: another mechanism for host protein synthesis shutoff? J Virol 1999;73:709-717.

173. Badorff C, Lee GH, Lamphear BJ, Martone ME, Campbell KP, Rhoads RE, Knowlton KU. Enteroviral protease 2A cleaves dystrophin: evidence of cytoskeletal disruption in an acquired cardiomyopathy. Nat Med 1999;5:320-326.

174. Beck MA, Levander OA. Effects of nutritional antioxidants and other dietary constituents on coxsackievirus-induced myocarditis. Curr Top Microbiol Immunol 1997;223:81-96.

175. Liu P, Aitken K, Kong YY, Opavsky MA, Martino T, Dawood F, Wen WH, Kozieradzki I, Bachmaier K, Straus D, Mak TW, Penninger JM. The tyrosine kinase p56^{lck} is essential in coxsackievirus B3-mediated heart disease. Nat Med 2000;6:429-434.

176. Yang D, Yu J, Luo Z, Carthy CM, Wilson JE, Liu Z, McManus BM. Viral myocarditis: identification of five differentially expressed genes in coxsackievirus B3-infected mouse heart. Circ Res 1999;84:704-712.

177. Christian HA. Nearly ten decades of interest in idiopathic pericarditis. Am Heart J 1951;42:645-651.

The Primary Viruses of Myocarditis

Kyung-Soo Kim, Ph.D., Katja Höfling, M.D.,
Steven D. Carson, Ph.D., Nora M. Chapman, Ph.D.,
and Steven Tracy, Ph.D.

INTRODUCTION

In any review of the viruses responsible for causing human myocarditis, one naturally focuses on the 6 serotypes of the group B coxsackieviruses (CVB1-6) (Table 2-1), human enteroviruses that have been well-established as primary causes of the disease since the mid-1950s. However, data from the mid-1990s suggested 2 other players whose roles seem also to be significant in the causation of this disease. Human adenovirus (Ad) DNA, specifically from adenovirus type 2 (Ad2) (Table 2-1), has been detected in a large proportion of human myocarditis cases. To date, there are no confirmed data suggesting that other Ad serotypes are involved, but it is not clear whether sufficient work has been done to screen for and so eliminate the possibility of other genotypes. Hepatitis C virus (HCV) (Table 2-1), a flavivirus, has been identified as a potential cause of human myocarditis, especially in studies of Japanese patients, although the evidence for a causal link elsewhere is less sound. Many viruses other than these 3 distinct viruses have been named as real or potential agents of viral inflammatory cardiomyopathy, but these 3—CVB, Ad2 and maybe other Ad, and HCV—seem, at present, to be the primary viral causes of the disease on the basis of isolation of virus from diseased tissue, serologic studies, or some type of

Table 2-1
Three Viruses Closely Linked as Agents of Human Myocarditis

Virus and classification	Virus description
Coxsackievirus, group B; genus *Enterovirus*, family Picornaviridae	Nonenveloped, icosahedral capsid, single-stranded RNA genome, positive sense, 7.4 kb (http://life.anu.edu.au/viruses/Ictv/fs_picor.htm#Genus1)
Adenovirus, genus *Mastadenovirus*, family Adenoviridae	Nonenveloped, icosahedral capsid, double-stranded linear DNA genome, 36-38 kbp (http://www.ncbi.nlm.nih.gov/ICTVdb/Ictv/fs_adeno.htm#Genus1)
Hepatitis C virus, genus *Hepacivirus*, family Flaviviridae	Enveloped capsid, linear, single-stranded RNA, positive sense, 9.4 kb (http://life.anu.edu.au/viruses/ICTVdB/26030001.htm)

Data from International Committee on the Taxonomy of Viruses, Virology Division, International Union of Microbiological Societies. http://www.ncbi.nlm.nih.gov/ICTV/ (February, 2000). Murphy FA, Fauquet CM, Bishop DK, Ghabrial SA, Jarvis AW, Martelli GP, Mayo MA, Summers MD. Virus taxonomy: the sixth report of the International Committee on Taxonomy of Viruses. Vienna: Springer-Verlag, 1995.
All the Virology on the World Wide Web at http://www.virology.net
To view images of these viruses online, see All the Virology on the World Wide Web, The Big Picture Book of Viruses, http://www.virology.net/Big_Virology/BVHomePage.html
Fields BN, Knipe DM, Howley PM, Chanock RM, Melnick JL, Monath TP, Roizman B, Straus SE, eds. Fields virology. 3rd ed. Philadelphia: Lippincott-Raven, 1996.

molecular detection method such as reverse transcription polymerase chain reaction (RT-PCR) or nucleic acid hybridization. Although this review deals with these 3 groups of viruses specifically, the reader should understand that these are not the sole agents of viral myocarditis but those for which strong cases have been or can be made for a primary etiologic role. This review examines papers published mainly since 1996; we direct the reader to earlier[1-4] and more recent[5-11] reviews for other references.

GROUP B COXSACKIEVIRUSES: INTRODUCTION

The CVB are human enteroviruses (family Picornaviridae), a genus that includes the well-studied and closely related polioviruses.[12] There are 6 CVB serotypes (CVB1-6); by definition, immunity against 1 serotype does not confer immunity against any of the other 5 serotypes. The CVB are typical enteroviruses and, after the polioviruses, are the best studied enterovirus group.[1,7]

The CVB genome is a single strand of positive (message) sense RNA, 7,400 nucleotides in length.[13] The 5' end of the genome is not capped but is linked covalently to the viral protein, VPg. The single open reading frame is preceded by the 5' nontranslated region (5' NTR), which at 741 nucleotides represents 10% of the viral genome. As in all picornaviruses, the enterovirus 5' NTR is a highly structured RNA sequence[14] whose functions include both viral protein translation and viral genome replication.[15-19] Although the primary structure (nucleotide sequence) of enteroviral or different CVB serotype 5' NTRs differs significantly, the overall higher-order RNA structures that are predicted to form are sufficiently similar to permit artificially engineered viruses, in which the 5' NTR from one enterovirus is replaced by that from another, to replicate and function in cell culture at near wild-type levels.[20,21] The CVB ORF encodes 11 proteins within a polyprotein of 2,185 amino acids. Two viral proteases process the CVB polyprotein cotranslationally so that, as in polioviruses and other picornaviruses, no full-length viral polyprotein is observed. The structure of the CVB3 capsid has been solved[22] and it, like other picornaviruses, is an icosahedron, made up of 60 copies each of the 4 viral capsid proteins. The virus receptor, human coxsackievirus and adenovirus receptor (CAR), a protein of the immunoglobulin superfamily,[23-25] most likely interacts with the virus capsid in the depressions (called canyons) that surround the 5-fold axes of symmetry. Interestingly, CAR is also a primary receptor for the Ad (see below).

EVIDENCE FOR CVB INVOLVEMENT IN MYOCARDITIS

Strong evidence supports an etiologic role for the CVB in myocarditis and dilated cardiomyopathy. From the mid-1950s onward, coxsackieviruses had been repeatedly isolated from myocarditic hearts;[26-31] furthermore, models of the disease were being established that indicated the virus could cause myocarditis in mice. The first demonstration that entero-viral RNA could be detected in myocarditic hearts was published by Bowles and colleagues;[32] these workers used slot blot detection of human heart RNA that was probed with radioactively labeled complementary DNA (cDNA) transcribed from CVB3 RNA. Much interest was generated by the findings that claimed as positive for viral RNA more than 50% of the myocarditic heart samples assayed. The claim that the viral RNA detected was specifically coxsackieviral represented a misunderstanding of the technique, which as designed was sufficiently generic to enable the detection of RNAs from many different enteroviruses. Numerous subsequent studies used filter hybridization, in situ hybridization, and RT-PCR to probe for the presence of enterovirus RNA in human heart tissues (reviewed in references 2 and 5). While some studies failed to detect any samples that were positive for enteroviral RNA, most detected enteroviral RNA in approximately 20% to 25% of hearts examined. Unfortunately, no multicenter study—to avoid possible biases or errors specific to a single laboratory and to screen samples from around the world—has yet rigorously defined by sequence the enteroviral genotypes detected in numerous endomyo-cardial biopsy or explanted heart muscle samples.

As representatives of all the CVB genomes have been sequenced and as there is a deep database of enteroviral genomic sequences, the design of the appropriate primers for the identification and characterization of the primary enteroviruses by sequence analysis is straightforward. The diagnostic sequence to target should be the region encompassing the junction of the capsid protein 1D with the viral protease 2Apro.[33-35] The strong molec-ular evidence of enteroviral involvement with myocarditis combined with the earlier findings of various CVB serotypes in diseased hearts and the excellent models of murine myocarditis that recapitulate many of the human disease symptoms make it highly likely that the CVB are the enterovirus most often responsible for causing human myocarditis.

THE COXSACKIEVIRUS-ADENOVIRUS RECEPTOR

Evidence that several of the coxsackieviruses and Ad use a common cell surface receptor was provided initially by experiments that tested the abilities of different viruses (CVB1, CVB3, and Ad2) to interfere with one another for binding to and infecting target cells.[36,37] These early results have now been confirmed in detail. The shared receptor is commonly referred to as CAR (HCAR and MCAR are used to denote CAR of human or mouse origin, respec-tively). The CAR has been shown to function as the cellular receptor for Ad subgroups A, C, D, E, and F as well as the CVB.[38]

Three laboratories concurrently reported the isolation and identification of CAR as a unique new membrane protein in 1997.[23-25] All 3 of these groups used reagents or methods developed earlier in Crowell's laboratory.[39,40] The CAR amino acid sequence has been determined both by partial amino-terminal sequencing and by sequence analysis of the cloned cDNAs. The CAR is a member of the immunoglobulin superfamily of proteins, containing an amino-terminal V-like domain (frequently referred to as D1), followed by a C2-like domain (D2), a single membrane-spanning sequence, and a 107-residue cytoplasmic domain (Fig. 2-1; see color plate 1). The amino acid sequence provides a calculated molecular weight for the polypeptide chain of 37,969 after removal of the signal sequence. The mature protein that is expressed in cultured cells is glycosylated; there are 2 AsnXSer/Thr sites, 1 in each extracellular domain, which potentially contain N-linked carbohydrate. By sodium dodecyl sulfate-polyacyl-amide gel electrophoresis, the mature protein has an apparent mass near 46 kDa. Neither the cytoplasmic domain nor the membrane-spanning domain are required for CAR to function as a receptor for Ad or CVB: viruses of both groups can infect cells which express only the extracellular domain anchored to the membrane by either the native membrane-spanning sequence or glycophosphatidylinositol[43,44] (Carson S, Chapman N, unpublished data).

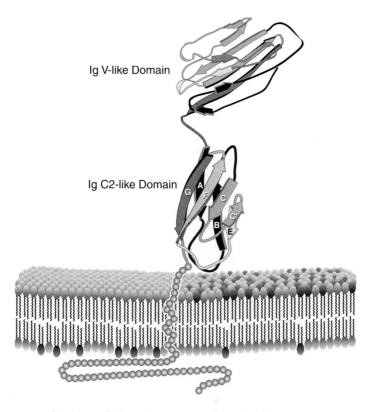

Fig. 2-1. Human coxsackievirus and adenovirus receptor. See color plate 1.

Adenoviruses bind the V-like domain of CAR. The structure of the Ad12 fiber knob complexed with the V-like domain, produced in *Escherichia coli*, has been solved.[41] Three CAR V-like domains bind a single fiber knob. The structure of the C2-like domain and the overall CAR structure remain to be determined, but similarity to C2 domains of other members of the immunoglobulin superfamily is anticipated. Although several groups have expressed the individual V-like and C2-like domains, the binding site for CVB has not been reported. The silence on this issue suggests that CVB binding may require contributions from both domains or that carbohydrate moieties, present on the native protein but absent from protein that is artificially expressed in *E coli*, play a role in CVB association with the CAR. The potential importance of glycosylation on CVB binding was suggested by experiments that predate the isolation and characterization of CAR.[45] Although virus overlay blots use radiolabeled CVB to detect CAR isolated directly from cultured cells, such approaches fail to demonstrate CVB3 binding to the glycosylation-deficient extracellular domain of CAR expressed in *E coli* (Carson S, Chapman N, unpublished data).

Interestingly, the CAR has a high degree of sequence homology to A33, a protein known for its prevalence on colon carcinoma cells, and CTX, a *Xenopus laevis* protein expressed on thymocytes; the chicken and human equivalents of CTX have also been cloned and are quite similar.[46] This group of closely related proteins has an unusual second disulfide bond in the C2-like domain that is not present in other immunoglobulin superfamily proteins, indicating that they represent a subgroup that has been conserved during evolution. The degree of evolutionary conservation from amphibians to humans portends an important but unknown physiologic function for CAR.

The localization of the CAR gene to chromosome 21 was inferred by matching the CAR sequence data with sequences in the Expressed Sequence Tag database that had been assigned to chromosome 21.[23-25] Subsequently, mapping studies localized the CAR gene to 21q11.2 and identified 3 pseudogenes located on chromosomes 15, 18, and 21. The CAR gene has been characterized further in the context of genomic organization and shown to be divided into 7 exons.[47] Regulatory elements that control CAR transcription and translation remain to be identified, and evidence suggesting that CAR expression is highly regulated (discussed below) indicates that such elements will be interesting and important.

With rare exceptions (see below), CVB infect only cultured cells which express CAR (eg, HeLa cells but not RD cells). It may, therefore, be anticipated that CAR should be expressed in tissues and organs that are infected by CVB. Similar expectations may hold for Ad infection, but established roles for coreceptor proteins and for secondary receptors indicate that simple interpretations of infection-receptor expression association may not be generally appropriate with Ad (eg, alpha V integrins[48] and glycosaminoglycans[49]). The CVB are appreciated for their ability to infect brain, pancreas, and heart. Northern blot analyses readily detected CAR mRNA in human pancreas, heart, prostate, testis, intestine, and brain.[25,50] The CAR mRNA was also present in murine kidney, liver, and lung. Although northern blot analyses failed to detect CAR mRNA from human lung, human airway epithelial cells in culture have been shown to express CAR on the basolateral aspects of the cell surface.[51]

Consistent with decreasing susceptibility of both mice and humans after the early neonatal period, recent studies have found decreased expression of CAR in muscle cells of adult rats and mice.[52,53] Similar results were obtained in vivo in mice.[54] In rats, immuno-histochemical analysis revealed broad neural and epithelial distribution of CAR during development, with expression more pronounced in epithelial cells of adult animals.[55] Significantly, CAR was reexpressed in adult hearts during myocarditis and could also be induced in cultured cardiomyocytes treated with supernatants from phytohemagglutinin-stimulated leukocytes.[52] We have shown that human umbilical vein endothelial cells increased the expression of CAR per cell as the density of cultured cells increased, in sharp contrast to HeLa cells in which CAR expression per cell was constant at all densities.[56] Expression of CAR by HeLa cells is down-regulated by an unknown mechanism when the cells are transfected for expression of plasminogen activator inhibitor 2.[57] These findings, considered in context of the epidemiology of CVB disease, suggest that susceptibility to CVB diseases and the pathology of the viral infection will be closely tied to the regulated expression of CAR. Because males are more susceptible to viral myocarditis than females, it will be interesting to determine whether androgenic hormones increase the expression of CAR, especially in tissues associated with CVB pathologies, as was suggested by Lyden et al.[58]

Much of the work predating the discovery and characterization of CAR was reviewed in 1997 by Kuhn.[59] In the course of efforts to identify and isolate CAR, other proteins that bind CVB have been identified, including decay accelerating factor (DAF, CD55), a complement regulatory protein on the cell surface, and nucleolin, an intracellular protein that had not previously been observed on the cell surface.[60,61] The roles of DAF and nucleolin with regard to receptor-associated functions during CVB infection remain unclear. Findings published since the initial reports that these proteins bind CVB have largely served to increase our confidence that CAR is the principal receptor for CVB (and Ad). Although nucleolin appears to bind CVB on virus overlay blots,[61] it does not support infection of Chinese hamster ovary cells,[62] cells that are refractory to CVB infection owing to lack of a suitable receptor.

In contrast to the sparse data on nucleolin, several reports provide compelling evidence that DAF binds not only strains of CVB that have been selected for growth on RD cells (which lack CAR and are generally refractory to CVB replication) but that DAF also binds CVB in general.[63,64] Although DAF-binding strains of CVB3 require CAR to productively infect and lyse RD cells,[65] demonstrating that binding DAF alone is insufficient for CVB to enter RD cells, a combination of antibodies against DAF and CAR is required to block infection of HeLa cells by strains of CVB3, which differ in their DAF-binding affinity.[66] Moreover, CVB which bind human DAF fail to bind DAF from rat and mouse,[67] but CVB do infect mouse 3T3 cells, which express human CAR[25] (Carson S, Chapman N, unpublished data). Overall, the data clearly show that CVB bind DAF, and probably nucleolin, but that neither of these proteins is necessary and sufficient for infection. Current data, however, do indicate that CAR is both necessary and sufficient for CVB infection of cells on which it is expressed, either naturally or after transfection. While it is tempting to accept CAR as the singular receptor for CVB, other data show that antibodies to DAF or removal of DAF from cells with phospholipase diminishes CVB infectivity.[63,66] Consequently, we speculate that DAF and CAR may be closely associated on the cell surface, that DAF may serve to provide a cell-associated reservoir of virus thereby increasing access to CAR, and that the optimally functional CVB receptor may be a complex of proteins in which CAR is the principal and key component. Resolution of this issue awaits detailed structural analysis of CVB bound to CAR, to DAF, and to the putative DAF-CAR complex and molecular description of the participation of these proteins in virus binding and cell entry.

Proteins other than CAR can bind Ad2 and Ad5, including integrins, MHC-1, and glycosaminoglycans.[48,49,68] The role of glycosaminoglycans remains to be studied, and the involvement of major histocompatibility complex-1 in Ad infection is controversial following reports that CAR, and not major histocompatibility complex-1, is required for Ad infection.[69,70] In contrast, it appears that CAR functions as a primary receptor for Ad binding to cells, but alpha (v) integrins are required for viral uptake and infection.[68] Viral tropism, however, depends on other factors in addition to the expression of CAR and integrins.[71]

The different protein-virus interactions required for infection indicate that the mechanisms of cell entry, or at least the determinants for cell entry, differ for CVB and Ad, and that CAR does not provide equivalent access to the cell for these different viruses. Although mice are readily infectable by CVB, human Ad do not replicate in mice. If the primary component in the CVB infection of murine tissues is the presence of MCAR, a protein closely similar to HCAR, then MCAR alone must be insufficient for human Ad replication. This may be due to differences in the abilities of equivalent coreceptor proteins from mouse and human to support viral entry into cells, or it may be the result of subtle differences between the HCAR and MCAR structures important for Ad binding. Because mutation of L54→A can abrogate Ad binding to HCAR, it is possible that apparently minor differences between HCAR and MCAR are sufficient to render MCAR incapable of binding human Ad. The Ad12 fiber knob contacts HCAR in the C, C′, C″, and F strands of the V-like domain.[41] Although key contact residues are conserved in MCAR, 3 of the 9 amino acid differences found in this domain occur in the C′ and C″ strands (A93→S, K97→I, and D63→N).

From studies published since 1997, one can conclude that the predicted human receptor shared by Ad and CVB has been isolated and partially characterized. Although the Ad12 binding site on HCAR has been defined at near atomic detail, these details have not illuminated the molecular mechanisms of Ad infection of cells, especially in view of requirements for secondary receptor (or coreceptor) proteins. Details of the molecular interaction between CAR and Ad may provide new avenues for pharmacologic interventions in infection and approaches for targeting Ad-based gene therapy vectors to target tissues that do not express CAR. At this writing, the fine details of CVB binding to CAR are not yet known. It has been suggested that the CAR-CVB association may require glycosylation of the receptor or features contributed from both of the extracellular protein subdomains. The few reports of CAR expression in different tissues support the idea that CVB tropism may be directed by receptor expression. This interpretation may be simplistic because prostate, testis, kidney, and lung have been reported to express CAR, yet the pathologic feature of CVB-associated disease is associated primarily with pancreas, heart, and brain. The findings that CAR is expressed in cultured endothelial cells, which can harbor chronic CVB infections, and that CAR can be regulated by inflammatory mediators indicate that understanding the epidemiology and pathology of CVB and Ad infections depends on elucidating the cell biology and physiology of CAR expression and function.

THE GENETICS OF CVB CARDIOVIRULENCE

The genetics of viral virulence phenotypes have not been worked out for any of the picornaviruses, with the exception of the CVB, in which work has just begun. We distinguish here between the genetics of *artificially altered* virulence phenotypes (as, for example, by mutation or animal passage) and the genetics of *naturally occurring* virulence phenotypes, such as are found in clinical viral isolates. In the former case, the genetics and the mechanism of artificially induced attenuation have been worked out for the Sabin poliovirus vaccine strains,[12,72-77] but the natural genetic determinants of the poliovirus neurovirulence phenotype were never mapped. With poliovirus approaching worldwide eradication as a cause of disease,[78-81] it is doubtful that this mapping will occur for poliovirus.

ARTIFICIAL ATTENUATION VERSUS NATURALLY OCCURRING VIRULENCE PHENOTYPES

The CVB are, however, not under a cloud of eradication like the related polioviruses and are an excellent model system with which to study the genetics that underlie naturally occurring virulence phenotypes and approaches to artificial attenuation. A distinct advantage to the study of CVB virulence phenotypes is the ability of these viruses to replicate well and to high titers in mice and the ability to induce diseases, such as acute myocarditis and pancreatitis, that are close counterparts to the human disease.[4,82-84] Another key aspect is the availability of numerous clinical isolates of the 6 CVB serotypes that permit sorting by virulence phenotype in mice. Finally, the genomes of all CVB serotypes have been cloned as infectious cDNA copies, permitting ready mapping of viral genetics by comparative sequence analysis and by chimeric genome construction.

Until recently, the studies that have dealt with the topic of cardiovirulence have focused on the genetics of artificially induced attenuation; the exception has been a series of studies mapping sites of CVB4 pancreovirulence. In 1995, we[85] reported the mapping and identification of the single nucleotide mutation that was responsible for the attenuation of the cardiovirulent phenotype of a well-characterized noncardiovirulent CVB3 strain called CVB3/0.[86] The U234C mutation in the CVB3 5' NTR attenuated CVB3/0 for replication in murine heart cells in culture and in the mouse and was responsible for attenuating the myocarditic phenotype in mice. This work also showed that replication of CVB3/0 in severe combined immunodeficient mice that lack functional T- and B-cell immune responses resulted in the rapid acquisition of a cardiovirulent phenotype and that this was linked to a C to U reversion at nucleotide (nt) 234.

Our findings have been extended by inducing transversion mutations within the 5mer.[87] Transversion mutations (Py/Pu or Pu/Py) more deleteriously affect the replicative vigor of the resulting progeny viral strains in cell culture; the strains are effectively unable to replicate successfully in mice. As opposed to the key attenuating 5' NTR mutations of the Sabin poliovirus strains that slowed viral translation in cells of neural origin,[88] we found that the 5mer mutations altered the positive-to-negative viral RNA strand ratio in infected cells, a finding that suggests a lesion in positive strand viral RNA synthesis. Subsequent investigation demonstrated that the nt234C mutation was unique to CVB3/0 and that nt234 existed always as U in a completely conserved 5mer defined by nt232-236 (5'-CGUUA) in all enteroviruses known. Therefore, the 234C was most likely an artificial mutation and not a naturally occurring determinant of a noncardiovirulent phenotype.[89]

Much attention was drawn by a report that CVB3/0 rapidly became virulent on replication in selenium-deficient mice,[90] data that suggested a correlation between selenium deficiency and the possibility of a normally benign CVB3 infection causing Keshan disease,[91] with greater implications for nutrition and viral diseases. The data were generated by using the artificially attenuated CVB3/0 strain, a strain that reverts even in well-fed mice. These findings have not been tested, however, with a series of avirulent CVB strains to determine whether a naturally occurring avirulent strain will become virulent during replication under conditions of selenium deficiency. Recently, CVB-induced murine myocarditis has been shown to be linked to murine pancreatitis, and myocarditis does not apparently exist in the absence of pancreatitis.[84] The noncardiovirulent CVB3/0 is nonetheless partially pancreovirulent in mice, inducing pancreatitis (acinar tissue destruction). Replication of CVB in the murine pancreas occurs soon after inoculation and reaches titers higher than those observed in sera during viremia. This work has also shown that CVB strains exist that replicate well in mice, yet cause no detectable disease in murine pancreas or heart. Such naturally occurring avirulent strains are potentially valuable candidates for naturally stable vaccine strains. Knowlton and colleagues[92] identified a mutation in the capsid protein 1B (also termed "VP2") that attenuated a highly cardiovirulent CVB3 strain; however, like the mutation characterized by Tu et al.,[85] the capsid protein mutation has not been found in any other CVB strains and must be considered artificial.

Ramsingh and co-workers[83,93-97] have focused on CVB4 involvement as an agent of pancreatitis. They used an avirulent strain of CVB4 and a derivative of the same strain passed in mice that acquired a pancreovirulent and cardiovirulent phenotype to map 2 primary sites that determine the pancreovirulent phenotype to the capsid proteins. Although in this case the phenotype that was acquired was a virulent rather than an attenuated one, experiments to show that the mutations are not murine adaptations (for example, by mapping pancreovirulence of clinical CVB4 isolates) have yet to be performed. Iizuka and colleagues[98] deleted approximately 100 nt of the CVB1 5′ NTR from just upstream of the translational start site and demonstrated that the resultant virus was less virulent in mice. All of these artificially altered genomes, especially the chimeric and deletion strains, also represent potentially useful models for the study of viral quasispecies and viral evolution in cell cultures and in mice.

A key set of experiments mapped cardiovirulence of clinical isolates of CVB3 to the 5′ NTR. Using several different CVB3 strains that naturally varied in their cardiovirulence phenotypes and the CVB3/20 infectious clone (a virus that is both pancreovirulent and cardiovirulent in mice[13]) as the background, Dunn[99] and others constructed several genomic chimera and tested their virulence phenotype in mice. The capsid protein coding region or the 3′ half of different CVB3 genomes (encoding the nonstructural proteins) in the CVB3/20 background caused no change in the cardiovirulent phenotype, regardless of whether the donated sequences were obtained from cardiovirulent or noncardiovirulent strains. However, when the 5′ NTR of the noncardiovirulent strain CVB3/CO was used to replace its homolog in CVB3/20, the resultant virus was no longer cardiovirulent. Replacement of the CVB3/CO 5′ NTR with that from the parental CVB3/20 or from another, different cardiovirulent strain (CVB3/AS) restored the cardiovirulent phenotype. These data are strong evidence that the CVB3 5′ NTRs naturally encode cardiovirulence. The site that controls the cardiovirulent phenotype has been more finely mapped to the stem-loop II region of the 5′ NTR. Although these exciting results are unique and for the first time indicate where in the genome cardiovirulence is likely encoded, many questions remain. Are these results applicable to other CVB3 strains and other CVB serotypes? Does this same site control pancreovirulence and avirulence? Although the pancreovirulent and cardiovirulent phenotypes appear to be linked,[84] similar chimeric cDNA constructs are needed using pancreovirulent and avirulent strains to determine the answer. How does stem-loop II interact with the infected host cell to set the chain of events in motion that culminates in clinically describable disease?

The importance attached to understanding the natural genetics of CVB virulence is understandable. Different attenuating approaches may be taken to reduce the replicative fitness of CVB strains and thus generate a potentially useful vaccine strain. However, as evident from Sabin poliovirus vaccine strains (reviewed in reference 77) and an attenuating mutation in CVB3,[85] the attenuated phenotype can rapidly revert during replication in the host, resulting in reacquisition of a virulent phenotype. It can be argued that, were the Sabin poliovirus strains developed today to fight poliomyelitis, this rapidity of reversion would not be commercially acceptable in a vaccine. A vaccine against the 6 CVB types would be useful to reduce the incidence of viral myocarditis and virus-induced dilated cardiomyopathy but, given the relatively small market (about 10% of that for poliovirus during the epidemic years of the 1940s and 1950s), it is unlikely that any company will spend the funds necessary to bring such a vaccine to market.

It is possible that CVB will be used in the future as chimeric vaccine and virus expression vectors as well as therapeutic vectors. Much evidence, obtained using polioviruses as vectors, has shown that enteroviruses could succeed as chimeric vectors against other diseases of viral and bacterial origin and perhaps even cancer.[100-107] Höfling and colleagues[108] demonstrated that an attenuated strain of CVB3, expressing an antigenic polypeptide from adenovirus type 2 (Ad2) hexon protein, induced both anti-Ad2 and anti-CVB3 immunity in mice. These workers demonstrated that the chimeric virus induced anti-Ad2 immunity even in mice that had been immunized previously with CVB3 to mimic preexisting immunity in humans, suggesting the potential for reuse of the viral vector and expression of multiple epitopes. In another demonstration of the potential clinical utility of chimeric CVB vectors, Chapman et al.[109] showed that an attenuated strain of CVB3 can express biologically active murine interleukin-4 and that its replication in mice can induce CVB3-binding IgG1 antibodies. These results cumulatively raise many interesting questions. For example, can a different cytokine, interleukin-2, when linked to virus-expressed antigens, potentiate the host immune response to the foreign vector and to the foreign antigen, as has been shown for nonviral systems?[110] Can CVB be used to express polyvalent epitope arrays, similar to those that have been studied for use as immunogens against *Plasmodium falciparum* (malaria) infection?[111]

PROGRESS TOWARD UNDERSTANDING THE MOLECULAR MECHANISMS OF CVB-INDUCED INFLAMMATORY HEART DISEASE

The molecular and immunologic mechanisms that determine CVB inflammatory heart disease are being studied. The first step in pathogenesis once the virus has entered the body (ie, entry into the cell) has been resolved through the discovery and characterization of the receptor that the virus uses to gain entry into cells (see above).

Two findings have made important strides in the overall understanding of intracellular molecular mechanisms of viral heart disease. The src kinase p56lck plays a role in CVB3 heart disease in knock-out mice: mice lacking p56lck did not develop CVB3-induced disease.[112] Although the mechanism of this finding has not been derived, the findings suggest that p56lck might be targeted to intervene in CVB-caused disease. Importantly, these findings extended to other organs besides the heart, making the possibility of an anti-p56lck compound of significant interest.

How CVB3 replication interacts with components of the infected cell is the subject of 2 further papers. Lloyd's[113] and Knowlton's[114] groups showed that 1 of the 2 CVB proteases, termed "2Apro," cleaves poly A binding protein; Knowlton showed it also cleaves dystrophin. Dystrophin and the dystrophin-associated glycoproteins alpha-sarcoglycan and beta-dystroglycan were morphologically disrupted in infected myocytes. They also determined that there was a closer relationship between the kinetics of cleavage of poly A binding protein and HeLa cell host cell capped mRNA translational shutoff and viral protein synthesis than for the cleavage of eIF4G1, traditionally named as the key intracellular protein inhibited by 2Apro during enterovirus cleavage (primarily from poliovirus studies).

In other work, using mice with the inducible nitric oxide synthase gene knocked out, Zaragoza and colleagues[115] have demonstrated that CVB3-induced heart disease is worse than in normal mouse controls; similar results hold for pancreatitis,[116] a likely precursor to CVB-induced myocarditis.[84] The inflammatory response defines myocarditis; the inducible nitric oxide synthase gene can be induced by Th1-type cytokines such as interferon-γ and tumor necrosis factor-α, cytokines associated with CVB infection. The relationship of the extent of inducible nitric oxide synthase induction and the phenotype of the CVB strain used to inoculate mice needs, however, to be investigated; to date, the viruses used are all cardiovirulent and such strains are a minority of those that circulate naturally.[84] Is inducible nitric oxide synthase induced even during infections by avirulent strains of CVB? Heim and others[117] showed that proinflammatory cytokines interleukin-6 and interleukin-8 are transiently up-regulated in myocardial fibroblasts immediately after exposure to CVB3, consistent with others' findings that proinflammatory cytokines can also be expressed in the murine model of CVB3-induced myocarditis.[118] Huber and colleagues[119,120] demonstrated that $\gamma\delta+$ T cells modulate the major histocompatibility complex class II susceptibility to CVB3-induced heart disease, and that these cells primarily induce Fas-mediated killing and are more effective in inducing cardiomyocyte apoptosis than $\alpha\beta+$ T cells.

ADENOVIRUSES: INTRODUCTION

Human Ad have been highlighted as probable causes of human myocarditis. The Ad are double-stranded DNA viruses with linear genomes of approximately 40 kbp.[121,122] Like picornaviruses, their capsids consist of proteins arranged in an icosahedral design.[123] The discovery of the receptor protein, CAR, used by the CVB to enter human cells (see above) and subsequent work has shown that CAR is also the primary receptor used by Ad. Because the ability of a virus to enter cells represents a primary first step toward causing a disease in a given tissue, the ability of both CVB and Ad to use CAR as their receptor and their linkage to human inflammatory heart disease are perhaps not surprising. Nonetheless, viral pathogenesis requires more than mere cell access; many viruses can infect various tissues but cause no disease. Thus, much remains to be done to understand the propensity for Ad to replicate and cause disease in myocardial cells.

THE ADENOVIRUS GENOME AND REPLICATION

The human Ad are members of the genus *Mastadenovirus* (family Adenoviridae), which contains the nonavian Ad (reviewed in reference 122). Forty-nine serotypes of human Ad are organized into 6 subgroups by red blood cell agglutination. Human Ad2 and 5 of subgenus C are the best studied because of their ease of replication in HeLa or KB cell culture. The human Ad have a 30- to 38-kb linear double-stranded DNA genome with inverted terminal repeats of about 100 to 140 bp and are packaged in an icosahedral protein capsid containing 240 hexon and 12 penton proteins enclosing the core of the genome complexed with 4 viral proteins.

Ad of all but the B subgenus[38] have been shown to use either CAR[23-25] with high affinity or the $\alpha2$ domain of major histocompatibility complex class I[124] with low affinity as a human cell receptor via binding of the fiber protein of the capsid. However, Ad37 of the D subgenus has been shown to use sialic acid, not CAR, as a receptor.[125] Adenovirus entry into cells appears to be greatly stimulated by internalization receptors, the vitronectin-binding integrins $\alpha V\beta3$ and $\alpha V\beta5$, which are bound by RGD (arg-gly-asp) motifs of the penton base protein of the capsid.[48] This binding results in signal transduction required for endocytosis of the virus.[126] On entry into the cell, the virus escapes the endocytic vacuoles[127] and uncoats, and the core reaches the nucleus[128] in which the viral DNA serves as a transcriptional template for viral RNAs and is replicated.

Three temporal classes of RNAs encoding proteins are transcribed from Ad DNA: early (including E1A, E2, and E3 among others), delayed early, and late (mostly proteins of the virion) (reviewed in reference 122). Transcribed RNAs are spliced to generate mRNAs of multiple viral proteins.[129] The E1A proteins activate viral RNA transcription, affect cellular gene expression, induce entry of infected cells into the S phase (optimal for viral DNA replication), and prevent viral-induced apoptosis of infected cells. E1A and

E3 proteins have effects that decrease major histocompatibility complex class I expression on infected cells, thus decreasing the ability of cytotoxic T lymphocytes to eliminate infected cells (reviewed in reference 122). In addition, E3 and E1B proteins have antagonistic effects toward the antiviral activities of tumor necrosis factor-α.

The E2 proteins are involved in Ad DNA replication and include the precursor termination protein, the DNA polymerase, and DNA binding protein. These proteins and cellular transcription factors (Oct-1 and NFII) are necessary for viral DNA replication (reviewed in reference 130), a process that occurs by binding a replication complex to the terminal 5′ end of the repeated region of the genome, initiating transcription at nucleotide 4-6, jumping back to the initial 3 nucleotides (which have the identical sequence) and elongating the nascent strand of DNA. The precursor termination protein remains covalently attached to the 5′ end of the nascent DNA. The displaced strand of DNA can form base pairs at the terminal inverted repeats, generating a "panhandle" with a suitable 5′ end for initiation of DNA replication of a second strand. Alternatively, 2 replication forks from opposite ends of a replicating genome can meet, allowing the 2 parental strands to separate and nascent strands to be completed on them.

Replication of the viral genome results in increased activation of the major late promoter for expression of late RNAs (many different transcripts are produced by splicing and differential use of poly [A] sites), a process that involves binding of multiple cellular factors and adenovirus protein IVa2. Production of these late proteins depends on controlled elongation of the viral RNAs. Host cell protein synthesis is curtailed in Ad-infected cells: cellular RNAs are blocked from transport to the cytoplasm[131] and an initiation factor that is required for translation of most cellular RNAs is inactivated.[132] Adenovirus late RNAs use a different cap-dependent form of translational initiation, ribosome shunting,[133] which is functional with the late RNA tripartite leader. In addition to these processes, activation of the cellular protein kinase R by interferon or double-stranded RNA (produced during Ad infection), which stops translation by phosphorylation of eIF-2 to block initiation of translation, is prevented by the production of small viral RNAs, VAI RNA and VAII RNA (reviewed in reference 122). As late proteins accumulate, penton-hexon complexes are transported to the nucleus where Ad DNA is encapsidated in a process dependent on a packaging signal in the genome. Activity of the L3-encoded viral protease results in maturation of viral proteins in the virion, generating an infectious particle. Virus particles are released by lysis of the cell.

EVIDENCE FOR ADENOVIRUS INVOLVEMENT IN MYOCARDITIS

Relatively little evidence links human Ad to myocarditis, and it is primarily molecular in nature. Towbin's laboratory has promoted Ad as potential causes of human heart disease, beginning with the detection of Ad DNA by PCR in 15 of 38 pediatric heart samples.[134]

Concurrently, the detection of Ad DNA in the hearts of 2 patients with clinically unsuspected but histologically proven myocarditis was described by another group,[135] and Ad DNA was also detected by using PCR in the myocardium of an infant with myocarditis and pericarditis.[136] Matsumori[137] detected enteroviral RNA in 1 patient of 36 with cardiomyopathy and myocarditis; no other virus, including Ad, of those assayed was detected. Human heart biopsy samples from patients with dilated cardiomyopathy were probed with PCR; Ad DNA was detected in 17% of samples with inflammation and in 15% of samples without inflammation.[138]

Only in 1999 was sequence analysis applied to answer the question of which Ad serotype was being detected in human heart tissues.[139] With PCR and sequence analysis of the amplified fragments, 94 heart samples were examined from patients with left ventricular dysfunction; 13% were positive for Ad, and these were consistent with Ad serotype 2 (Ad2). To date, no other report has confirmed another serotype in the heart, but this is itself interesting, for 3 Ad serotypes are closely related: 1, 2, and 5 (previously called type C Ad). Is Ad2 the only cardiotropic and cardiovirulent Ad? If so, why? It is clear that a concerted effort is needed to resolve this question. Also in 1999, another group probed 31 samples from patients with myocarditis (n = 15) and dilated cardiomyopathy (n = 16) for enteroviral and Ad sequences.[140] These workers failed to find evidence for Ad DNA in their samples, although enteroviral RNA was detected in 27% of the patients. Towbin's group published another study on the use of tracheal aspirates as an approach to the detection of viruses in pediatric myocarditis and pneumonia.[141] Comparison of findings with the PCR analysis of endomyocardial biopsies showed 3 children with Ad and the confirmation of Ad2 in another patient who had both myocarditis and pneumonia.

Cumulatively, these reports suggest that similar problems exist for the detection of Ad DNA as for enteroviral RNA. Primarily, these are believed to revolve about the sensitivity of any specific group's enzymatic amplification assay and the as yet unresolved issue of prevalence of a specific virus at any time in a specific population. The results are highly inferential, however, that human Ad are involved as etiologic agents of human heart disease. At present, there is no small animal model with which to study Ad involvement in heart disease. Although there are murine adenoviruses (Mav) that replicate in their natural host and these viruses have been reasonably well characterized (reviewed in references 142 and 143), there is no Mav-induced mouse myocarditis model, although reports exist regarding myocarditis and endocarditis in mice induced by Mav type 1.[144,145] Given the apparent etiologic connection in humans, the molecular understanding of much of the Ad and Mav genomes, and the ready availability of inbred mouse strains, refinement of these early results into a working model of Mav-induced heart disease has merit.

HEPATITIS C VIRUSES: INTRODUCTION

Infection by HCV (family Flaviviridae, genus *Hepacivirus*), the cause of most cases of non-A, non-B viral hepatitis, is a major cause of chronic hepatitis, resulting in liver cirrhosis and hepatocellular carcinoma worldwide[146] and infects 175 million people globally. More than 80% of infected patients develop chronic disease while remaining essentially asymptomatic.[147] In the United States, an estimated 2 to 3 million people are currently infected and more than 150,000 new cases of HCV infection occur per year. The sequelae of HCV-induced and serious chronic liver disease result in 8,000 to 10,000 deaths annually.[147] Since the first report of viral genomic sequences from HCV in 1989, a greater understanding of the HCV infection has been achieved.

HCV infection usually develops after direct blood-borne percutaneous exposure. High risk of HCV infection has been reported often after blood transfusion.[148] Epidemiologic evidence exists for the transmission of HCV to renal dialysis patients, among intravenous drug users, during heterosexual sex, from mother to baby, and even by needle-stick victims.[149] With anti-HCV screening tests for blood donors, advanced assay techniques (eg, RT-PCR and in situ hybridization) have made it possible to detect early infection before the progression to acute disease.

THE HCV GENOME AND REPLICATION

Hepatitis C does not easily replicate to usable titers in cell culture, a fact that has hindered the study of the molecular biology of this virus. The viral genome is a positive-sense, single-stranded, 9.6-kb RNA molecule with highly conserved 5′ and 3′ NTR, approximately 341 and 500 nt, respectively, and is encapsidated with a core protein, C, that is enclosed in a membrane containing at least 2 envelope proteins, E1 and E2.[150] The 5′ NTR is a complex secondary structure, indicating the function of an internal ribosomal entry site,[151] whereas the 3′ NTR contains a highly conserved 98-nt sequence with a secondary structure which in combination with other sequences and the viral polymerase, NS5B, is necessary for the replication of the minus strand viral RNA.[152,153] The genome's single large open reading frame produces a polyprotein that is cotranslationally and post-translationally processed by the combination of host signal peptidases and viral proteinases, resulting in all 11 known viral proteins, including the nonstructural proteins NS2, NS3, NS4A, NS4B, NS5A, and NS5B (reviewed in reference 154). Viral proteases include NS2 acting in complex with NS3 and NS3 in complex with NS4A. NS3 also has RNA-stimulated NTPase and RNA helicase activities and has the potential to transform cells in culture. The functions of the protein p7, which is derived from processing of the structural region by signal peptidases, NS4B and NS5A, is currently unknown.

A host signal peptidase associated with transport into the endoplasmic reticulum is responsible for maturation of the structural proteins located in the N-terminal one-third of the polyprotein, whereas viral proteinases process the mature nonstructural proteins, NS2 to NS5B.[155] Thus far, 4 enzymatic activities encoded by the nonstructural proteins have been reported. The NS2-NS3 region codes for an autoproteinase responsible for cleavage at the 2/3 site.[156] Cleavage at the NS2/NS3 junction is accomplished by a metal-dependent, autocatalytic proteinase encoded within NS2 and the N-terminus of NS3. The remaining cleavages downstream from this site are effected by a serine proteinase also contained within the N-terminal region of NS3 (reviewed in reference 157). The N-terminal one-third of NS3 functions as the catalytic subunit of a serine proteinase, which cleaves at the NS3/4A, NS4A/4B, NS4B/5A, and NS5A/5B sites; NS4A is a membrane protein that acts as a cofactor of the proteinase.[155] NS3 in a heterodimeric complex with NS4A also encodes an RNA-stimulated NTPase/RNA helicase domain at its C-terminus.[158] To date, no functions have been reported for NS4B or NS5A in RNA replication; however, NS5A has been implicated in modulating the sensitivity of HCV to interferon.[159]

EVIDENCE FOR HCV INVOLVEMENT IN MYOCARDITIS

The literature on HCV involvement in heart disease is not vast and can be divided by results from Japanese and European groups. Matsumori and colleagues[160] initially suggested that HCV may play an etiologic role in the development of heart disease. Thirty-six patients with dilated cardiomyopathy were screened for anti-HCV antibodies in serum; 16.7% of the patients and 2.5% of controls ($n = 40$) were positive. HCV type II RNA was detectable by RT-PCR analysis in 4 of the 6 patients with antibodies against HCV, and RNA was detected in 3 of the positive patients' heart muscle. Matsumori et al.[161] then reported finding serologic evidence of HCV infection in 6 of 35 patients with hypertrophic cardiomyopathy versus 2% to 3% of patients with ischemic heart disease; HCV RNA was detected in the heart RNA from 3 of the 6 positive patients who had hypertrophic cardiomyopathy. This was followed by another group's findings that HCV RNA could be detected in the hearts and livers of 3 patients with chronic active myocarditis.[162] A multicenter study in Japan published in 1998 had examined 697 patients with hypertrophic cardiomyopathy and 663 patients with dilated cardiomyopathy for the presence of anti-HCV antibodies in sera:[163] 10% to 11% of the former and 6% of the latter were positive. In normal blood donors 2% to 3% were positive. In another Japanese study, 9 of 65 patients with hypertrophic cardiomyopathy tested positive for anti-HCV antibodies (13%-14%) versus 2% to 3% of the control population;[164] HCV RNA was also detected in 5 of the HCV positive patients.

In contrast to these findings of about 10% to 15% HCV positivity in patients with heart disease in Japan, Figulla and colleagues in Germany found a much lower percentage of dilated cardiomyopathy or myocarditis patients (n = 73) with anti-HCV sera: 1%-2% as opposed to 6% in the control group.[165] These workers concluded there was little obvious correlation between HCV exposure and heart disease. Another European study found no correlation in the sera or by PCR analysis between HCV or other microorganisms and end-stage idiopathic dilated cardiomyopathy (n = 37); 39 patients with end-stage dilated cardiomyopathy of known etiology were used as controls.[166] Prati and colleagues[167] studied HCV involvement in 752 patients with dilated cardiomyopathy and other heart diseases (along with 443 control samples) and found a lower percentage of anti-HCV antibodies in sera from heart patients (3% to 4%) than in the control group (6% to 7%), concluding that HCV exposure did not correlate with myocarditis or dilated cardiomyopathy. A study in Greece also found no evidence for linkage between HCV infection and dilated cardiomyopathy.[168] Patients with chronic HCV infection (n = 102) and dilated cardiomyopathy (n = 55) were assayed for exposure to HCV serologically and by RT-PCR. No chronic HCV patients had evidence of dilated cardiomyopathy, and no dilated cardiomyopathy patients showed serologic or molecular evidence of HCV infection.

The possible etiologic role of HCV infection in the development of myocarditis is still debatable: the reasons for the disparity in results between the Japanese and European studies are not evident. A difference in viral strains that circulate locally may represent a key factor.[169] HCV is a long-term persistent infection, permitting quasispecies variations to occur[170,171] and be selected within the unique environment of any human; such viral quasispecies might not be dominant in a general viral population.[172] This has been well-documented in HIV-infected patients. Individual variations or those endemic in a population as a locally dominant quasispecies can be postulated to influence disease outcome in those infected.[173] Therefore, it might be illuminating to determine whether significant differences in HCV sequences exist between those strains isolated from diseased heart tissues in Japan and those from HCV strains circulating generally in Japan and in Europe.

The problematic correlation of HCV infection with heart disease might also be said to exist for enteroviral infections and myocarditis, although the weight of the cumulative evidence makes for an extremely strong inferential argument for enterovirus causation of human myocarditis despite some reports in which enteroviral RNA has not been detected in diseased hearts. However, a similar weight of evidence does not exist at present supporting the role of HCV as a key agent of myocarditis. One primary aspect of the argument for enteroviral, specifically CVB, involvement in heart disease derives from correlative animal studies; it is clear that human CVB can cause acute myocarditis in mice and that this is both virus strain (eg, reference 84) and mouse strain[174] dependent. As for Ad involvement in heart disease, there is no current murine model as easily used for HCV heart disease as that available for the CVB, but this may be changing. A report offers a murine model of flavivirus infection,[175] thus raising the possibility of eventually deriving a murine model for flavivirus-induced myocarditis. Use of a transgenic mouse model[176] to model anti-HCV protection using vaccinia virus-HCV chimeric vaccines has also been reported. GB virus-B is a member of the flavivirus family and is closely related to HCV. Bukh and colleagues[177] have shown that GBV-B can replicate in tamarins and induce hepatitis, demonstrating a potential small primate model for HCV infection that might be adapted to heart disease.

REMAINING QUESTIONS

Although a review of the literature reveals known, suspected, or potential viral causes of human myocarditis, only the 6 serotypes of CVB and Ad2 appear at present to be the primary etiologic agents. The involvement of HCV may be important, especially in Japan and perhaps elsewhere on the western Pacific rim, but this is not yet clear. Other viruses come and go in reports, but none with the regularity of detection of enteroviruses and Ad. With enzymatic amplification and genetic arrays now commonplace, permitting rapid and sensitive detection of specific nucleic acids, a well-designed multicenter study is needed to determine which viruses (and other microorganisms) might be detected in myocarditis. Such studies would be expected to confirm and extend current knowledge, providing a stronger rationale for the targeting of key infectious agents as subjects of prophylactic, and possibly therapeutic, vaccine development. Clearly, a side but significant benefit of such vaccines would be the reduction in other diseases associated with these agents.

Much of what is understood about enteroviral involvement in human myocarditis stems from the availability and exploitation of excellent murine models of CVB-induced myocarditis. It makes sense to pursue such a model for adenovirus, using murine Ad because human Ad do not replicate in mice. This effort should also be linked with an effort to understand the role of CAR in the development of viral disease in mice and humans. Clearly, entry to cells is a prerequisite of viral disease but, conversely, the mere presence of the viral receptor does not imply that a specific tissue promotes productive viral infection that leads to disease. What is the natural purpose and ligand of CAR? Interventional therapy such as blocking CAR might be considered in severe cases of CVB disease such as in neonatal and pediatric patients.

For none of the 3 virus groups examined in this review is there complete consensus on the involvement of the specific virus in myocarditis. Viral antibodies have been found in sera or viral nucleic acid sequences in cells from diseased heart tissue; this contrasts with other studies that have failed to find significant linkage between viral exposure and heart disease. The efficacy and diligence of specific detection methods can always be argued as one cause of this variance, but, in general, serology and molecular detection techniques are now so well developed and so widely used that their credibility can no longer be raised as a fundamental issue. (Of course, how such data are interpreted will always remain problematic for some.) All viruses, far from being single entities, are better understood as populational swarms of related yet distinguishable strains termed "quasispecies."[178,179] With this concept firmly in mind, one can more easily cope with the idea that a specific "virus" in one part of the world may differ signficantly from its counterpart elsewhere or from one person to another in the same community. Studies of virus involvement in human disease, such as those discussed in this review and elsewhere, must also consider which viruses are in common circulation in the community in which the patients live. Is the failure to find virus nucleic acid in diseased hearts due to a limited circulation of virus for a specific time in a specific community? Serologic data are more telling in this respect: antibodies persist for long periods and represent a longer view. The 2 techniques—serology and molecular analysis—are complementary in defining the relationship of humans, viruses, and the diseases they cause.

Evidence suggests that vaccines can be created that can immunize humans against the primary viral agents of myocarditis—CVB and Ad2. The initial step in that direction has already been taken with the demonstration that an antigenic fragment of Ad2 hexon protein can be expressed by CVB3 and the replication of this chimeric virus in mice induces anti-Ad2 and anti-CVB3 neutralizing antibodies, even in the face of preexisting mouse anti-CVB3 immunity.[108] Unlike the Ad, which are also potential chimeric vaccine vectors, we understand much more about attenuating CVB for disease, primarily because of the advantage of a relevant disease system in mice.[20,85-87,180] Also, the CVB are closely related to the polioviruses against which excellent vaccines have been made. So successful have these vaccines been that poliovirus should soon be an extinct pathologic agent. Work in progress shows that multiantigenic chimeric CVB strains can induce protective immunity in mice against virulent challenge by CVB and Ad (the latter can be modeled by using Mav-1).[143] Coxsackievirus constructs can express cytokines and redirect the host immune response,[109] a finding that suggests therapeutic and immunomodulatory possibilities similar to what has been demonstrated by viral and subunit vaccines.[110,181,182]

REFERENCES

1. Bendinelli M, Friedman H, eds. Coxsackieviruses: a general update. New York: Plenum Press, 1988.
2. Martino TA, Liu P, Petric M, Sole MJ. Enteroviral myocarditis and dilated cardiomyopathy: a review of clinical and experimental studies. In: Rotbart HA, ed. Human enterovirus infections. Washington, DC: ASM Press, 1995:291-352.

3. Savoia MC, Oxman MN. Myocarditis, pericarditis and mediastinitis. In: Mandell GL, Douglas RG Jr, Bennett JE, eds. Principles and practice of infectious diseases. New York: Churchill Livingstone, 1990:721-732.

4. Woodruff JF. Viral myocarditis. A review. Am J Pathol 1980;101:425-484.

5. Baboonian C, Davies MJ, Booth JC, McKenna WJ. Coxsackie B viruses and human heart disease. Curr Top Microbiol Immunol 1997;223:31-52.

6. Melnick JL. Enteroviruses: polioviruses, coxsackieviruses, echoviruses, and newer enteroviruses. In: Fields BN, Knipe DM, Howley PM, Chanock RM, Melnick JL, Monath TP, Roizman B, Straus SE, eds. Fields virology. 3rd ed. Vol. 1. Philadelphia: Lippincott-Raven, 1996:655-712.

7. Tracy S, Chapman NM, Mahy BWJ. The coxsackie B viruses. Curr Top Microbiol Immunol 1997;223:1-303.

8. Bowles NE, Towbin JA. Molecular aspects of myocarditis. Curr Opin Cardiol 1998;13:179-184.

9. Kawai C. From myocarditis to cardiomyopathy: mechanisms of inflammation and cell death; learning from the past for the future. Circulation 1999;99:1091-1100.

10. Liu P, Martino T, Opavsky MA, Penninger J. Viral myocarditis: balance between viral infection and immune response. Can J Cardiol 1996;12:935-943.

11. Matsumori A. Cytokines in myocarditis and cardiomyopathies. Curr Opin Cardiol 1996;11:302-309.

12. Racaniello VR, Ren R. Poliovirus biology and pathogenesis. Curr Top Microbiol Immunol 1996;206:305-325.

13. Tracy S, Chapman NM, Tu Z. Coxsackievirus B3 from an infectious cDNA copy of the genome is cardiovirulent in mice. Arch Virol 1992;122:399-409.

14. Palmenberg AC, Sgro J-Y. Topological organization of picornaviral genomes: statistical prediction of RNA structural signals. Semin Virol 1997;8:231-241.

15. Agol VI, Paul AV, Wimmer E. Paradoxes of the replication of picornaviral genomes. Virus Res 1999;62:129-147.

16. Blyn LB, Swiderek KM, Richards O, Stahl DC, Semler BL, Ehrenfeld E. Poly(rC) binding protein 2 binds to stem-loop IV of the poliovirus RNA 5′ noncoding region: identification by automated liquid chromatography-tandem mass spectrometry. Proc Natl Acad Sci U S A 1996;93:11115-11120.

17. Parsley TB, Towner JS, Blyn LB, Ehrenfeld E, Semler BL. Poly (rC) binding protein 2 forms a ternary complex with the 5′-terminal sequences of poliovirus RNA and the viral 3CD proteinase. RNA 1997;3:1124-1134.

18. Shiroki K, Ishii T, Aoki T, Kobashi M, Ohka S, Nomoto A. A new cis-acting element for RNA replication within the 5′ noncoding region of poliovirus type 1 RNA. J Virol 1995;69:6825-6832.

19. Xiang W, Harris KS, Alexander L, Wimmer E. Interaction between the 5′-terminal cloverleaf and 3AB/3CDpro of poliovirus is essential for RNA replication. J Virol 1995;69:3658-3667.

20. Chapman NM, Ragland A, Leser JS, Hofling K, Willian S, Semler BL, Tracy S. A group B coxsackievirus/poliovirus 5′ nontranslated region chimera can act as an attenuated vaccine strain in mice. J Virol 2000;74:4047-4056.

21. Semler BL, Johnson VH, Tracy S. A chimeric plasmid from cDNA clones of poliovirus and coxsackievirus produces a recombinant virus that is temperature-sensitive. Proc Natl Acad Sci U S A 1986;83:1777-1781.

22. Muckelbauer JK, Kremer M, Minor I, Diana G, Dutko FJ, Groarke J, Pevear DC, Rossmann MG. The structure of coxsackievirus B3 at 3.5 Å resolution. Structure (London) 1995;3:653-667.

23. Bergelson JM, Cunningham JA, Droguett G, Kurt-Jones EA, Krithivas A, Hong JS, Horwitz MS, Crowell RL, Finberg RW. Isolation of a common receptor for Coxsackie B viruses and adenoviruses 2 and 5. Science 1997;275:1320-1323.

24. Carson SD, Chapman NN, Tracy SM. Purification of the putative coxsackievirus B receptor from HeLa cells. Biochem Biophys Res Commun 1997;233:325-328.

25. Tomko RP, Xu R, Philipson L. HCAR and MCAR: the human and mouse cellular receptors for subgroup C adenoviruses and group B coxsackieviruses. Proc Natl Acad Sci U S A 1997;94:3352-3356.

26. Dalldorf G. The coxsackie viruses. Annu Rev Microbiol 1955;9:277-296.

27. Disney ME, Howard EM, Wood BSB. Myocarditis in children. Br Med J 1953;1:1351-1354.

28. Fechner RE, Smith MG, Middlekamp JN. Coxsackie B virus infection of the newborn. Am J Pathol 1963;42:493-505.

29. Kibrick S, Benirschke K. Severe generalized disease (encephalohepatomyocarditis) occurring in the newborn period and due to infection with coxsackie virus, group B: evidence of intrauterine infection with this agent. Pediatrics 1958;22:857-875.

30. Nezelof C, LeSec G. Multifocal myocardial necrosis and fibrosis in pancreatic diseases of children. Pediatrics 1979;63:361-368.

31. Verlinde J, Van Tongeren H, Kret A. Myocarditis in newborns due to group B coxsackievirus: virus studies. Acta Pediatr 1956;187:113-118.

32. Bowles NE, Richardson PJ, Olsen EG, Archard LC. Detection of Coxsackie-B-virus-specific RNA sequences in myocardial biopsy samples from patients with myocarditis and dilated cardiomyopathy. Lancet 1986;1:1120-1123.

33. Mulders MN, Lipskaya GY, van der Avoort HG, Koopmans MP, Kew OM, van Loon AM. Molecular epidemiology of wild poliovirus type 1 in Europe, the Middle East, and the Indian subcontinent. J Infect Dis 1995;171:1399-1405.

34. Mulders MN, Salminen M, Kalkkinen N, Hovi T. Molecular epidemiology of coxsackievirus B4 and disclosure of the correct VP1/2A(pro) cleavage site: evidence for high genomic diversity and long-term endemicity of distinct genotypes. J Gen Virol 2000;81 Part 3:803-812.

35. Rico-Hesse R, Pallansch MA, Nottay BK, Kew OM. Geographic distribution of wild poliovirus type 1 genotypes. Virology 1987;160:311-322.

36. Crowell RL. Specific cell-surface alteration by enteroviruses as reflected by viral-attachment interference. J Bacteriol 1966;91:198-204.

37. Lonberg-Holm K, Crowell RL, Philipson L. Unrelated animal viruses share receptors. Nature 1976;259:679-681.

38. Roelvink PW, Lizonova A, Lee JG, Li Y, Bergelson JM, Finberg RW, Brough DE, Kovesdi I, Wickham TJ. The coxsackievirus-adenovirus receptor protein can function as a cellular attachment protein for adenovirus serotypes from subgroups A, C, D, E, and F. J Virol 1998;72:7909-7915.

39. Hsu KH, Lonberg-Holm K, Alstein B, Crowell RL. A monoclonal antibody specific for the cellular receptor for the group B coxsackieviruses. J Virol 1988;62:1647-1652.

40. Mapoles JE, Krah DL, Crowell RL. Purification of a HeLa cell receptor protein for group B coxsackieviruses. J Virol 1985;55:560-566.

41. Bewley MC, Springer K, Zhang YB, Freimuth P, Flanagan JM. Structural analysis of the mechanism of adenovirus binding to its human cellular receptor, CAR. Science 1999;286:1579-1583.

42. Barclay AN, Birkeland ML, Brown ML, Beyers MH, Davis AD, Somoza A, Williams AF. The leucocyte antigen factsbook. London: Academic Press, 1993.

43. Leon RP, Hedlund T, Meech SJ, Li S, Schaack J, Hunger SP, Duke RC, DeGregori J. Adenoviral-mediated gene transfer in lymphocytes. Proc Natl Acad Sci U S A 1998;95:13159-13164.

44. Wang X, Bergelson JM. Coxsackievirus and adenovirus receptor cytoplasmic and transmembrane domains are not essential for coxsackievirus and adenovirus infection. J Virol 1999;73:2559-2562.

45. Krah DL, Crowell RL. Properties of the deoxycholate-solubilized HeLa cell plasma membrane receptor for binding group B coxsackieviruses. J Virol 1985;53:867-870.

46. Chretien I, Marcuz A, Courtet M, Katevuo K, Vainio O, Heath JK, White SJ, Du Pasquier L. CTX, a Xenopus thymocyte receptor, defines a molecular family conserved throughout vertebrates. Eur J Immunol 1998;28:4094-4104.

47. Bowles KR, Gibson J, Wu J, Shaffer LG, Towbin JA, Bowles NE. Genomic organization and chromosomal localization of the human Coxsackievirus B-adenovirus receptor gene. Hum Genet 1999;105:354-359.

48. Wickham TJ, Mathias P, Cheresh DA, Nemerow GR. Integrins alpha v beta 3 and alpha v beta 5 promote adenovirus internalization but not virus attachment. Cell 1993;73:309-319.

49. Dechecchi MC, Tamanini A, Bonizzato A, Cabrini G. Heparan sulfate glycosaminoglycans are involved in adenovirus type 5 and 2-host cell interactions. Virology 2000;268:382-390.

50. Bergelson JM, Krithivas A, Celi L, Droguett G, Horwitz MS, Wickham T, Crowell RL, Finberg RW. The murine CAR homolog is a receptor for coxsackie B viruses and adenoviruses. J Virol 1998;72:415-419.

51. Walters RW, Grunst T, Bergelson JM, Finberg RW, Welsh MJ, Zabner J. Basolateral localization of fiber receptors limits adenovirus infection from the apical surface of airway epithelia. J Biol Chem 1999;274:10219-10226.

52. Ito M, Kodama M, Masuko M, Yamaura M, Fuse K, Uesugi Y, Hirono S, Okura Y, Kato K, Hotta Y, Honda T, Kuwano R, Aizawa Y. Expression of coxsackievirus and adenovirus receptor in hearts of rats with experimental autoimmune myocarditis. Circ Res 2000;86:275-280.

53. Nalbantoglu J, Pari G, Karpati G, Holland PC. Expression of the primary coxsackie and adenovirus receptor is downregulated during skeletal muscle maturation and limits the efficacy of adenovirus-mediated gene delivery to muscle cells. Hum Gene Ther 1999;10:1009-1019.

54. Xu R, Crowell RL. Expression and distribution of the receptors for coxsackievirus B3 during fetal development of the Balb/c mouse and of their brain cells in culture. Virus Res 1996;46:157-170.

55. Tomko RP, Johansson CB, Totrov M, Abagyan R, Frisen J, Philipson L. Expression of the adenovirus receptor and its interaction with the fiber knob. Exp Cell Res 2000;255:47-55.

56. Carson SD, Hobbs JT, Tracy SM, Chapman NM. Expression of the coxsackievirus and adenovirus receptor in cultured human umbilical vein endothelial cells: regulation in response to cell density. J Virol 1999;73:7077-7079.

57. Shafren DR, Gardner J, Mann VH, Antalis TM, Suhrbier A. Picornavirus receptor down-regulation by plasminogen activator inhibitor type 2. J Virol 1999;73:7193-7198.

58. Lyden DC, Olszewski J, Feran M, Job LP, Huber SA. Coxsackievirus B-3-induced myocarditis. Effect of sex steroids on viremia and infectivity of cardiocytes. Am J Pathol 1987;126:432-438.

59. Kuhn RJ. Identification and biology of cellular receptors for the coxsackie B viruses group. Curr Top Microbiol Immunol 1997;223:209-226.

60. Bergelson JM, Mohanty JG, Crowell RL, St John NF, Lublin DM, Finberg RW. Coxsackievirus B3 adapted to growth in RD cells binds to decay-accelerating factor (CD55). J Virol 1995;69:1903-1906.

61. de Verdugo UR, Selinka HC, Huber M, Kramer B, Kellermann J, Hofschneider PH, Kandolf R. Characterization of a 100-kilodalton binding protein for the six serotypes of coxsackie B viruses. J Virol 1995;69:6751-6757.

62. Kramer B, Huber M, Kern C, Klingel K, Kandolf R, Selinka HC. Chinese hamster ovary cells are non-permissive towards infection with coxsackievirus B3 despite functional virus-receptor interactions. Virus Res 1997;48:149-156.

63. Martino TA, Petric M, Brown M, Aitken K, Gauntt CJ, Richardson CD, Chow LH, Liu PP. Cardiovirulent coxsackieviruses and the decay-accelerating factor (CD55) receptor. Virology 1998;244:302-314.

64. Shafren DR, Bates RC, Agrez MV, Herd RL, Burns GF, Barry RD. Coxsackieviruses B1, B3, and B5 use decay accelerating factor as a receptor for cell attachment. J Virol 1995;69:3873-3877.

65. Shafren DR, Williams DT, Barry RD. A decay-accelerating factor-binding strain of coxsackievirus B3 requires the coxsackievirus-adenovirus receptor protein to mediate lytic infection of rhabdomyosarcoma cells. J Virol 1997;71:9844-9848.

66. Pasch A, Kupper JH, Wolde A, Kandolf R, Selinka HC. Comparative analysis of virus-host cell interactions of haemagglutinating and non-haemagglutinating strains of coxsackievirus B3. J Gen Virol 1999;80:3153-3158.

67. Spiller OB, Goodfellow IG, Evans DJ, Almond JW, Morgan BP. Echoviruses and coxsackie B viruses that use human decay-accelerating factor (DAF) as a receptor do not bind the rodent analogues of DAF. J Infect Dis 2000;181:340-343.

68. Nemerow GR, Stewart PL. Role of alpha(v) integrins in adenovirus cell entry and gene delivery. Microbiol Mol Biol Rev 1999;63:725-734.

69. Davison E, Kirby I, Elliott T, Santis G. The human HLA-A*0201 allele, expressed in hamster cells, is not a high-affinity receptor for adenovirus type 5 fiber. J Virol 1999;73:4513-4517.

70. McDonald D, Stockwin L, Matzow T, Zajdel MB, Blair G. Coxsackie and adenovirus receptor (CAR)-dependent and major histocompatibility complex (MHC) class I-independent uptake of recombinant adenoviruses into human tumour cells. Gene Ther 1999;6:1512-1519.

71. Fechner H, Haack A, Wang H, Wang X, Eizema K, Pauschinger M, Schoemaker RG, van Veghel R, Houtsmuller AB, Schultheiss H-P, Lamers JMJ, Poller W. Expression of coxsackie adenovirus receptor and alpha$_v$-integrin does not correlate with adenovector targeting in vivo indicating anatomical vector barriers. Gene Ther 1999;6:1520-1535.

72. Evans DM, Dunn G, Minor PD, Schild GC, Cann AJ, Stanway G, Almond JW, Currey K, Maizel JV. Increased neurovirulence associated with a single nucleotide change in a noncoding region of the Sabin type 3 poliovaccine genome. Nature 1985;314:548-550.

73. Kawamura N, Kohara M, Abe S, Komatsu T, Tago K, Arita M, Nomoto A. Determinants in the 5′ noncoding region of poliovirus Sabin 1 RNA that influence the attenuation phenotype. J Virol 1989;63:1302-1309.

74. Macadam AJ, Ferguson G, Burlison J, Stone D, Skuce R, Almond JW, Minor PD. Correlation of RNA secondary structure and attenuation of Sabin vaccine strains of poliovirus in tissue culture. Virology 1992;189:415-422.

75. Macadam AJ, Pollard SR, Ferguson G, Skuce R, Wood D, Almond JW, Minor PD. Genetic basis of attenuation of the Sabin type 2 vaccine strain of poliovirus in primates. Virology 1993;192:18-26.

76. Modlin J. Poliomyelitis and poliovirus immunization. In: Rotbart HA, ed. Human enterovirus infections. Washington, DC: ASM Press, 1995:195-220.

77. Racaniello VR. Poliovirus neurovirulence. Adv Virus Res 1988;34:217-246.

78. Dove AW, Racaniello VR. The polio eradication effort: should vaccine eradication be next? Science 1997;277:779-780.

79. Dowdle WR, Birmingham ME. The biologic principles of poliovirus eradication. J Infect Dis 1997;175 Suppl 1:S286-S292.

80. Dowdle WR, Featherstone DA, Birmingham ME, Hull HF, Aylward RB. Poliomyelitis eradication. Virus Res 1999;62:185-192.

81. Smith J, Aylward RB, Salisbury D, Wassilak S, Oblapenko G. Certifying the elimination of polio-myelitis from Europe: advancing towards global eradication. Eur J Epidemiol 1998;14:769-773.

82. Gomez RM, Cui X, Castagnino CG, Berria MI. Differential behaviour in pancreas and heart of two coxsackievirus B3 variants. Intervirology 1993;36:153-160.

83. Ramsingh AI. Coxsackieviruses and pancreatitis. Front Biosci 1997;2:53-62.

84. Tracy S, Hofling K, Pirruccello S, Lane PH, Reyna SM, Gauntt CJ. Group B coxsackievirus myocarditis and pancreatitis: connection between viral virulence phenotypes in mice. J Med Virol 2000;62:70-81.

85. Tu Z, Chapman NM, Hufnagel G, Tracy S, Romero JR, Barry WH, Zhao L, Currey K, Shapiro B. The cardiovirulent phenotype of coxsackievirus B3 is determined at a single site in the genomic 5′ nontranslated region. J Virol 1995;69:4607-4618.

86. Chapman NM, Tu Z, Tracy S, Gauntt CJ. An infectious cDNA copy of the genome of a non-cardiovirulent coxsackievirus B3 strain: its complete sequence analysis and comparison to the genomes of cardiovirulent coxsackieviruses. Arch Virol 1994;135:115-130.

87. Willian S, Tracy S, Chapman N, Leser S, Romero J, Shapiro B, Currey K. Mutations in a conserved enteroviral RNA oligonucleotide sequence affect positive strand viral RNA synthesis. Arch Virol 2000;145:2061-2086.

88. Svitkin YV, Maslova SV, Agol VI. The genomes of attenuated and virulent poliovirus strains differ in their in vitro translation efficiencies. Virology 1985;147:243-252.

89. Chapman NM, Romero JR, Pallansch MA, Tracy S. Sites other than nucleotide 234 determine cardiovirulence in natural isolates of coxsackievirus B3. J Med Virol 1997;52:258-261.

90. Beck MA, Shi Q, Morris VC, Levander OA. Rapid genomic evolution of a non-virulent coxsackie-virus B3 in selenium-deficient mice results in selection of identical virulent isolates. Nat Med 1995;1:433-436.

91. Levander OA, Beck MA. Interacting nutritional and infectious etiologies of Keshan disease. Insights from coxsackie virus B-induced myocarditis in mice deficient in selenium or vitamin E. Biol Trace Elem Res 1997;56:5-21.

92. Knowlton KU, Jeon ES, Berkley N, Wessely R, Huber S. A mutation in the puff region of VP2 attenuates the myocarditic phenotype of an infectious cDNA of the Woodruff variant of coxsackie-virus B3. J Virol 1996;70:7811-7818.

93. Caggana M, Chan P, Ramsingh A. Identification of a single amino acid residue in the capsid protein VP1 of coxsackievirus B4 that determines the virulent phenotype. J Virol 1993;67:4797-4803.

94. Halim S, Ramsingh AI. A point mutation in VP1 of coxsackievirus B4 alters antigenicity. Virology 2000;269:86-94.

95. Ramsingh A, Hixson A, Duceman B, Slack J. Evidence suggesting that virulence maps to the P1 region of the coxsackievirus B4 genome. J Virol 1990;64:3078-3081.

96. Ramsingh AI, Lee WT, Collins DN, Armstrong LE. T cells contribute to disease severity during coxsackievirus B4 infection. J Virol 1999;73:3080-3086.

97. Ramsingh AI, Collins DN. A point mutation in the VP4 coding sequence of coxsackievirus B4 influences virulence. J Virol 1995;69:7278-7281.

98. Iizuka N, Yonekawa H, Nomoto A. Nucleotide sequences important for translation initiation of enterovirus RNA. J Virol 1991;65:4867-4873.

99. Dunn JJ. Identification of the primary genomic determinant of cardiovirulence for clinical coxsackievirus B3 isolates. Doctoral thesis. University of Nebraska Medical Center, Omaha, Nebraska, 2000.

100. Anderson MJ, Porter DC, Moldoveanu Z, Fletcher TM, McPherson S, Morrow CD. Characterization of the expression and immunogenicity of poliovirus replicons that encode simian immunodeficiency virus SIVmac239 Gag or envelope SU proteins. AIDS Res Hum Retroviruses 1997;13:53-62.

101. Choi WS, Pal-Ghosh R, Morrow CD. Expression of human immunodeficiency virus type 1 (HIV-1) gag, pol, and env proteins from chimeric HIV-1-poliovirus minireplicons. J Virol 1991;65:2875-2883.

102. Crotty S, Lohman BL, Lu FX, Tang S, Miller CJ, Andino R. Mucosal immunization of cynomolgus macaques with two serotypes of live poliovirus vectors expressing simian immunodeficiency virus antigens: stimulation of humoral, mucosal, and cellular immunity. J Virol 1999;73:9485-9495.

103. Mandl S, Sigal LJ, Rock KL, Andino R. Poliovirus vaccine vectors elicit antigen-specific cytotoxic T cells and protect mice against lethal challenge with malignant melanoma cells expressing a model antigen. Proc Natl Acad Sci U S A 1998;95:8216-8221.

104. Moldoveanu Z, Porter DC, Lu A, McPherson S, Morrow CD. Immune responses induced by

administration of encapsidated poliovirus replicons which express HIV-1 gag and envelope proteins. Vaccine 1995;13:1013-1022.

105. Novak MJ, Smythies LE, McPherson SA, Smith PD, Morrow CD. Poliovirus replicons encoding the B subunit of *Helicobacter pylori* urease elicit a Th1 associated immune response. Vaccine 1999;17:2384-2391.

106. Porter DC, Ansardi DC, Choi WS, Morrow CD. Encapsidation of genetically engineered poliovirus minireplicons which express human immunodeficiency virus type 1 Gag and Pol proteins upon infection. J Virol 1993;67:3712-3719.

107. Yim TJ, Tang S, Andino R. Poliovirus recombinants expressing hepatitis B virus antigens elicited a humoral immune response in susceptible mice. Virology 1996;218:61-70.

108. Höfling K, Tracy S, Chapman N, Kim KS, Smith Leser J. Expression of an antigenic adenovirus epitope in a group B coxsackievirus. J Virol 2000;74:4570-4578.

109. Chapman NM, Kim K-S, Tracy S, Jackson J, Hofling K, Leser JS, Malone J, Kolbeck P. Coxsackievirus expression of the murine secretory protein interleukin-4 induces increased synthesis of immunoglobulin G1 in mice. J Virol 2000;74:7952-7962.

110. Chen TT, Tao MH, Levy R. Idiotype-cytokine fusion proteins as cancer vaccines. Relative efficacy of IL-2, IL-4, and granulocyte-macrophage colony-stimulating factor. J Immunol 1994;153:4775-4787.

111. Shi YP, Hasnain SE, Sacci JB, Holloway BP, Fujioka H, Kumar N, Wohlhueter R, Hoffman SL, Collins WE, Lal AA. Immunogenicity and in vitro protective efficacy of a recombinant multistage *Plasmodium falciparum* candidate vaccine. Proc Natl Acad Sci U S A 1999;96:1615-1620.

112. Liu P, Aitken K, Kong YY, Opavsky MA, Martino T, Dawood F, Wen WH, Kozieradzki I, Bachmaier K, Straus D, Mak TW, Penninger JM. The tyrosine kinase p56lck is essential in coxsackievirus B3-mediated heart disease. Nat Med 2000;6:429-434.

113. Joachims M, Van Breugel PC, Lloyd RE. Cleavage of poly(A)-binding protein by enterovirus proteases concurrent with inhibition of translation in vitro. J Virol 1999;73:718-727.

114. Badorff C, Lee GH, Lamphear BJ, Martone ME, Campbell KP, Rhoads RE, Knowlton KU. Enteroviral protease 2A cleaves dystrophin: evidence of cytoskeletal disruption in an acquired cardiomyopathy. Nat Med 1999;5:320-326.

115. Zaragoza C, Ocampo C, Saura M, Leppo M, Wei XQ, Quick R, Moncada S, Liew FY, Lowenstein CJ. The role of inducible nitric oxide synthase in the host response to Coxsackievirus myocarditis. Proc Natl Acad Sci U S A 1998;95:2469-2474.

116. Zaragoza C, Ocampo CJ, Saura M, Bao C, Leppo M, Lafond-Walker A, Thiemann DR, Hruban R, Lowenstein CJ. Inducible nitric oxide synthase protection against coxsackievirus pancreatitis. J Immunol 1999;163:5497-5504.

117. Heim A, Zeuke S, Weiss S, Ruschewski W, Grumbach IM. Transient induction of cytokine production in human myocardial fibroblasts by coxsackievirus B3. Circ Res 2000;86:753-759.

118. Seko Y, Takahashi N, Yagita H, Okumura K, Yazaki Y. Expression of cytokine mRNAs in murine hearts with acute myocarditis caused by coxsackievirus b3. J Pathol 1997;183:105-108.

119. Huber SA. T cells expressing the gamma delta T cell receptor induce apoptosis in cardiac myocytes. Cardiovasc Res 2000;45:579-587.

120. Huber SA, Stone JE, Wagner DH, Kupperman J, Pfeiffer L, David C, O'Brien RL, Davis GS, Newell MK. Gamma delta+ T cells regulate major histocompatibility complex class II (IA and IE)-dependent susceptibility to coxsackievirus B3-induced autoimmune myocarditis. J Virol 1999;73:5630-5636.

121. Berencsi G, Nasz I. Molecular biological characterization of adenovirus DNA. Acta Microbiol Immunol Hung 1998;45:297-304.

122. Shenk T. Adenoviridae: the viruses and their replication. In: Fields BN, Knipe DM, Howley PM, Chanock RM, Melnick JL, Monath TP, Roizman B, Straus SE, eds. Virology. 3rd ed. Vol. 2. Philadelphia: Lippincott-Raven Publishers, 1996:2111-2148.

123. Sander DM, Garry RF. On-line virology. The "All the virology on the WWW" experience. (XIIth International Congress of Virology, Sydney, Australia, August 8-13, 1999.) (http://www.Tulane.EDU:80/~dmsander/Abstracts/atvwww99.htn), 2000.

124. Hong SS, Karayan L, Tournier J, Curiel DT, Boulanger PA. Adenovirus type 5 fiber knob binds to MHC class I alpha2 domain at the surface of human epithelial and B lymphoblastoid cells. EMBO J 1997;16:2294-2306.

125. Arnberg N, Edlund K, Kidd AH, Wadell G. Adenovirus type 37 uses sialic acid as a cellular receptor. J Virol 2000;74:42-48.

126. Li E, Stupack D, Klemke R, Cheresh DA, Nemerow GR. Adenovirus endocytosis via alpha(v) integrins requires phosphoinositide-3-OH kinase. J Virol 1998;72:2055-2061.

127. Wang K, Guan T, Cheresh DA, Nemerow GR. Regulation of adenovirus membrane penetration by the cytoplasmic tail of integrin beta5. J Virol 2000;74:2731-2739.

128. Chardonnet Y, Dales S. Early events in the interaction of adenoviruses with HeLa cells. I. Penetration of type 5 and intracellular release of the DNA genome. Virology 1970;40:462-477.

129. Berget SM, Moore C, Sharp PA. Spliced segments at the 5' terminus of adenovirus 2 late mRNA. Proc Natl Acad Sci U S A 1977;74:3171-3175.

130. de Jong RN, van der Vliet PC. Mechanism of DNA replication in eukaryotic cells: cellular host factors stimulating adenovirus DNA replication. Gene 1999;236:1-12.

131. Babiss LE, Ginsberg HS, Darnell JE. Adenovirus E1B proteins are required for accumulation of late viral mRNA and for effects on cellular mRNA translation and transport. Mol Cell Biol 1985;5:2552-2558.

132. Huang JT, Schneider RJ. Adenovirus inhibition of cellular protein synthesis involves inactivation of cap-binding protein. Cell 1991;65:271-280.

133. Jackson RJ. A comparative view of initiation site selection mechanisms. In: Hershey WB, Mathews MB, Sonenberg N, eds. Translational control. Cold Spring Harbor, NY: Cold Spring Harbor Laboratory Press, 1996:71-112.

134. Martin AB, Webber S, Fricker FJ, Jaffe R, Demmler G, Kearney D, Zhang Y-H, Bodurtha J, Gelb B, Ni J, Bricker JT, Towbin JA. Acute myocarditis: rapid diagnosis by PCR in children. Circulation 1994;90:330-339.

135. Lozinski GM, Davis GG, Krous HF, Billman GF, Shimizu H, Burns JC. Adenovirus myocarditis: retrospective diagnosis by gene amplification from formalin-fixed, paraffin-embedded tissues. Hum Pathol 1994;25:831-834.

136. Shimizu C, Rambaud C, Cheron G, Rouzioux C, Lozinski GM, Rao A, Stanway G, Krous HF, Burns JC. Molecular identification of viruses in sudden infant death associated with myocarditis and pericarditis. Pediatr Infect Dis J 1995;14:584-588.

137. Matsumori A. Molecular and immune mechanisms in the pathogenesis of cardiomyopathy—role of viruses, cytokines, and nitric oxide. Jpn Circ J 1997;61:275-291.

138. Pankuweit S, Hufnagel G, Eckhardt H, Herrmann H, Uttecht S, Maisch B. Cardiotropic DNA viruses and bacteria in the pathogenesis of dilated cardiomyopathy with or without inflammation. [German.] Med Klin 1998;93:223-228.

139. Pauschinger M, Bowles NE, Fuentes-Garcia FJ, Pham V, Kuhl U, Schwimmbeck PL, Schultheiss HP, Towbin JA. Detection of adenoviral genome in the myocardium of adult patients with idiopathic left ventricular dysfunction. Circulation 1999;99:1348-1354.

140. Grumbach IM, Heim A, Pring-Akerblom P, Vonhof S, Hein WJ, Muller G, Figulla HR. Adenoviruses and enteroviruses as pathogens in myocarditis and dilated cardiomyopathy. Acta Cardiol 1999;54:83-88.

141. Akhtar N, Ni J, Stromberg D, Rosenthal GL, Bowles NE, Towbin JA. Tracheal aspirate as a substrate for polymerase chain reaction detection of viral genome in childhood pneumonia and myocarditis. Circulation 1999;99:2011-2018.

142. Guida JD, Fejer G, Pirofski LA, Brosnan CF, Horwitz MS. Mouse adenovirus type 1 causes a fatal hemorrhagic encephalomyelitis in adult C57BL/6 but not BALB/c mice. J Virol 1995;69:7674-7681.

143. Smith K, Spindler KR. Murine adenovirus. In: Ahmed R, Chen ISY, eds. Persistent viral infections. New York: John Wiley & Sons, 1999:477-484.

144. Blailock ZR, Rabin ER, Melnick JL. Adenovirus endocarditis in mice. Science 1967;157:69-70.

145. Blailock ZR, Rabin ER, Melnick JL. Adenovirus myocarditis in mice. An electron microscopic study. Exp Mol Pathol 1968;9:84-96.

146. Nagayama K, Kurosaki M, Enomoto N, Miyasaka Y, Marumo F, Sato C. Characteristics of hepatitis C viral genome associated with disease progression. Hepatology 2000;31:745-750.

147. Sarbah SA, Younossi ZM. Hepatitis C: an update on the silent epidemic. J Clin Gastroenterol 2000;30:125-143.

148. Kao JH, Heptonstall J, Chen DS. Molecular methods of measurement of hepatitis B virus, hepatitis C virus, and human immunodeficiency virus infection: implications for occupational health practice. Occup Environ Med 1999;56:730-734.

149. Houghton M. Hepatitis C viruses. In: Fields BN, Knipe DM, Howley PM, Chanock RM, Melnick JL, Monath TP, Roizman B, Straus SE, eds. Fields virology. 3rd ed. Vol. 1. Philadelphia: Lippincott-Raven Publishers, 1996:1035-1058.

150. Baumert TF, Ito S, Wong DT, Liang TJ. Hepatitis C virus structural proteins assemble into virus-like particles in insect cells. J Virol 1998;72:3827-3836.

151. Reynolds JE, Kaminski A, Kettinen HJ, Grace K, Clarke BE, Carroll AR, Rowlands DJ, Jackson RJ. Unique features of internal initiation of hepatitis C virus RNA translation. EMBO J 1995;14:6010-6020.

152. Oh JW, Ito T, Lai MM. A recombinant hepatitis C virus RNA-dependent RNA polymerase capable of copying the full-length viral RNA. J Virol 1999;73:7694-7702.

153. Oh J-W, Sheu G-T, Lai MMC. Template requirement and initiation site selection by hepatitis C virus polymerase on a minimal viral RNA template. J Biol Chem 2000;275:17710-17717.

154. De Francesco R. Molecular virology of the hepatitis C virus. J Hepatol 1999;31 Suppl 1:47-53.

155. Blight KJ, Kolykhalov AA, Reed KE, Agapov EV, Rice CM. Molecular virology of hepatitis C virus: an update with respect to potential antiviral targets. Antivir Ther 1998;3 Suppl:71-81.

156. Pieroni L, Santolini E, Fipaldini C, Pacini L, Migliaccio G, La Monica N. In vitro study of the NS2-3 protease of hepatitis C virus. J Virol 1997;71:6373-6380.

157. De Francesco R, Steinkuhler C. Structure and function of the hepatitis C virus NS3-NS4A serine proteinase. Curr Top Microbiol Immunol 2000;242:149-169.

158. Kwong AD, Kim JL, Lin C. Structure and function of hepatitis C virus NS3 helicase. Curr Top Microbiol Immunol 2000;242:171-196.

159. Gale M, Blakely CM, Kwieciszewski B, Tan SL, Dossett M, Tang NM, Korth MJ, Polyak SJ, Gretch DR, Katze MG. Control of PKR protein kinase by hepatitis C virus nonstructural 5A protein: molecular mechanisms of kinase regulation. Mol Cell Biol 1998;18:5208-5218.

160. Matsumori A, Matoba Y, Sasayama S. Dilated cardiomyopathy associated with hepatitis C virus infection. Circulation 1995;92:2519-2525.

161. Matsumori A, Matoba Y, Nishio R, Shioi T, Ono K, Sasayama S. Detection of hepatitis C virus RNA from the heart of patients with hypertrophic cardiomyopathy. Biochem Biophys Res Commun 1996;222:678-682.

162. Okabe M, Fukuda K, Arakawa K, Kikuchi M. Chronic variant of myocarditis associated with hepatitis C virus infection. Circulation 1997;96:22-24.

163. Matsumori A, Ohashi N, Hasegawa K, Sasayama S, Eto T, Imaizumi T, Izumi T, Kawamura K, Kawana M, Kimura A, Kitabatake A, Matsuzaki M, Nagai R, Tanaka H, Hiroe M, Hori M, Inoko H, Seko Y, Sekiguchi M, Shimotohno K, Sugishita Y, Takeda N, Takihara K, Tanaka M, Tokuhisa T, Toyo-oka T, Yokoyama M, and co-research workers. Hepatitis C virus infection and heart diseases: a multicenter study in Japan. Jpn Circ J 1998;62:389-391.

164. Matsumori A, Ohashi N, Nishio R, Kakio T, Hara M, Furukawa Y, Ono K, Shioi T, Hasegawa K, Sasayama S. Apical hypertrophic cardiomyopathy and hepatitis C virus infection. Jpn Circ J 1999;63:433-438.

165. Grumbach IM, Heermann K, Figulla HR. Low prevalence of hepatitis C virus antibodies and RNA in patients with myocarditis and dilated cardiomyopathy. Cardiology 1998;90:75-78.

166. de Leeuw N, Melchers WJ, Balk AH, de Jonge N, Galama JM. Study on microbial persistence in end-stage idiopathic dilated cardiomyopathy. Clin Infect Dis 1999;29:522-525.

167. Prati D, Poli F, Farma E, Picone A, Porta E, De Mattei C, Zanella A, Scalamogna M, Gamba A, Gronda E, Faggian G, Livi U, Puricelli C, Vigano M, Sirchia G. Multicenter study on hepatitis C virus infection in patients with dilated cardiomyopathy. North Italy Transplant Program (NITP). J Med Virol 1999;58:116-120.

168. Dalekos GN, Achenbach K, Christodoulou D, Liapi GK, Zervou EK, Sideris DA, Tsianos EV. Idiopathic dilated cardiomyopathy: lack of association with hepatitis C virus infection. Heart 1998;80:270-275.

169. Miyakawa Y, Okamoto H, Mayumi M. Classifying hepatitis C virus genotypes. Mol Med Today 1995;1:20-25.

170. Farci P, Shimoda A, Coiana A, Diaz G, Peddis G, Melpolder JC, Strazzera A, Chien DY, Munoz SJ, Balestrieri A, Purcell RH, Alter HJ. The outcome of acute hepatitis C predicted by the evolution of the viral quasispecies. Science 2000;288:339-344.

171. Pessoa MG, Bzowej N, Berenguer M, Phung Y, Kim M, Ferrell L, Hassoba H, Wright TL. Evolution of hepatitis C virus quasispecies in patients with severe cholestatic hepatitis after liver transplantation. Hepatology 1999;30:1513-1520.

172. Sakai A, Kaneko S, Honda M, Matsushita E, Kobayashi K. Quasispecies of hepatitis C virus in serum and in three different parts of the liver of patients with chronic hepatitis. Hepatology 1999;30:556-561.

173. Colina R, Azambuja C, Uriarte R, Mogdasy C, Cristina J. Evidence of increasing diversification of hepatitis C viruses. J Gen Virol 1999;80:1377-1382.

174. Rose NR, Neumann DA, Herskowitz A, Traystman MD, Beisel KW. Genetics of susceptibility to viral myocarditis in mice. Pathol Immunopathol Res 1988;7:266-278.

175. Neyts J, Leyssen P, De Clercq E. Infections with flaviviridae. Verh K Acad Geneeskd Belg 1999;61:661-697.

176. Arichi T, Saito T, Major ME, Belyakov IM, Shirai M, Engelhard VH, Feinstone SM, Berzofsky JA. Prophylactic DNA vaccine for hepatitis C virus (HCV) infection: HCV-specific cytotoxic T lymphocyte induction and protection from HCV-recombinant vaccinia infection in an HLA-A2.1 transgenic mouse model. Proc Natl Acad Sci U S A 2000;97:297-302.

177. Bukh J, Apgar CL, Yanagi M. Toward a surrogate model for hepatitis C virus: an infectious molecular clone of the GB virus-B hepatitis agent. Virology 1999;262:470-478.

178. Domingo E, Escarmis C, Sevilla N, Moya A, Elena SF, Quer J, Novella IS, Holland JJ. Basic concepts in RNA virus evolution. FASEB J 1996;10:859-864.

179. Holland JJ, De La Torre JC, Steinhauer DA. RNA virus populations as quasispecies. Curr Top Microbiol Immunol 1992;176:1-20.

180. Dunn JJ, Chapman NM, Tracy S, Romero JR. Genomic determinants of cardiovirulence in coxsackievirus B3 clinical isolates: localization to the 5' nontranslated region. J Virol 2000;74:4787-4794.

181. Ruby J, Brinkman C, Jones S, Ramshaw I. Response of monkeys to vaccination with recombinant vaccinia virus which coexpress HIV gp160 and human interleukin-2. Immunol Cell Biol 1990;68:113-117.

182. Xin KQ, Hamajima K, Sasaki S, Honsho A, Tsuji T, Ishii N, Cao XR, Lu Y, Fukushima J, Shapshak P, Kawamoto S, Okuda K. Intranasal administration of human immunodeficiency virus type-1 (HIV-1) DNA vaccine with interleukin-2 expression plasmid enhances cell-mediated immunity against HIV-1. Immunology 1998;94:438-444.

Cellular Autoimmunity in Myocarditis

Sally A. Huber, Ph.D.

HOST DEFENSE MECHANISMS

To understand how autoimmunity occurs, one first needs to review the basic processes of immune response and immune regulation. Host defense mechanisms can be broadly defined as 2 types: innate and adaptive (or antigen-specific) immunity.[1,2] Although adaptive immunity is usually the most effective mechanism for eliminating invading organisms, this response is relatively slow, taking up to 7 to 10 days for effective primary immune responses and 2 to 3 days for anamnestic or memory responses. During this time, rapidly proliferating infectious agents could produce significant tissue injury and possibly death of the organism if left uncontrolled. For this reason, broadly reactive host responses, which are constantly maintained or can be rapidly induced, are essential in containing infections until the adaptive immune response "kicks in."

INNATE IMMUNITY

Innate immunity takes many forms and may play a significant role in the host response to cardiotropic viruses. Most viruses make double-stranded RNA (dsRNA) as part of their replicative cycle, and this dsRNA initiates profound alterations in cell physiology. For picornaviruses, the major family associated with clinical myocarditis and dilated cardiomyopathy, production of dsRNA occurs during the replicative intermediate stage. This is when negative strand RNA is produced from genomic RNA templates.[3] The dsRNA induces interferon-α/β, which in turn up-regulates expression of interferon-inducible protein kinase (PKR) and $2',5'$-oligoadenylate synthetase. Activated PKR phosphorylates many cellular proteins, including the protein synthesis inhibitory factor, eIF-2, which subsequently could inhibit virus protein synthesis. Phosphorylation of cytoplasmic IκB activates NFκB/Rel family members, transcription factors involved in synthesis of cytokines (interleukin [IL]-1; IL-2; tumor necrosis factor-α; IL-6; macrophage, granulocyte, and macrophage-granulocyte colony-stimulating factors; IL-2 receptor; chemotactic protein MCP-1/JE; and inducible nitric oxide synthetase [iNOS]). iNOS up-regulation increases nitric oxide (NO) concentration. NO has important antimicrobial activity and may also damage tissues.[4-7]

During bacterial infections, endotoxin also initiates activation of NFκB/Rel family members, including a unique member called RelB.[8] RelB is primarily expressed in mature dendritic cells but not in macrophages/monocytes or precursor (immature) dendritic cells. Thus, RelB may have an essential role in mature dendritic cell function, such as initiation of immunity and negative selection (deletion) of autoreactive T cells.

Other major aspects of the innate immune response include natural killer (NK) cells and T cells expressing a T-cell receptor (TCR) composed of a gamma and a delta polypeptide chain ($\gamma\delta$+ T cells). NK cells usually recognize either infected or transformed cells in the body and kill these targets through predominantly perforin-mediated mechanisms.

The basis for NK cell recognition of valid target cells is poorly understood, but likely involves 2 receptorlike molecules called LY-49 and NKR-P1.[9] Target cell sensitivity to NK cell killing is inversely related to major histocompatibility complex (MHC) class I antigen expression. Thus, NK cell killing should be greatest before adaptive immunity induction and decrease subsequent to CD8 cytolytic T-lymphocyte (CTL) activation, because up-regulation of MHC antigens is a common consequence of adaptive immunity and is mediated through the release of interferon gamma (IFN-γ).

γδ+T cells are an intriguing population of lymphocytes. Lymphocytes are often categorized according to characteristics or functions, such as expression of cell surface molecules (CD4, CD8) or production of specific types of cytokines. One way in which T lymphocytes are categorized is through the type of TCR they express. TCRs contain 2 polypeptide chains[10,11] (Fig. 3-1). Most T lymphocytes in peripheral lymphoid tissues and blood contain TCRs consisting of an alpha (α) and a beta (β) chain. These are the classic antigen-restricted T cells that react to processed antigenic epitopes presented by either class I or class II MHC molecules. A second population of T lymphocytes have TCRs consisting of a gamma (γ) and a delta (δ) chain. γδ+ T cells constitute a minor subpopulation in normal peripheral lymphoid tissues (1%-5% of T cells in the spleen or lymph node), but they account for more than 50% of the T cells in mucosal tissues and skin.

As with αβ+ T cells, the polypeptide chains of γδ+ T cells consist of constant and variable (V) regions that undergo somatic rearrangements to give the antigen-specificity of

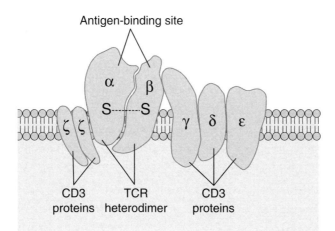

Fig. 3-1. The T-cell receptor complex. Schematic illustration of T-cell (*TCR*) and TCRα and TCRβ polypeptide chains linked to the CD3 molecular complex. (From Cotran RS, Kumar V, Collins T. Robbins pathologic basis of disease. 6th ed. Philadelphia: WB Saunders Company, 1999:189. By permission of the publisher.)

the cell. Because the δ locus is situated within the α locus, successful rearrangement of either the δ or α genes precludes rearrangement of the other locus. Thus, any T cell can make only a δ or an α polypeptide chain. Successful rearrangement of the δ or α gene subsequently induces rearrangement, respectively, of the β or γ loci, meaning that αβ and γδ rearrangements are mutually exclusive and any T cell can express only an αβ or a γδ TCR, but not both.

Both αβ+ and γδ+ T cells mature in the thymus from prethymocyte precursors and undergo positive and negative clonal selection. γδ+ T cells exit the thymus in waves during ontogeny as a function of their V gene usage and generally populate distinct tissues. For example, Vγ7+ cells predominate in intestinal epithelium; Vγ3+ cells, in skin; and Vγ1+ and Vγ4+ cells, in peripheral lymphoid tissues.

Antigenic specificity of γδ+ cells is poorly understood. Heat shock or stress proteins (hsp) represent one type of antigen recognized by at least some γδ+ T cells.[12] Other γδ+ T cells recognize small phosphorylated nonpeptide antigens, which are frequently produced by microbial pathogens such as mycobacteria;[13-15] human MHC class I-related molecules MICA and MICB, which may have broad stress- or tumor-associated expression;[16] and virus-specific antigens.[17] Unlike antigens recognized by αβ+ T cells, molecules stimulating γδ+ lymphocytes usually do not require processing by antigen-presenting cells (APCs) or interaction with MHC proteins.

ADAPTIVE IMMUNITY

Adaptive immunity or antigen-specific immunity involves clones of either T or B lymphocytes that are committed to respond to a single antigen. Antigens are molecules that can both stimulate an immune response and interact with the products of that immune response. Antigens must exceed a minimum size (usually greater than 1,000 daltons). Molecular composition, shape, and ability to be catabolized all influence antigenicity. Usually, proteins and carbohydrates make the best antigens, but just about any compound can induce an immune response under the appropriate conditions.[18] Small molecules might also be recognized by the immune system, but these "haptens" cannot induce immunity unless they are bound to carrier molecules. The minimum size requirement basically reflects the necessity of antigens to be phagocytosed or pinocytosed by APCs. Binding of haptens to carrier molecules, even self-molecules such as serum albumin, provides the minimum size for uptake by APC. In this way, antibiotics, such as penicillin, or metals, such as nickel, can induce allergic reactions.[19]

Exogenous molecules entering an APC are degraded in phagosomes and the small peptides, carbohydrates, or lipids (usually 5-6 sugar residues or 10-15 amino acid residues) are loaded into the groove of class II MHC molecules as these MHC molecules are transported to the APC cell surface through the endosome pathway (Fig. 3-2). When class II MHC

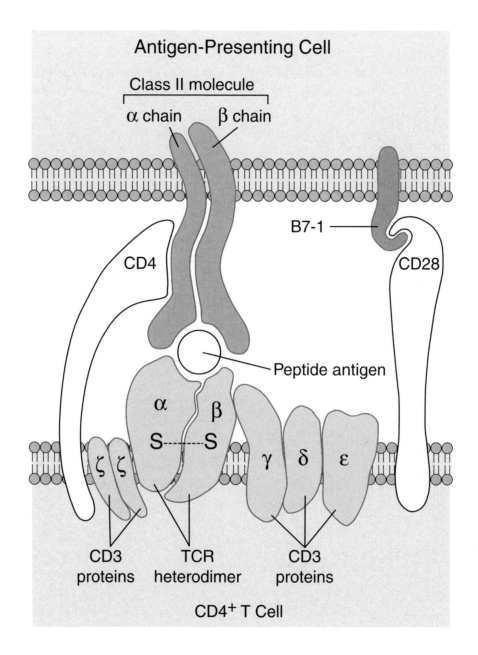

Fig. 3-2. Antigen recognition by CD4+ T cells. Schematic representation of antigen recognition by CD4+ T cells. Note that the T-cell receptor (*TCR* heterodimer) recognizes a peptide fragment of antigen bound to the major histocompatibility complex (MHC) class II molecule. The CD4 molecule binds to the nonpolymorphic portion of the class II molecule. The interaction between the TCR and the MHC-bound antigen provides signal 1 for T-cell activation. Signal 2 is provided by the interaction of the CD28 molecule with the costimulatory molecules (B7-1 and B7-2) expressed on antigen presenting cell. (From Cotran RS, Kumar V, Collins T. Robbins pathologic basis of disease. 6th ed. Philadelphia: WB Saunders Company, 1999:190. By permission of the publisher.)

molecules are synthesized in the endoplasmic reticulum (ER), an invariant or "I-chain" caps the MHC groove and prevents uptake of endogenous peptides. When the endosome carrying the class II MHC molecule to the APC surface fuses with the phagosome, the low pH of the fused vesicle degrades the I-chain and opens the groove for antigen binding.[20] In contrast to class II MHC molecules, class I molecules usually bind endogenously produced molecules. Some of the endogenous proteins are degraded in proteosomes and transported through TAP (transporter associated with antigen processing) to the ER where the class I MHC polypeptide and β_2-microglobulin actually fold around the epitope during their synthesis.[21] Once made, the MHC-peptide complex passes through the Golgi complex and is transported to the cell surface. The class I and class II MHC locus is highly polymorphic, but nearly all variation between alleles is located in the groove region or is located in areas of the polypeptide which when folded into the tertiary structure of the MHC molecule impact the morphology or ionic character of the groove.

Whereas each distinct MHC molecule can bind many different peptides in its groove, allelic MHC molecules usually bind different peptides from any one antigen. For example, individuals expressing human class II DR4 would not present the same epitopes of cox-sackievirus as individuals having DR2. Because of the complexity of the MHC locus (each human codes for 3 classic class I and 3 classic class II on each chromosome, and the genes on both chromosomes are codominantly expressed), 2 unrelated individuals will not likely "see" a pathogen at the molecular level in exactly the same way. In other words, virtually everyone makes an anticoxsackievirus immune response, but nearly everyone's specific immune response is unique at the epitope level.

THE MAJOR HISTOCOMPATIBILITY COMPLEX

The MHC-peptide complex is recognized by T lymphocytes using the variable regions on the $\alpha\beta$ + TCR (Fig. 3-3; see color plate 2). Because each TCR is basically specific for a different antigenic epitope, and individuals generally possess the ability to respond to between 10^7 and 10^9 different antigens, individuals begin with few naïve antigen-specific T cells in any clone. Once antigen is introduced into the individual, clonal expansion of this initial naïve population occurs relatively rapidly. Dendritic cells (DCs) are the most potent of the APCs, and the only APCs capable of stimulating naïve T cells. There may be many subtypes of dendritic cells, but 2 subtypes are presently best recognized[8,22-24]: a myeloid (CD8α-, DEC205-, CD11c+, CD11b+ in the mouse)-derived subpopulation and a lymphoid (CD8α+, DEC205+)-derived subpopulation. The CD8α-subtype induces Th2 cell responses and the CD8α+ DC induces Th1 responses. Immature DCs are present in many tissues and act as a sentinel network for invading microbes or other antigens capable of stimulating the immune system. Immature DCs are highly endocytic and use various receptors to internalize antigen.[25] Various stimuli (including double-

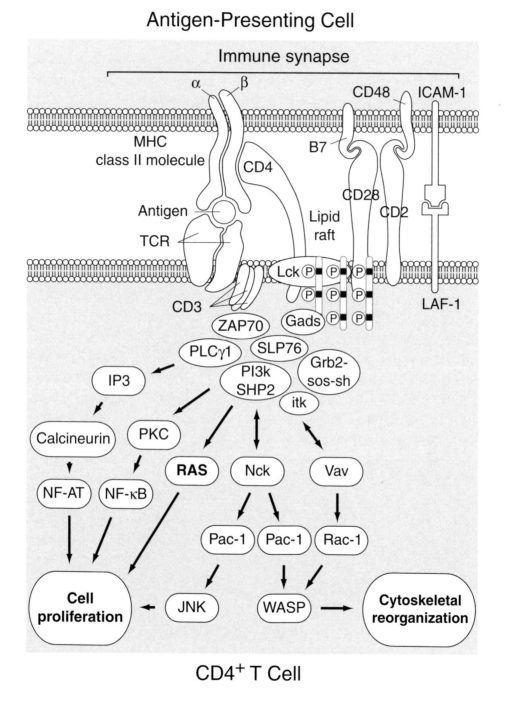

Fig. 3-3. Signaling pathways in T cells after T-cell receptor engagement leads to cell proliferation and cytoskeleton reorganization. See color plate 2. (Modified from Lanzavecchia and Sallusto.[29] By permission of Excerpta Medica.)

stranded RNA, bacterial metabolic products, ultraviolet light, and tissue injury) cause the immature DCs to migrate out of peripheral tissues to lymph nodes or spleen[26,27] and mature. During this migration, DCs mature and lose their phagocytic potential, preventing them from capturing more antigen. DCs increase expression of peptide-loaded MHC molecules and accessory proteins, such as CD40, CD80 (B7-1), and CD86 (B7-2), making the mature DC a potent APC. Actual interaction of the MHC-peptide-TCR between the APC and T cell results in redistribution of cell surface molecules in both the APC and T cell and the formation of supramolecular activation complexes (SMACs) or immune synapses.

Immune synapses consist of the MHC, TCR/CD3, CD4 or CD8, and protein kinase C (PKC)-θ with integrin and adhesion molecules such as intercellular adhesion molecule (ICAM)-1/leukocyte function-associated antigen (LFA)-1 and (CD80,CD86)/CD28 (APC ligand/T-cell ligand) in the outer ring.[28,29] Engagement of CD28 recruits lipid rafts containing Lck and LAT to the synapse where Lck phosphorylates CD3 and ζ chains, followed by recruitment and activation of ZAP-70.[29,30] ZAP-70 phosphorylates LAT, which links the TCR signal to the Ras signal pathway by using Grb2-SOS and to the JNK pathway by using SLP-76, ultimately leading to T-cell proliferation.[29,31] Additional linkages of LAT to Nck and Pak1 through the SLP-76 adapter molecule activate WASP and result in actin polymerization and reorganization of the cytoskeleton. Naïve T cells require extended TCR signaling of at least 20 hours to commit these cells to proliferation. Accessory molecules such as CD28 are essential in naïve T-cell responses because of their augmentation of the TCR signal. After the first division, T-cell proliferation becomes more rapid, with each cell cycle requiring only 6 hours. Activated and memory cells contain substantially greater numbers of lipid rafts in their membranes, which also amplify the cell signal. Thus, memory cells require less costimulation to initiate T-cell proliferation and can use less potent APCs such as macrophages, B lymphocytes, activated fibroblasts, or endothelial cells to maintain the T-cell response. Once generated, differentiated CTLs also require a relatively short interaction time (30 min) to transmit the "lethal hit" to the target cell. Thus, a major impediment to the activation of T-cell clones is the strength (avidity) and duration of the TCR-MHC interaction.

AUTOIMMUNITY

Basically, autoimmunity can be defined as an immune response to self-tissues. Initiation of autoimmunity has 3 components: development or maintenance of an autoreactive repertoire of lymphocytes, activation of the autoimmune cells, and failure of the immune system to suppress or regulate this autoreactivity.[32]

AUTOREACTIVE REPERTOIRE

Self-reactive T-cell clones should be deleted in the thymus during ontogeny (central toler-ance) or inactivated peripherally through anergy by inappropriate antigen presentation (peripheral tolerance). High-affinity interactions of self-reactive T cells in the thymus with self-epitope-loaded MHC molecules on thymic epithelium or medullary dendritic cells result in clonal deletion of the autoreactive clones (negative selection). Interactions between T cells and self-MHC with nonspecific epitopes are not of high enough avidity to cause apoptosis of the developing T cell but provide sufficient signal to retain the lympho-cyte in the thymus (positive selection) for further differentiation. The problem with this form of tolerance is that it depends on self-antigens being present in the thymus during T-cell ontogeny. This could be true for common cellular molecules present in all cells, but would not necessarily be true for specialized or sequestered antigens, such as thyroglobulin, cardiac myosin, or myelin basic protein, the presumed autoantigens in autoimmune thyroiditis, myocarditis, and multiple sclerosis, respectively. Furthermore, autoreactive T-cell clones having low avidity TCR for MHC self-antigen would not be deleted. Peripheral tolerance can be induced either by deleting autoreactive T cells through high-dose antigen exposure in tissues[22,33-35] or by exposing self-reactive T cells to antigen-loaded MHC molecules without appropriate secondary signals (cytokines or adhesion molecules such as CD28 and B7) (anergy).[36-38] Finally, self-reactive T cells may not be deleted or anergized. Immunologic "ignorance" occurs because the self-antigen is either sequestered or present at concentrations below threshold levels required to initiate immunity.[22,33,34,39,40] If these antigens become available to the immune system under conditions favoring normal immune responses, autoimmunity should result.

"Cryptic" antigen is one form of sequestered antigen.[41,42] These are antigenic epitopes that are not readily available to T lymphocytes either because of low concentration, poor MHC binding avidity, or destruction of the epitope during antigen processing under nor-mal circumstances. In the first case, certain molecules may be present in limited amounts in healthy tissues. However, extensive tissue damage, such as might occur during virus infection or traumatic injury, could release substantial quantities of these self-molecules and raise concentrations of the relevant epitope to immunogenic levels. Furthermore, antigen might be concentrated during antigen processing. Although antigen presentation usually begins with basically "nonspecific" phagocytosis or pinocytosis of materials in the extra-cellular milieu, uptake of antigens can become more "directed," provided antibodies to these self-molecules are present. APCs having Fc receptors could selectively bind antigen-antibody complexes causing disproportional uptake of these antigens.

Furthermore, B lymphocytes, which also have the potential to process and present antigens to T lymphocytes, would preferentially internalize antigens to which they react via the immunoglobulin on their cell surface. Autoreactive B cells are relatively common, and their numbers actually increase with age. The frequency of autoreactive B cells likely reflects the fact that tolerance of B cells is usually difficult to accomplish and easily overcome. Thus, the autoreactive B lymphocyte might have a crucial role in autoimmunity induction.

A second form of cryptic epitope reflects epitopes that are not readily seen in whole proteins, but which become immunogenic as individual peptides.[43] Use of different proteases by the various APC cell types or induction of new proteases during activation of APC can change the way protein antigens are processed and result in either destruction of some epitopes or production of new ones by changing cleavage sites during protein degradation.[42,44] Cryptic epitopes have been found in several human autoimmune diseases and in animal disease models: autoimmune hemolytic anemia,[45] multiple sclerosis,[46] myasthenia gravis,[47] and Graves disease,[48] among others.[49,50]

AUTOIMMUNE T-CELL ACTIVATION

Antigenic mimicry is one mechanism for infectious diseases to trigger autoimmunity. Antigenic mimicry is defined as a cross-reactivity between the epitopes of an infectious organism and one or more self-antigens.[51,52] The self-antigens themselves are incapable of inducing an immune response because they are sequestered, are presented by APC in the absence of appropriate accessory molecules or sufficient cytokines required for adequate immune stimulation, or induce autoimmune T cells having low avidity TCR, which cannot maintain contact with the MHC-peptide in the immune synapse for the 20 hours required to initiate cell proliferation. Infections induce such potent immunity to the invading organism, and the infection usually results in tissue damage with accompanying release of cellular molecules, that self-proteins may be taken up by professional APCs and presented to the low-avidity autoreactive T cell under conditions favoring their activation. Also, infection will have a stronger effect on the immature DC than self-antigens alone, such as the dsRNA associated with picornavirus infection stimulating DC migration to secondary lymphoid tissues and maturation into highly potent APC. Thus, even low-avidity TCR would have an improved chance of stimulating autoreactive T-cell proliferation.

Sequestered antigens would also be released in greater quantity during virus infections as a result of tissue damage. These sequestered antigens would be taken up by the immature DC simultaneously with virus proteins and transported to secondary lymphoid tissues. Antigen presentation requirements for effector cells or for reactivation of memory cells is far less stringent in terms of secondary signals and TCR-MHC interactions. This means that once autoreactive T cells proliferate, maintenance of the autoimmune response and production of autoimmune damage occur even when the infectious agent has been eliminated.[53,54]

Infectious agents could additionally activate memory autoimmune T cells in a non–antigen-specific manner through superantigens and through the induction of class I interferons.[55] Thus, throughout the lifetime of an individual, multiple infections with any virus could continuously stimulate autoimmune T-cell clonal expansion even when the subsequent infectious agents lack cross-reactive epitopes with the self-molecule.

FAILURE TO REGULATE THE AUTOIMMUNE RESPONSE

Immune responses are usually strictly controlled. One control mechanism is the elimination of stimulated T or B lymphocytes by apoptosis once the antigen has been cleared. In this way, total lymphocyte numbers in the body are restricted, which conserves resources. Memory cells, however, are readily available to expand the antigen-specific clone if the pathogen is encountered again. Individuals with defective apoptotic pathways (such as the Fas-deficient *lpr/lpr* mouse)[56] can develop autoimmunity as part of generalized lymphadenopathy because their autoreactive T cells are never eliminated.

A second mechanism of losing control is through epitope spread. Prolonged in situ inflammatory responses may give rise to sequential autoimmune responses directed toward different self-antigens. Epitope spreading as a component of autoimmunity has been shown in both experimental allergic and Theiler virus-induced encephalomyelitis.[32,57,58] Finally, chronic infections, such as might occur with persistent virus, could kill terminally differentiated cells, like cardiac myocytes, through continuous stimulation of immune responses. The loss of sufficient numbers of terminally differentiated cells could result in organ failure. Because a major mechanism for clearing virus is through immune-mediated lysis of infected cells, widespread distribution of the virus in an organ could easily result in serious immune damage.

AUTOIMMUNITY IN MYOCARDITIS AND DILATED CARDIOMYOPATHY

HUMORAL AUTOIMMUNITY

Heart reactive autoantibodies are found in a high percentage of patients with myocarditis and in a somewhat lower proportion of patients with dilated cardiomyopathy.[59-69] Autoantibodies are relatively rare in patients with ischemic heart disease or normal (non-cardiovascular disease) individuals. Severity of cardiac impairment often correlates with concentrations of autoantibodies eluted from the heart,[60,67,70] and patients in remission often show a corresponding decrease in serum autoantibody concentrations.[63]

Identified autoantigens include the β1 adrenoreceptor adenine nucleotide translocator (ANT), branched-chain keto acid dehydrogenase (BCKD), cardiac myosin, sarcolemmal and myolemmal proteins, connective tissue, and extracellular matrix proteins including laminin.[68,69,71,72] These autoantibodies have been shown to alter cardiac function (nucleoside transport, contractility, calcium modulation) or directly cause myocyte lysis in the presence of complement.[68,73]

Adsorption of sera containing heart-reactive antibodies with coxsackievirus B3 or B4 substantially reduces autoantibody titers and cytolytic activity, suggesting cross-reactivity between viruses that are frequently associated with triggering clinical myocarditis and autoantibodies often found in myocarditis patients.[68] This strongly implicates antigenic mimicry as an initiating factor in the humoral autoimmune response. Studies in experimental models of myocarditis further confirm cross-reactivity between coxsackieviral epitopes and heart antigens. Autoantibodies to cardiac myosin, ANT, and BCKD are found in myocarditis-susceptible mice infected with coxsackievirus B3, but these autoantibodies are generally absent in infected mice that fail to develop myocarditis.[74-79] Severity of cardiac injury correlates with the autoantibody titers found in the heart.[77,80]

Monoclonal antibody clones making coxsackievirus-neutralizing antibodies have been described; they react to the cardiac isoform of myosin and to mouse laminin, actin, elastin, vimentin, and phosphorylase b.[74,81-83] Although these cross-reactive antiviral antibodies usually fail to induce myocardial damage when adoptively transferred into most healthy mice, they can exacerbate injury when given to coxsackievirus-infected animals.[74,82] One reason why antimyosin antibodies are minimally pathogenic when directly transferred into mice is that cardiac myosin is an intracellular molecule that would not normally be accessible to autoantibodies in healthy heart tissue. Unlike T lymphocytes, which react to processed antigens, antibodies usually respond to native molecules. DBA/2 mice represent an interesting exception to the inability of antimyosin antibodies to cause myocarditis directly. These animals apparently have native cardiac myosin in the extracellular matrix of the heart. Thus, adoptive transfer of antimyosin antibodies in this mouse strain results in substantial myocarditis.[84,85] In contrast to antimyosin antibodies, antibodies to ANT may be directly injurious to cardiac function.[86]

CELLULAR AUTOIMMUNITY

Many immunopathogenic diseases are associated with specific MHC haplotypes.[87,88] Often, the disease susceptibility can be linked to specific subtypes of MHC molecules, even to a particular mutation at a specific location of an MHC allele. Several studies suggested that individuals with particular class II MHC haplotypes, including HLA-DR4/1, HLA-DQ beta 1 (histadine at position 36), and HLA-DQ5, have increased susceptibility to myocarditis or dilated cardiomyopathy or both.[89,90] In a more recent study, production of "humanized" mice (transgenic mice expressing the human CD4 and HLA-DQ6 genes) allowed induction of heart disease through immunization with cardiac myosin.[91] This last report provides strong evidence that an MHC class II allele known to be implicated in myocarditis actually induces autoimmunity to a heart protein long suspected of being a major autoantigen in this disease.

Lymphocytes isolated from hearts of patients with myocarditis or dilated cardiomy-opathy proliferate in response to ANT and coxsackievirus. Furthermore, adoptive transfer of lymphocytes from myocarditis patients into severe combined immunodeficient (SCID) mice induces myocarditis.[86,92] ANT, BCKD, and especially cardiac myosin are all capable of inducing autoimmune myocarditis when injected into susceptible strains of mice.[69,93-95] Immunization of mice with skeletal myosin does not induce myocarditis.[75,94] Cardiac myosin epitopes are expressed in heart class II MHC molecules before the observance of inflammation,[96] and distinct immunogenic myosin epitopes have been identified in different strains of mice.[97,98] These include the myosin heavy chain alpha (mhcα) peptide 334-352 that binds to the mouse MHC class II antigen IA^k and is highly pathogenic in mice expressing this MHC allele and peptides 614-643, 735-747, and 947-960 of mhcα, which cause myocarditis in H-2d mice. As indicated earlier, different peptides should induce disease in mice having distinct MHC haplotypes, because each MHC molecule binds a separate set of peptides having the distinctive binding motif for that particular MHC groove.

Figure 3-4 (see color plate 3) demonstrates several hypothetical mechanisms by which myocarditis can be induced. Virus infection is undoubtedly a major trigger in this disease. How much of the myocardial damage results from autoimmune, let alone immune-mediated, mechanisms is far from certain. Although autoantibodies are found in the majority of myocarditis patients, this autoimmunity might reflect a relatively late event in the disease process and result from epitope spreading.

The studies mentioned above clearly indicate that antigenic mimicry exists between the major pathogens implicated in myocarditis (coxsackievirus) and the major cellular antigens associated with the disease (cardiac myosin, ANT, and BCKD). However, because one would assume that there are restricted peptides within the whole cardiac proteins that could cross-react with virus, autoimmunity initiated in response to antigenic mimicry ought to be limited to individuals with specific MHC haplotypes. Although there is an increased risk of myocarditis associated with some MHC haplotypes, individuals with other haplotypes develop myocarditis. This must mean either that there are a great number of cross-reactive epitopes between the common heart antigens and myocarditis-inducing pathogens or that antigenic mimicry is only one of several different methods of inducing myocarditis.

There is a second problem with depending on antigenic mimicry as a major component in the pathogenesis of myocarditis. Sustainable autoimmunity usually requires a large number of autoreactive T cells stimulated over an extended time.[32] The precursor frequency, or number of lymphocytes belonging to any one clone, is likely to be small in antigen-specific responses. Frequencies of antigen-specific T cells in the murine model of myocarditis often are about 0.02%, or about 1/5,000 cells,[102] yet various studies indicate that a

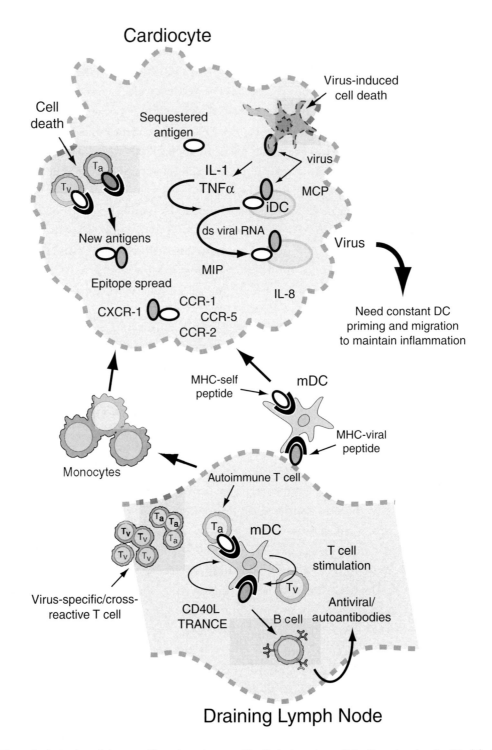

Fig. 3-4. Activation of virus-specific and autoimmune T cells during myocarditis. See color plate 3. (Modified from Lanzavecchia and Sallusto.[29] By permission of Excerpta Medica.)

threshold of about 1/1,500 reactive cells is required for induction of clinical disease.[32,103,104] Thus, it is highly unlikely that antigenic mimicry alone could induce myocarditis. However, antigenic mimicry could initiate a cascade of immune responses that results in epitope spread (activation of waves of autoimmune T cells to various self-antigens as tissue is destroyed in the heart and sequestered antigens are made available to the immune system). The combined frequencies of many autoreactive clones could accumulate to the threshold level required for clinical disease. Additionally, cytokines and chemokines elicited by the specific immune response could induce cardiac dysfunction directly[105,106] or indirectly through the induction of other molecules such as iNOS.[7,106,107] Furthermore, existence of autoreactive T-cell clones would be insufficient unless homing of these cells to the heart could be accomplished. During active virus infection, substantial up-regulation of chemokine and chemotactic factors should be produced as part of the host defense response to draw pathogen-reactive T cells to the heart. These chemotactic factors could also draw the autoreactive cell populations to the myocardium. The importance of such chemotaxis is shown by the ability to suppress myocarditis and cardiac injury by interfering with specific chemokine mediators like MIP-1, RANTES,[108] MIP-2,[109] and MCP-1.[110,111]

The above discussion is simply meant to caution investigators about assuming that autoimmunity is solely responsible for myocarditis and dilated cardiomyopathy. This is undoubtedly a complex disease with multiple pathogenic mechanisms, and various combinations of pathogenic mechanisms are likely to be important in different patients. Any disease that is defined primarily by a single characteristic, such as the presence of inflammatory cells in the heart, is apt to represent a mixed bag of diseases sharing this particular characteristic.

CONCLUSIONS

Myocarditis is likely to be a complex disease. Viruses, especially the coxsackie B viruses, are major etiologic agents for clinical myocarditis, but many other infectious and noninfectious agents are also capable of inducing heart damage.[112] The evidence that autoimmunity occurs in many myocarditis and dilated cardiomyopathy patients is quite strong. It implicates a relatively restricted number of autoantigens, including cardiac myosin, ANT, and BCKD. Many other cellular (sarcolemmal, myolemmal, and endothelial cell), connective tissue, and extracellular matrix molecules (laminin, actin, vimentin) can also act as auto-antigens. Given the number of different antigen-specific responses frequently detected during myocarditis and dilated cardiomyopathy, some form of epitope spreading is probable as a foundation for cardiac injury. However, antigenic mimicry between the dominant self-molecules (myosin, ANT, and BCKD) and the infectious agents also contributes to the disease process and may even dominate in some proportion of patients. An initial infection might commence autosensitization by releasing sequestered antigens in the heart and stimulating uptake of virus and self-antigens by dendritic cells for presentation of antigen in secondary lymphoid tissues. Just as important, subsequent infections of the heart with totally unrelated viruses might augment the autoimmunity through restimulation of memory autoimmune cells. Studies by Yu et al.[100] demonstrate that sequential infection of mice with 2 different viruses significantly augments tissue injury and inflammation, although whether this augmentation of disease reflects reactivation of memory autoimmune T cells was not determined.

ACKNOWLEDGMENTS

This work was supported by R01 HL 58583 and AHA 97508IN (Sally A. Huber).

REFERENCES

1. Fearon DT, Locksley RM. The instructive role of innate immunity in the acquired immune response. Science 1996;272:50-53.
2. Mantegazza R, Bernasconi P, Confalonieri P, Cornelio F. Inflammatory myopathies and systemic disorders: a review of immunopathogenetic mechanisms and clinical features. J Neurol 1997;244:277-287.
3. Gribaudo G, Lembo D, Cavallo G, Landolfo S, Lengyel P. Interferon action: binding of viral RNA to the 40-kilodalton 2′-5′-oligoadenylate synthetase in interferon-treated HeLa cells infected with encephalomyocarditis virus. J Virol 1991;65:1748-1757.
4. Hiraoka Y, Kishimoto C, Takada H, Nakamura M, Kurokawa M, Ochiai H, Shiraki K. Nitric oxide and murine coxsackievirus B3 myocarditis: aggravation of myocarditis by inhibition of nitric oxide synthase. J Am Coll Cardiol 1996;28:1610-1615.
5. Hirasawa K, Jun HS, Maeda K, Kawaguchi Y, Itagaki S, Mikami T, Baek HS, Doi K, Yoon JW. Possible role of macrophage-derived soluble mediators in the pathogenesis of encephalomyocarditis virus-induced diabetes in mice. J Virol 1997;71:4024-4031.
6. Huot AE, Hacker MP. Nitric oxide. In: Craighead JE, ed. Pathology of environmental and occupational disease. St. Louis: Mosby, 1995:357-372.
7. Lowenstein CJ, Hill SL, Lafond-Walker A, Wu J, Allen G, Landavere M, Rose NR, Herskowitz A. Nitric oxide inhibits viral replication in murine myocarditis. J Clin Invest 1996;97:1837-1843.
8. Lo D, Feng L, Li L, Carson MJ, Crowley M, Pauza M, Nguyen A, Reilly CR. Integrating innate and adaptive immunity in the whole animal. Immunol Rev 1999;169:225-239.
9. Yokoyama WM, Seaman WE. The Ly-49 and NKR-P1 gene families encoding lectin-like receptors on natural killer cells: the NK gene complex. Annu Rev Immunol 1993;11:613-635.
10. Ferrick DA, Braun RK, Lepper HD, Schrenzel MD. Gamma delta T cells in bacterial infections. Res Immunol 1996;147:532-541.
11. Haas W, Pereira P, Tonegawa S. Gamma/delta cells. Annu Rev Immunol 1993;11:637-685.

12. Born W, Happ MP, Dallas A, Reardon C, Kubo R, Shinnick T, Brennan P, O'Brien R. Recognition of heat shock proteins and gamma delta cell function. Immunol Today 1990;11:40-43.

13. Belmant C, Espinosa E, Poupot R, Peyrat MA, Guiraud M, Poquet Y, Bonneville M, Fournié J-J. 3-Formyl-1-butyl pyrophosphate A novel mycobacterial metabolite-activating human $\gamma\delta$ T cells. J Biol Chem 1999;274:32079-32084.

14. Constant P, Davodeau F, Peyrat MA, Poquet Y, Puzo G, Bonneville M, Fournie JJ. Stimulation of human gamma delta T cells by nonpeptidic mycobacterial ligands. Science 1994;264:267-270.

15. Morita CT, Lee HK, Leslie DS, Tanaka Y, Bukowski JF, Marker-Hermann E. Recognition of nonpeptide prenyl pyrophosphate antigens by human gammadelta T cells. Microbes Infect 1999;1:175-186.

16. Groh V, Rhinehart R, Secrist H, Bauer S, Grabstein KH, Spies T. Broad tumor-associated expression and recognition by tumor-derived gamma delta T cells of MICA and MICB. Proc Natl Acad Sci U S A 1999;96:6879-6884.

17. Sciammas R, Johnson RM, Sperling AI, Brady W, Linsley PS, Spear PG, Fitch FW, Bluestone JA. Unique antigen recognition by a herpesvirus-specific TCR-gamma delta cell. J Immunol 1994;152:5392-5397.

18. Sell S. Immunology, immunopathology, and immunity. 4th ed. New York: Elsevier, 1987.

19. Huber SA. Immunopathology. In: Craighead JE, ed. Pathology of environmental and occupational disease. St. Louis: Mosby, 1995:397-409.

20. Castellino F, Zhong G, Germain RN. Antigen presentation by MHC class II molecules: invariant chain function, protein trafficking, and the molecular basis of diverse determinant capture. Hum Immunol 1997;54:159-169.

21. York IA, Goldberg AL, Mo XY, Rock KL. Proteolysis and class I major histocompatibility complex antigen presentation. Immunol Rev 1999;172:49-66.

22. Ludewig B, Odermatt B, Ochsenbein AF, Zinkernagel RM, Hengartner H. Role of dendritic cells in the induction and maintenance of autoimmune diseases. Immunol Rev 1999;169:45-54.

23. Masurier C, Pioche-Durieu C, Colombo BM, Lacave R, Lemoine FM, Klatzmann D, Guigon M. Immunophenotypical and functional heterogeneity of dendritic cells generated from murine bone marrow cultured with different cytokine combinations: implications for anti-tumoral cell therapy. Immunology 1999;96:569-577.

24. Reid SD, Penna G, Adorini L. The control of T cell responses by dendritic cell subsets. Curr Opin Immunol 2000;12:114-121.

25. Cella M, Sallusto F, Lanzavecchia A. Origin, maturation and antigen presenting function of dendritic cells. Curr Opin Immunol 1997;9:10-16.

26. Banchereau J, Steinman RM. Dendritic cells and the control of immunity. Nature 1998;392:245-252.

27. Bell D, Young JW, Banchereau J. Dendritic cells. Adv Immunol 1999;72:255-324.

28. Kane LP, Lin J, Weiss A. Signal transduction by the TCR for antigen. Curr Opin Immunol 2000;12:242-249.

29. Lanzavecchia A, Sallusto F. From synapses to immunological memory: the role of sustained T cell stimulation. Curr Opin Immunol 2000;12:92-98.

30. Janes PW, Ley SC, Magee AI, Kabouridis PS. The role of lipid rafts in T cell antigen receptor (TCR) signalling. Semin Immunol 2000;12:23-34.

31. Pivniouk VI, Geha RS. The role of SLP-76 and LAT in lymphocyte development. Curr Opin Immunol 2000;12:173-178.

32. Horwitz MS, Sarvetnick N. Viruses, host responses, and autoimmunity. Immunol Rev 1999;169:241-253.

33. Ferber I, Schonrich G, Schenkel J, Mellor AL, Hammerling GJ, Arnold B. Levels of peripheral T cell tolerance induced by different doses of tolerogen. Science 1994;263:674-676.

34. Kurts C, Miller JF, Subramaniam RM, Carbone FR, Heath WR. Major histocompatibility complex class I-restricted cross-presentation is biased towards high dose antigens and those released during cellular destruction. J Exp Med 1998;188:409-414.

35. Lo D, Freedman J, Hesse S, Brinster RL, Sherman L. Peripheral tolerance in transgenic mice: tolerance to class II MHC and non-MHC transgene antigens. Immunol Rev 1991;122:87-102.

36. Gimmi CD, Freeman GJ, Gribben JG, Gray G, Nadler LM. Human T-cell clonal anergy is induced by antigen presentation in the absence of B7 costimulation. Proc Natl Acad Sci U S A 1993;90:6586-6590.

37. Rocha B, Tanchot C, Von Boehmer H. Clonal anergy blocks in vivo growth of mature T cells and can be reversed in the absence of antigen. J Exp Med 1993;177:1517-1521.

38. Theofilopoulos AN. The basis of autoimmunity: Part I. Mechanisms of aberrant self-recognition. Part II. Genetic predisposition. Immunol Today 1995;16:90-98, 150-159.

39. Barker CF, Billingham RE. Immunologically privileged sites. Adv Immunol 1977;25:1-54.

40. Oldstone MB, Nerenberg M, Southern P, Price J, Lewicki H. Virus infection triggers insulin-dependent diabetes mellitus in a transgenic model: role of anti-self (virus) immune response. Cell 1991;65:319-331.

41. Chan LS, Vanderlugt CJ, Hashimoto T, Nishikawa T, Zone JJ, Black MM, Wojnarowska F, Stevens SR, Chen M, Fairley JA, Woodley DT, Miller SD, Gordon KB. Epitope spreading: lessons from autoimmune skin diseases. J Invest Dermatol 1998;110:103-109.

42. Warnock MG, Goodacre JA. Cryptic T-cell epitopes and their role in the pathogenesis of auto-immune diseases. Br J Rheumatol 1997;36:1144-1150.

43. Sercarz EE, Lehmann PV, Ametani A, Benichou G, Miller A, Moudgil K. Dominance and crypticity of T cell antigenic determinants. Annu Rev Immunol 1993;11:729-766.

44. Diment S. Different roles for thiol and aspartyl proteases in antigen presentation of ovalbumin. J Immunol 1990;145:417-422.

45. Barker RN, Elson CJ. Multiple self epitopes on the Rhesus polypeptides stimulate immunologically ignorant human T cells in vitro. Eur J Immunol 1994;24:1578-1582.

46. Markovic-Plese S, Fukaura H, Zhang J, al-Sabbagh A, Southwood S, Sette A, Kuchroo VK, Hafler DA. T cell recognition of immunodominant and cryptic proteolipid protein epitopes in humans. J Immunol 1995;155:982-992.

47. Matsuo H, Batocchi AP, Hawke S, Nicolle M, Jacobson L, Vincent A, Newsom-Davis J, Willcox N. Peptide-selected T cell lines from myasthenia gravis patients and controls recognize epitopes that are not processed from whole acetylcholine receptor. J Immunol 1995;155:3683-3692.

48. Quaratino S, Feldmann M, Dayan CM, Acuto O, Londei M. Human self-reactive T cell clones expressing identical T cell receptor beta chains differ in their ability to recognize a cryptic self-epitope. J Exp Med 1996;183:349-358.

49. Casciola-Rosen L, Wigley F, Rosen A. Scleroderma autoantigens are uniquely fragmented by metal-catalyzed oxidation reactions: implications for pathogenesis. J Exp Med 1997;185:71-79.

50. Goodacre JA, Middleton S, Lynn S, Ross DA, Pearson J. Human cartilage aggrecan CS1 region contains cryptic T-cell recognition sites. Immunology 1993;78:586-591.

51. Baum H, Davies H, Peakman M. Molecular mimicry in the MHC: hidden clues to autoimmunity? Immunol Today 1996;17:64-70.

52. von Herrath MG, Oldstone MB. Virus-induced autoimmune disease. Curr Opin Immunol 1996;8:878-885.

53. Oldstone MB, von Herrath M. Virus-induced autoimmune diseases: transgenic approach to mimic insulin-dependent diabetes mellitus and other autoimmune diseases. APMIS 1996;104:689-697.

54. Wang R, Wang-Zhu Y, Gabaglia CR, Kimachi K, Grey HM. The stimulation of low-affinity, non-

tolerized clones by heteroclitic antigen analogues causes the breaking of tolerance established to an immunodominant T cell epitope. J Exp Med 1999;190:983-994.

55. Tough DF, Borrow P, Sprent J. Induction of bystander T cell proliferation by viruses and type I interferon in vivo. Science 1996;272:1947-1950.

56. Matsuzawa A, Katagiri T, Ogata Y, Kominami R, Kimura M. Lymphadenopathy induced by the cooperation between lpr^{cg} and gld genes is of lpr but not of gld phenotype. Eur J Immunol 1994;24:1714-1716.

57. McRae BL, Vanderlugt CL, Dal Canto MC, Miller SD. Functional evidence for epitope spreading in the relapsing pathology of experimental autoimmune encephalomyelitis. J Exp Med 1995;182:75-85.

58. Miller SD, Vanderlugt CL, Begolka WS, Pao W, Yauch RL, Neville KL, Katz-Levy Y, Carrizosa A, Kim BS. Persistent infection with Theiler's virus leads to CNS autoimmunity via epitope spreading. Nat Med 1997;3:1133-1136.

59. Anderson J, Hammond E, Menlove R. Determining humoral and cellular-immune components in myocarditis: complementary diagnostic role of immunofluorescence microscopy in the evaluation of endomyocardial biopsy specimens. In: Kawai C, Abelmann WH, eds. Pathogenesis of myocarditis and cardiomyopathy: recent experimental and clinical studies. Tokyo: University of Tokyo Press, 1987:233-244.

60. Bolte HD, Schultheiss P. Immunological results in myocardial diseases. Postgrad Med J 1978;54:500-504.

61. Caforio AL, Bauce B, Boffa GM, De Cian F, Angelini A, Melacini P, Razzolini R, Fasoli G, Chioin R, Schiaffino S, Thiene G, Dalla Volta S. Autoimmunity in myocarditis and dilated cardiomyopathy: cardiac autoantibody frequency and clinical correlates in a patient series from Italy. G Ital Cardiol 1997;27:106-112.

62. Caforio ALP, Goldman JH, Haven AJ, Baig KM, Libera LD, McKenna WJ, and the Myocarditis Treatment Trial Investigators. Circulating cardiac-specific autoantibodies as markers of autoimmunity in clinical and biopsy-proven myocarditis. Eur Heart J 1997;18:270-275.

63. Limas CJ, Limas C. Immune-mediated modulation of beta-adrenoceptor function in human dilated cardiomyopathy. Clin Immunol Immunopathol 1993;68:204-207.

64. Maisch B. Autoreactivity to the cardiac myocyte, connective tissue and the extracellular matrix in heart disease and postcardiac injury. Springer Semin Immunopathol 1989;11:369-395.

65. Maisch B, Herzum M, Hufnagel G, Bethge C, Schonian U. Immunosuppressive treatment for myocarditis and dilated cardiomyopathy. Eur Heart J 1995;16 Suppl O:153-161.

66. Neumann DA, Allen GS, Narins CR, Rose NR, Herskowitz A. Idiopathic dilated cardiomyopathy. In: Figulla H-R, Kandolf R, McManus B, eds. Idiopathic dilated cardiomyopathy. Berlin: Springer-Verlag, 1993:325-334.

67. Neumann DA, Burek CL, Baughman KL, Rose NR, Herskowitz A. Circulating heart-reactive antibodies in patients with myocarditis or cardiomyopathy. J Am Coll Cardiol 1990;16:839-846.

68. Schultheiss HP. The significance of autoantibodies against the ADP/ATP carrier for the pathogenesis of myocarditis and dilated cardiomyopathy—clinical and experimental data. Springer Semin Immunopathol 1989;11:15-30.

69. Schwimmbeck PL, Schwimmbeck NK, Schultheiss HP, Strauer BE. Mapping of antigenic determinants of the adenine-nucleotide translocator and coxsackie B3 virus with synthetic peptides: use for the diagnosis of viral heart disease. Clin Immunol Immunopathol 1993;68:135-140.

70. Wallukat G, Kayser A, Wollenberger A. The beta 1-adrenoceptor as antigen: functional aspects. Eur Heart J 1995;16 Suppl O:85-88.

71. Gauntt CJ, Sakkinen PA, Rose NR, Huber SA. Picornaviruses: immunopathology and autoimmunity. In: Cunningham MW, Fujinami RS, eds. Effects of microbes on the immune system. Philadelphia: Lippincott Williams & Wilkins, 2000:313-329.

72. Wolff PG, Kuhl U, Schultheiss HP. Laminin distribution and autoantibodies to laminin in dilated cardiomyopathy and myocarditis. Am Heart J 1989;117:1303-1309.

73. Maisch B, Bauer E, Cirsi M, Kochsiek K. Cytolytic cross-reactive antibodies directed against the cardiac membrane and viral proteins in coxsackievirus B3 and B4 myocarditis. Characterization and pathogenetic relevance. Circulation 1993;87 Suppl 4:IV49-IV65.

74. Gauntt CJ, Arizpe HM, Higdon AL, Wood HJ, Bowers DF, Rozek MM, Crawley R. Molecular mimicry, anti-coxsackievirus B3 neutralizing monoclonal antibodies, and myocarditis. J Immunol 1995;154:2983-2995.

75. Neu N, Beisel KW, Traystman MD, Rose NR, Craig SW. Autoantibodies specific for the cardiac myosin isoform are found in mice susceptible to Coxsackievirus B3-induced myocarditis. J Immunol 1987;138:2488-2492.

76. Neumann DA, Lane JR, Wulff SM, Allen GS, LaFond-Walker A, Herskowitz A, Rose NR. In vivo deposition of myosin-specific autoantibodies in the hearts of mice with experimental autoimmune myocarditis. J Immunol 1992;148:3806-3813.

77. Neumann DA, Rose NR, Ansari AA, Herskowitz A. Induction of multiple heart autoantibodies in mice with coxsackievirus B3- and cardiac myosin-induced autoimmune myocarditis. J Immunol 1994;152:343-350.

78. Rose N, Neu N, Neumann D, Herskowitz A. Myocarditis: a postinfectious autoimmune disease. In: Schultheiss H-P, ed. New concepts in viral heart disease: virology, immunology, and clinical management. Berlin: Springer-Verlag, 1988:139-147.

79. Schwimmbeck PL, Schultheiss H-P, Strauer BE. Identification of a main autoimmunogenic epitope of the adenine nucleotide translocator which cross-reacts with Coxsackie B3 virus: use in the diagnosis of myocarditis and dilative cardiomyopathy (abstract). Circulation 1989;80 Suppl 2:II665.

80. Traystman MD, Beisel KW. Genetic control of Coxsackievirus B3-induced heart-specific autoantibodies associated with chronic myocarditis. Clin Exp Immunol 1991;86:291-298.

81. Gauntt CJ, Higdon AL, Arizpe HM, Tamayo MR, Crawley R, Henkel RD, Pereira ME, Tracy SM, Cunningham MW. Epitopes shared between coxsackievirus B3 (CVB3) and normal heart tissue contribute to CVB3-induced murine myocarditis. Clin Immunol Immunopathol 1993;68:129-134.

82. Gauntt C, Higdon A, Bowers D, Maull E, Wood J, Crawley R. What lessons can be learned from animal model studies in viral heart disease? Scand J Infect Dis Suppl 1993;88:49-65.

83. Saegusa J, Prabhakar BS, Essani K, McClintock PR, Fukuda Y, Ferrans VJ, Notkins AL. Monoclonal antibody to coxsackievirus B4 reacts with myocardium. J Infect Dis 1986;153:372-373.

84. Kuan AP, Chamberlain W, Malkiel S, Lieu HD, Factor SM, Diamond B, Kotzin BL. Genetic control of autoimmune myocarditis mediated by myosin-specific antibodies. Immunogenetics 1999;49:79-85.

85. Liao L, Sindhwani R, Rojkind M, Factor S, Leinwand L, Diamond B. Antibody-mediated autoimmune myocarditis depends on genetically determined target organ sensitivity. J Exp Med 1995;181:1123-1131.

86. Schwimmbeck PL, Badorff C, Schultheiss HP, Strauer BE. Transfer of human myocarditis into severe combined immunodeficiency mice. Circ Res 1994;75:156-164.

87. Horn GT, Bugawan TL, Long CM, Erlich HA. Allelic sequence variation of the HLA-DQ loci: relationship to serology and to insulin-dependent diabetes susceptibility. Proc Natl Acad Sci U S A 1988;85:6012-6016.

88. Tiwari JL, Terasaki PI. HLA and disease associations. New York: Springer-Verlag, 1985.

89. Limas CJ. Autoimmunity in dilated cardiomyopathy and the major histocompatibility complex. Int J Cardiol 1996;54:113-116.

90. Lozano MD, Rubocki RJ, Wilson JE, McManus BM, Wisecarver JL. Human leukocyte antigen class II associations in patients with idiopathic dilated cardiomyopathy. Myocarditis Treatment Trial Investigators. J Card Fail 1997;3:97-103.

91. Bachmaier K, Neu N, Yeung RS, Mak TW, Liu P, Penninger JM. Generation of humanized mice susceptible to peptide-induced inflammatory heart disease. Circulation 1999;99:1885-1891.

92. Schwimmbeck P, Badorff C, Schulze K, Schultheiss H-P. The significance of T cell responses in human myocarditis. In: Schultheiss H-P, Schwimmbeck P, eds. The role of immune mechanisms in cardiovascular disease. Berlin: Springer-Verlag, 1997:65-76.

93. Liao L, Sindhwani R, Leinwand L, Diamond B, Factor S. Cardiac alpha-myosin heavy chains differ in their induction of myocarditis. Identification of pathogenic epitopes. J Clin Invest 1993;92:2877-2882.

94. Neu N, Rose NR, Beisel KW, Herskowitz A, Gurri-Glass G, Craig SW. Cardiac myosin induces myocarditis in genetically predisposed mice. J Immunol 1987;139:3630-3636.

95. Smith SC, Allen PM. Myosin-induced acute myocarditis is a T cell-mediated disease. J Immunol 1991;147:2141-2147.

96. Smith SC, Allen PM. Expression of myosin-class II major histocompatibility complexes in the normal myocardium occurs before induction of autoimmune myocarditis. Proc Natl Acad Sci U S A 1992;89:9131-9135.

97. Donermeyer DL, Beisel KW, Allen PM, Smith SC. Myocarditis-inducing epitope of myosin binds constitutively and stably to I-A^k on antigen-presenting cells in the heart. J Exp Med 1995;182:1291-1300.

98. Pummerer CL, Luze K, Grassi G, Bachmaier K, Offner F, Burrell SK, Lenz DM, Zamborelli TJ, Penninger JM, Neu N. Identification of cardiac myosin peptides capable of inducing autoimmune myocarditis in BALB/c mice. J Clin Invest 1996;97:2057-2062.

99. Shi Y, Radvanyi LG, Sharma A, Shaw P, Green DR, Miller RG, Mills GB. CD28-mediated signaling in vivo prevents activation-induced apoptosis in the thymus and alters peripheral lymphocyte homeostasis. J Immunol 1995;155:1829-1837.

100. Yu JZ, Wilson JE, Wood SM, Kandolf R, Klingel K, Yang D, McManus BM. Secondary heterotypic versus homotypic infection by Coxsackie B group viruses: impact on early and late histopathological lesions and virus genome prominence. Cardiovasc Pathol 1999;8:93-102.

101. Kandolf R, Klingel K, Zell R, Selinka HC, Raab U, Schneider-Brachert W, Bultmann B. Molecular pathogenesis of enterovirus-induced myocarditis: virus persistence and chronic inflammation. Intervirology 1993;35:140-151.

102. Huber SA, Polgar J, Schultheiss P, Schwimmbeck P. Augmentation of pathogenesis of coxsackievirus B3 infections in mice by exogenous administration of interleukin-1 and interleukin-2. J Virol 1994;68:195-206.

103. Oldstone MB. Molecular mimicry and autoimmune disease. Cell 1987;50:819-820.

104. von Herrath MG, Dockter J, Oldstone MB. How virus induces a rapid or slow onset insulin-dependent diabetes mellitus in a transgenic model. Immunity 1994;1:231-242.

105. Finkel MS, Oddis CV, Jacob TD, Watkins SC, Hattler BG, Simmons RL. Negative inotropic effects of cytokines on the heart mediated by nitric oxide. Science 1992;257:387-389.

106. Freeman GL, Colston JT, Zabalgoitia M, Chandrasekar B. Contractile depression and expression of proinflammatory cytokines and iNOS in viral myocarditis. Am J Physiol 1998;274:H249-258.

107. Liu P. The role of cytokines in the pathogenesis of myocarditis. In: Schultheiss H-P, Schwimmbeck P, eds. The role of immune mechanisms in cardiovascular disease. Berlin: Springer-Verlag, 1997:44-56.

108. Song HK, Lin TH, Noorchashm H, Greeley SA, Moore DJ. Specialized CC-chemokine secretion by heart-specific CD4+ T cells contributes to their pathogenic potential in a novel model of autoimmune myocarditis (abstract). Circulation 1999;100 Suppl 1:I-614.

109. Kishimoto C, Kawamata H, Sakai S, Shinohara H, Ochiai H. Role of MIP-2 in coxsackievirus B3 myocarditis. J Mol Cell Cardiol 2000;32:631-638.

110. Cook DN, Beck MA, Coffman TM, Kirby SL, Sheridan JF, Pragnell IB, Smithies O. Requirement of MIP-1 alpha for an inflammatory response to viral infection. Science 1995;269:1583-1585.

111. Kolattukudy PE, Quach T, Bergese S, Breckenridge S, Hensley J, Altschuld R, Gordillo G, Klenotic S, Orosz C, Parker-Thornburg J. Myocarditis induced by targeted expression of the MCP-1 gene in murine cardiac muscle. Am J Pathol 1998;152:101-111.

112. Friman G, Wesslen L, Fohlman J, Karjalainen J, Rolf C. The epidemiology of infectious myocarditis, lymphocytic myocarditis and dilated cardiomyopathy. Eur Heart J 1995;16 Suppl O:36-41.

Humoral Immune Response in Viral Myocarditis

Bernhard Maisch, M.D., and
Arsen D. Ristić, M.D., M.Sc.

INTRODUCTION

DEFINITIONS AND TERMINOLOGY
First Biopsy
Subsequent Biopsies
Expert Committee on the Definition of Viral Cardiomyopathy

PATHOGENESIS OF MYOCARDIAL INJURY IN VIRAL
AND POSTVIRAL MYOCARDITIS
The Postviral Autoimmunity Hypothesis
Antigenic Mimicry Hypothesis
Direct Viral Injury Hypothesis
Direct Immune Injury Hypothesis

HUMORAL IMMUNE MECHANISMS
Myocardial Antigens in Autoreactive and Postviral Heart Disease
Functional Aspects
Specific Antibodies to the Cardiac Membrane and Its
Constituents
Antibodies to Intracellular Antigens
Antibodies to the Extracellular Matrix and to Endothelial Cells
Circulating Immune Complexes

CYTOKINES

ADHESION MOLECULES
Cellular Effector Mechanisms in Humans

CONCLUSION

INTRODUCTION

Viral and postviral autoimmune myocarditis are important causes of cardiac morbidity. The spectrum of the infectious agents varies with geographic region, age of the patient, application of different therapeutic procedures, and additional diseases. In many cases, dilated cardiomyopathy may be the consequence of a secondary immunopathogenesis after viral disease or unknown agents. This chapter deals with our knowledge of the humoral immune response in the myocarditis-perimyocarditis syndrome and its interplay with the viral agents and with the immune system. A more detailed definition of terms is used for the histologic and immunologic diagnosis of myocarditis.

DEFINITIONS AND TERMINOLOGY

Classically, histologically validated myocarditis is defined as active, healing, or healed myocarditis according to Daly et al.[1] or to the almost identical Dallas criteria.[2] It has been suggested that acute forms of myocarditis be subclassified clinically and histologically in fulminant forms with severe acute complications (cardiogenic shock) and either acute death or almost complete recovery and in chronic forms with incomplete recovery or worse long-term prognosis.[3,4] Japanese authors suggested a set of criteria to separate acute from chronic forms of myocarditis. However, these criteria were not widely accepted.

To resolve this problem, the World Heart Federation's Council on Cardiomyopathies formed 2 task forces: the first dedicated to viral cardiomyopathies and the second dedicated to the histology of dilated inflammatory cardiomyopathy (DCMI).[5] The task forces included numerous international experts who convened in 2 separate sessions and formulated new definitions of chronic myocarditis and DCMI and of viral cardiomyopathies, which were reported in brief [5] and will be published in full.

According to the task force on DCMI, active myocarditis was quantitatively defined as ≥ 14 infiltrative lymphocytes $\pm$ macrophages/mm^2 (reference 6) accompanied by necrosis or degeneration (Table 4-1) (Fig. 4-1; see color plate 4). In chronic myocarditis, necrosis is not an obligatory feature by definition. When referring to the Dallas criteria,[2] the term "acute myocarditis" corresponds to active myocarditis; chronic myocarditis may be defined as comprising borderline or healing myocarditis.

The inflammatory infiltrate should be subclassified as lymphocytic, eosinophilic, neutrophilic, giant cell, granulomatous, or mixed. The distribution should be classified as focal, confluent, or diffuse. The panel has chosen for the definition of myocarditis a minimum of 14 infiltrating leukocytes/mm^2, preferably T lymphocytes (T200) or activated T cells (eg, CD45RO), and up to 4 macrophages may be included in this total amount. The total number is more than 2 standard deviations above the number of leukocytes found in con-

Table 4-1
Histologic Criteria for the Diagnosis of Myocarditis According
to the Dallas Classification[7] and World Heart Federation Criteria

Biopsy	Dallas terminology	Histopathology			WHF classification	
		Infiltrate	Myocytolysis	Edema	Infiltrate, cells/mm^2	Terminology
1st	Active myocarditis	+	+	+	≥ 14	Active myocarditis
	Borderline myocarditis	+	–	–	≥ 14	Chronic myocarditis or DCMI
2nd	Ongoing myocarditis	+	+	+	≥ 14	Ongoing myocarditis
	Resolving or healing myocarditis	+	–	–	≥ 14	Resolving or chronic myocarditis or DCMI
	Resolved myocarditis	–	–	–	< 14	Resolved myocarditis

DCMI, dilated inflammatory cardiomyopathy; WHF, World Heart Federation.
From Maisch et al.[5] By permission of Urban & Vogel.

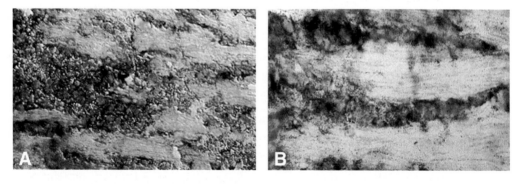

Fig. 4-1. Cryostat sections demonstrate CD4-positive lymphocytes in chronic myocarditis by using monoclonal antibodies to CD4 (Becton Dickinson, NJ, USA). *A*, Low magnification (x80). *B*, High magnification (x400). See color plate 4. (From Maisch et al.[5] By permission of Urban & Vogel.)

trol tissue (2-4). In case of nests of leukocytes (ie, 3 lymphocytes, preferably T cells) located outside the lumen of a vessel, a focal inflammatory process (myocarditis) is diagnosed. If foci of T lymphocytes are present, myocarditis can be diagnosed owing to the nature of the infiltrate, even when the critical number of 14 leukocytes/mm^2 is not reached. If the focal or diffuse leukocytes are localized in fibrotic areas, the process may be termed "reparative."

The amount and distribution of fibrosis should be described similarly as no (grade 0), mild (grade 1), moderate (grade 2), or severe (grade 3). Localization or formation of fibrosis should be outlined as endocardial, replacement, or interstitial. Thus, the following terminology was adopted.

FIRST BIOPSY

1. **Acute (active) myocarditis.** A clear-cut infiltrate (diffuse, focal, or confluent) of ≥ 14 leukocytes/mm^2 (preferably activated T cells). The amount of the infiltrate should be quantitated by immunohistochemistry. Necrosis or degeneration is compulsory; fibrosis may be absent or present and should be graded.
2. **Chronic myocarditis.** An infiltrate of ≥ 14 leukocytes/mm^2 (diffuse, focal, or confluent, preferably activated T cells). Quantification should be made by immunohistochemistry. Necrosis or degeneration is usually not evident; fibrosis may be absent or present and should be graded.
3. **No myocarditis.** No infiltrating cells or < 14 leukocytes/mm^2.

SUBSEQUENT BIOPSIES

1. **Ongoing (persistent) myocarditis.** Criteria as in 1 or 2 (features of an acute or chronic myocarditis).
2. **Resolving (healing) myocarditis.** Criteria as in 1 or 2 but the immunologic process is sparser than in the first biopsy.
3. **Resolved (healed) myocarditis.** Corresponds to the Dallas classification.

Chronic myocarditis in its histologic sense remains controversial in international histopathology, although histologic features of chronicity have been known for a long time.[8] Studies on the secondary immunopathogenesis in protracted forms of (peri)myocarditis and in enteroviral heart disease with viral persistence suggest that an effort to reintroduce this term in a clinical context may be worthwhile.[9] Further subclassification into chronic and chronic persistent forms[3,10] was not generally accepted.

The World Heart Federation Task Force on the histologic features of inflammatory cardiomyopathy introduced chronic myocarditis as a histologically defined independent category (presence of a diffuse or focal leukocytic infiltrate or foci of lymphocytes associated with the presence of myocellular hypertrophy, focal or diffuse interstitial, replacement or perivascular fibrosis, and nonobligatory microvascular changes) for dilated cardiomyopathies. The presence of chronic inflammatory cells (eg, lymphocytes, monocytes, or macrophages) defined by histologic features or immunohistochemistry in association with the cardiomyopathic changes defines chronic myocarditis or DCMI. Chronic myocarditis was defined interchangeably with DCMI. A minimum of 14 infiltrating cells/mm^2 is obligatory; necrosis or apoptosis is not.

EXPERT COMMITTEE ON THE DEFINITION OF VIRAL CARDIOMYOPATHY

Because isolation of the virus from swabs or tissue is possible in only the acute phase of infection, it is unlikely to succeed in patients with longer-lasting diseases or chronic infections. Enteroviruses, therefore, have been isolated effectively in pediatric patients only. A higher sensitivity is achieved with molecular techniques (eg, gene amplification), which are significantly more sensitive than standard histochemical techniques for the detection of viral proteins. Except for human immunodeficiency virus, hepatitis C, and cytomegalovirus, serologic assessment of antiviral antibodies appeared to be of limited diagnostic value with respect to the actual disease status of the patients and for the critical issue of whether the viral genome is present in the myocardium.

The World Heart Federation expert panel reached a consensus on current diagnostic approaches to viral heart disease by means of an international, multicenter, and blinded interlaboratory study. The assessment of viral nucleic acid in the myocardium with the polymerase chain reaction (PCR) technique was the first choice of methods because of its rapidity, wide availability, high sensitivity, and specificity.

The highest sensitivity and reproducibility for the detection of enteroviral genomes were achieved with frozen tissue (100%) in 5 of 9 centers. Reverse transcription (RT) PCR of enterovirus RNA from fixed embedded tissue was less reliable. Detection of enterovirus sequences in formalin-fixed samples was not convincing. The incidence of hepatitis C virus in formalin-fixed tissue (15%) was remarkable. PCR for the genomic sequences of DNA viruses in formalin-fixed tissue is less critical, and adenovirus (12.5%-22.5%), cytomegalovirus (5%), and Epstein-Barr virus (2.5%) could also be detected in formalin-fixed tissue. New data from several laboratories indicate that parvovirus B19 should also be included in the list of cardiotropic viruses with a prevalence well over or in the range of enterovirus.[11] An overview of the incidence of a positive viral PCR in the literature and our own myocarditis registry is given in Table 4-2.

On the basis of the interlaboratory analysis, the World Heart Federation expert panel on viral cardiomyopathies has given for the first time a reliable comparative analysis of cardiac tissue samples infected in part with cardiotropic viruses.

Perimyocarditis is defined as pericardial effusion and cardiomegaly or segmental wall motion abnormality. Demonstration of pericardial effusion (in the absence of neoplastic, postirradiation, or postinjury syndromes; systemic disorders; metabolic disorders; or uremia) ascertains the inflammatory epicardial or pericardial process; cardiac dilatation or wall motion abnormality shows the myocardial involvement.[12-14] Viral pericarditis is nearly always associated with underlying epicardial and myocardial lesions,[15] which lead to the use of myopericarditis[16] or more precisely perimyocarditis.[12] Because myocarditis is not associated regularly with pericardial effusion, the clinical entities overlap but are not identical. For these patients, a biopsy with demonstration of active inflammation is helpful.

Table 4-2
Bacterial and Viral Etiology of Myocarditis, Dilated Cardiomyopathy, and Pericarditis

Pathogen	Type	Patients positive, %		
		Myocarditis	DCM	Pericarditis
Bacteria	Staphylococci	0	0	1
	Streptococci	0	0	1
	Mycobacterium tuberculosis	~0	0	1 (Europe)-50 (Asia)
	Borrelia burgdorferi	0.5	1	3
	Chlamydia pneumoniae	0	~1	~1
Rickettsia	*Coxiella burnetii*		< 1	< 1
Viruses				
Picornavirus (RNA)	Coxsackie A and B virus	5-50	5-50	4
	Echovirus	?	?	?
	Hepatitis A virus	?	?	?
	Hepatitis C virus	0-15	0-10	?
Orthomyxovirus (RNA)	Influenza A and B	?	?	< 5
Paramyxovirus (RNA)	RSV, mumps, measles virus	?	< 1	< 1
Rubivirus/Toga virus (RNA)	Rubella virus	?	< 1	< 1
Rhabdovirus (RNA)	Rabies virus	?	?	?
Arbovirus/Tahyna (RNA)	Dengue, yellow fever virus	?	?	?
Retrovirus/Lenti (RNA)	HIV (reverse transcriptase)	Variable	?	?
Herpesvirus (DNA)	Varicella-zoster virus	1-2	1-2	2
	Cytomegalovirus	1-15	1-10	< 5
	Epstein-Barr virus	1-3	1-3	1-3
	Human herpesvirus 6	0-5	0-5	?
	Herpes simplex virus	0-3	?	?
Mastadenovirus (DNA)	Adenovirus	5-20	10-12	5-9
Parvovirus (DNA)	Parvo B 19 virus	10-30	10-25	10-15

DCM, dilated cardiomyopathy; RSV, respiratory syncytial virus.
Data from Marburg University hospital registry, Fairweather et al.,[84] Goin et al.,[30] Pankuweit et al.,[11] and
  Brooks GF, Butel JS, Morse SA. Jawetz, Melnick, & Adelberg's medical microbiology. 21st ed. Stamford,
  CT: Appleton & Lange, 1998.

PATHOGENESIS OF MYOCARDIAL INJURY IN VIRAL
AND POSTVIRAL MYOCARDITIS

THE POSTVIRAL AUTOIMMUNITY HYPOTHESIS

According to this hypothesis, the initial viral infection of the myocardium produces limited myocardial lesions but triggers an adverse immune response that is primarily responsible for myocyte damage and resultant heart failure. Rose and Hill[17] built a strong case for such a mechanism in a murine model. Coxsackie B3 viral infection causes initial myocyte damage, releasing myosin into the circulation. The viral infection then clears but is followed by a second phase of disease mediated largely by antibodies to myosin heavy chain and CD4 T lymphocytes. The latter may produce myocyte damage not only by inducing B cells to produce antimyosin antibodies but also by stimulating cytokine accumulation and by inciting production of cytotoxic CD8 T lymphocytes. Although this mechanism has not been demonstrated in humans, antimyosin antibodies have been found in patients with myocarditis,[13,14,18,19] which supports the possibility that it occurs clinically. A delay of 1 to several weeks is commonly reported between recovery from a viral infection and development of heart failure. This time lag is consistent with development of a postinfectious autoimmune phase. A similar mechanism has been proposed by Maisch[20] for antisarcolemmal and antimyolemmal antibodies that can be induced in antibody-producing mice strains (DBA, NMRI).

ANTIGENIC MIMICRY HYPOTHESIS

Antigenic mimicry is another postinfectious autoimmune mechanism documented in animal models and in humans.[21] The infectious agent carries an antigen identical to normal myocyte antigens. The antibody response to the antigen cross-reacts with the infecting agent and the myocyte. Cellular immune responses also may be induced by cross-reactive epitopes. Antigenic mimicry has evolved as an important pathomechanism by sensitized T cells and autoantibodies, which could cause cardiac damage independent from any viral infection of the myocardium.[20] In humans, cytolytic antibodies against the myolemma and sarcolemma of isolated myocytes cross-react with enteroviral proteins. By absorption experiments with the virus or a human heart membrane extract or a pellet of isolated myocytes, the antibody fluorescence on isolated human and rat myocytes vanished. Consequently, the cytolytic properties of absorbed sera, which previously needed the presence of complement to work, were completely abolished.

DIRECT VIRAL INJURY HYPOTHESIS

In certain animal models, viral proliferation alone is sufficient to initiate severe myocarditis with resultant heart failure. After successful replication within the myocyte, highly lytic viruses may destroy the host cell in the process of separation from the cell. This damage can occur in the complete absence of host immune defenses.[22] It is likely that this mechanism occurs in humans, explaining why some patients who are clearly still viremic are seen with heart failure after a short period of viral symptoms.

If antibodies induced by the viral infection injure the myocardium directly, homologies between cardiac cellular antigens and the offending viruses must be recognized. Antibodies that recognize discontinuous epitopes on Coxsackie B virus capsid proteins induce cytopathologic alterations in adolescent male mice.[21] Additionally, the anti-idiotypic antibodies that are generated nonspecifically during humoral immune responses inhibit the expression of CVB3-induced myocarditis in syngeneic mice.[23] Cardiac myocyte injury, as a result of viral antibody production, is one possible mechanism for the cardiac dysfunction of myocarditis.

Horwitz et al.[24] used a transgenic nonobese diabetic (NOD) mouse myocarditis model to study the mechanism behind virus-induced autoimmunity. In these mice, pancreatic islet cells express interferon (IFN)-gamma under the influence of the insulin promoter. Pancreatic expression of IFN-gamma protects mice from lethal infection by a diabetogenic coxsackievirus—CB4. Transgenic expression of IFN-gamma by pancreatic beta cells protected mice from lethal infection with CB3, decreased the amount of the virus in the heart, and prevented myocarditis. Nontransgenic NOD littermates, on the other hand, all died promptly. Although autoantibodies against cardiac myosin were present in the transgenic CB3-infected NOD mice as well as in the nontransgenic infected NOD mice, the authors concluded that molecular mimicry was not likely to be a mechanism, because cardiac damage induced by CB3 was required to initiate disease, probably by exposing heart antigens. They favored the hypothesis of virus-mediated damage. However, there are also several studies that have failed to confirm this hypothesis.[25-27]

DIRECT IMMUNE INJURY HYPOTHESIS

Less lytic viruses may continue to infect the cell without killing it, but they nevertheless cause its destruction by inducing a virus-specific immune response. Nonspecific responses may also be involved. Nitric oxide and several endogenous cytokines have been implicated in animal models[28,29] (Table 4-3).

HUMORAL IMMUNE MECHANISMS

MYOCARDIAL ANTIGENS IN AUTOREACTIVE AND POSTVIRAL HEART DISEASE

Various cardiac antigens can be identified as targets of humoral and cellular autoreactivity. They include components to be identified by light microscopy on cryostat sections (Fig. 4-2; see color plate 6) or antigens characterized biochemically or defined by monoclonal antibodies. Many of these antigens have been associated with the major cardiotropic viruses for possible cross-reactivity (Table 4-4). These antigens have more or less precisely defined epitopes, but in some cases they are simply assigned according to the involved anatomic structure (eg, components of the conduction system). Table 4-5 for myocarditis, Table 4-6 for pericarditis, and Table 4-7 for DCM give an overview of the organ-specific and non–organ-specific antibodies.

Table 4-3
Immunologic Classification of Dilated Heart Muscle Diseases

Disease	Endomyocardial biopsy Lymphocytic infiltrate	IgG, M, A, C3 binding	Peripheral blood Class II M	Cardio-LC	NK cell	AMLAs	Anti-ANT ab	AFA ab	Matrix ab/AEA
Myocarditis	++	++	+	+	Reduced	++		+	
Perimyocarditis	++	++	+	+	Reduced		++		+
Pericarditis	−	+	+/−	−*	=		+		−
Postmyocarditis									
HMD	−	++	−	+	Reduced		++/+		+
DCM	−	+/−	−	+/−	Reduced/=	+		+	

AEA, antiendothelial antibodies; AFA, antifibrillary antibodies mostly from the antimyosin type; AMLAs, antimyolemmal antibodies; ANT, adenine nucleotide translocator; DCM, dilated cardiomyopathy; HMD, heart muscle disease; LC, lymphocytotoxicity to isolated rat heart cells by peripheral blood lymphocytes (non-major histocompatibility complex controlled lymphocytotoxicity); M, (expression on) myocytes; NK, natural killer cell activity to K562 erythroblast cell line; =, unchanged; −, negative; +, positive finding in more than 50% of patients; ++, positive finding in more than 80% of patients.
*No cardiocytotoxicity of peripheral blood lymphocytes but strong lymphocytotoxicity from lymphocytes of the pericardial fluid.

Myolemma and sarcolemma are antigens with different subepitopes, which have been extensively analyzed in our laboratory.[9,12-14,20,31,39,49,50,56,57,59-62] Various receptors such as the acetylcholine receptor, the β_1-receptor, and the Ca^{2+} channel have been studied by others (see Table 4-4). Contractile and other intracellular or extracellular proteins such as myosin, actin, laminin, vimentin, and desmin can be identified immunohistochemically and by enzyme-linked immunosorbent assay or radioimmunoassay with the defined protein or by functional in vitro assays (beta-receptor antibodies).[34] For aconitate hydratase, pyruvate kinase, dihydrolipoamide dehydrogenase, creatine kinase, nicotinamide adenine dinucleotide dehydrogenase, ubiquinol–cytochrome-c reductase, adenine nucleotide translocator, carnitine, and heat shock proteins, 2-dimensional western blots and protein sequencing are necessary to define antibodies and their binding sites. For nuclear antigens, established methods are needed. For extracellular matrix and endothelial cell antigens, proteins in blots or the total number of cells is used for antibody identification. All the above-mentioned epitopes have been postulated to be involved in an antigenic mimicry process or in the cross-reactivity with viral antigens. Except for the sarcolemmal and myolemmal and myosin epitopes and some mitochondrial proteins, the evidence for cross-reactivity is either hypothetical or has yet to be reproduced.

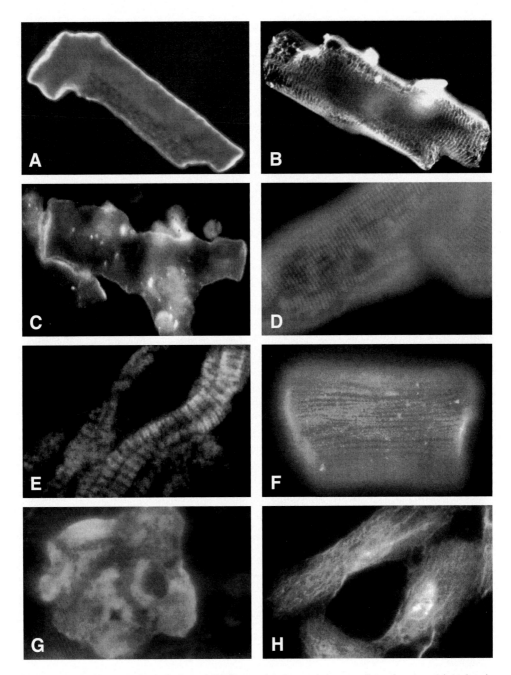

Fig. 4-2. Demonstration of circulating antibodies to the *A*, sarcolemma and myolemma with isolated rat cardiocytes; *B*, laminin with isolated rat cardiocytes; *C*, specific positive staining of the sarcolemma with isolated Purkinje (dog) fibers; *D*, myosin with isolated rat cardiocytes; *E*, actin with isolated rat cardiocytes; *F*, anti-interfibrillary staining (eg, antimitochondrial or anticytoplasmic antibodies against isolated rat cardio-myocytes; *G*, intracellular staining of Purkinje fibers in bovine false tendon; and *H*, antiendothelial staining on Hep2 cells. (Magnification x400.) See color plate 6. (2 *A* and *C-H* from Maisch et al.[5] By permission of Urban & Vogel. 2 *B* from Maisch.[9] By permission of Springer-Verlag.)

Table 4-4
Antibodies to Cardiac Antigen and Their Possible Cross-Reactivity and Pathomechanism

Antigen	Antibody	Cross-reactivity	Pathomechanism	Reference
ACh-receptor	Anti-ACh	Unknown	Bradycardia*	Goin et al.[30]
Actin	Antiactin	Unknown	Unknown	Maisch et al.[31]
AH, PK, DLD, CK	Anti-AH, anti-PK, anti-DLD, anti-CK	Unknown	Impairment of energy metabolism*	Pankuweit et al.[32]
ANT	Anti-ANT	Enterovirus*	Impairment of energy metabolism	Schulze and Schultheiss[33]
β_1-receptor	Anti-β_1	Enterovirus*	Positive chronotropic[†]	Wallukat et al.[34]
β_1-receptor	Anti-β_1	Unknown	Negative inotropic*	Limas et al.[35]
Ca^{2+} channel	Anti-Ca^{2+}	ANT,* enterovirus*	Unknown	Schulze et al.[36]
Carnitine	Anticarnitine	Unknown	Unknown	Otto et al.[37]
Conduction system	Antisinus, anti-AV node, anti-Purkinje	Unknown	Conduction defect*	Maisch et al.[38]
Desmin	Antidesmin	Unknown	Unknown	Maisch et al.[9,39] Obermayer et al.[40]
Hsp60, hsp70, vimentin	Anti-hsp60, anti-hsp70, antivimentin	Multiple	Unknown	Portig et al.[41]
Laminin	Antilaminin	Unknown	Unknown	Maisch et al.[42]
Mitochondria/ microsomes	AMA	Multiple[†]	Inhibition of sarcosine dehydrogenase	Klein et al.[43] Pohlner et al.[44]
Myolemma	AMLA	Enterovirus[†]	Lytic[†]	Maisch et al.[31]
Myosin	Antimyosin	Unknown	Negative inotropic*	Maisch[14]
Myosin	Antimyosin	Enterovirus*	Negative inotropic*	Caforio et al.[18]
NADD, UCR	Anti-NADD, anti-UCR	Unknown	Impairment of energy metabolism*	Pohlner et al.[44]
Nuclear antigen, ENA	ANA, ENA, ANCA Anti-SS-A, Anti-SS-B	Unknown	Immune complex-mediated, degranulation of neutrophils* AV-block	Naparstek and Plotz[45]
Sarcolemma	ASA	Enterovirus[†]	Lytic[†]	Maisch et al.[31]
SR-Ca-ATPase	Anti-cardiac SR-Ca^{2+} ATPase antibody	Unknown	Metabolic interactions	Khaw et al.[46]

ACh, acetylcholine; AH, aconitate hydratase; AMA, antimitochondrial antibody; AMLA, antimyolemmal antibody; ANA, antinuclear antigen; ANCA, antineutrophil cytoplasmic antigen; ANT, adenine nucleotide translocator; ASA, antisarcolemmal antibody; AV, atrioventricular; CK, creatine kinase; DLD, dihydrolipoamide dehydrogenase; ENA, extractable nuclear antigen; hsp, heat shock protein; NADD, nicotinamide adenine dinucleotide dehydrogenase; PK, pyruvate kinase; SR-Ca-ATPase, sarcoplasmic reticulum calcium ATPase; SS-A, skin-sensitizing antibody A; SS-B, skin-sensitizing antibody B; UCR, ubiquino–cytochrome-c reductase.
*Hypothetical.
[†]Experimentally proven.

Table 4-5

Circulating Antibodies to the Sarcolemma, Extracellular Matrix, and Intermediate Filaments in Myocarditis (% of Sample Positive)*

Reference	N	AMLA (homol)	ASA (homol)	A-ALA	A-fibron bands	Z-bands	A-actin	A-myosin	A-tubulin	AIDA	A-desmin	A-vimentin	A-M7	AEA	A-collagen type			
															I	II	III	IV
De Scheerder et al.[47]	12	100	12	ND	ND	ND	58	67	ND	ND	ND	ND	ND	91	35	40	35	35
Klein et al.[43,48]	ND	ND	ND	ND	ND	ND	ND	ND	ND	ND	ND	ND	13	ND	ND	ND	ND	ND
Maisch et al., [12,14,49,50] viral myocarditis (adults)	44	79-90	ND	ND	ND	15	7	10-50	0	0	ND	ND	ND	80	ND	ND	ND	ND
Idiopathic myocarditis	144	59	45	ND	ND	ND	0	23	9	0	ND	ND	ND	40	ND	ND	ND	ND
Myocarditis in children (Maisch et al.[51])[43]	100	100	ND	ND	0	0	0	0	0	ND	ND	ND	91	ND	ND	ND	ND	
Maisch et al.[39]	132	ND	30-35	ND	ND	ND	ND	ND	ND	ND	ND	ND	ND	ND	ND	ND	ND	ND
Obermayer et al.[40]	25	64	72	ND	ND	16	0	4	0	ND	0	0	ND	72	ND	ND	ND	ND
Schultheiss and Kühl[52,53]	29	ND	ND	60	20	ND	ND	ND	ND	ND	ND	ND	ND	ND	35	40	35	35

A, anti; AEA, antiendothelial antibody; AIDA, anti-intercalated disk antibody; ALA, antilaminin antibody; AMLA, antimyolemmal antibody; ASA, antisarcolemmal antibody; fibron, fibronectin; homol, homologous; ND, not done.
*Anti-β receptor and antinucleotide translocator were not tested for in any of these studies.
Modified from Maisch.[9] By permission of Springer-Verlag.

Table 4-6
Circulating Antibodies to the Sarcolemma, Extracellular Matrix, and Intermediate Filaments in Pericarditis (% of Sample Positive)*

Reference	N	AMLA (homol)	ASA (homol)	ALA	A-fibron	Z-bands	A-actin	A-myosin	A-tubulin	AIDA	A-desmin	A-vimentin	ANT	A-M7	AEA
De Scheerder et al.[47]	10	10	60	60	ND	ND	10	10	ND	ND	ND	ND	ND	ND	70
Maisch et al.,[54] tuberculous pericarditis	10	100	100	ND	ND	0	8	67	ND	0	ND	ND	ND	ND	42
Maisch and Kochsiek,[55] uremic pericarditis	41	30-83	50-100	ND	ND	0	0	0	ND	0	ND	ND	ND	ND	20-50
Obermayer et al.,[40] idiopathic pericarditis	10	80	50	ND	ND	0	0	ND	0	ND	0	0	0	ND	ND

A, anti; AEA, antiendothelial antibody; AIDA, anti-intercalated disk antibody; ALA, antilaminin antibody; AMLA, antimyolemmal antibody; ANT, anti-nucleotide translocator; ASA, antisarcolemmal antibody; fibron, fibronectin; homol, homologous; ND, not done.
*Anti-β receptor and A-collagen type I through IV were not tested for in any of these studies.
From Maisch.[9] By permission of Springer-Verlag.

Table 4-7
Circulating Antibodies to the Sarcolemma, Extracellular Matrix, and Intermediate Filaments in Dilated Cardiomyopathy (% of Sample Positive)*

Reference	N	AMLA (homol)	ASA (homol)	ALA	A-fibron	Z-bands	A-actin	A-myosin	A-tubulin	AIDA	A-vimentin	A-M7	AEA	A-collagen type			
														I	II	III	IV
Klein et al.[43]	ND	ND	ND	ND	ND	ND	ND	ND	ND	ND	ND	30	ND	ND	ND	ND	ND
Maisch et al.[56]	79	9	10	ND	ND	ND	4	20	ND	2	ND	ND	13	ND	ND	ND	ND
Maisch et al.[57]	30	33	42	ND	ND	ND	10	33	ND	2	ND	ND	45	ND	ND	ND	ND
Schultheiss et al.[53,58]	51	ND	ND	72	ND	ND	ND	ND	ND	ND	ND	ND	ND	1	2	6	2
														2	4		4
Obermayer et al.[40]	36	42	31	ND	ND	8	0	8	0	ND	0	ND	31	ND	ND	ND	ND

A, anti; AEA, antiendothelial antibody; AIDA, anti-intercalated disk antibody; ALA, antilaminin antibody; AMLA, antimyolemmal antibody; ASA, antisarcolemmal antibody; fibron, fibronectin; homol, homologous; ND, not done.

*Antidesmin, antinucleotide, and anti-β receptor were not tested for in any of these studies.

From Maisch.[9] By permission of Springer-Verlag.

Important information on cross-reactive epitopes comes from 1- and 2-dimensional immunoblots followed by N-terminal amino acid sequencing. These methods have been used to identify corresponding antigens of autoantibodies in the serum of patients with myocarditis and dilated cardiomyopathy.[32,41,44] It appears from these studies that no one antibody is the sole causative agent, but that sarcolemmal and mitochondrial epitopes play key roles in the humoral immune damage and antibody response in humans. This occurs in the context of a polyclonal stimulation of the immune system after the initial viral assault that may have been cleared already when the autoreactive B- and T-cell response occurs.

In a large series of patients from Italy,[63] cardiac antimyosin autoantibodies were found in 25% to 35% of patients with myocarditis and dilated cardiomyopathy. The frequency of organ-specific cardiac autoantibodies was higher ($P = 0.0001$) in myocarditis (45%) and in dilated cardiomyopathy (20%) than in other cardiac disease (1%), in ischemic heart failure (1%), or in normals (2.5%). Cross-reactive antibodies were detected in similar proportions of study patients and controls. Both patients with giant cell myocarditis were antibody positive. Myocarditis patients with cardiac antibodies had a shorter duration of symptoms than those who were antibody negative (0.4 ± 0.3 vs. 4 ± 1 months, $P = 0.004$). In dilated cardiomyopathy, antibody status was not associated with any clinical or diagnostic feature.

FUNCTIONAL ASPECTS

Experiments in animals or in in vitro models have shown that autoantibodies may well have a role in compromising myocardial function. For example, antimyolemmal antibodies, detected by direct immunofluorescence, exhibit lytic properties toward isolated rat cardiomyocytes in the presence of complement or lymphocytes.[31] Antibodies to receptors of the sympathetic and parasympathetic nervous systems have been shown to modulate myocardial performance in vitro.[30,34,64] Antibodies to the Ca^{2+} channel cross-reacting with the adenine nucleotide translocator may depress myocardial function.[33,36]

Antibodies binding to mitochondrial and microsomal proteins are believed to impair the energy metabolism of myocardial cells.[43,44,65] Antibodies binding to nuclear antigens (antinuclear antibody, extractable nuclear antigen) have been shown to form immune complexes, and antineutrophil cytoplasmic antibodies are thought to degranulate activated neutrophils, thereby leading to vasculitis in small vessels. Moreover, recent data on the improvement of myocardial function of patients with dilated cardiomyopathy after plasmapheresis to eliminate circulating antibodies show that we may still underestimate the role of autoantibodies in dilated cardiomyopathy, with and without inflammation.[66]

SPECIFIC ANTIBODIES TO THE CARDIAC MEMBRANE AND ITS CONSTITUENTS

Antimembrane Antibodies

Circulating and biopsy-specimen–bound antibodies to the membrane of the cardiomyocyte, the sarcolemma and myolemma, which may be cytolytic and complement-fixing (antimyolemmal antibodies [AMLAs] (Fig. 4-2 *A*; see color plate 6), have been demonstrated in coxsackievirus B, mumps, and influenza myocarditis.[12,20,49,57,59,60,67] Antigenic mimicry may play an important role: epitopes on the sarcolemmal surface[31] cross-reacted with Coxsackie B viruses. In absorption experiments, it could be shown that in viral myocarditis the sarcolemmal fluorescence was greatly diminished, and the cytolytic serum activity could be absorbed by the respective viruses. This could be done for Coxsackie B and influenza viruses.[12,14,39,49,61] In addition, AMLA titer and cytolytic serum activity correlated nicely, demonstrating the presence of a complement-fixing cytolytic antimembrane antibody. It could be shown by western blot analysis that they are cross-reactive to enteroviral core proteins (Fig. 4-3).

For the first time, adult human myocytes isolated from atrial appendages during open heart surgery were used in the study by Maisch et al.[31] as antigen in the indirect immunofluorescence test: 9 of 10 serum samples from patients with coxsackievirus B myocarditis demonstrated AMLAs of the homologous type in titers of 1:40 to 1:320, whereas 8 of 10 reacted with rat myocytes (heterologous type) only. Circulating AMLAs fixed complement component C4 in the majority of cases. During the in vitro assay of antibody-mediated cytolysis with vital heart cells, fixation of components C3 and C4 to the myolemma in all, of C1q in 7, and of the C3b9 complex in 8 of 10 sera was demonstrated after addition of a fresh complement source, indicating the potential of a complement-mediated cytolysis being operative. In vitro cardiocytolysis of isolated adult rat heart cells is present in the untreated sera of patients with enteroviral myocarditis and is abolished after adsorption of sera with coxsackievirus B and with isolated rat heart cells. This indicates functional cross-reactivity of the antimembrane antibodies.

To analyze the cross-reactive epitopes further, sodium dodecyl sulfate gel electrophoresis of human and rat sarcolemma and consecutive immunoblots were performed. Cross-reactivity between viral and sarcolemmal epitopes could be demonstrated to bands of 220 kDa in 10%, 110 kDa in 50%, 48 kDa in 40%, 35 kDa in 40%, and 31 kDa and 28 kDa in 30% each. Cardiospecific, non–cross-reactive epitopes for antisarcolemmal antibodies or AMLAs were membrane proteins of 90 kDa and 78 kDa in 50%, 72 kDa in 90%, 67 kDa in 40%, and 45 kDa in 50%. Virus-specific antibody binding sites for sera included proteins of 33 kDa and 34 kDa. The cytolytic property of the patients' sera in vitro suggests, in contrast to the findings from Horwitz et al.,[24] that humoral autoreactivity

Immunoblot

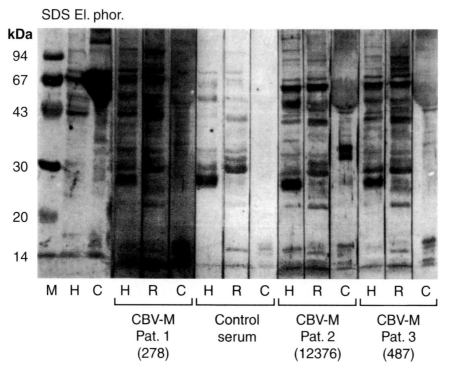

Fig. 4-3. Demonstration of cardiospecific, virus-specific, and cross-reactive epitopes in Coxsackie B myocarditis with sera of different patients. *M*, marker proteins; *H*, human membrane proteins; *R*, rat membrane proteins; *C*, Coxsackie B preparation. The broad band between 55 and 65 kDa does not stain when incubated with the patients' sera (fetal calf serum stabilizing medium). Cross-reactivity to enteroviral proteins could be demonstrated at 35 (VP1), 31 (VP2), and 28 (VP3) kDa in myocarditis patients to different percentages; virus-specific antibody sites were 33- and 34-kDa proteins; cardiospecific antibodies included 90-, 72-, 67-, and 45-kDa proteins. (From Maisch et al.[31] By permission of the American Heart Association.)

and antigenic mimicry are major pathogenetic mechanisms operating in human enteroviral myocarditis and its sequelae.[31]

Antibodies to the beta-adrenoceptor have been shown to exist in patients with dilated cardiomyopathy[63,68] and were postulated to possess beta-blocking activity. In contrast, beta-receptor antibodies that increased the beating frequency of isolated fetal heart cells have also been demonstrated.[69] These antibodies induce a Mg^{+2}-dependent conformational change to the receptor, independent of coupling to the guanosine triphosphate regulatory protein but similar to that induced by the agonist isoproterenol.[70]

Inomata et al.[71] investigated the effect of a monoclonal antibody against CD2 molecules (OX34) in preventing the induction of experimental autoimmune myocarditis by immunizing Lewis rats with cardiac myosin. Administration of OX34 before immunization, on days -6, -4, -2, and 0, completely prevented myocarditis occurrence. On the other hand, treatment with OX34 just before the appearance of myocardial lesions, on days 9, 11, 13, and 15, only partially prevented the disease. Flow cytometric analysis of lymph node cells showed that CD^{3+} T cells were immediately depleted with the administration of OX34 but had largely recovered on day 21. Ultimate production of the antimyosin antibody was not inhibited by the treatment with OX34. These results suggest that the prevention of experimental autoimmune myocarditis by administering the anti-CD2 monoclonal antibody OX34 resulted from T-cell depletion during the induction phase and might, in addition, result from T-cell anergy of Th1, but not Th2, cells.

Bound Antimembrane Antibodies in Endomyocardial Biopsy Specimens

Antimembrane antibodies not only circulate in the peripheral blood but are also bound to the sarcolemma (Fig. 4-4; see color plate 5) and the interstitial tissue[49,50,56,72] in the endomyocardial biopsy specimens of patients. In a multicenter study,[50] IgG fixation is found in more than 80% of patients with myocarditis and DCMI. IgM, IgA, and C3 or C1q fixation, however, are of particular diagnostic value indicating secondary immuno-pathogenesis in the course of an inflammatory or postinflammatory process.

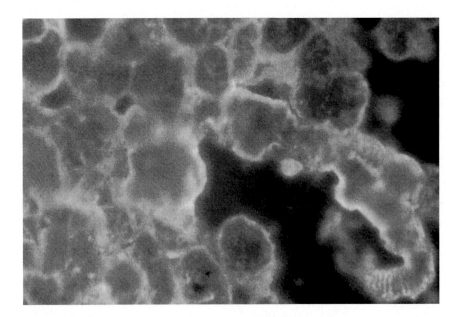

Fig. 4-4. Demonstration of IgG binding (fluorescein isothiocyanate-labeled F[ab]2 antihuman IgG) in dilated cardiomyopathy with inflammation. See color plate 5. (From Maisch et al.[5] By permission of Urban & Vogel.)

ANTIBODIES TO INTRACELLULAR ANTIGENS

Antimitochondrial Antibodies

Antibodies to mitochondrial proteins include the M7 protein[43,48] and its relevant constituent sarcosin dehydrogenase[44] and the antinucleotide translocator (ANT),[52,53,58,64,73,74] which have been demonstrated in patients with myocarditis and dilated cardiomyopathy.

The adenosine diphosphate/adenosine triphosphate (ADP/ATP) carrier protein is responsible for the transport of high-energy phosphates across (mitochondrial and other) cell membranes. Antibodies to the carrier have been identified in human and animal models.[64,75,76] Guinea pigs immunized to ADP/ATP carrier protein develop autoantibodies that penetrate into the cell and bind to the mitochondrial membrane.[77] Cytosolic ATP is decreased in immunized animals, with a subsequent increase in the ADP/ATP ratio in the mitochondria. ADP/ATP carrier antibodies from patients with myocarditis and dilated cardiomyopathy enhanced calcium influx by enhancing the calcium current—an effect not mediated by beta-adrenergic receptors.[78] These antibodies also decreased the external work of isolated, perfused, spontaneously beating hearts.[79]

The ANT antibodies have also been shown to interfere with the energy metabolism in vitro of the myocardial cells from experimental animals. It has been suggested[80,81] that the ANT antibody may cross-react with the calcium channel. In animal models of CVB3 infection, Schultheiss and Bolte[58] reported that there was an inhibition of nucleotide transport and reductions in stroke volume and work in animals with anti-ANT antibodies compared with controls. By using synthetic peptides, evidence of cross-reactivity has been demonstrated between peptides from the adenine nucleotide translocator of the inner mitochondrial membrane and peptides from coxsackievirus B3.[74]

There are 2 isoforms of ANT. An increase in the ANT1 isoform was detected in patients together with a concomitant decrease in ANT2. Further, in patients with enterovirus infection, this was more pronounced than in patients in whom no enterovirus was detected.

Antisarcoplasmic Antibodies

Khaw et al.[46] investigated the development of autoimmunity to cardiac sarcoplasmic reticulum calcium ATPase (SR-Ca^{2+} ATPase) in experimental myocarditis. Immunization of CAF1/J mice with 4C11-20.21-affinity-column-purified cardiac SR-ATPase produced a time-dependent induction of myocardial injury consistent with the diagnosis of myocarditis. Furthermore, the antibody 4C11-20.21 alone can induce myonecrosis in severe combined immunodeficiency mice, indicating a mechanism of cardiomyopathy independent of the cytotoxic T-cell–mediated autoimmunopathy. Administration of 4C11-20.21 into immunocompetent CAF1/J mice resulted in minimal myocardial abnormality (40% with perivascular or interstitial [or both] mononuclear lymphoplasmacytoid aggregates, 10% with borderline myocarditis, and 10% with lesions consistent with focal myocarditis). Immunoperoxidase electron microscopic examination of the involved cardiac tissues showed antibody localization in the subsarcolemmal myotubular system and focal staining of the immediately adjacent sarcolemma in mice injected with 4C11-20.21 but not in mice injected with 2C12.1B5.

Antimicrosomal Antibodies

An antigen-specific immune response to cardiac epitopes was demonstrated by our group[32] in 73% of 54 patients with histologically proven myocarditis utilizing the indirect immunofluorescence test with human myocardium and adult heterologous cardiocytes. By immunoblot, 44% of sera from patients reacted with cardiac tissue. These antibodies were directed preferentially against 43- to 67-kDa proteins. One of these proteins was dihydrolipoamide dehydrogenase.

Antibodies to Fibrils

Antibodies to fibrils, particularly antibodies to myosin and actin, have been described in human[82] and murine myocarditis.[83]

In a large series, Caforio et al.[63] described cardiac antimyosin autoantibodies in 25% to 35% of patients with myocarditis and dilated cardiomyopathy. The frequency of organ-specific cardiac autoantibodies was higher ($P = 0.0001$) in myocarditis (45%) and in dilated cardiomyopathy (20%) than in other cardiac disease (1%), in ischemic heart failure (1%), or in normals (2.5%). Myosin antibodies were also detected in family members of the patients with enteroviral heart disease. This might point to an infectious pathway via cross-reactive antibodies in patients, but it could indicate a familial predisposition to antibody production (as marker or cause) of autoreactive postviral heart disease. It will be of interest to follow up the antibody-carrying family members and to see whether cardiomyopathy develops.

The true pathogenetic relevance of antimyosin antibodies in viral heart disease is a matter of investigation. Cross-reactivity to the coxsackievirus proteins is less likely but not entirely excluded; cross-reactivity to mitochondrial proteins has been postulated but not yet conclusively demonstrated. Because fibrils lie intracellularly, antibodies directed to them are more likely to be a secondary phenomenon unless true sequence homologies to sarcolemmal proteins are demonstrated.

Lauer et al.[19] found antimyosin autoantibodies in 17 of 33 patients (52%) with chronic myocarditis proven on endomyocardial biopsy at the initial presentation. After 6 months, antimyosin autoantibodies were still found in 13 (76%) initially antibody-positive patients. No initially antibody-negative patient ($n = 16$) developed antimyosin autoantibodies during follow-up. Clinical symptoms improved slightly in antibody-negative patients and remained stable in antibody-positive patients. Left ventricular ejection fraction developed significantly better in antibody-negative patients (+8.9 ± 10.1%) compared with antibody-positive patients (-0.1 ± 9.4%). The constant of myocardial stiffness "b" also improved significantly in antibody-negative patients (-6.1 ± 10.8) compared with antibody-positive patients (+7.3 ± 22.6).

Fairweather et al.[84] investigated the occurrence of autoantibodies to cardiac myosin after inoculation of K181 strain of murine cytomegalovirus (MCMV), causing chronic myocarditis in susceptible BALB/c mice. The degrees of myocarditis induced by the wild isolates during the chronic phase of the disease (days 32-56 postinfection) were low in contrast to the K181 strain. Interestingly, 30% of wild-trapped mice showed histologic evidence of myocarditis, and all were seropositive to MCMV. Sera from BALB/c mice infected with wild MCMV isolates and from wild-trapped mice contained antibodies that cross-reacted with MCMV and cardiac myosin (S2 region). The cross-reactive region of MCMV was a 50,000 to 55,000 molecular weight viral polypeptide. These findings suggest that molecular mimicry may be involved in the pathogenesis of autoimmune myocarditis after infection with laboratory and wild MCMV strains.

Schwimmbeck et al.[85] identified regions of high homology between Coxsackie B3 virus and rabbit cardiac myosin heavy chain. However, the antimyosin autoantibodies produced in coxsackievirus B3-induced murine myocarditis did not cross-react with the virus.[27] Another possibility is the exposition of sequestered antigens to the immune system in the course of myocarditis.

When cardiac myocytes undergo necrosis, their cell membrane integrity will be lost and myosin heavy chains inside the cells will be exposed to the circulation. Then, antimyosin antibody specifically binds to these exposed myosin molecules when they are injected into the patients. Myocardial imaging using indium-111-labeled antimyosin monoclonal antibody was established for the assessment of the disease activity and the extent of myocardial damage in patients with myocarditis and dilated cardiomyopathy.[86]

An antigen-specific immune response to cardiac epitopes was demonstrated by our group[32] in 73% of 54 patients with histologically proven myocarditis by the indirect immunofluorescence test with human myocardium and adult heterologous cardiocytes. By immunoblot, 44% of sera from patients reacted with cardiac tissue. These antibodies were directed preferentially against proteins with a molecular mass of 43 up to 67 kDa. One of these proteins was dihydrolipoamide dehydrogenase and one was identified as a sarcomere-specific creatine kinase.

Other antibodies directed to antigenic intracellular enzymes such as branched chain alpha-keto-acid dehydrogenase have also been identified.[87] Antibody-mediated interference with metabolic activity without alteration of cell viability is a plausible explanation for reversible myocardial dysfunction after myocarditis.

ANTIBODIES TO THE EXTRACELLULAR MATRIX AND TO ENDOTHELIAL CELLS

Further non–organ-specific but defined antigens include desmin (in myocytes), vimentin (which is a marker of fibroblasts and histiocytes), collagen (particularly type III), laminin,[88] and fibronectin.[9]

Vimentin Autoantibodies

These arise in the murine encephalomyocarditis virus model of myocarditis within 9 days after initial infection.[89] When an extract of cardiac C-protein was used to immunize syngeneic mice, autoimmune myocarditis characterized by severe inflammation resulted.[90]

Ubiquitous antigens such as the microfilaments and intermediate filaments, the macrofilaments, or the extracellular matrix constituents may evoke non–organ-specific immune responses in contrast to species-specific or even individually unique epitopes, such as the major histocompatibility complex constituents, or to organ-specific autoreactivity. The tissue-specific epitopes could be of greater importance in immune diseases restricted to the myocardium, whereas in systemic disease, in which the myocardium may also be involved, these or nonspecific proteins (eg, parts of the cytoskeleton, the extracellular matrix, and the microfilaments) could also be involved. Antibodies to the extracellular matrix components occur frequently in endomyocardial biopsy specimens[9,12,72,80] and less frequently circulating in the serum of patients with myocarditis.[40]

Antiendothelial Antibodies

Renewed interest has also been paid to the vascular endothelium. De novo expression of class I and II antigens of the major histocompatibility complex was found in myocarditis.[91,92] In addition, antiendothelial antibodies were demonstrated in myocarditis, which may be cytolytic to living cultured human endothelial cells. These antibodies can also be demonstrated in the endomyocardial biopsy specimens of patients with biopsy-proven myocarditis.

CIRCULATING IMMUNE COMPLEXES

Immune complexes composed of a soluble antigen and specific antibody are formed in the circulation and may deposit in vessel walls anywhere in the body. This leads to local activation of leukocytes and the complement system with resultant tissue injury. In myocarditis, circulating immune complexes may be present at the time of the myocarditic viral illness in the majority of patients.[93] They may be in part responsible for some of the systemic features during this viral illness (eg, proteinuria or hematuria and even myalgia). Immune complex deposition can be seen in the endomyocardial biopsy specimen of patients. However, with light microscopy and indirect immunofluorescence, the immune complex cannot be easily distinguished from bound antiendothelial antibodies.

In patients with DCMI, immune complexes have been found more frequently than in normals and in patients with dilated cardiomyopathy without inflammation.[62] These circulating immune complexes consisted of IgG, IgM, C3, and C4; in myocarditis, IgM predominated.[94] The nature of the soluble antigen (foreign or self) has not been determined. Although detectable, immune complex deposition does not seem to play a major role in the pathogenesis of dilated cardiomyopathy.

CYTOKINES

Cytokines may induce or exacerbate myocarditis through several mechanisms. They may activate cytotoxic T cells. They may induce cell adhesion molecule (CAM) expression and other proinflammatory phenomena. They may induce nitric oxide synthetase (NOS), resulting in increased local nitric oxide. Nitric oxide and some cytokines can directly damage myocytes and cause reversible depression of contractility.

Cytokines mediate activation and the effector phase of innate and specific immunity, which are both important in controlling viral infection. The innate immune response not only has an important protective function but also serves to initiate and regulate subsequent specific immune responses. There are 2 principal mechanisms of innate immunity against viruses. 1) Viral infection directly stimulates the production of type I IFN (IFN-alfa and -beta) by infected cells. Type I IFN inhibits viral replication by initiating the synthesis of enzymes, which collectively interfere with replication of viral RNA or DNA. 2) Natural killer cells lyse a wide variety of virally infected cells and are probably one of the principal mechanisms of immunity against viruses early in the course of infection, before specific immune responses have developed.[95]

In specific immunity, various cytokines, chemokines, and adhesion molecules are involved in regulating migration and activation of T- and B-cell responses, including migration and activity of macrophages. Interest has focused on tumor necrosis factor (TNF)-α, interleukin (IL)-1, and IL-6, because increased concentrations have been reported in plasma of patients with myocarditis. Moreover, plasma values of TNF-α and IL-6 correlate with clinical signs of heart insufficiency in patients with dilated cardiomyopathy.[96]

Increased concentrations of TNF-α have been reported in the serum of patients with chronic heart disease,[97] including a subset of patients with myocarditis or DCMI.[96] TNF-α is able to potentiate the immune response and induce apoptosis in cells, both of which appear to hold special importance in the pathogenesis of myocarditis. Other inflammatory mediators, including IL-1 and granulocyte colony-stimulating factor, also have increased values in myocarditis patients.[96]

Kubota et al.[98] described a transgenic mouse model of myocarditis in which TNF-α is expressed specifically in the myocardium, under the control of the α-myosin heavy-chain promoter. These animals developed gross lymphocytic infiltrates in the myocardium and interstitial edema. In addition, globular dilation of the heart and cardiomegaly were noted.

Satoh et al.[99] reported the expression of IL-6, IL-8, IL-10, and TNF-α in all myocardial samples of 6 patients with acute myocarditis. In the same patients, however, analysis of repeated biopsy samples, at the time when DCM with enteroviral RNA persistence had developed, identified IL-6 (3 patients) and IL-8 (4 patients). In 21 DCM patients studied, only IL-6 (5 patients), IL-8 (8 patients), and TNF-α (12 patients) were detected, and enteroviral RNA was detected in 9 patients.

The ability of IL-12 to protect mice from encephalomyocarditis virus-induced myocarditis has also been reported.[100] IL-12 has been shown to augment cytotoxic activity and induction of Th1-specific immune responses. Shioi et al.[100] used IL-12 treatment in mice with encephalomyocarditis virus-induced myocarditis and this therapy reduced viral replication, inflammation, and myocyte necrosis, with a concomitant increase in survival. Successive administration of 10 ng of IL-12 from the day of virus inoculation to 5 days thereafter decreased mortality, myocardial damage, and viral replication in the heart tissue. The gene expression of IL-12p35 and IL-12p40 was enhanced in the hearts of mice inoculated with encephalomyocarditis virus. Treatment with neutralizing anti-IL-12 resulted in increased mortality of inoculated mice. Because both Th1 and Th2 immune responses were augmented, it was not possible to associate recovery with a predominant type of response. Further, it would be interesting to know if the virus was completely cleared after IL-12 treatment and whether dilated cardiomyopathy subsequently developed, as has been shown in an encephalomyocarditis virus model of myocarditis.[101] In this model, persistent expression of IL-1β and TNF-α occurred during the development of DCM after myocarditis healing.

One possible effect of cytokine expression is the activation of inducible nitric oxide synthase (iNOS). Increased expression of NOS has been proposed to account for some of the dilation associated with DCMI[102] and has been demonstrated in a murine CVB3-induced myocarditis model.[103] In a study of a cardiac myosin-induced myocarditis model in mice, NOS expression was induced in macrophages and cardiomyocytes.[104] However, nitric oxide synthesis did not appear to be essential for the development of pathologic conditions because myocarditis developed in mice lacking interferon regulatory transcription factor (IRF)-l, a transcription factor that controls iNOS expression. Despite the failure to synthesize NOS in the myocardium, the prevalence and severity of disease in IRF-1-deficient animals were similar to those in control animals. In addition, no difference was detected in animals lacking the *IRF-2* gene, a negative regulator of IRF-l-induced transcription.

In contrast to these data, Ishiyama et al.[105] found nitric oxide expression played a critical role in the resultant pathologic condition produced in a rat model of autoimmune myocarditis, after induction with cardiac myosin. Rats treated with aminoguanidine, an inhibitor of iNOS, had only focal mononuclear infiltration and reduced numbers of cardiomyocytes positive for iNOS compared with untreated animals that had considerable inflammatory infiltration and myocyte damage. In addition, serum concentrations of creatine kinase were significantly decreased in the treated animals, indicating decreased muscle damage. In a separate study of autoimmune myocarditis in the rat,[106] IL-2 appeared early, whereas IL-3, TNF-α, and iNOS were present later, during the period of peak inflammation. IL-10 was detected only once inflammation began to subside and persisted during recovery. These data support the notion that changes in the Th1 and Th2 responses are important for controlling outcome, as previously suggested for CVB3-induced myocarditis.

ADHESION MOLECULES

The integrin family of heterodimeric leukocyte proteins functions primarily as adhesion molecules, although they may serve signaling functions as well. In DCM with and without inflammation, the following adhesion molecules responsible for leukocyte adhesion to resting or cytokine-activated endothelium and for mediation of inflammatory reactions have been studied extensively: E-selectin, E-selectin ligand, lymphocyte function-associated (glycoprotein)-1, very late activation (antigen)-4, ICAM-1, -2, and -3, and VCAM-1. Inflammatory endothelial activation is present in a large percentage of patients with dilated cardiomyopathy. A correlation was demonstrated between the expression of CAMs and the immunohistologic diagnosis of inflammatory dilated cardiomyopathy and counterreceptor-bearing intramyocardial infiltrates.[107,108]

The mechanisms leading to the expression of cytokine-induced CAMs on endothelium in patients with dilated cardiomyopathy preceding the inflammatory response are still not fully understood. In myosin-induced myocarditis, a mouse model, the expression of class II antigen of the major histocompatibility complex or endothelial ICAM-1 (or both), induced by the administration of lipopolysaccharide, is a prerequisite for emigration of passively transferred myosin-reactive T cells.[109] Similar mechanisms could be involved in humans during the systemic phase of viral infection.

CELLULAR EFFECTOR MECHANISMS IN HUMANS

Natural Killer Cell Activity

Natural killer cell activity in patients with perimyocarditis is markedly decreased in the acute state in all 3 lymphocyte/target cell ratios examined. In postmyocarditic dilated muscle heart disease, natural killer cell activity returns to normal (Table 4-3). In primary dilated cardiomyopathy, however, a significant decrease in natural killer cell activity can be observed again.[12,110]

Target Cell-specific Non-major Histocompatibility Complex-restricted Lymphocytotoxicity

In myocarditis, target cell-specific non–major histocompatibility complex-restricted lysis of living adult allogeneic rat myocytes by patients' circulating lymphocytes is sustained or slightly enhanced (Table 4-5). This also applies to postmyocarditic dilated heart disease and primary dilated cardiomyopathy in which one-third of patients demonstrated an increase of target cell-specific cytotoxicity. Analysis of antibody-dependent cellular cytotoxicity showed little variation from normal.[49]

CONCLUSION

Humoral autoimmunity in postviral heart disease remains an attractive but complicated hypothesis. Antigenic mimicry with or without cytolytic antibody properties has been shown to play a role in the immunopathogenesis of myocarditis with respect to sarcolemmal/myolemmal epitopes (including the β-receptor), myosin, and some mitochondrial proteins, including the ANT-carrier and dihydrolipoamide dehydrogenase. Today, refined two-dimensional western blots are able to identify receptors and enzymes that are targets of a humoral immune response or the consequence of an "immunization process." The former will indicate immunodestruction and the latter will demonstrate a healing or healed process.

ACKNOWLEDGMENT

With support from the German Science Foundation for B. Maisch and the European Society of Cardiology and the World Heart Federation (Twin Center Program) for A. D. Ristić.

REFERENCES

1. Daly K, Richardson PJ, Olsen EG, Morgan-Capner P, McSorley C, Jackson G, Jewitt DE. Acute myocarditis. Role of histological and virological examination in the diagnosis and assessment of immunosuppressive treatment. Br Heart J 1984;51:30-35.
2. Aretz HT, Billingham ME, Edwards WD, Factor SM, Fallon JT, Fenoglio JJ Jr, Olsen EG, Schoen FJ.

Myocarditis. A histopathologic definition and classification. Am J Cardiovasc Pathol 1987;1:3-14.

3. Fenoglio JJ Jr, Ursell PC, Kellogg CF, Drusin RE, Weiss MB. Diagnosis and classification of myocarditis by endomyocardial biopsy. N Engl J Med 1983;308:12-18.

4. Kawai S, Okada R. A histopathological study of dilated cardiomyopathy—with special reference to clinical and pathological comparisons of the degeneration-predominant type and fibrosis-predominant type. Jpn Circ J 1987;51:654-660.

5. Maisch B, Portig I, Ristić A, Hufnagel G, Pankuweit S. Definition of inflammatory cardiomyopathy (myocarditis): on the way to consensus. A status report. Herz 2000;25:200-209.

6. Maisch B, Bültman B, Factor S, Gröne H-J, Hufnagel G, Kawamura K, Kühl U, Olsen EJ, Pankuweit S, Virmani R, McKenna W, Richardson PJ, Thiene G, Schultheiss H-P, Sekiguchi M, Aepinus C, Aitken K, Arbustini E, Archard L, Baboonian C, Bowles N, Broor S, Kandolf R, Liu P, Matsumori A, Pauschinger M, Slenczka W, Sole M, Talwar KK, Towbin J, Tracy S, Bayes de Luna A, Goodwin JF. World Heart Federation consensus conferences' definition of inflammatory cardiomyopathy (myocarditis): report from two expert committees on histology and viral cardiomyopathy. Heartbeat 1999;4:3-4.

7. Aretz HT. Myocarditis: the Dallas criteria. Hum Pathol 1987;18:619-624.

8. Doerr W. Morphology of myocarditis. [German.] Verh Dtsch Ges Inn Med 1971;77:301-335.

9. Maisch B. Autoreactivity to the cardiac myocyte, connective tissue and the extracellular matrix in heart disease and postcardiac injury. Springer Semin Immunopathol 1989;11:369-395.

10. Fowles RE, Bieber CP, Stinson EB. Defective in vitro suppressor cell function in idiopathic congestive cardiomyopathy. Circulation 1979;59:483-491.

11. Pankuweit S, Portig I, Eckhardt H, Crombach M, Hufnagel G, Maisch B. Prevalence of viral genome in endomyocardial biopsies from patients with inflammatory heart muscle disease. Herz 2000;25:221-226.

12. Maisch B. Immunologic regulator and effector functions in perimyocarditis, postmyocarditic heart muscle disease and dilated cardiomyopathy. Basic Res Cardiol 1986;81 Suppl 1:217-241.

13. Maisch B. Immunological mechanisms in human cardiac injury. In: Spry CJF, ed. Immunology and molecular biology of cardiovascular diseases. Lancaster, England: MTP Press, 1987:225-252.

14. Maisch B. The sarcolemma as antigen in the secondary immunopathogenesis of myopericarditis. Eur Heart J (Suppl J) 1987;8:155-165.

15. Woodruff JF. Viral myocarditis. A review. Am J Pathol 1980;101:425-484.

16. Smith WG. Coxsackie B myopericarditis in adults. Am Heart J 1970;80:34-46.

17. Rose NR, Hill SL. The pathogenesis of postinfectious myocarditis. Clin Immunol Immunopathol 1996;80:S92-S99.

18. Caforio AL, Goldman JH, Haven AJ, Baig KM, McKenna WJ. Evidence for autoimmunity to myosin and other heart-specific autoantigens in patients with dilated cardiomyopathy and their relatives. Int J Cardiol 1996;54:157-163.

19. Lauer B, Schannwell M, Kuhl U, Strauer BE, Schultheiss HP. Antimyosin autoantibodies are associated with deterioration of systolic and diastolic left ventricular function in patients with chronic myocarditis. J Am Coll Cardiol 2000;35:11-18.

20. Maisch B. The heart in rheumatic disease. Rheumatology 1992;16:81-117.

21. Gauntt CJ, Arizpe HM, Higdon AL, Wood HJ, Bowers DF, Rozek MM, Crawley R. Molecular mimicry, anti-coxsackievirus B3 neutralizing monoclonal antibodies, and myocarditis. J Immunol 1995;154:2983-2995.

22. McManus BM, Chow LH, Wilson JE, Anderson DR, Gulizia JM, Gauntt CJ, Klingel KE, Beisel KW, Kandolf R. Direct myocardial injury by enterovirus: a central role in the evolution of murine myocarditis. Clin Immunol Immunopathol 1993;68:159-169.

23. Paque RE. Role of anti-idiotypic antibodies in induction, regulation, and expression of coxsackie-virus-induced myocarditis. Prog Med Virol 1992;39:204-227.

24. Horwitz MS, La Cava A, Fine C, Rodriguez E, Ilic A, Sarvetnick N. Pancreatic expression of interferon-gamma protects mice from lethal coxsackievirus B3 infection and subsequent myocarditis. Nat Med 2000;6:693-697.

25. Hill SL, Rose NR. Molecular pathology of autoimmune myocarditis. In: Theofilopoulos AN, Bona CA, eds. The molecular pathology of autoimmune diseases. 2nd ed. Amsterdam: Harwood Academic Publishers (in press).

26. Miller SD, Vanderlugt CL, Begolka WS, Pao W, Yauch RL, Neville KL, Katz-Levy Y, Carrizosa A, Kim BS. Persistent infection with Theiler's virus leads to CNS autoimmunity via epitope spreading. Nat Med 1997;3:1133-1136.

27. Neu N, Craig SW, Rose NR, Alvarez F, Beisel KW. Coxsackievirus induced myocarditis in mice: cardiac myosin autoantibodies do not cross-react with the virus. Clin Exp Immunol 1987;69:566-574.

28. Matsumori A. Cytokines in myocarditis and cardiomyopathies. Curr Opin Cardiol 1996;11:302-309.

29. Matsumori A. Molecular and immune mechanisms in the pathogenesis of cardiomyopathy—role of viruses, cytokines, and nitric oxide. Jpn Circ J 1997;61:275-291.

30. Goin JC, Borda ES, Auger S, Storino R, Sterin-Borda L. Cardiac m_2 muscarinic cholinoceptor activation by human chagasic autoantibodies: association with bradycardia. Heart 1999;82:273-278.

31. Maisch B, Bauer E, Cirsi M, Kochsiek K. Cytolytic cross-reactive antibodies directed against the cardiac membrane and viral proteins in coxsackievirus B3 and B4 myocarditis. Characterization and pathogenetic relevance. Circulation 1993;87 Suppl 4:IV49-IV65.

32. Pankuweit S, Portig I, Lottspeich F, Maisch B. Autoantibodies in sera of patients with myocarditis: characterization of the corresponding proteins by isoelectric focusing and N-terminal sequence analysis. J Mol Cell Cardiol 1997;29:77-84.

33. Schulze K, Schultheiss HP. The role of the ADP/ATP carrier in the pathogenesis of viral heart disease. Eur Heart J 1995;16 Suppl O:64-67.

34. Wallukat G, Wollenberger A, Morwinski R, Pitschner HF. Anti-beta 1-adrenoceptor autoantibodies with chronotropic activity from the serum of patients with dilated cardiomyopathy: mapping of epitopes in the first and second extracellular loops. J Mol Cell Cardiol 1995;27:397-406.

35. Limas CJ, Limas C, Kubo SH, Olivari MT. Anti-beta-receptor antibodies in human dilated cardiomyopathy and correlation with HLA-DR antigens. Am J Cardiol 1990;65:483-487.

36. Schulze K, Heineman FW, Schultheiss HP, Balaban RS. Impairment of myocardial calcium homeostasis by antibodies against the adenine nucleotide translocator. Cell Calcium 1999;25:361-370.

37. Otto LR, Boriack RL, Marsh DJ, Kum JB, Eng C, Burlina AB, Bennett MJ. Long-chain L 3-hydroxyacyl-CoA dehydrogenase (LCHAD) deficiency does not appear to be the primary cause of lipid myopathy in patients with Bannayan-Riley-Ruvalcaba syndrome (BRRS). Am J Med Genet 1999;83:3-5.

38. Maisch B, Lotze U, Schneider J, Kochsiek K. Antibodies to human sinus node in sick sinus syndrome. Pacing Clin Electrophysiol 1986;9:1101-1109.

39. Maisch B, Wedeking U, Kochsiek K. Quantitative assessment of antilaminin antibodies in myocarditis and perimyocarditis. Eur Heart J (Suppl J) 1987;8:233-235.

40. Obermayer U, Scheidler J, Maisch B. Antibodies against micro- and intermediate filaments in carditis and dilated cardiomyopathy—are they a diagnostic marker? Eur Heart J (Suppl J) 1987;8:181-186.

41. Portig I, Pankuweit S, Maisch B. Antibodies against stress proteins in sera of patients with dilated cardiomyopathy. J Mol Cell Cardiol 1997;29:2245-2251.

42. Maisch B, Drude L, Hengstenberg C, Herzum M, Hufnagel G, Kochsiek K, Schmaltz A, Schonian U, Schwab MD. Are antisarcolemmal (ASAs) and antimyolemmal antibodies (AMLAs) "natural" antibodies? Basic Res Cardiol 1991;86 Suppl 3:101-114.

43. Klein R, Maisch B, Kochsiek K, Berg PA. Demonstration of organ specific antibodies against heart

mitochondria (anti-M7) in sera from patients with some forms of heart diseases. Clin Exp Immunol 1984;58:283-292.

44. Pohlner K, Portig I, Pankuweit S, Lottspeich F, Maisch B. Identification of mitochondrial antigens recognized by antibodies in sera of patients with idiopathic dilated cardiomyopathy by two-dimensional gel electrophoresis and protein sequencing. Am J Cardiol 1997;80:1040-1045.

45. Naparstek Y, Plotz PH. The role of autoantibodies in autoimmune disease. Annu Rev Immunol 1993;11:79-104.

46. Khaw BA, Narula J, Sharaf AR, Nicol PD, Southern JF, Carles M. SR-Ca^{2+} ATPase as an autoimmunogen in experimental myocarditis. Eur Heart J 1995;16 Suppl O:92-96.

47. De Scheerder I, De Buyzere M, Algoed L, De Lange M, Delanghe J, Bogaert AM, Clement DL. Characteristic anti-heart antibody patterns in post-cardiac injury syndrome, endocarditis and acute myocarditis. Eur Heart J (Suppl J) 1987;8:237-238.

48. Klein R, Seipel L, Kleemann U, Hassenstein P, Berg PA. Relevance of antimitochondrial antibodies (anti-M7) in cardiac diseases. Eur Heart J (Suppl J) 1987;8:223-226.

49. Maisch B, Trostel-Soeder R, Stechemesser E, Berg PA, Kochsiek K. Diagnostic relevance of humoral and cell-mediated immune reactions in patients with acute viral myocarditis. Clin Exp Immunol 1982;48:533-545.

50. Maisch B, Bauer E, Hufnagel G, Pfeifer U, Rohkamm R. The use of endomyocardial biopsy in heart failure. Eur Heart J (Suppl H) 1988;9:59-71.

51. Maisch B, Schwab D, Bauer E, Sandhage K, Schmaltz AA, Wimmer M. Antimyolemmal antibodies in myocarditis in children. Eur Heart J (Suppl J) 1987;8:167-173.

52. Schultheiss H-P. The mitochondrium as antigen in inflammatory heart disease. Eur Heart J (Suppl J) 1987;8:203-210.

53. Schultheiss H-P, Kühl U. Charakterisierung verschiedener Autoantikörper gegen myokardiale Matrixproteine bei Myokarditis und Dilativer Kardiomyopathie (abstract). Klin Wochenschr (Suppl IX) 1987;65:263-264.

54. Maisch B, Maisch S, Kochsiek K. Immune reactions in tuberculous and chronic constrictive pericarditis. Clinical data and diagnostic significance of antimyocardial antibodies. Am J Cardiol 1982;50:1007-1013.

55. Maisch B, Kochsiek K. Humoral immune reactions in uremic pericarditis. Am J Nephrol 1983;3:264-271.

56. Maisch B, Deeg P, Liebau G, Kochsiek K. Diagnostic relevance of humoral and cytotoxic immune reactions in primary and secondary dilated cardiomyopathy. Am J Cardiol 1983;52:1072-1078.

57. Maisch B, Buschel G, Izumi T, Eigel P, Regitz V, Deeg P, Pfeifer U, Schmaltz A, Herzum M, Liebau G, Kochsiek K. Four years of experience in endomyocardial biopsy—an immunohistologic approach. Heart Vessels Suppl 1985;1:59-67.

58. Schultheiss HP, Bolte HD. Immunological analysis of auto-antibodies against the adenine nucleotide translocator in dilated cardiomyopathy. J Mol Cell Cardiol 1985;17:603-617.

59. Maisch B. Diagnostic relevance of humoral and cell-mediated immune reactions in patients with acute myocarditis and congestive cardiomyopathy. In: Chazov EI, Smirnov VN, Organov RG, eds. Cardiology: an international perspective. New York: Plenum Press, 1984:1327-1338.

60. Maisch B. Surface antigens of adult heart cells and their use in diagnosis. Basic Res Cardiol 1985;80 Suppl 1:47-51.

61. Maisch B, Trostel-Soeder R, Berg PA, Kochsiek K. Assessment of antibody mediated cytolysis of adult cardiocytes isolated by centrifugation in a continuous gradient of Percoll in patients with acute myocarditis. J Immunol Methods 1981;44:159-169.

62. Maisch B. Immunologic regulator and effector mechanisms in myocarditis and perimyocarditis. Heart Vessels Suppl 1985;1:209-217.

63. Caforio AL, Bauce B, Boffa GM, De Cian F, Angelini A, Melacini P, Razzolini R, Fasoli G, Chioin R, Schiaffino S, Thiene G, Dalla Volta S. Autoimmunity in myocarditis and dilated cardiomyopathy: cardiac autoantibody frequency and clinical correlates in a patient series from Italy. G Ital Cardiol 1997;27:106-112.

64. Limas CJ, Goldenberg IF, Limas C. Autoantibodies against beta-adrenoceptors in human idiopathic dilated cardiomyopathy. Circ Res 1989;64:97-103.

65. Schultheiss HP. The significance of autoantibodies against the ADP/ATP carrier for the pathogenesis of myocarditis and dilated cardiomyopathy—clinical and experimental data. Springer Semin Immunopathol 1989;11:15-30.

66. Müller J, Wallukat G, Dandel M, Bieda H, Brandes K, Spiegelsberger S, Nissen E, Kunze R, Hetzer R. Immunoglobulin adsorption in patients with idiopathic dilated cardiomyopathy. Circulation 2000;101:385-391.

67. Kirsner AB, Hess EV, Fowler NO. Immunologic findings in idiopathic cardiomyopathy: a prospective serial study. Am Heart J 1973;86:625-630.

68. Limas CJ, Goldenberg IF. Autoantibodies against cardiac β-adrenoceptors in human dilated cardiomyopathy (abstract). Circulation 1987;76 Suppl 4:262.

69. Wallukat G, Boewer V. Stimulation of chronotropic beta-adrenoceptors of cultures neonatal rat heart myocytes by the serum of gammaglobulin fraction of patients with dilated cardiomyopathy and myocarditis. In: International Symposium: heart failure, pathogenesis and therapy, Berlin 28.2.-2.3, 1988. [Book of abstracts.] Berlin: Universitätsverlag, 1988:A24.

70. Magnusson Y, Wallukat G, Guillet JG, Hjalmarson A, Hoebeke J. Functional analysis of rabbit anti-peptide antibodies which mimic autoantibodies against the beta 1-adrenergic receptor in patients with idiopathic dilated cardiomyopathy. J Autoimmunol 1991;4:893-905.

71. Inomata T, Watanabe T, Haga M, Hirahara H, Abo T, Okura Y, Hanawa H, Kodama M, Izumi T. Anti-CD2 monoclonal antibodies prevent the induction of experimental autoimmune myocarditis. Jpn Heart J 2000;41:507-517.

72. Hammond EH, Menlove RL, Anderson JL. Immunofluorescence microscopy in the diagnosis and follow-up of patients suspected of having inflammatory heart disease. In: Schultheiss H-P, ed. New concepts in viral heart disease: virology, immunology and clinical management. Berlin: Springer-Verlag, 1988:303-311.

73. Schulze K, Becker BF, Schauer R, Schultheiss HP. Antibodies to ADP-ATP carrier—an autoantigen in myocarditis and dilated cardiomyopathy—impair cardiac function. Circulation 1990;81:959-969.

74. Schwimmbeck PL, Schultheiss H-P, Strauer BE. Identification of a main autoimmunogenic epitope of the adenine nucleotide translocator which cross-reacts with coxsackie B3 virus: use in the diagnosis of myocarditis and dilative cardiomyopathy (abstract). Circulation 1989;80 Suppl 2:II-665.

75. Takemoto M, Kusachi S, Urabe N, Inoue K, Tsuji T. Auto-antibody against adenine nucleotide translocator in dilated cardiomyopathy and myocarditis—incidence and relation to cardiac function and morphology. Jpn Circ J 1993;57:1150-1158.

76. Liao YH. Functional analysis of autoantibodies against ADP/ATP carrier from dilated cardiomyopathy. Int J Cardiol 1996;54:165-169.

77. Schulze K, Becker BF, Schultheiss HP. Antibodies to the ADP/ATP carrier, an autoantigen in myocarditis and dilated cardiomyopathy, penetrate into myocardial cells and disturb energy metabolism in vivo. Circ Res 1989;64:179-192.

78. Morad M, Nabauer M, Schultheiss H-P. Antibodies and autoantibodies against ADP/ATP carrier enhance calcium current in isolated ventricular myocytes. In: Schultheiss H-P, ed. New concepts in viral heart disease: virology, immunology and clinical management. Berlin: Springer-Verlag, 1988:236-242.

79. Schultheiss HP, Schulze K, Schauer R, Witzenbichler B, Strauer BE. Antibody-mediated imbalance

of myocardial energy metabolism. A causal factor of cardiac failure? Circ Res 1995;76:64-72.

80. Kühl U, Ulrich G, Melzner B, Schoeber B, Morad M, Schultheiss HP. Characterization of autoantibodies against the Ca2+-channel inducing cytotoxicity by enhancement of calcium permeability. In: Seventh International Congress of Immunology, July 30-August 5, 1989: Abstracts. Stuttgart: Gustav Fischer, 1989:116-117.

81. Kühl U, Ulrich G, Schultheiss H-P. Cross-reactivity of antibodies to the ADP/ATP translocator of the inner mitochondrial membrane with the cell surface of cardiac myocytes. Eur Heart J (Suppl J) 1987;8:219-222.

82. Wittner B, Maisch B, Kochsiek K. Quantification of antimyosin antibodies in experimental myocarditis by a new solid phase fluorometric assay. J Immunol Methods 1983;64:239-247.

83. Beisel KW. Immunogenetic basis of myocarditis: role of fibrillary antigens. Springer Semin Immunopathol 1989;11:31-42.

84. Fairweather D, Lawson CM, Chapman AJ, Brown CM, Booth TW, Papadimitriou JM, Shellam GR. Wild isolates of murine cytomegalovirus induce myocarditis and antibodies that cross-react with virus and cardiac myosin. Immunology 1998;94:263-270.

85. Schwimmbeck PL, Bland NK, Schultheiss HP, Strauer BE. The possible value of synthetic peptides in the diagnosis and therapy of myocarditis and dilated cardiomyopathy. Eur Heart J 1991;12 Suppl D:76-80.

86. Matsumori A, Yamada T, Sasayama S. Antimyosin antibody imaging in clinical myocarditis and cardiomyopathy: principle and application. Int J Cardiol 1996;54:183-190.

87. Ansari AA, Wang YC, Danner DJ, Gravanis MB, Mayne A, Neckelmann N, Sell KW, Herskowitz A. Abnormal expression of histocompatibility and mitochondrial antigens by cardiac tissue from patients with myocarditis and dilated cardiomyopathy. Am J Pathol 1991;139:337-354.

88. Wolff PG, Kuhl U, Schultheiss HP. Laminin distribution and autoantibodies to laminin in dilated cardiomyopathy and myocarditis. Am Heart J 1989;117:1303-1309.

89. Sato Y, Matsumori A, Sasayama S. Autoantibodies against vimentin in a murine model of myocarditis. Autoimmunity 1994;18:145-148.

90. Kasahara H, Itoh M, Sugiyama T, Kido N, Hayashi H, Saito H, Tsukita S, Kato N. Autoimmune myocarditis induced in mice by cardiac C-protein. Cloning of complementary DNA encoding murine cardiac C-protein and partial characterization of the antigenic peptides. J Clin Invest 1994;94:1026-1036.

91. Hufnagel G, Maisch B. Expression of MHC class I and II antigens and the Il-2 receptor in rejection, myocarditis and dilated cardiomyopathy. Eur Heart J 1991;12 Suppl D:137-140.

92. Herskowitz A, Neumann DA, Rose NR, Beschorner WE, Sell KL, Ansari AA, Baughman KL. Histocompatibility (MHC) antigens in human myocarditis: new markers of immune-mediated disease (abstract). Circulation 1989;80 Suppl 2:II-676.

93. Herzum M, Maisch B, Kochsiek K. Circulating immune complexes in perimyocarditis and infective endocarditis. Eur Heart J (Suppl J) 1987;8:323-325.

94. Cristea A, Rus H, Niculescu F, Bedeleanu D, Vlaicu R. Characterization of circulating immune complexes in heart disease. Immunol Lett 1986;13:45-49.

95. Zinkernagel RM. Immunology taught by viruses. Science 1996;271:173-178.

96. Matsumori A, Yamada T, Suzuki H, Matoba Y, Sasayama S. Increased circulating cytokines in patients with myocarditis and cardiomyopathy. Br Heart J 1994;72:561-566.

97. Levine B, Kalman J, Mayer L, Fillit HM, Packer M. Elevated circulating levels of tumor necrosis factor in severe chronic heart failure. N Engl J Med 1990;323:236-241.

98. Kubota T, McTiernan CF, Frye CS, Demetris AJ, Feldman AM. Cardiac-specific overexpression of tumor necrosis factor-alpha causes lethal myocarditis in transgenic mice. J Card Fail 1997;3:117-124.

99. Satoh M, Tamura G, Segawa I, Tashiro A, Hiramori K, Satodate R. Expression of cytokine genes and presence of enteroviral genomic RNA in endomyocardial biopsy tissues of myocarditis and dilated cardiomyopathy. Virchows Arch 1996;427:503-509.

100. Shioi T, Matsumori A, Nishio R, Ono K, Kakio T, Sasayama S. Protective role of interleukin-12 in viral myocarditis. J Mol Cell Cardiol 1997;29:2327-2334.

101. Shioi T, Matsumori A, Sasayama S. Persistent expression of cytokine in the chronic stage of viral myocarditis in mice. Circulation 1996;94:2930-2937.

102. de Belder AJ, Radomski MW, Why HJ, Richardson PJ, Martin JF. Myocardial calcium-independent nitric oxide synthase activity is present in dilated cardiomyopathy, myocarditis, and postpartum cardiomyopathy but not in ischaemic or valvular heart disease. Br Heart J 1995;74:426-430.

103. Mikami S, Kawashima S, Kanazawa K, Hirata K, Katayama Y, Hotta H, Hayashi Y, Ito H, Yokoyama M. Expression of nitric oxide synthase in a murine model of viral myocarditis induced by coxsackievirus B3. Biochem Biophys Res Commun 1996;220:983-989.

104. Bachmaier K, Neu N, Pummerer C, Duncan GS, Mak TW, Matsuyama T, Penninger JM. iNOS expression and nitrotyrosine formation in the myocardium in response to inflammation is controlled by the interferon regulatory transcription factor 1. Circulation 1997;96:585-591.

105. Ishiyama S, Hiroe M, Nishikawa T, Abe S, Shimojo T, Ito H, Ozasa S, Yamakawa K, Matsuzaki M, Mohammed MU, Nakazawa H, Kasajima T, Marumo F. Nitric oxide contributes to the progression of myocardial damage in experimental autoimmune myocarditis in rats. Circulation 1997;95:489-496.

106. Okura Y, Yamamoto T, Goto S, Inomata T, Hirono S, Hanawa H, Feng L, Wilson CB, Kihara I, Izumi T, Shibata A, Aizawa Y, Seki S, Abo T. Characterization of cytokine and iNOS mRNA expression in situ during the course of experimental autoimmune myocarditis in rats. J Mol Cell Cardiol 1997;29:491-502.

107. Noutsias M, Seeberg B, Schultheiss H-P, Kühl U. Expression of cell adhesion molecules in dilated cardiomyopathy: evidence for endothelial activation in inflammatory cardiomyopathy. Circulation 1999;99:2124-2131.

108. Devaux B, Scholz D, Hirche A, Klovekorn WP, Schaper J. Upregulation of cell adhesion molecules and the presence of low grade inflammation in human chronic heart failure. Eur Heart J 1997;18:470-479.

109. Pummerer CL, Grassl G, Sailer M, Bachmaier KW, Penninger JM, Neu N. Cardiac myosin-induced myocarditis: target recognition by autoreactive T cells requires prior activation of cardiac interstitial cells. Lab Invest 1996;74:845-852.

110. Anderson JL, Carlquist JF, Hammond EH. Deficient natural killer cell activity in patients with idiopathic dilated cardiomyopathy. Lancet 1982;2:1124-1127.

Cytokines in Experimental Myocarditis

Akira Matsumori, M.D., Ph.D.

INTRODUCTION

Several viruses are known to cause myocarditis, and a link between viral myocarditis and the subsequent development of dilated cardiomyopathy is becoming increasingly evident. Besides coxsackieviruses, the importance of hepatitis C virus infection has been noted in patients with myocarditis and cardiomyopathy.[1-5] Cytokines play an important role in the pathogenesis and pathophysiology of these disorders.

Cytokines consist of peptide or glycoprotein mediators, with molecular weights ranging from 6,000 to 60,000, which act as intercellular signals, although they may also act systemically, in an endocrine manner. Cytokines include lymphokines produced by T and B lymphocytes, monokines produced by monocytes, hematopoietic colony-stimulating factors (CSFs), interferons (IFNs), and connective tissue growth factors.

Cytokines stimulate the growth, differentiation, and miscellaneous functions of a wide variety of target cells, and a given cytokine may activate several cell types. Consequently, most cytokines have multiple overlapping biologic activities, and their actions are notably redundant. The activity of immune and inflammatory leukocytes can be up- or down-regulated by cytokines, which also exert a marked influence on the activities of connective tissue and neural, epithelial, endothelial, cardiac, and other cell types engaged in tissue repair and restoration of homeostasis (Fig. 5-1).[6]

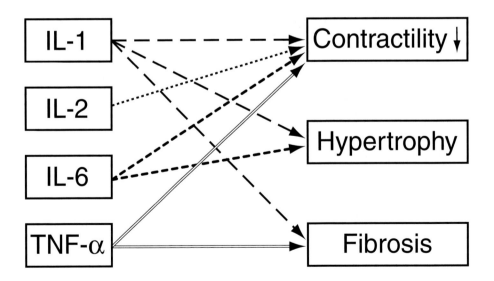

Fig. 5-1. Cytokines and the heart. Interleukin (*IL*)-1, IL-2, IL-6, and tumor necrosis factor (*TNF*)-α may depress myocardial contractility; IL-1 and IL-6 may induce hypertrophy of myocytes; and IL-1 and TNF-α may play a role in the development of myocardial fibrosis.

INCREASED CIRCULATING LEVELS
OF CYTOKINES IN PATIENTS WITH HEART DISEASES

Several clinical studies have confirmed the expression of excessive concentrations of tumor necrosis factor (TNF)-α in the plasma of patients with congestive heart failure.[7-9] There is disagreement with regard to the correlation between severity of symptoms and magnitude of increase in cytokine concentrations. We found increased TNF-α concentrations in asymptomatic patients with dilated or hypertrophic cardiomyopathy.[8] In that study, increased concentrations of interleukin (IL)-1α and IL-1β were detected in patients with acute myocarditis. Similarly, granulocyte CSF (G-CSF) was often increased in myocarditis, cardiomyopathies, acute myocardial infarction, and angina pectoris, suggesting activation of macrophages or endothelial cells (or both), although this increase was not disease specific.

CYTOKINES AND MYOCARDIAL INJURY

Cytokines have effects on myocytes, although it remains unclear whether their negative inotropic effect is direct, from blunting of the effects of catecholamines, or from stimulation of nitric oxide production. Studies in isolated cardiac myocytes have shown that cytokines generated by activated immune cells cause an increase in nitric oxide via the induction of nitric oxide synthase,[10] resulting in a direct negative inotropic effect and a modulation of inotropic responsiveness.[11-13]

The effect of IL-1 on cardiac function is controversial. IL-1 decreased cardiac contractility in isolated perfused rat hearts,[14] isolated ferret papillary muscles,[12] and cultured mouse cardiac myocytes.[15] In contrast, recombinant human IL-1α had little inotropic effect on isolated Syrian hamster papillary muscles.[16] In guinea pig ventricular myocytes, IL-1 prolonged action potential duration, increased L-type Ca^{2+} current, and enhanced contractility.[17] In cultured rat ventricular myocytes, IL-1β suppressed Ca^{2+} current via a pertussis toxin-insensitive G protein.[18] In addition to its effects on myocytes, IL-1β activates fibroblasts,[19] which may significantly influence cardiac remodeling.[20] Furthermore, IL-1β, TNF-α, and IFN-γ have cytotoxic effects on cultured cardiac myocytes.[21] Besides these humoral effects, these cytokines may activate cytotoxic T cells, which may cause direct myocyte injury[22] as well as induce cell adhesion molecules, which may promote the persistent traffic of inflammatory cells within the myocardium.[23] IL-1β has been shown to cause myocyte hypertrophy via a nitric oxide-independent mechanism, with induction of fetal genes and down-regulation of calcium regulatory genes.[24]

Depression of myocardial function and myocarditis have been reported after administration of high chemotherapeutic doses of IL-2.[25,26] In addition, IL-2-stimulated cultured human mononuclear cells produce a soluble factor, which causes the reversible depression of isolated perfused rat heart contractility.[27]   However, Yokoyama et al.[28] showed that TNF-α also has a direct negative inotropic effect in the isolated adult cat heart and in isolated adult cat ventricular myocytes.   This effect was associated with a decrease in Ca^{2+} transient, without change in L-type Ca^{2+} current, and was not inhibited by blockers of nitric oxide production or of arachidonic acid metabolism.   In addition, the overexpression of TNF-α by a murine α-myosin heavy chain promoter caused myocarditis and heart failure in a transgenic mouse model.[29]

IL-6 may exert a negative inotropic effect and lower the concentration of intracellular Ca^{2+} through nitric oxide-cyclic guanosine monophosphate pathways in cultured chick embryonic ventricular myocytes and isolated hamster papillary muscles.[16]   Mice overexpressing both IL-6 and its receptor have been reported to develop cardiac hypertrophy.[30]

A transgenic mouse model has been developed that expresses monocyte chemoattractant protein-1 (MCP-1) with the α-cardiac myosin heavy chain promoter.[31]   MCP-1 values in the transgenic hearts increased up to age 45 days, and leukocytic infiltration into the interstitium between cardiomyocytes increased up to age 75 days.   The infiltrate consisted mainly of macrophages rather than T cells.   Comparisons of the echocardiographic findings in 1-year-old mice, which expressed MCP-1 in the myocardium, and in age-matched control animals revealed the presence of cardiac hypertrophy and dilatation and of increases in left ventricular mass and systolic and diastolic internal diameters.   A significant decline in M-mode fractional shortening indicated depressed contractile function.   Hearts from transgenic mice were 65% heavier than hearts from control mice, and histologic examination showed moderate myocarditis, edema, and some degree of fibrosis.   Thus, MCP-1 expression in the heart muscle may represent a useful experimental model of myocarditis and cardiomyopathy.

CYTOKINES IN EXPERIMENTAL MODELS OF ENCEPHALOMYOCARDITIS VIRUS

We have developed a mouse model infected by the encephalomyocarditis virus (EMCV), in which a high incidence of severe myocarditis, congestive heart failure, and dilated cardiomyopathy is observed.[32]   From these models, we have learned the natural history and pathogenesis of viral myocarditis and tested new diagnostic, therapeutic, and preventive methods.

The expression of cytokine messenger RNA (mRNA) was recently examined in our EMCV model (Fig. 5-2).[33]   IL-1β and TNF-α mRNAs were induced 3 days after virus inoculation, when few cell infiltrates were present, suggesting that, at that stage, these cytokines were produced by cells belonging to the heart itself.   Immunohistochemical analysis confirmed that endothelial cells and interstitial macrophages were positive for

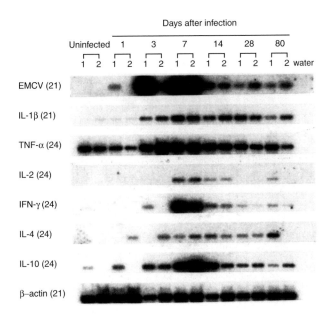

Fig. 5-2. Photograph of a representative analysis of interleukin (*IL*)-1β, tumor necrosis factor (*TNF*)-α, IL-2, IL-4, IL-10, interferon (*IFN*)-γ and β-actin mRNA, and encephalomyocarditis virus (*EMCV*) genome RNA by semiquantitative polymerase chain reaction (PCR). RNA was extracted from control hearts and hearts obtained at days 1 through 80 after EMCV inoculation. The cDNA was synthesized, amplified by PCR, and probe hybridized. Two representative samples from each group are shown. The number of amplification cycles in the PCR reaction is given in parentheses. (Modified from Shioi et al.[33] By permission of the American Heart Association.)

IL-1β and TNF-α immunoreactivity 3 days after virus inoculation (Fig. 5-3). The expression of such cytokines is likely to influence the induction of the local inflammatory process.[34]

IFN-γ mRNA appeared 3 days and IL-2 mRNA 7 days after viral inoculation, whereas T-cell infiltration into the heart peaked between 7 and 14 days. The temporal correlation between cellular infiltration and IL-2 and IFN-γ mRNA production suggests that infiltrating cells, rather than resident heart cells, account for the appearance of IFN-γ and IL-2 mRNA in the heart. IFN-γ and IL-2 protein are likely to be produced, because the production of IFN-γ and IL-2 is regulated mainly at the transcriptional level.[35,36]

One of our study's most important findings was the persistent expression of IFN-γ, IL-1β, IL-2, and TNF-α for as long as 80 days after virus inoculation. IL-2, which is produced exclusively by T lymphocytes, probably originates from infiltrating mononuclear cells, occasionally seen 80 days after inoculation. The presence of IL-2 mRNA suggests that T cells, activated in a major histocompatibility complex-dependent manner, are present in myocardium in the chronic stage. The temporal expression of IL-2 and IFN-γ mRNA in the chronic phase correlated with that of the EMCV genome RNA. This suggests that, in

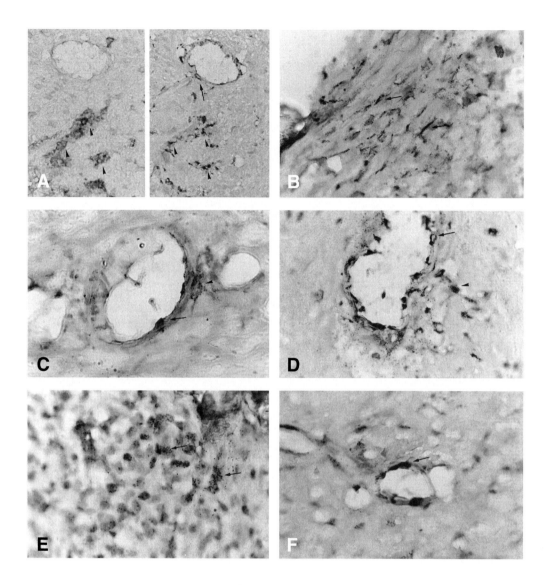

Fig. 5-3. Localization of interleukin (IL)-1β and tumor necrosis factor (TNF)-α protein by immuno-histochemical analysis in encephalomyocarditis virus (EMCV) myocarditis. At 3 days after EMCV inoculation, serial section of heart tissue stained with antibody to IL-1 (*A, right*) and antibody to macrophages (*A, left*). Interstitial cells (*arrowheads*) positive for IL-1β were predominantly macrophages. Endothelial cells (*arrow*) were also positive for IL-1β. (x80.) At 80 days after inoculation, fibroblasts (*arrows*), infiltrating mononuclear cells (*B*), endothelial cells (*arrow*), and interstitial cells (*arrowhead*) (*C*) were positive for IL-1β. (x400.) TNF-α protein was positive in endothelial cells (*arrow*) and interstitial cells (*arrowhead*) at 3 days after inoculation (*D*). (x400.) At 80 days, mononuclear cells (*arrows*) (*E*) (x400.) and endothelial cells (*arrow*) (*F*) are positive for TNF-α. (x400.) (From Shioi et al.[33] By permission of the American Heart Association.)

this experimental model, the expression of IL-2 and IFN-γ is triggered by persistent viral infection. However, since focal accumulation of mononuclear cells was preceded by myosin-induced autoimmune myocarditis in a rat model, autoimmune mechanisms should also be considered.[37]

In the chronic phase of our experiments, IL-1β gene expression was relatively high compared with that of other cytokines and correlated positively with the heart weight/body weight ratio and extent of fibrotic lesions, suggesting a role played by IL-1β in the pathogenesis of cardiomyopathic changes in this model. IFN-γ, IL-2, and TNF-α gene expression in the chronic stage did not correlate with the heart weight/body weight ratio or extent of fibrosis. The expression of the IL-4 and IL-10 genes, so-called inhibitory cytokines, was also enhanced during the acute phase and persisted into the chronic stage. These observations are consistent with the general activation of a cytokines network (Fig. 5-2).

CYTOKINES IN EXPERIMENTAL MODELS OF COXSACKIEVIRUS B MYOCARDITIS

The expression of various cytokine mRNAs has also been studied in coxsackievirus myocarditis.[38] IL-1α, IL-1β, IL-6, TNF-α, and TNF-β were expressed throughout the early phase. IL-2, IL-3, IL-4, IL-10, IFN-γ, granulocyte-macrophage CSF (GM-CSF), and IL-2 receptor (IL-2R) were mainly expressed by the infiltrating cells. TNF-α, TNF-β, and IL-1β were also expressed in part by the infiltrating cells. T-helper (Th)1-related cytokines (IL-2, IFN-γ, and TNF-α) were more strongly expressed than Th2-related cytokines (IL-4 and IL-10) in vivo, indicating that the Th cells that infiltrated the heart and mediated the immune responses in the early phase of acute myocarditis were mainly of the Th1-type.

Different responses to coxsackievirus infection have been observed in different strains of mice.[39] IL-6 and TNF-α levels were increased at 7 days in CD-1 and in C3H mice, had returned to near control values in CD-1 mice by 21 days, but remained increased in C3H mice. IL-1β concentration hardly increased in CD-1 mice, but it increased steadily in C3H mice. An increased expression of proinflammatory cytokines was associated with a reduced contractile performance.

Modulation of cytokine expression by CD4[+] T cells during coxsackievirus B3 infection is initiated by cells expressing the gamma delta + T-cell receptor.[40] The influence of T-cell subpopulations on the host susceptibility to coxsackievirus B3 myocarditis has been studied in knockout mice lacking CD4 and CD8.[41] The severity of the disease was magnified in CD8(-/-) and attenuated in CD4(-/-) mice, consistent with a pathogenic role played by CD4[+] lymphocytes. Elimination of both CD4 and CD8 molecules from T lymphocytes by genetic knockout offered the animals greater protection against myocarditis, confirming that both CD4$^+$ and CD8$^+$ T cells contribute to the host susceptibility.

The same benefit was conferred to T-cell receptor β(-/-) mice, which survived longer and developed minimal myocardial disease after coxsackievirus B3 infection. Increased IFN-γ expression and decreased TNF-α expression were associated with attenuated myocardial injury in CD4(-/-) and CD8(-/-) mice. These results confirm that the presence of T-cell receptor αβ (+) T cells enhances the host susceptibility to myocarditis. The severity of myocardial injury and associated mortality depend on the predominant T-cell type available to respond to the coxsackievirus B3 infection. Thus, CD4$^+$ and CD8$^+$ T-cell subsets may influence specific cytokine expression patterns.

CYTOKINES IN EXPERIMENTAL MODEL OF MYOCARDITIS

INTERFERONS

In an animal model of EMCV myocarditis, human leukocyte IFN-α A/D administered 1 day before or at the time of virus inoculation inhibited viral multiplication in the heart and protected the mice against myocarditis. The preventive effect depended on dosage and on the time of initiation of treatment. When treatment was initiated before or at the time of virus inoculation, IFN-α A/D, 10^7 units/kg per day, effectively attenuated the inflammatory response and myocardial injury.[42]

IFN-β inhibits the replication of coxsackievirus B3 in cultured cells from human heart. Murine IFN-β reduces the number of coxsackievirus B3-induced myocardial lesions in CD-1 mice but does not lower the viral infectivity in heart tissue. Murine IFN-α/β administered at the time of or soon after inoculation effectively protected mice against the fatal consequences of coxsackievirus A16 and enterovirus 71 infections. In an animal model of coxsackievirus myocarditis, human leukocyte IFN-α A/D administered 1 day before or at the time of inoculation inhibited viral multiplication in the heart and protected the mice from coxsackievirus B3 myocarditis.

Ribavirin is a synthetic nucleoside analog, structurally related to inosine and guanosine, which has a broad activity against RNA and DNA viruses. Clinically, its efficacy has been confirmed in measles, influenza, and respiratory syncytial virus infections. Because the mode of action of interferon may differ from that of ribavirin, a possible synergism of recombinant IFN-α A/D and ribavirin was studied. Plaque reduction assays in tissue cultures showed a synergistic inhibition of EMCV replication by ribavirin and IFN-α A/D.

Ribavirin, 100 mg/kg, or IFN, 10^6 units/kg, did not separately inhibit EMCV replication in the heart.[32] However, when used daily together, ribavirin, 100 mg/kg, and IFN,

10^6 units/kg, had a pronounced synergistic effect, apparent in a prolonged survival of the animals, a considerable decrease in myocardial virus titers, and a significant attenuation of inflammatory response and myocardial injury. Combined therapy achieved its effects in lower doses than when either preparation was used alone. Such drug combinations may reduce the incidence of adverse effects caused by either drug used in higher doses. A synergistic effect of IFN and ribavirin was also shown against coxsackievirus infection.[43] Furthermore, combined IFN-α and ribavirin have been effective in chronic hepatitis C.[44,45] The use of antiviral agent combinations deserves careful studies in other serious viral infections.

TUMOR NECROSIS FACTOR-α

To examine the role of TNF-α in our model of EMCV myocarditis, plasma TNF-α levels were measured by enzyme-linked immunosorbent assay, and the effects of recombinant human TNF-α[46] and of antimurine TNF-α monoclonal antibody were tested in vivo.[47] Plasma TNF-α concentrations were increased in the blood of infected mice 3, 5, and 7 days after virus inoculation. The myocardial virus content was higher in the TNF-α-treated group than in the control group. Histopathologic analysis revealed that myocardial necrosis and cellular infiltration were more prominent in the TNF-α-treated group than in the control group. Treatment with the anti-TNF-α antibody prolonged survival of the animals and attenuated the myocardial lesions if it was initiated 1 day before virus inoculation (Fig. 5-4). In contrast, it had no therapeutic effect when initiated at the time of virus inoculation or the next day. TNF-α may play an important role in the early stage of the immune response, and anti-TNF-α monoclonal antibody may block the early pathway of acute viral myocarditis.[47]

INTERLEUKIN-2

IL-2 is a lymphokine produced by activated T cells. It plays an important role in the immune system, inducing differentiation and proliferation of T and B cells, proliferation of natural killer cells, and induction of antigen-specific killer cells. IL-2 also has an antiviral effect induced by activation of natural killer cells and cytotoxic T cells. The effects of recombinant human (rh) IL-2 were studied in our mouse model of EMCV myocarditis. rhIL-2 was administered intravenously on the day before virus inoculation and then continued daily intraperitoneally in the same dose until day 5, when the mice were sacrificed. No significant difference was observed in histopathologic findings in treated and control mice. Thus, no protective effect of rhIL-2 against EMCV infection was demonstrable in mice.[46]

We[46] studied the effects of the anti-IL-2 receptor antibody M7/20 in EMCV myocarditis. BALB/c mice were inoculated with EMCV and injected with M7/20 intraperitoneally

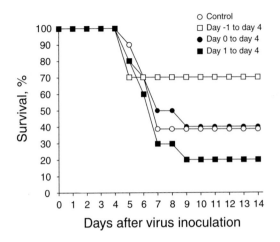

Fig. 5-4. The effect of anti-tumor necrosis factor-α on survival in viral myocarditis in DBA/2 mice. A significant increase in survival rates was measured in the anti-tumor necrosis factor-α Ab-treated mice compared with the saline-treated control group when treatment was initiated 1 day before virus inoculation. (From Yamada et al.[47] By permission of the American Heart Association.)

daily for 14 days. There was no significant difference in mortality or cardiac histopathologic findings between treated and control mice. These observations suggest that treatment with an anti-IL-2 receptor monoclonal antibody is ineffective.

INTERLEUKIN-10

The current understanding of the immune responses focuses on the cross-regulation between the 2 types of Th cells. Th1 cells produce proinflammatory cytokines and contribute to cell-mediated immunity, whereas the Th2-associated cytokines enhance humoral immunity. The cytokines produced by one type of Th cell regulate the others. IL-10, a Th2-associated cytokine, possesses immunomodulatory properties involving the inhibition of Th1 cells and macrophage function and the production of proinflammatory cytokines. It inhibits the inflammatory response by inhibiting the activation of NF-κB through the preservation of IκBα. The profound immunosuppression associated with IL-10 may be effective against the rejection of transplanted organs, immune complex diseases, and sepsis,[48] and clinical trials of IL-10 are being conducted in patients with these conditions.

We studied the effects of rhIL-10 fully active on mouse cells in a mouse experimental model of EMCV myocarditis.[49] The survival rate of mice treated with rhIL-10 was significantly higher than that of control animals (Fig. 5-5). Treatment with rhIL-10 attenuated myocardial lesions and suppressed TNF-α and IL-2 in the heart, but it had little effect on virus concentrations in the myocardium. The expression level of myocardial inducible nitric oxide synthase mRNA was significantly decreased in the group treated with rhIL-10 (Fig. 5-5). Thus, IL-10 administration suppressed inflammation without altering virus replication, suggesting that it does not impair the host defense against intracellular pathogens in vivo. In this model of viral myocarditis, administration of IL-12[50] and IFN-γ[51] also lowered mortality and attenuated myocardial injury.

These observations provide new insights into the in vivo effects of IL-10 on viral infection and suggest a therapeutic effect of IL-10 in viral myocarditis. However, they do not allow us to conclude whether these effects are associated with a predominant response of Th1 or Th2. They merely point to the important role of these cytokines in the immune response and to their potential clinical applications.

Exogenous cytokines or neutralizing antibodies influence several effectors of the immune response in vivo, including the induction or suppression of other endogenous cytokines. In addition, it has been reported that IL-10 acts in a Th-subset-independent fashion. A simple Th1-Th2 dichotomy may not explain the mechanisms of viral myocarditis. The immune system may be inherently toxic to the host, and the negative regulation of an immune response prevents the toxicity caused by excessive inflammation. This study shows that IL-10 may be a key regulatory cytokine that protects the organism against noxious inflammatory responses.

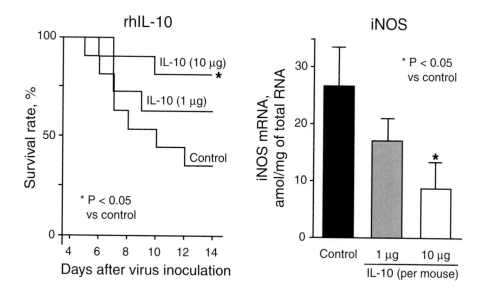

Fig. 5-5. Effect of interleukin (*IL*)-10 on encephalomyocarditis virus myocarditis. Recombinant human (*rh*) IL-10 prolonged the survival of mice and decreased the expression of myocardial inducible nitric oxide synthase (*iNOS*) mRNA. (Modified from Nishio et al.[49] By permission of the American Heart Association.)

INTERLEUKIN-12

IL-12, which is induced in response to various infections, mediates a broad range of effects on innate and acquired immunity, including augmentation of cytotoxic activity and IFN-γ production by NK and T cells and induction of Th1-specific immune responses.[51-54] Its protective role in parasitic infections is rapidly being confirmed,[51,52,55] whereas its importance in the induction of protective immune responses to viral infections is still uncertain.[56-58] A protection against lethal EMCV infection by the exogenous administration of IL-12 in mice was reported.[59] However, the expression and role of endogenous IL-12 produced during the course of viral myocarditis have not been studied.

To further examine the role of cytokines in the modulation of viral clearance by the host and in the recovery from myocarditis, we administered a neutralizing anti-IL-12 antibody and recombinant IL-12 in mice inoculated with the EMCV.[50] Exogenously administered IL-12 markedly reduced mortality, myocardial injury, and viral replication in the hearts of the treated animals (Fig. 5-6). The gene expression of IL-12p35 and IL-12p40 was enhanced in the hearts of inoculated mice. Treatment with the neutralizing anti-IL-12 antibody increased mortality, suggesting a critical role of endogenous IL-12 in murine viral myocarditis.

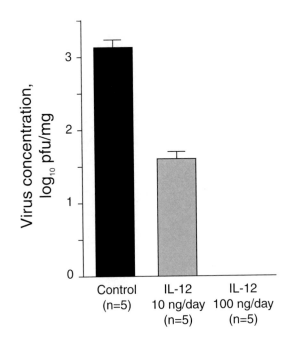

Fig. 5-6. Effect of interleukin (*IL*)-12 on viral replication in the heart. There was a dose-dependent reduction in virus concentration in the hearts of mice treated with IL-12. (Data from Shioi et al.[50])

The roles of IL-12 in vivo may be IFN-γ dependent or independent.[60-62] The effect of exogenous recombinant human IL-12 in EMCV infection is almost completely IFN-γ dependent.[59] No significant difference in the amount of IFN-γ mRNA was measured in inoculated mice treated with saline and those treated with IL-12. This might be explained by the induction of IFN-γ by virus-induced inflammation and IL-12 treatment and by the nearly complete inhibition of viral replication and tissue inflammation by IL-12 treatment. The effects of endogenous IL-12 may be mediated by IFN-γ: 1) the effect of exogenously administered IL-12 is IFN-γ dependent; 2) IL-12 has no direct antiviral activity,[59] whereas IFN-γ exerts potent antiviral activity in vivo and in vitro;[63,64] and 3) the decreased resistance to *Listeria* infection by neutralization of endogenous IL-12 was reversed by IFN-γ.[61]

Two subsets of Th cells have been characterized according to the cytokines they produce.[65] The differential activation of Th1 and Th2 cells during infection may substantially influence the course of the disease.[66] IL-12 regulates the development of human and murine Th1 cells.[67,68] We have examined the gene expression of IFN-γ and IL-10, respective representative cytokines for Th1 and Th2, in heart tissue. IL-12-induced IFN-γ and IL-10 in the heart tissue of noninfected mice, as previously reported.[69] It may limit its own effects by inducing the production of IL-10, which down-regulates the production of IL-12 and IL-12-induced IFN-γ.[65] IL-4, another important Th2 cytokine, was not detected in all groups under our experimental conditions. From these data, we cannot ascertain whether the attenuation of myocardial injury is attributable to a predominant response from Th1 or Th2. However, in experimental autoimmune myocarditis, IL-12 potentiated the expansion of cardiac myosin-specific Th1 cells and hastened the development of myocarditis.[70]

THERAPEUTIC MODIFICATIONS OF CYTOKINE PRODUCTION IN EXPERIMENTAL MYOCARDITIS

PHOSPHODIESTERASE INHIBITOR

Several orally active phosphodiesterase III inhibitors have been developed for the treatment of heart failure. Although their short-term use results in marked hemodynamic improvements, long-term treatment with most of these agents has had an adverse effect on survival. In contrast, vesnarinone, a synthetic quinolinone derivative, improved the quality of life and overall prognosis of patients with heart failure.[71,72] However, an unexplained increase in mortality was measured in the group of patients treated with the highest dose of vesnarinone.[73]

In the hope of clarifying the mechanisms of this adverse result, my colleagues and I[74] studied the effects of vesnarinone in our animal model of myocarditis. Cumulative survival was significantly prolonged in a dose-dependent manner in mice treated with vesnarinone. In contrast, equivalent molar doses of amrinone, an inotropic agent that did not prolong survival in clinical trials, had no effect on survival in our experiments. Although the virus concentration in the heart of mice treated with vesnarinone was the same as that measured in control animals, myocardial necrosis was significantly less in the actively treated mice. Vesnarinone suppressed TNF-α production from spleen cells stimulated with lipopolysaccharide in a dose-dependent manner. Thus, we hypothesize that vesnarinone exerts its beneficial effects by inhibiting the production of TNF-α and that it serves as an immuno-modulator offering new therapeutic options for the treatment of viral myocarditis and immunologic disorders. Vesnarinone attenuated myocardial injury and decreased the induction of cytokines and inducible nitric oxide synthase in experimental autoimmune myocarditis in rats.[75]

We studied the different modulations of the production of cytokines by the phosphodi-esterase III inhibitors amrinone, pimobendan, and vesnarinone.[76] We also studied the effects of amrinone, pimobendan, vesnarinone, and the cell-permeable cyclic nucleotide analog, 8-bromoadenosine-3'5'-cyclic monophosphate (8-Br-cAMP), on the induction of nitric oxide synthase by lipopolysaccharide in J774A.1 macrophages in vitro. Although the 3 inotropic agents inhibited the accumulation of nitrite, the degree of inhibition varied, pimobendan being the most and amrinone the least potent inhibitor. 8-Br-cAMP in high concentrations increased nitrite production, suggesting that the inhibitory effects of the inotropes were not due to an increase in cAMP.[77] Thus, the variable inhibition of inducible nitric oxide synthase by inotropic agents suggested different effects of these drugs in patients with heart failure.

In our murine model of heart failure due to viral myocarditis, pimobendan prolonged survival, attenuated inflammatory lesions, and decreased the production of intracardiac IL-1β, IL-6, TNF-α, and nitric oxide[78] (Fig. 5-7). However, the inhibitory mechanism of pimobendan on these mediators was not clarified. In a study from our laboratory, pimobendan, but not the other phosphodiesterase III inhibitors, inhibited activation of NF-κB[79] (Fig. 5-8). Like forskolin, NKH477 directly activates the catalytic unit of adenylate cyclase and increases cAMP. Because NKH did not suppress the activation of NF-κB either, inhibition of NF-κB activation by pimobendan was apparently not attributable to an increase in cAMP. The mechanism by which pimobendan inhibits NF-κB remains unclear.

The importance of intracellular free calcium in the regulation of cytokine expression has been established in human monocytes, and changes in calcium levels modulate the phosphorylation of IκB, which regulates the activation of NF-κB.[80] Because pimobendan possesses calcium-sensitizing properties, it may inhibit the activation of NF-κB by modu-lating these signal transduction pathways. Activation of NF-κB is critical for the expression

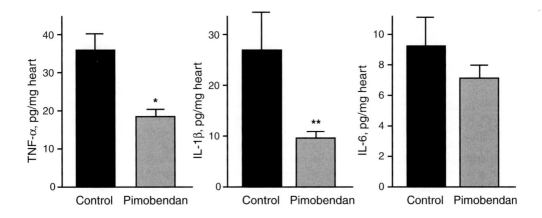

Fig. 5-7. Effects of pimobendan on the intracardiac production of tumor necrosis factor (*TNF*)-α, interleukin (*IL*)-1β, and IL-6 measured on day 7 after encephalomyocarditis virus inoculation. The intracardiac TNF-α and IL-1β levels in animals treated with pimobendan, 1 mg/kg, were significantly lower than in the control group. The intracardiac IL-6 level in the animals treated with pimobendan, 1 mg/kg, was also less than in the control group, but the difference did not reach statistical significance. *P < 0.001 versus control. **P < 0.01 versus control. (From Iwasaki et al.[78] By permission of Excerpta Medica.)

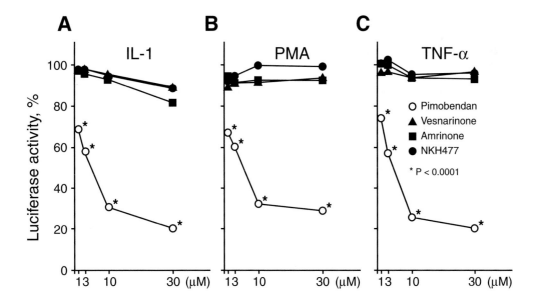

Fig. 5-8. Effects of pimobendan, vesnarinone, amrinone, and NKH477 on the transcriptional responses of NF-κB stimulated with interleukin (*IL*)-1 (*A*), phorbol myristate acetate (*PMA*) (*B*), and tumor necrosis factor (*TNF*)-α (*C*). Pimobendan decreased the expression of luciferase protein in a concentration-dependent manner. (From Matsumori et al.[79] By permission of Excerpta Medica.)

of proinflammatory cytokines (such as IL-1β, IL-6, and TNF-α) and inducible nitric oxide synthase, and it plays an important role in the pathogenesis of inflammation and immunologic diseases.[81,82] Thus, the inhibitory effect of pimobendan on the production of proinflammatory cytokines and nitric oxide is explained by its inhibitory effect on the activation of NF-κB. The effect of pimobendan in heart failure may also be partially explained by this effect.

DIGITALIS

Digitalis has been a controversial drug since its introduction more than 200 years ago. Although its efficacy in patients with heart failure and atrial fibrillation is clear, its value in patients with heart failure and sinus rhythm has often been questioned. The results of the multicenter trial by the Digitalis Investigation Group indicate that, in a large population of patients with heart failure, long-term treatment with digoxin had no significant effect on overall mortality, although it reduced the overall rate of hospital admissions and the rate for worsening heart failure.

In another study, digoxin had an adverse effect on ventricular remodeling after myocardial infarction, despite an increase in ejection fraction. The growing awareness of neurohumoral activation as a contributing factor in the progression of chronic heart failure has redirected the attention of investigators toward the modulating effects of digoxin on neurohumoral and autonomic states.

My colleagues and I[83] found that the cardiac glycoside ouabain induces the production of IL-1β, IL-6, and TNF-α in human peripheral blood mononuclear cells. Ouabain induced mRNA of these cytokines, and the induction appeared to be at the transcriptional level. When peripheral blood mononuclear cells were stimulated with lipopolysaccharide, however, ouabain suppressed the production of IL-6 and TNF-α. Thus, cardiac glycosides may have different effects on the production of cytokines among individuals with or without immune activation.

In other experiments in a mouse model of EMCV-induced myocarditis, digoxin in high doses increased the mortality of the animals, extent of myocardial necrosis, amount of cellular infiltration, and production of intracardiac IL-1β and TNF-α[84] (Fig. 5-9). The shorter survival did not seem attributable to direct toxicity, because none of the uninfected mice treated with digoxin, 10 mg/kg, died. My colleagues and I[83] found that 1 mg/kg of ouabain protected against lipopolysaccharide-induced lethal toxicity in mice and suppressed circulating IL-6 and TNF-α. However, 1 mg/kg of digoxin increased myocardial IL-1β and TNF-α in viral myocarditis. Thus, digitalis may have different effects on heart diseases caused by bacterial or viral infection as a result of its variable modulation of cytokine production. Digoxin appears to exacerbate viral myocarditis, and its use in high doses is contraindicated in patients who have heart failure due to viral myocarditis.

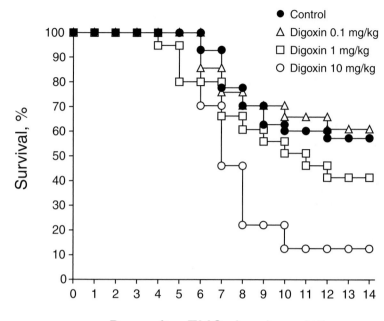

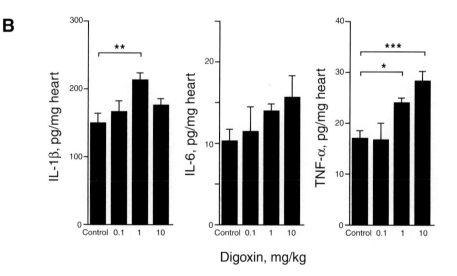

Fig. 5-9. *A,* Effects of digoxin on survival after encephalomyocarditis (*EMC*) virus inoculation. Survival decreased in a dose-dependent manner. Treatment with digoxin, 10 mg/kg per day, significantly increased the 14-day mortality (*P* < 0.0001 vs. control). *B,* Effect of digoxin on myocardial interleukin (*IL*)-1β, IL-6, and tumor necrosis factor (*TNF*)-α production measured on day 5 after EMC virus inoculation. In the animals treated with digoxin, 1 mg/kg, IL-1β was significantly higher than in the control group. **P* < 0.01. Intracardiac TNF-α levels increased in a dose-dependent manner. **P* < 0.05 and ****P* < 0.001. (From Matsumori et al. [84] By permission of the Japanese Circulation Society.)

We[85] have also reported that amlodipine had a protective effect against myocardial injury in an animal model of heart failure due to viral myocarditis, and that its therapeutic effect may be partially attributable to inhibition of overproduction of nitric oxide. Inducible nitric oxide is a type of calcium-independent nitric oxide synthase, and its inhibition is probably by inhibition of the cytokine production that mediates the induction of nitric oxide synthase. In a study from our laboratory,[86] amlodipine inhibited the ouabain-induced production of IL-1α, IL-1β, and IL-6 in a concentration-dependent manner. An earlier study has suggested that the mechanism of ouabain-induced production of cytokines was calcium dependent.[83] Thus, amlodipine may block calcium entry into mononuclear cells. The mechanism of its inhibition of cytokine production remains to be clarified.

DENOPAMINE

Denopamine is an orally active, selective β_1-adrenergic agonist, which has no catecholamine moiety in its chemical structure. We[87] found that denopamine directly suppressed lipopolysaccharide-induced TNF-α production from murine spleen cells. In splenic tissue, TNF-α is synthesized mainly by macrophages and lymphocytes. Agents that act via β_1-adrenoceptors inhibit lipopolysaccharide-induced TNF-α production from the promonocytic leukemia cell line THP-1 by increasing intracellular cAMP levels. On the other hand, lymphocytes have β_2- but not β_1-adrenergic receptors. Because denopamine does not increase cAMP via β_2-adrenergic receptors, even in a dose of 100 μmol/L, it probably does not act on lymphocytes through their β_2-receptors. To determine whether the effect of denopamine on TNF-α is mediated by β_1-adrenoceptors, the selective β_1-antagonist metoprolol was administered with denopamine. Metoprolol significantly blocked the effect of denopamine. Thus, denopamine seems to inhibit lipopolysaccharide-induced TNF-α production by macrophages via β_1-adrenoceptors in murine spleen cells.[87]

We have also shown, in our murine model of viral myocarditis, that denopamine inhibits TNF-α production in the heart. When we examined the effects of denopamine combined with metoprolol in our in vivo model, metoprolol blocked the action of denopamine. Denopamine significantly prolonged survival and attenuated myocardial lesions. These results suggest that the therapeutic effects of denopamine are partially attributable to the suppression of TNF-α production.

AMIODARONE

Amiodarone is now widely used to prevent life-threatening ventricular arrhythmias in patients with heart failure. Although amiodarone did not decrease mortality in large-scale clinical trials, a significant reduction was measured in the combined end points of cardiac death and worsening heart failure.[88] When human peripheral blood mononuclear cells were cultured with amiodarone in the presence of lipopolysaccharide, cytokine levels in the culture supernatants decreased significantly.[89] Because amiodarone blocks the inward rectifier K^+ channel, inhibition of the K^+ current-mediated T-cell activation may be involved in this effect.

ENDOTHELIN ANTAGONISTS

An increase in circulating endothelin (ET)-1 has been reported in patients with heart failure, and higher concentrations have been measured in the failing left ventricle than in plasma. In our animal model of heart failure, extensive inflammation develops in the heart, and myocardial and plasma ET-1 levels increase in parallel with the progression of myocardial injury.[90] The finding of higher ET-1 concentrations in myocardium than in plasma suggests that the heart is a major ET-1-producing organ in myocarditis. Our immunohistochemical studies were performed to identify the cellular origin of ET-1. Although we found it localized in failing cardiac myocytes, as observed in previous studies, infiltrating mononuclear cells were also positive for ET-1, a finding specific to this model. However, tissue ET-1 concentration had already increased by day 5 after virus inoculation, when few infiltrating cells were present. Therefore, myocytes and endothelial cells seem to produce ET-1 mostly before cellular infiltration occurs.

The development of specific ET receptor antagonists enables the study of important physiologic and pathophysiologic roles of ETs and of their receptors. Little information is available, however, regarding the effects of ET-1 receptor antagonists in acute myocarditis. Bosentan, a mixed ET_A and ET_B ET receptor antagonist, was chosen for our experiments because of recent conflicting results obtained with the continuous intravenous infusion of BQ-123, which reduced infarct size in dogs, and those of FR13937, which had no effects in rabbits. We hypothesized that mixed ET_A and ET_B ET receptor antagonism would be more effective in limiting myocardial injury because ET_A and ET_B receptors are present in arterial and venous smooth muscle and in cardiac tissue, and coronary vasoconstriction via ET_B receptors had been demonstrated. Treatment with bosentan was associated with a lower heart weight/body weight ratio and lower histologic scores for myocardial necrosis and cellular infiltration, suggesting that ET-1 plays an important pathophysiologic role in viral myocarditis (Fig. 5-10 C). Treatment with bosentan had a cardioprotective effect without modifying viral replication.

ACKNOWLEDGMENTS

This work was supported, in part, by a research grant from the Japanese Ministry of Health and Welfare and by a Grant-in-Aid for General Scientific Research from the Japanese Ministry of Education, Science and Culture. We thank Drs. I. Okada, T. Yamada, Y. Sato, T. Shioi, S. Matsui, Y. Furukawa, K. Ono, R. Nishio, and A. Iwasaki for their collaborations.

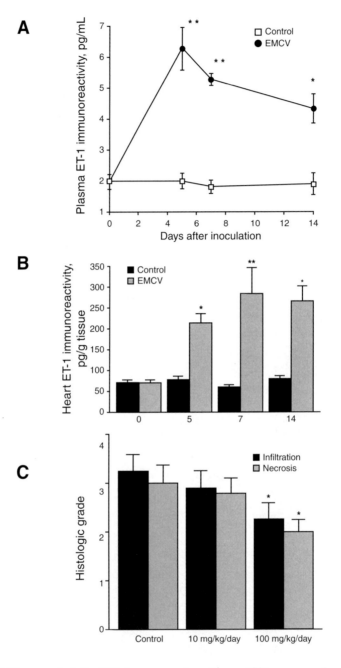

Fig. 5-10. *A*, Plasma endothelin (*ET*)-1 concentration. Plasma ET-1 concentration peaked at day 5 and remained increased until day 14 after encephalomyocarditis virus (*EMCV*) inoculation. *B*, ET-1 concentration in the heart. Myocardial ET-1 concentration peaked at day 7 and remained increased until day 14. *C*, Histologic scores at 14 days after virus inoculation. The histologic scores for myocardial necrosis and cellular infiltration were significantly lower in mice treated with bosentan, 100 mg/kg per day, than in the control group. *P < 0.05, **P < 0.01 vs. control. (From Ono et al.[90] By permission of the American Heart Association.)

REFERENCES

1. Matsumori A, Matoba Y, Sasayama S. Dilated cardiomyopathy associated with heptitis C virus infection. Circulation 1995;92:2519-2525.

2. Matsumori A, Matoba Y, Nishio R, Shioi T, Ono K, Sasayama S. Detection of hepatitis C virus RNA from the heart of patients with hypertrophic cardiomyopathy. Biochem Biophys Res Commun 1996;222:678-682.

3. Matsumori A. Molecular and immune mechanisms in the pathogenesis of cardiomyopathy—role of viruses, cytokines, and nitric oxide. Jpn Circ J 1997;61:275-291.

4. Matsumori A, Ohashi N, Hasegawa K, Sasayama S, Eto T, Imaizumi T, Izumi T, Kawamura K, Kawana M, Kimura A, Kitabatake A, Matsuzaki M, Nagai R, Tanaka H, Hiroe M, Hori M, Inoko H, Seko Y, Sekiguchi M, Shimotohno K, Sugishita Y, Takeda N, Takihara K, Tanaka M, Tokuhisa T, Toyo-oka T, Yokoyama M, and Co-research workers. Hepatitis C virus infection and heart diseases: a multicenter study in Japan. Jpn Circ J 1998;62:389-391.

5. Matsumori A, Ytani C, Ikeda Y, Kawai S, Sasayama S. Hepatitis C virus from the hearts of patients with myocarditis and cardiomyopathy. Lab Invest 2000;80:1137-1142.

6. Oppenheim JJ, Saklatvala J. Cytokines and their receptors. In: Oppenheim JJ, Rossio JL, Gearing AJH, eds. Clinical applications of cytokines: role in pathogenesis, diagnosis, and therapy. New York: Oxford University Press, 1993:3-15.

7. Levine B, Kalman J, Mayer L, Fillit HM, Packer M. Elevated circulating levels of tumor necrosis factor in severe chronic heart failure. N Engl J Med 1990;323:236-241.

8. Matsumori A, Yamada T, Suzuki H, Matoba Y, Sasayama S. Increased circulating cytokines in patients with myocarditis and cardiomyopathy. Br Heart J 1994;72:561-566.

9. Katz SD, Rao R, Berman JW, Schwarz M, Demopoulos L, Bijou R, LeJemtel TH. Pathophysiological correlates of increased serum tumor necrosis factor in patients with congestive heart failure. Relation to nitric oxide-dependent vasodilation in the forearm circulation. Circulation 1994;90:12-16.

10. Tsujino M, Hirata Y, Imai T, Kanno K, Eguchi S, Ito H, Marumo F. Induction of nitric oxide synthase gene by interleukin-1 beta in cultured rat cardiocytes. Circulation 1994;90:375-383.

11. Balligand JL, Ungureanu D, Kelly RA, Kobzik L, Pimental D, Michel T, Smith TW. Abnormal contractile function due to induction of nitric oxide synthesis in rat cardiac myocytes follows exposure to activated macrophage-conditioned medium. J Clin Invest 1993;91:2314-2319.

12. Evans HG, Lewis MJ, Shah AM. Interleukin-1 beta modulates myocardial contraction via dexa-methasone sensitive production of nitric oxide. Cardiovasc Res 1993;27:1486-1490.

13. Kinugawa K, Takahashi T, Kohmoto O, Yao A, Aoyagi T, Momomura S, Hirata Y, Serizawa T. Nitric oxide-mediated effects of interleukin-6 on $(Ca2+)i$ and cell contraction in cultured chick ventricular myocytes. Circ Res 1994;75:285-295.

14. Hosenpud JD, Campbell SM, Mendelson DJ. Interleukin-1-induced myocardial depression in an isolated beating heart preparation. J Heart Transplant 1989;8:460-464.

15. Weisensee D, Bereiter-Hahn J, Schoeppe W, Low-Friedrich I. Effects of cytokines on the contrac-tility of cultured cardiac myocytes. Int J Immunopharmacol 1993;15:581-587.

16. Finkel MS, Oddis CV, Jacob TD, Watkins SC, Hattler BG, Simmons RL. Negative inotropic effects of cytokines on the heart mediated by nitric oxide. Science 1992;257:387-389.

17. Li YH, Rozanski GJ. Effects of human recombinant interleukin-1 on electrical properties of guinea pig ventricular cells. Cardiovasc Res 1993;27:525-530.

18. Liu S, Schreur KD. G protein-mediated suppression of L-type Ca^{2+} current by interleukin-1 beta in cultured rat ventricular myocytes. Am J Physiol 1995;268:C339-C349.

19. Libby P, Warner SJ, Friedman GB. Interleukin 1: a mitogen for human vascular smooth muscle cells that induces the release of growth-inhibitory prostanoids. J Clin Invest 1988;81:487-498.

20. Boluyt MO, O'Neill L, Meredith AL, Bing OH, Brooks WW, Conrad CH, Crow MT, Lakatta EG. Alterations in cardiac gene expression during the transition from stable hypertrophy to heart failure. Marked upregulation of genes encoding extracellular matrix components. Circ Res 1994;75:23-32.

21. Pinsky DJ, Cai B, Yang X, Rodriguez C, Sciacca RR, Cannon PJ. The lethal effects of cytokine-induced nitric oxide on cardiac myocytes are blocked by nitric oxide synthase antagonism or transforming growth factor beta. J Clin Invest 1995;95:677-685.

22. Woodley SL, McMillan M, Shelby J, Lynch DH, Roberts LK, Ensley RD, Barry WH. Myocyte injury and contraction abnormalities produced by cytotoxic T lymphocytes. Circulation 1991;83:1410-1418.

23. Seko Y, Ishiyama S, Nishikawa T, Kasajima T, Hiroe M, Kagawa N, Osada K, Suzuki S, Yagita H, Okumura K, Yazaki Y. Restricted usage of T cell receptor V alpha-V beta genes in infiltrating cells in the hearts of patients with acute myocarditis and dilated cardiomyopathy. J Clin Invest 1995;96:1035-1041.

24. Thaik CM, Calderone A, Takahashi N, Colucci WS. Interleukin-1 beta modulates the growth and phenotype of neonatal rat cardiac myocytes. J Clin Invest 1995;96:1093-1099.

25. Truica CI, Hansen CH, Garvin DF, Meehan KR. Idiopathic giant cell myocarditis after autologous hematopoietic stem cell transplantation and interleukin-2 immunotherapy: a case report. Cancer 1998;83:1231-1236.

26. Beck AC, Ward JH, Hammond EH, Wray RB, Samlowski WE. Cardiomyopathy associated with high-dose interleukin-2 therapy. West J Med 1991;155:293-296.

27. Sobotka PA, McMannis J, Fisher RI, Stein DG, Thomas JX. Effects of interleukin 2 on cardiac function in the isolated rat heart. J Clin Invest 1990;86:845-850.

28. Yokoyama T, Vaca L, Rossen RD, Durante W, Hazarika P, Mann DL. Cellular basis for the negative inotropic effects of tumor necrosis factor-alpha in the adult mammalian heart. J Clin Invest 1993;92:2303-2312.

29. Kubota T, McTiernan CF, Frye CS, Slawson SE, Lemster BH, Koretsky AP, Demetris AJ, Feldman AM. Dilated cardiomyopathy in transgenic mice with cardiac-specific overexpression of tumor necrosis factor-alpha. Circ Res 1997;81:627-635.

30. Hirota H, Yoshida K, Kishimoto T, Taga T. Continuous activation of gp130, a signal-transducing receptor component for interleukin 6-related cytokines, causes myocardial hypertrophy in mice. Proc Natl Acad Sci U S A 1995;92:4862-4866.

31. Kolattukudy PE, Quach T, Bergese S, Breckenridge S, Hensley J, Altschuld R, Gordillo G, Klenotic S, Orosz C, Parker-Thornburg J. Myocarditis induced by targeted expression of the MCP-1 gene in murine cardiac muscle. Am J Pathol 1998;152:101-111.

32. Matsumori A. Animal models: pathological findings and therapeutic consideration. In: Banatvala JE, ed. Viral infections of the heart. London: Edward Arnold, 1993:110-137.

33. Shioi T, Matsumori A, Sasayama S. Persistent expression of cytokine in the chronic stage of viral myocarditis in mice. Circulation 1996;94:2930-2937.

34. Jaattela M. Biologic activities and mechanisms of action of tumor necrosis factor-alpha/cachectin. Lab Invest 1991;64:724-742.

35. Taniguchi T. Regulation of cytokine gene expression. Annu Rev Immunol 1988;6:439-464.

36. Efrat S, Pilo S, Kaempfer R. Kinetics of induction and molecular size of mRNAs encoding human interleukin-2 and gamma-interferon. Nature 1982;297:236-239.

37. Kodama M, Hanawa H, Saeki M, Hosono H, Inomata T, Suzuki K, Shibata A. Rat dilated cardio-myopathy after autoimmune giant cell myocarditis. Circ Res 1994;75:278-284.

38. Seko Y, Takahashi N, Yagita H, Okumura K, Yazaki Y. Expression of cytokine mRNAs in murine hearts with acute myocarditis caused by coxsackievirus B3. J Pathol 1997;183:105-108.

39. Freeman GL, Colston JT, Zabalgoitia M, Chandrasekar B. Contractile depression and expression

of proinflammatory cytokines and iNOS in viral myocarditis. Am J Physiol 1998;274:H249-H258.

40. Huber SA, Mortensen A, Moulton G. Modulation of cytokine expression by CD4$^+$ T cells during coxsackievirus B3 infections of BALB/c mice initiated by cells expressing the gamma delta + T-cell receptor. J Virol 1996;70:3039-3044.

41. Opavsky MA, Penninger J, Aitken K, Wen WH, Dawood F, Mak T, Liu P. Susceptibility to myocarditis is dependent on the response of α-β T lymphocytes to coxsackieviral infection. Circ Res 1999;85:551-558.

42. Matsumori A, Crumpacker CS, Abelmann WH. Prevention of viral myocarditis with recombinant human leukocyte interferon alpha A/D in a murine model. J Am Coll Cardiol 1987;9:1320-1325.

43. Okada I, Matsumori A, Matoba Y, Tominaga M, Yamada T, Kawai C. Combination treatment with ribavirin and interferon for coxsackievirus B3 replication. J Lab Clin Med 1992;120:569-573.

44. Reichard O, Norkrans G, Fryden A, Braconier JH, Sonnerborg A, Weiland O. Randomised, double-blind, placebo-controlled trial of interferon alpha-2b with and without ribavirin for chronic hepatitis C. The Swedish Study Group. Lancet 1998;351:83-87.

45. McHutchison JG, Gordon SC, Schiff ER, Shiffman ML, Lee WM, Rustgi VK, Goodman ZD, Ling MH, Cort S, Albrecht JK. Interferon alfa-2b alone or in combination with ribavirin as initial treatment for chronic hepatitis C. Hepatitis Interventional Therapy Group. N Engl J Med 1998;339:1485-1492.

46. Matsumori A, Yamada T, Kawai C. Immunomodulating therapy in viral myocarditis: effects of tumour necrosis factor, interleukin 2 and anti-interleukin-2 receptor antibody in an animal model. Eur Heart J 1991;12 Suppl D:203-205.

47. Yamada T, Matsumori A, Sasayama S. Therapeutic effect of anti-tumor necrosis factor-α antibody on the murine model of viral myocarditis induced by encephalomyocarditis virus. Circulation 1994;89:846-851.

48. Furukawa Y, Becker G, Stinn JL, Shimizu K, Libby P, Mitchell RN. Interleukin-10 (IL-10) augments allograft arterial disease: paradoxical effects of IL-10 in vivo. Am J Pathol 1999;155:1929-1939.

49. Nishio R, Matsumori A, Shioi T, Ishida H, Sasayama S. Treatment of experimental viral myocarditis with interleukin-10. Circulation 1999;100:1102-1108.

50. Shioi T, Matsumori A, Nishio R, Ono K, Kakio T, Sasayama S. Protective role of interleukin-12 in viral myocarditis. J Mol Cell Cardiol 1997;29:2327-2334.

51. Yamamoto N, Shibamori M, Ogura M, Seko Y, Kikuchi M. Effects of intranasal administration of recombinant murine interferon-gamma on murine acute myocarditis caused by encephalomyocarditis virus. Circulation 1998;97:1017-1023.

52. Hendrzak JA, Brunda MJ. Interleukin-12. Biologic activity, therapeutic utility, and role in disease. Lab Invest 1995;72:619-637.

53. Bost KL, Clements JD. In vivo induction of interleukin-12 mRNA expression after oral immunization with *Salmonella dublin* or the B subunit of *Escherichia coli* heat-labile enterotoxin. Infect Immun 1995;63:1076-1083.

54. Ma Y, Seiler KP, Tai KF, Yang L, Woods M, Weis JJ. Outer surface lipoproteins of *Borrelia burgdorferi* stimulate nitric oxide production by the cytokine-inducible pathway. Infect Immun 1994;62:3663-3671.

55. Heinzel FP, Schoenhaut DS, Rerko RM, Rosser LE, Gately MK. Recombinant interleukin 12 cures mice infected with *Leishmania major*. J Exp Med 1993;177:1505-1509.

56. Bi Z, Quandt P, Komatsu T, Barna M, Reiss CS. IL-12 promotes enhanced recovery from vesicular stomatitis virus infection of the central nervous system. J Immunol 1995;155:5684-5689.

57. Kanangat S, Thomas J, Gangappa S, Babu JS, Rouse BT. Herpes simplex virus type 1-mediated up-regulation of IL-12 (p40) mRNA expression. Implications in immunopathogenesis and protection. J Immunol 1996;156:1110-1116.

58. Orange JS, Wolf SF, Biron CA. Effects of IL-12 on the response and susceptibility to experimental viral infections. J Immunol 1994;152:1253-1264.

59. Ozmen L, Aguet M, Trinchieri G, Garotta G. The in vivo antiviral activity of interleukin-12 is mediated by gamma interferon. J Virol 1995;69:8147-8150.

60. Car BD, Eng VM, Schnyder B, LeHir M, Shakhov AN, Woerly G, Huang S, Aguet M, Anderson TD, Ryffel B. Role of interferon-gamma in interleukin 12-induced pathology in mice. Am J Pathol 1995;147:1693-1707.

61. Tripp CS, Gately MK, Hakimi J, Ling P, Unanue ER. Neutralization of IL-12 decreases resistance to *Listeria* in SCID and C.B-17 mice. Reversal by IFN-gamma. J Immunol 1994;152:1883-1887.

62. Wang ZE, Zheng S, Corry DB, Dalton DK, Seder RA, Reiner SL, Locksley RM. Interferon gamma-independent effects of interleukin 12 administered during acute or established infection due to *Leishmania major*. Proc Natl Acad Sci U S A 1994;91:12932-12936.

63. Ozmen L, Gribaudo G, Fountoulakis M, Gentz R, Landolfo S, Garotta G. Mouse soluble IFN gamma receptor as IFN gamma inhibitor. Distribution, antigenicity, and activity after injection in mice. J Immunol 1993;150:2698-2705.

64. Heim A, Canu A, Kirschner P, Simon T, Mall G, Hofschneider PH, Kandolf R. Synergistic interaction of interferon-beta and interferon-gamma in coxsackievirus B3-infected carrier cultures of human myocardial fibroblasts. J Infect Dis 1992;166:958-965.

65. Street NE, Mosmann TR. Functional diversity of T lymphocytes due to secretion of different cytokine patterns. FASEB J 1991;5:171-177.

66. Scott P, Kaufmann SH. The role of T-cell subsets and cytokines in the regulation of infection. Immunol Today 1991;12:346-348.

67. Sieling PA, Wang X-H, Gately MK, Oliveros JL, McHugh T, Barnes PF, Wolf SF, Golkar L, Yamamura M, Yogi Y, Uyemura K, Rea TH, Modlin RL. IL-12 regulates T helper type 1 cytokine responses in human infectious disease. J Immunol 1994;153:3639-3647.

68. Sypek JP, Chung CL, Mayor SE, Subramanyam JM, Goldman SJ, Sieburth DS, Wolf SF, Schaub RG. Resolution of cutaneous leishmaniasis: interleukin 12 initiates a protective T helper type 1 immune response. J Exp Med 1993;177:1797-1802.

69. Morris SC, Madden KB, Adamovicz JJ, Gause WC, Hubbard BR, Gately MK, Finkelman FD. Effects of IL-12 on in vivo cytokine gene expression and Ig isotype selection. J Immunol 1994;152:1047-1056.

70. Okura Y, Takeda K, Honda S, Hanawa H, Watanabe H, Kodama M, Izumi T, Aizawa Y, Seki S, Abo T. Recombinant murine interleukin-12 facilitates induction of cardiac myosin-specific type 1 helper T cells in rats. Circ Res 1998;82:1035-1042.

71. Sasayama S. What do the newer inotropic drugs have to offer? Cardiovasc Drugs Ther 1992;6:15-18.

72. Feldman AM, Bristow MR, Parmley WW, Carson PE, Pepine CJ, Gilbert EM, Strobeck JE, Hendrix GH, Powers ER, Bain RP, White BG, for the Vesnarinone Study Group. Effects of vesnarinone on morbidity and mortality in patients with heart failure. N Engl J Med 1993;329:149-155.

73. Cohn JN, Goldstein SO, Greenberg BH, Lorell BH, Bourge RC, Jaski BE, Gottlieb SO, McGrew F, DeMets DL, White BG. A dose-dependent increase in mortality with vesnarinone among patients with severe heart failure. Vesnarinone Trial Investigators. N Engl J Med 1998;339:1810-1816.

74. Matsui S, Matsumori A, Matoba Y, Uchida A, Sasayama S. Treatment of virus-induced myocardial injury with a novel immunomodulating agent, vesnarinone. Suppression of natural killer cell activity and tumor necrosis factor-alpha production. J Clin Invest 1994;94:1212-1217.

75. Ishiyama S, Hiroe M, Nishikawa T, Shimojo T, Hosokawa T, Ikeda I, Toyosaki T, Kasajima T, Marumo F. Inhibitory effects of vesnarinone in the progression of myocardial damage in experimental autoimmune myocarditis in rats. Cardiovasc Res 1999;43:389-397.

76. Matsumori A, Ono K, Sato Y, Shioi T, Nose Y, Sasayama S. Differential modulation of cytokine production by drugs: implications for therapy in heart failure. J Mol Cell Cardiol 1996;28:2491-2499.

77. Matsumori A, Okada I, Shioi T, Furukawa Y, Nakamura T, Ono K, Iwasaki A, Sasayama S. Inotropic agents differentially inhibit the induction of nitric oxide synthase by endotoxin in cultured macrophages. Life Sci 1996;59:L121-L125.

78. Iwasaki A, Matsumori A, Yamada T, Shioi T, Wang W, Ono K, Nishio R, Okada M, Sasayama S. Pimobendan inhibits the production of proinflammatory cytokines and gene expression of inducible nitric oxide synthase in a murine model of viral myocarditis. J Am Coll Cardiol 1999;33:1400-1407.

79. Matsumori A, Nunokawa Y, Sasayama S. Pimobendan inhibits the activation of transcription factor NF-kappa B: a mechanism which explains its inhibition of cytokine production and inducible nitric oxide synthase. Life Sci 2000;67:2513-2519.

80. Asea A, Kraeft SK, Kurt-Jones EA, Stevenson MA, Chen LB, Finberg RW, Koo GC, Calderwood SK. HSP70 stimulates cytokine production through a CD14-dependent pathway, demonstrating its dual role as a chaperone and cytokine. Nat Med 2000;6:435-442.

81. Baldwin AS. The NF-kappa B and I kappa B proteins: new discoveries and insights. Annu Rev Immunol 1996;14:649-683.

82. Baeuerle PA, Baichwal VR. NF-kappa B as a frequent target for immunosuppressive and anti-inflammatory molecules. Adv Immunol 1997;65:111-137.

83. Matsumori A, Ono K, Nishio R, Igata H, Shioi T, Matsui S, Furukawa Y, Iwasaki A, Nose Y, Sasayama S. Modulation of cytokine production and protection against lethal endotoxemia by the cardiac glycoside ouabain. Circulation 1997;96:1501-1506.

84. Matsumori A, Igata H, Ono K, Iwasaki A, Miyamoto T, Nishio R, Sasayama S. High doses of digitalis increase the myocardial production of proinflammatory cytokines and worsen myocardial injury in viral myocarditis: a possible mechanism of digitalis toxicity. Jpn Circ J 1999;63:934-940.

85. Wang WZ, Matsumori A, Yamada T, Shioi T, Okada I, Matsui S, Sato Y, Suzuki H, Shiota K, Sasayama S. Beneficial effects of amlodipine in a murine model of congestive heart failure induced by viral myocarditis. A possible mechanism through inhibition of nitric oxide production. Circulation 1997;95:245-251.

86. Matsumori A, Ono K, Nishio R, Nose Y, Sasayama S. Amlodipine inhibits the production of cytokines induced by ouabain. Cytokine 2000;12:294-297.

87. Nishio R, Matsumori A, Shioi T, Wang W, Yamada T, Ono K, Sasayama S. Denopamine, a beta$_1$-adrenergic agonist, prolongs survival in a murine model of congestive heart failure induced by viral myocarditis: suppression of tumor necrosis factor-alpha production in the heart. J Am Coll Cardiol 1998;32:808-815.

88. Massie BM, Fisher SG, Radford M, Deedwania PC, Singh BN, Fletcher RD, Singh SN. Effect of amiodarone on clinical status and left ventricular function in patients with congestive heart failure. CHF-STAT investigators. Circulation 1996;93:2128-2134.

89. Matsumori A, Ono K, Nishio R, Nose Y, Sasayama S. Amiodarone inhibits production of tumor necrosis factor-alpha by human mononuclear cells: a possible mechanism for its effect in heart failure. Circulation 1997;96:1386-1389.

90. Ono K, Matsumori A, Shioi T, Furukawa Y, Sasayama S. Contribution of endothelin-1 to myocardial injury in a murine model of myocarditis: acute effects of bosentan, an endothelin receptor antagonist. Circulation 1999;100:1823-1829.

Nitric Oxide Signaling in Myocarditis

Joshua M. Hare, M.D., and Charles J. Lowenstein, M.D.

NITRIC OXIDE IN THE FAILING HEART

NITRIC OXIDE KILLS CARDIAC PATHOGENS

INFECTIOUS CAUSES OF MYOCARDITIS

PATHOGENESIS OF VIRAL MYOCARDITIS
Direct Viral Damage
Cytolytic T-lymphocyte Damage
Autoimmune Responses

NITRIC OXIDE AND THE INNATE IMMUNE SYSTEM
OF THE HEART
Adaptive Immunity
NO and Innate Immunity

NITRIC OXIDE AND VIRAL MYOCARDITIS
NO Inhibits Viral Replication in the Heart
NO Inhibits Viral Disruption of the Myocyte Cytoskeleton

NITRIC OXIDE AND CHAGAS DISEASE

NITRIC OXIDE AND AUTOIMMUNE MYOCARDITIS

NITRIC OXIDE AND APOPTOSIS

CONCLUSION

INTRODUCTION

The nitric oxide (NO) signaling pathway plays important roles in the regulation of most organ systems. NO participates in physiologic regulation and pathophysiologic organ dysfunction. The latter is often mediated by induction of the high-output NO synthase isoform, NOS2, induced by cytokines. Myocarditis represents a prototypic clinical scenario for the induction of NOS2 within the heart. In this chapter, we review the physiologic roles for NOS1 and NOS3 in cardiac function and the various consequences of NOS2 induction, which influences organ function, antiviral immunity, and apoptosis.

NITRIC OXIDE SIGNALING

NO is produced by 3 NO synthase (NOS) enzymes, which oxidize the terminal guanidino nitrogen of L-arginine to form NO and the amino acid L-citrulline.[1] The NOS isoforms—neuronal NOS (nNOS or NOS1), inducible NOS (iNOS or NOS2), and endothelial NOS (eNOS or NOS3)—are found and play modulatory roles in most organ systems, including the nervous, immune, respiratory, urologic, and cardiovascular systems. NOS1 and NOS3 are activated by calcium and calmodulin, whereas NOS2 is calcium independent by virtue of its high Ca^{2+} and calmodulin affinity. NO activates soluble guanylyl cyclase (S-GC) by binding to its heme moiety, forming an Fe-nitrosyl complex.[2] This activation leads to the production of 3',5'-cyclic guanosine monophosphate (cGMP), which in turn activates protein kinase G and a cascade of biologic signaling events[3,4] (Fig. 6-1; see color plate 7).

Other NO reactions may participate in biologic signaling. NO may covalently react with nucleophilic centers in a nitrosation reaction. This reaction can occur with sulfhydryl moieties (termed "S-nitrosylation"[8]) on either low molecular weight compounds[9,10] or proteins.[8,11] Protein nitrosylation has been shown in vitro to activate various proteins involved in the regulation of myocardial contractility. NO may activate the L-type calcium channel[12] and the sarcoplasmic reticulum (SR) calcium-release channel (CRC).[13,14] The physiologic relevance of S-nitrosylation reactions is less well established than those due to cGMP formation. Nevertheless, there is growing support for the notion that there are both cGMP dependent and independent mechanisms by which NO may influence myocardial contractility.[15]

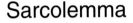

Sarcolemma

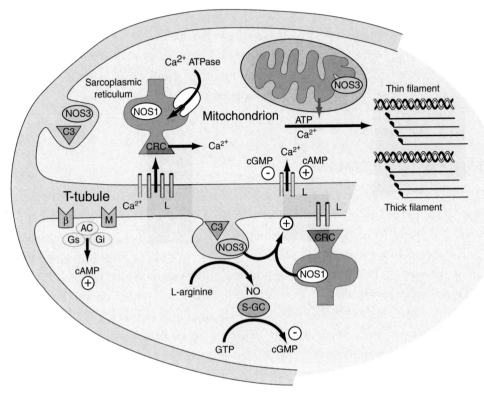

Fig. 6-1. Location and action of nitric oxide synthase (*NOS*) isoforms in the cardiac myocyte. The action potential initiated in the sinoatrial node opens a sarcolemmal Ca^{2+} pore (L-type channel). Ca^{2+} entering the myocyte (I_{Ca}) binds to the sarcoplasmic reticulum (SR) calcium release channel (*CRC*) and triggers a large release of Ca^{2+}, which in turn initiates myofilament contraction (excitation-contraction coupling). Systole (contraction phase) terminates when Ca^{2+} is actively pumped back into the SR by the calcium reuptake pump (Ca^{2+}-ATPase). Cyclic AMP (*cAMP*) stimulates contraction, partly by activation of the L-type Ca^{2+} channel. Increases in cAMP are produced by β-adrenergic coupling to adenylyl cyclase via a stimulatory G protein. cAMP effects are offset by inhibitory G proteins and cGMP, which is produced by particulate and soluble guanylyl cyclases, sensitive to natriuretic peptides and nitric oxide (*NO*), respectively. NO or related molecules also activate the L-type Ca^{2+} channel and CRC and inhibit the Ca^{2+}-ATPase by S-nitrosylation, thiol oxidation, or both. Alternative isoforms of NOS subserve different functions by virtue of their subcellular localization: NOS1 localizes to the SR (with the Ca^{2+}-ATPase and the CRC)[5] and NOS3 to the sarcolemma/T-tubule network (in proximity to the L-type channel)[6] and to mitochondria (ie, with the respiratory complexes).[7] *AC*, adenylyl cyclase; *β*, β-adrenergic receptor; *C3*, caveolin-3; *G_i*, inhibitory G protein; *G_s*, stimulatory G protein; *L*, L-type Ca^{2+} channel; *M*, muscarinic receptor; *S-GC*, soluble guanylyl cyclase. See color plate 7. (From Hare JM, Stamler JS. NOS: modulator, not mediator of cardiac performance. Nat Med 1999;5:273-274. By permission of Nature America.)

CARDIAC PHYSIOLOGIC RESPONSE TO NITRIC OXIDE-STIMULATED cGMP

CHEMISTRY

The nature of NO-related reactions depends on the concentration and location of NO formation. NO activation of S-GC requires low NO concentrations (EC_{50} of 100 nM).[2] NO is produced by NOS3 in concentrations adequate to diffuse to adjacent cells and activate S-GC. Thus, NO produced in microvascular endothelium and myocytes themselves may contribute to myocyte cGMP production.

BIOCHEMICAL REGULATION

In the heart, NOS3 is activated by coupling to numerous receptors, including (but not limited to) muscarinic, β-adrenergic, and bradykinin (BK2). The prototypic mode of activation appears to occur via an agonist-stimulated increase in Ca^{2+}, which leads to Ca^{2+} and calmodulin activation of NOS3. NOS3 is localized to caveolae of the sarcolemma and T tubules, where the scaffolding protein caveolin-3 inactivates it until displaced by Ca^{2+} and calmodulin.[16-18] NOS3 can also be activated directly by phosphorylation by Akt, without intracellular increases in calcium.[19,20]

As mentioned above, NO produced at the membrane can activate S-GC. Subsequent cGMP-related actions include 1) negative inotropic effects,[21-23] 2) negative chronotropic effects,[24] 3) positive lusitropic effects,[25] and 4) inhibition of mitochondrial respiration.[26]

PHYSIOLOGIC RESPONSE (MYOCARDIAL CONTRACTILITY)

The negative inotropic effects of cGMP are more marked when contractility is stimulated by either β-adrenergic activation or heart rate, a finding reminiscent of the phenomenon of "accentuated antagonism" that is observed with vagal nerve stimulation.[27] For example, in isolated guinea pig ventricles, acetylcholine stimulation increased cGMP levels but did not affect contractility, whereas both acetylcholine and dibutyryl cGMP antagonized the positive inotropic response to β-adrenergic stimulation with isoproterenol.[28] Similarly, in ferret muscle strips, 8-bromo-cGMP had a small negative inotropic effect, but it markedly antagonized the contractile response to the calcium channel agonist Bay K 8644.[23]

The observation that NO inhibition of contractility is more apparent during β-adrenergic stimulation has led to the proposal that NO serves as a negative feedback mechanism over contractile reserve, a notion supported by the findings of Kanai and colleagues[29] that adrenergic agonists directly stimulate NO production. We[30] showed that the novel β$_3$-receptor, recently appreciated in myocardium,[31] is the adrenergic receptor linked to NO production.

The negative inotropic effects may be due to cGMP inhibition of the slow inward calcium current (I_{Ca}), which is stimulated by cAMP.[32,33] The mechanism of this effect may involve increased cAMP hydrolysis via a cGMP-stimulated cAMP-phosphodiesterase (in the frog)[33] or a direct effect of a cGMP-dependent protein kinase (in the rat)[32] or both. The NO donor, SIN-1, exerted an inhibitory effect on I_{Ca} identical to the effect of cGMP in the frog.[34] Studies performed using myocytes from NOS3 null mice greatly support participation of the myocyte isoform in cyclic nucleotide signaling. Patch clamp experiments demonstrate marked reduction in cholinergic inhibition of I_{Ca}.[35] Moreover, muscarinic inhibition of heart rate and ability to produce cGMP are absent in cells from these animals but can be reconstituted by transfection of a wild-type NOS3 cDNA.[6] Many studies confirm that similar cyclic nucleotide signaling appears to be involved in modulating heart rate.[36-38] Taken together, these studies suggest that one mechanism for NO inhibition of β-adrenergic receptor-stimulated contractility is cGMP-mediated inhibition of I_{Ca}.

POSSIBLE CONTRIBUTION OF cGMP TO BIPHASIC CONTRACTILE RESPONSES

cGMP may have a biphasic effect on contractility. In isolated myocytes, 8-bromo-cGMP enhanced contractility transiently in a subset of myocytes before causing a decrease.[25] A possible explanation for this effect may involve the presence of both cGMP-stimulated and cGMP-inhibited cAMP-phosphodiesterases in the myocardium. Thus, at low concentrations, cGMP might inhibit cAMP phosphodiesterases, thereby increasing cAMP-stimulatory effects. At higher concentrations, the negative inotropic effects predominate.

CARDIAC PHYSIOLOGIC RESPONSE TO NITROSYLATION REACTIONS

CHEMISTRY

NO can participate in a nitrosation reaction (defined as transfer of NO to a nucleophilic center). This reaction usually occurs through intermediary reactions with O_2, $\cdot O_2^-$, or metal centers (see reactions A, B, and C below). Nitrosation of thiol residues (S-nitrosylation) forms S-nitrosothiols (S-NO). Owing to the abundance of thiol moieties on cysteine residues, protein S-nitrosylation (RS-NO) reactions may be important in physiologic signaling. Numerous proteins have been characterized with regard to S-nitrosylation-dependent functional modification. Among those particularly relevant to the cardiovascular system are hemoglobin[39] and proteins involved in cardiac calcium cycling, the CRC,[13,14] and the L-type calcium channel.[12] Eu and co-workers[14] showed that CRC activation via nitrosylation is oxygen sensitive. Specifically, at physiologic tissue oxygen tensions, NO robustly activated calcium release via the CRC, whereas at high oxygen tensions (those typically used in experimental preparations), this effect was obscured.

BIOCHEMICAL REGULATION

Local control appears important in NO signaling, and NOS isoforms localize to subcellular organelles in which NO effects have been implicated. In the myocyte, NOS3 is found in caveolae of the sarcolemma and T-tubule network (in proximity to the L-type channel),[18] and myocardial NOS1 is present in the SR (adjacent to the CRC and Ca^{2+}-ATPase).[5] As discussed below, NOS3 is also found in myocardial mitochondria.

PHYSIOLOGIC CONTRACTILE RESPONSE

S-nitrosylation of the L-type Ca channel and the CRC leads to activation of these channels in vitro. This activity in vivo would be predicted to produce a positive inotropic response. An increased myocardial contractility with NO donors has been observed experimentally, but this observation has not been consistent.[40-42] Some of the variability in experimental observations has been attributed to species differences or NO concentration or both. Biphasic responses have been noted, with low NO concentrations stimulating contractility and high concentrations leading to cardiodepression.[34]

The variable responses noted in these studies are not surprising given that the chemistry of positive inotropic responses likely involves the S-NO reaction, which can be either prevented or enhanced depending on redox milieu or oxygen tension (see below), and that this was not specifically controlled for in experimental preparations. To establish that this reaction occurs reproducibly, we performed experiments using NO donors effective as nitrosating agents. In these experiments, we found that the NO donors SIN-1 and DEA/NO stimulated positive inotropic responses in isolated rat hearts and in intact mice in a manner that was cGMP independent.[15] Moreover, glutathione and superoxide dismutase (SOD), redox active agents likely to compete with or block nitrosylation, prevented the positive inotropic response to the NO donors.

NO activity has been shown by some[5] but not all[14] investigators to inhibit SR Ca^{2+} uptake; S-NO reactions have the potential to modify Ca^{2+}-ATPase via thiol reactions.[43,44] Previous studies have shown that thiol oxidation reduces Ca^{2+} pump activity. To the extent that nitrosative stress and oxidative stress compete for the same thiol,[2,45] it is possible that reversible S-NO of the Ca^{2+}-ATPase may also modulate pump activity to coordinate with S-NO regulation of the CRC.

ROLE OF NITRIC OXIDE IN MITOCHONDRIAL RESPIRATION

CHEMISTRY

NO actions in mitochondria involve both metal-nitrosyl and nitrosation reactions.

Although NO inhibits mitochondrial respiration in skeletal and cardiac muscle,[46,47] it does so reversibly, suggesting that NO modulation of respiration may also be physiologic. NO forms a dinitrosyl adduct with aconitase, a metal-containing protein involved in the citric acid cycle. In terms of the electron transport chain, NO can reversibly inhibit cytochrome c activity. Higher concentrations of NO result in irreversible (and probably toxic) inhibition of mitochondrial complexes I and II.

Another potential mechanism by which NO may inhibit myocardial energetics is to impair phosphoryl transfer by creatine kinase (CK).[48] NO donor S-nitrosoacetylcysteine prevented a Ca^{2+}-stimulated increase in rate pressure product in the isolated rat heart associated with a decline in ATP as measured by nuclear magnetic resonance. In vitro studies indicated that NO acted by reversibly modifying CK via S-nitrosylation.

BIOCHEMICAL REGULATION

NOS3 has been described in mitochondria of several organs, including the heart, providing compartmentalization with respiratory complexes and enzymes of the citric acid cycle.[7]

PHYSIOLOGIC ROLE

In studies measuring muscle oxygen consumption, NO donors and agonists suppressed tissue O_2 consumption in a fashion that could be attenuated by NOS inhibitors (in the case of NO agonists).[26] Two reports indicated that myocardial energetics are also inhibited by NO.[49,50] Suto and colleagues,[49] in anesthetized animals, and Recchia et al.,[50] in conscious animals, have demonstrated increases in myocardial oxygen consumption (MVO_2) in response to NOS inhibition.

Given that NO appears to modulate mitochondrial respiration on the one hand and Ca^{2+} cycling on the other, it is likely that NO influences myocardial energetics and excitation-contraction coupling. Moreover, NO concentration, which increases and decreases on millisecond time scales, appears to modulate activity of key proteins in a cyclical fashion. Given its ability to stimulate and to inhibit proteins reversibly, it is likely that NO may be involved in enhancing the efficiency of energy production and consumption, linking them to myocyte contraction.

IMPACT OF OXIDANT STRESS ON NITRIC OXIDE SIGNALING

CHEMISTRY

As previously mentioned, the nitrosation reaction occurs via intermediary reactions with O_2, or $^{\cdot}O_2^{-}$, or metal centers.

$$A \quad NO^{\cdot} + O_2 \longrightarrow NO_x + RS^- \longrightarrow RS\text{-}NO$$

$$B \quad NO^{\cdot} + {}^{\cdot}O_2^- \longrightarrow ONOO^- + RS^- \longrightarrow RS\text{-}NO$$

$$C \quad NO^{\cdot} + M \longrightarrow M\text{-}NO \longrightarrow RS\text{-}NO$$

With oxygen (reaction A), there is intermediary formation of nitrogen oxides (NO_x), whereas with ${}^{\cdot}O_2^-$ (reaction B), peroxynitrite ($ONOO^-$), a potent oxidizing or nitrosylating species, is formed. Whether nitrosylation or oxidation occurs depends on the relative flux of $NO^{\cdot}$ and ${}^{\cdot}O_2^-$.[2,10,45,51] The concentration of the latter depends on the balance of its production (as a result of endogenous xanthine oxidase or NADPH oxidase) and its consumption or quenching (eg, endogenous SOD or exogenous antioxidants).

Oxidant stress may have a critical influence on nitrosylation reactions,[45] because ${}^{\cdot}O_2^-$ can compete with thiol for NO reactivity. With low concentration ${}^{\cdot}O_2^-$, S-NO reactions predominate (equation B), but as ${}^{\cdot}O_2^-$ increases, other reactions may occur. First, increases in peroxynitrite may be directly toxic, and, second, $ONOO^-$ or ${}^{\cdot}O_2^-$ may oxidize thiol, thereby preventing its subsequent nitrosylation. Oxidative modification of protein function has been well characterized[52,53] and, in particular, shown to activate the CRC and block its nitrosylation.[13] Oxidation of the CRC irreversibly activates it, likely causing its dysfunction. This continual on-switch also occurs with low-concentration ryanodine and leads to a syndrome that has been termed "leaky SR." Locking the CRC in an open configuration reduces myocardial efficiency, leads to futile calcium cycling, and increases the oxygen cost of excitation-contraction coupling.[54] As previously mentioned, the SR Ca^{2+}-ATPase may be another potential target for oxidative or NO-related redox modulation.[43,44]

PEROXYNITRITE FORMATION

Another potential mechanism by which oxidant stress may damage tissue is by formation of toxic peroxynitrite. This is highly controversial, given the abundance of intracytoplasmic SOD.[2] Oyama et al.[55] demonstrated that cytokine induction of NOS2 is associated with evidence of nitrotyrosine formation, a marker of $ONOO^-$ production, in canine myocardium. In the setting of cytokine exposure, induction of superoxide-generating systems (eg, xanthine oxidase) has been demonstrated, enhancing the likelihood of peroxynitrite formation.[56] We demonstrated a 4-fold increase in xanthine oxidase concentration in dogs with pacing-induced dilated cardiomyopathy and an improvement in myocardial mechano-energetic efficiency in response to xanthine oxidase inhibition with allopurinol.[57] We demonstrated cross talk between NOS and xanthine oxidase signaling in the regulation of myocardial energetics (unpublished observations). Whether peroxynitrite formation contributes to these effects remains to be determined.

NITRIC OXIDE IN THE FAILING HEART

NO has been implicated as contributing to myocardial dysfunction in the failing heart.[58,59] A leading theory is that inflammation[60,61] or cytokine activation[62-64] causes induction of NOS2, a high-output isoform.[65] NOS2, not normally present in myocardium, has been detected by immunohistochemistry, western blot, polymerase chain reaction,[66] and arginine-to-citrulline conversion assays[67,68] in myocardium from patients with heart failure due to idiopathic dilated cardiomyopathy, ischemic cardiomyopathy, valvular heart disease, and myocarditis.[69,70] Functionally, patients with heart failure[58,59] and dogs with pacing-induced heart failure[18] are more responsive to L-N^G-monomethyl arginine (L-NMMA) augmentation of β-adrenergic contractility than are subjects with normal left ventricular function (Fig. 6-2). Augmentation of β-adrenergic inotropic responses has been used as a functional marker of NOS activity within the heart. In myocarditis and sepsis,[71] increased NO production due to induction of NOS2 clearly contributes to this process.

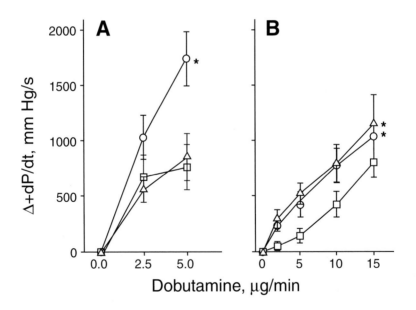

Fig. 6-2. Impact of the nitric oxide synthase (NOS) inhibitor L-N^G-monomethyl arginine (L-NMMA) on the positive inotropic response to dobutamine in conscious dogs. Dobutamine was infused intravenously in dogs before (*A*) and after (*B*) heart failure was induced by rapid pacing for 4 weeks. Dobutamine was infused at baseline (□)and after a 60-min infusion of L-NMMA at either 10 (△) or 20 (O) mg/kg. Before heart failure, 20 but not 10 mg/kg L-NMMA augmented the inotropic response to dobutamine. After heart failure, the lower infusion of L-NMMA (10 mg/kg) was equally effective at enhancing inotropic responses as the higher infusion. These data demonstrate an increased sensitivity to NOS-related influences over myocardial contractile regulation and are consistent with an increased biologic activity of NOS in heart failure. (Data from Hare et al.[18])

There are, however, mechanisms in addition to increased NO production that contribute to this phenomenon. Because β-adrenergic inotropic responses likely result from the balance between cGMP and cAMP, down-regulation in cAMP pathways, as occurs in heart failure,[72] could also lead to enhanced effects of NO. There is also the potential for abnormal signaling of NO with regard to S-NO reactions. To the extent that these reactions are the mode of NO signaling in the SR and mitochondria, they may contribute to the energetic abnormalities that are characteristic of the failing heart. Given that NO signaling appears to be locally regulated, it is plausible that one pathway may appear to have an increased or unchanged activity (sarcolemmal NOS3 influencing guanylyl cyclase activity or L-type function or both) while another is decreased or abnormal (SR NOS1 influencing the CRC or Ca^{2+}-ATPase or both).

NITRIC OXIDE KILLS CARDIAC PATHOGENS

In addition to its role as a signaling molecule in the heart, NO also serves as an effector of the innate immune system. NO kills or inhibits pathogens, including viruses, bacteria, fungi, and parasites, that cause myocarditis. However, NO may also play a role in the development of autoimmune myocarditis, by exacerbating inflammatory responses to cardiac infections.

INFECTIOUS CAUSES OF MYOCARDITIS

Various infections can cause myocarditis (Table 6-1). The most frequent cause of infectious myocarditis in the United States is viral myocarditis, and coxsackievirus infections account for more than 50% of viral myocarditides.[73] Myocarditis affects humans with clinically variable syndromes.[74,75] However, in Central and South America, the most frequent cause of myocarditis is the protozoan *Trypanosoma cruzi*, which causes Chagas disease.[76] NO plays an important role in defending the heart from both of these common causes of myocarditis.

PATHOGENESIS OF VIRAL MYOCARDITIS

DIRECT VIRAL DAMAGE

Viral infections can damage the heart by multiple pathways. Viruses can directly damage the heart by destroying cardiac myocytes: coxsackievirus infects cardiac myocytes and induces apoptosis in vitro.[77-81] The precise mechanism by which viruses cause apoptosis in

Table 6-1
Pathogens Reported to Cause Myocarditis

Viruses	Bacteria	Protozoa	Metazoa
Coxsackievirus	*Streptococcus*	*Trypanosoma*	*Trichinella*
Poliovirus	*Staphylococcus*	*Toxoplasma*	*Echinococcus*
Encephalomyocarditis virus	*Meningococcus*		
Cytomegalovirus	*Haemophilus*		
Varicella zoster virus	*Diphtheria*		
Epstein-Barr virus	*Salmonella*		
Adenovirus	*Mycobacterium*		
Arbovirus			
Echovirus			
Rubella virus			
Vaccinia virus			
Respiratory syncytial virus			
Rabies			
Influenza A			
Human immunodeficiency virus			

isolated cells is not clear. Coxsackievirus may activate inducers of apoptosis. For example, the coxsackievirus capsid protein VP2 activates the proapoptotic protein siva.[78] In addition, we discovered that a coxsackievirus protease can cleave intracellular mediators of apoptosis: the coxsackievirus protease 3Cpro can directly cleave BID, which then translocates to mitochondria, triggering release of cytochrome c and activating effector caspases (unpublished data).

Viral proteases can also interfere with cardiac myocyte signal transduction. The coxsackievirus protease 2Apro can cleave dystrophin.[82] Dystrophin is a polypeptide that forms a signaling complex on the cytoplasmic surface of the plasma membrane. Mutations in dystrophin cause Duchenne muscular dystrophy and Becker muscular dystrophy, diseases associated with dilated cardiomyopathy. Transgenic mice lacking dystrophin also develop cardiomyopathy. Important work by Knowlton and colleagues showed that cardiac expression of a large portion of the coxsackievirus genome in transgenic mice leads to cardiomyopathy.[83] This group then showed that the viral protease 2Apro cleaves dystrophin in vitro and in cardiac myocytes.[82] Finally, they showed that dystrophin is cleaved in mice infected with coxsackievirus.[82]

These important experiments suggest that coxsackievirus can also damage the heart by expressing a protease that cleaves a cytoskeletal protein. However, it is unclear whether or not this cleavage contributes to long-term cardiomyopathy in humans after viral infection, because viral infection usually leads to cell death within hours of infection.

CYTOLYTIC T-LYMPHOCYTE DAMAGE

Viral infections can damage the heart indirectly by inducing an inflammatory response that leads to cardiac myocyte death. As discussed above, an inflammatory infiltrate is one of the diagnostic criteria of myocarditis. Attracted by cytokines, cytolytic T lymphocytes infiltrate the heart, recognize infected myocytes, and kill them by the perforin and granzyme B pathway.[84-90]

AUTOIMMUNE RESPONSES

Finally, viral infections can induce an autoimmune myocarditis after the virus itself has been cleared. For example, Huber and colleagues showed that transfer of T lymphocytes from infected mice with myocarditis to healthy mice can induce myocarditis.[91] The precise mechanism by which viral infection stimulates autoimmunity is unclear. The theory of molecular mimicry postulates that coxsackievirus and other pathogens express peptides that resemble host peptides, provoking an immune response against the pathogen and the host epitopes.[92-95] The theory of cryptic epitopes states that viral infection induces abnormal processing of normal host proteins, and novel or cryptic epitopes to which the host is not tolerant are expressed on the surface of infected and noninfected cells.[96]

NITRIC OXIDE AND THE INNATE IMMUNE SYSTEM OF THE HEART

The immune response to infections of the heart is divided into 2 phases: the adaptive response and the innate response.

ADAPTIVE IMMUNITY

The adaptive response to infection of the heart is a slow but specific response. Developing within days after an infection, the adaptive response is mediated by CD4[+] T-helper lymphocytes, CD8[+] cytolytic lymphocytes, and B lymphocytes. Effector molecules of the adaptive immune response include the T-cell receptors and antibodies. The adaptive immune response achieves its specificity to each pathogen by selectively amplifying clones of B and T lymphocytes that express receptors that identify the pathogen.

NO AND INNATE IMMUNITY

In contrast, innate immunity is activated within hours of infection of the heart. Macrophages and natural killer cells mediate the innate immune response. Effector molecules of the innate immune system include complement and NO.

One hallmark of the innate immune response is its rapid activation. NOS2 expression and NO production are activated within hours of infection. Cytokines, such as tumor necrosis factor or interleukin-1β, or bacterial products, such as lipopolysaccharide or bacterial DNA, activate Toll-like receptors and CD14 receptors on macrophages. We[97] and others showed that innate immune system receptors are also present in tissues of the cardiovascular system, including cardiac myocytes.[98,99] Innate immune signaling through Toll-like receptors activates a signal cascade that releases nuclear factor kappa B (NF-κB). NF-κB translocates into the nucleus, interacts with other transcription factors, and induces transcription of NOS2.[100] Once NOS2 is expressed, it synthesizes NO.

Another hallmark of the innate immune system is its nonspecificity. NO can kill or inhibit a wide range of pathogens that cause myocarditis. Thus, NO is an ideal component of a rapid, nonspecific host response to myocardial infection.

NITRIC OXIDE AND VIRAL MYOCARDITIS

NO is an important component of the innate immune response to viral myocarditis. Our laboratory and others have used a mouse model of myocarditis to explore the role of NO in myocarditis. Coxsackievirus infection induces NOS activity in the heart of infected mice.[101-103] NOS2 appears to be expressed in infiltrating macrophages but not in cardiac myocytes.[102] NOS2 is expressed in the myocardium 3 days after infection, peaks 5 to 7 days after infection, and disappears 14 days after infection.[104]

NO plays a critical role in the innate response to viral myocarditis. Viral titers and viral RNA are greater in mice that lack NOS2 compared with wild-type mice.[104] Mice that lack NOS2 develop a myocarditis after coxsackievirus infection that is much more severe than infected wild-type mice.[104] An intact innate immune system controls viral replication to discrete inflammatory foci in the myocardium. However, an innate immune system lacking NOS2 permits widespread cardiac myocyte necrosis, resulting in dystrophic calcification (Fig. 6-3; see color plate 8).[104]

NO INHIBITS VIRAL REPLICATION IN THE HEART

We identified a key mechanism by which NO inhibits viral replication and inhibits viral myocarditis.[105] Coxsackievirus and many other viruses rely on viral proteases to process large viral polyproteins into smaller viral peptides. These viral proteases are critical to the viral life cycle (Fig. 6-4). NO targets 1 of the coxsackievirus proteases called 3Cpro.[106] 3Cpro is a cysteine protease. NO directly nitrosylates the cysteine in the catalytic site of 3Cpro, thereby inactivating it. With the 3C protease inactivated, the large coxsackievirus polyprotein cannot be processed into its components, and the virus cannot replicate. This is the first identification of a mechanism by which NO inhibits viral replication.

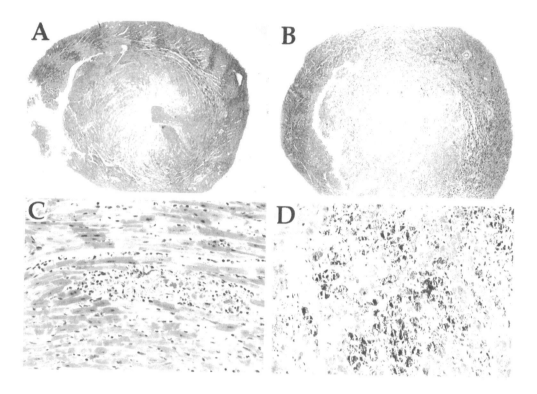

Fig. 6-3. Myocarditis in wild-type and NOS2 null mice. Wild-type mice (*A* and *C*) and NOS2 null mice (*B* and *D*) were infected with 107 pfu CVB3. Hearts were harvested and tissue sections were stained. (Hematoxylin and eosin; *A* and *B*, x40; *C* and *D*, x240.) See color plate 8.

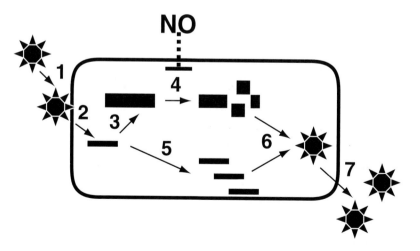

Fig. 6-4. Simplified scheme of the life cycle of picornaviruses. Picornavirus 1) binds to receptors, 2) enters cell and uncoats, 3) translates RNA genome into polyprotein, 4) autoprocesses polyprotein into viral polypeptides, 5) replicates RNA genome, 6) assembles virion, and 7) exits the cell. Nitric oxide (*NO*) blocks the viral protease in step 4.

NO INHIBITS VIRAL DISRUPTION OF THE MYOCYTE CYTOSKELETON

NO also inhibits the cardiac dysfunction caused by another viral protease. Knowlton and colleagues discovered that the coxsackievirus protease called 2Apro plays a role in viral cardiomyopathy by cleaving the cytoskeletal protein dystrophin.[82,107] Knowlton and colleagues extended this work, showing that NO inhibits coxsackievirus protease 2Apro; in particular, NO inhibits 2Apro cleavage of dystrophin.[108] The 2A protease also cleaves other cellular substrates, including the eukaryotic initiation factor 4F that is critical for host protein synthesis. Thus, NO can inhibit viral cleavage of dystrophin and other cellular substrates. This is another mechanism by which NO protects cardiac myocytes from damage during viral infection.

NITRIC OXIDE AND CHAGAS DISEASE

The protozoan *T cruzi* that causes Chagas disease infects more than 20 million people in Central and South America.[76] *T cruzi* is the most common cause of cardiomyopathy and death in South America. The natural history of Chagas disease is highly variable. Acute infection with *T cruzi* leads to hepatosplenomegaly but not myocarditis. The protozoan then enters a latent phase. Between 30% and 70% of patients with acute Chagas disease develop chronic Chagas disease 10 to 50 years after the initial infection. Fibrosis and inflammatory infiltrates of the gastrointestinal tract and the heart characterize chronic Chagas disease. However, *T cruzi* parasites are absent from the heart, suggesting that Chagas myocarditis is due to an autoimmune response.

NO plays a key role in the host immune response to *T cruzi* infection. *T cruzi* infection of macrophages in culture induces NOS2 expression.[109-111] Monocytes activated by cytokines can kill *T cruzi* in culture by producing NO.[112-114] *T cruzi* infection of mice induces NOS2, and NOS2 inhibitors increase mortality in infected mice.[109,115-118] Finally, NOS2 null mice are more vulnerable to *T cruzi* infection than wild-type mice.[119] Thus, NOS2 and NO play important roles in the host response to *T cruzi* infection in mice. Although this protective role has not been confirmed in humans, infected patients have higher serum levels of NO metabolites than noninfected controls.[120]

NITRIC OXIDE AND AUTOIMMUNE MYOCARDITIS

Pathogens are often not identified in patients with myocarditis. Unless a physical or chemical agent is identified, these patients are often assumed to have an autoimmune component to their myocarditis. The diagnosis of autoimmune myocarditis can be made by excluding other known causes of myocarditis. The diagnosis is more certain when autoantibodies are present in addition to an inflammatory infiltrate and myocyte necrosis. Patients with myocarditis have been found to produce antibodies against cardiac antigens, including cardiac myosin and the mitochondrial adenine nucleotide transporter.

The role of NO in autoimmune myocarditis is controversial. NOS2 and NO have been studied in a rodent model of autoimmune myocarditis, in which rats or mice are immunized with purified cardiac myosin. An autoimmune myocarditis develops within 2 to 4 weeks. NOS2 is expressed in cardiac myocytes and cardiac macrophages 2 to 4 weeks after immunization.[121-125] NO may exacerbate inflammation during autoimmune myocarditis, because NOS inhibitors appear to decrease the severity of the myocarditis.[121-125] However, NOS2 may not play a role in autoimmune myocarditis: mice that lack an inducer of NOS2 and cannot make NOS2 have an autoimmune myocarditis just as severe as in wild-type mice.[126] Thus, it is unclear whether or not NO damages the myocardium during autoimmune myocarditis or is merely a marker for inflammation.

NITRIC OXIDE AND APOPTOSIS

Cardiac myocytes undergo apoptosis in humans with dilated cardiomyopathies.[127,128] Cardiac myocyte apoptosis may also occur in humans with myocarditis. Because coxsackievirus can cause apoptosis in cardiac myocytes, directly triggering apoptosis and indirectly activating cytotoxic T lymphocytes, patients with viral myocarditis probably lose cardiac myocytes by apoptosis. Thus, apoptosis may be a prominent feature of infectious myocarditis.

NO may protect the heart by inhibiting apoptosis via different mechanisms. First, NO directly inhibits replication of pathogens such as the coxsackievirus that causes apoptosis. A lower viral burden means that fewer viral antigens are presented to cytotoxic T lymphocytes that kill infected cells through apoptosis. Second, NO can inhibit pathogen enzymes that trigger apoptosis. For example, NO inhibits the coxsackievirus 3C protease that cleaves BID and triggers the mitochondrial apoptosis pathway (unpublished data). Third, NO can inhibit caspases that are part of the intracellular apoptotic cascade. Caspases are cysteine proteases, and NO can nitrosylate cysteine residues, inactivating enzymes such as caspases that contain cysteine at their active site. Several groups have shown that NO can nitrosylate caspase-3, inhibit caspase activity, and inhibit apoptosis.[129-132] Thus, NO may protect the heart and preserve cardiac myocytes by inhibiting cardiac cell death.

CONCLUSION

All isoforms of NOS are found in the heart. In the healthy heart, NOS3 is the predominant isoform, and NO derived from NOS3 plays a critical role in regulation of cardiac signaling. During myocarditis, inflammatory mediators decrease expression of NOS3 in the cardiac vasculature and increase the expression of NOS2 in cardiac macrophages. Regulation of vascular tone is impaired by a decrease in NOS3. NO derived from NOS2 plays an important role in the innate immune response to infections. NO decreases pathogen replication and preserves cardiac myocytes by preventing apoptosis. However, excess NO can also decrease cardiac function, leading to severe but transient cardiomyopathy.

REFERENCES

1. Michel T, Feron O. Nitric oxide synthases: which, where, how, and why? J Clin Invest 1997;100:2146-2152.
2. Wink DA, Mitchell JB. Chemical biology of nitric oxide: insights into regulatory, cytotoxic, and cytoprotective mechanisms of nitric oxide. Free Radic Biol Med 1998;25:434-456.
3. Moncada S, Higgs A. The L-arginine-nitric oxide pathway. N Engl J Med 1993;329:2002-2012.
4. Hare JM, Colucci WS. Role of nitric oxide in the regulation of myocardial function. Prog Cardiovasc Dis 1995;38:155-166.
5. Xu KY, Huso DL, Dawson TM, Bredt DS, Becker LC. Nitric oxide synthase in cardiac sarcoplasmic reticulum. Proc Natl Acad Sci U S A 1999;96:657-662.
6. Feron O, Dessy C, Opel DJ, Arstall MA, Kelly RA, Michel T. Modulation of the endothelial nitric-oxide synthase-caveolin interaction in cardiac myocytes. Implications for the autonomic regulation of heart rate. J Biol Chem 1998;273:30249-30254.
7. Bates TE, Loesch A, Burnstock G, Clark JB. Mitochondrial nitric oxide synthase: a ubiquitous regulator of oxidative phosphorylation? Biochem Biophys Res Commun 1996;218:40-44.
8. Simon DI, Mullins ME, Jia L, Gaston B, Singel DJ, Stamler JS. Polynitrosylated proteins: characterization, bioactivity, and functional consequences. Proc Natl Acad Sci U S A 1996;93:4736-4741.
9. Scharfstein JS, Keaney JF Jr, Slivka A, Welch GN, Vita JA, Stamler JS, Loscalzo J. In vivo transfer of nitric oxide between a plasma protein-bound reservoir and low molecular weight thiols. J Clin Invest 1994;94:1432-1439.
10. Wink DA, Cook JA, Kim SY, Vodovotz Y, Pacelli R, Krishna MC, Russo A, Mitchell JB, Jourd'heuil D, Miles AM, Grisham MB. Superoxide modulates the oxidation and nitrosation of thiols by nitric oxide-derived reactive intermediates. Chemical aspects involved in the balance between oxidative and nitrosative stress. J Biol Chem 1997;272:11147-11151.
11. Stamler JS, Jaraki O, Osborne J, Simon DI, Keaney J, Vita J, Singel D, Valeri CR, Loscalzo J. Nitric oxide circulates in mammalian plasma primarily as an S-nitroso adduct of serum albumin. Proc Natl Acad Sci U S A 1992;89:7674-7677.
12. Campbell DL, Stamler JS, Strauss HC. Redox modulation of L-type calcium channels in ferret ventricular myocytes. Dual mechanism regulation by nitric oxide and S-nitrosothiols. J Gen Physiol 1996;108:277-293.
13. Xu L, Eu JP, Meissner G, Stamler JS. Activation of the cardiac calcium release channel (ryanodine receptor) by poly-S-nitrosylation. Science 1998;279:234-237.
14. Eu JP, Sun J, Xu L, Stamler JS, Meissner G. The skeletal muscle calcium release channel: coupled

O$_2$ sensor and NO signaling functions. Cell 2000;102:499-509.

15. Paolocci N, Ekelund UE, Isoda T, Ozaki M, Vandegaer K, Georgakopoulos D, Harrison RW, Kass DA, Hare JM. cGMP-independent inotropic effects of nitric oxide and peroxynitrite donors: potential role for nitrosylation. Am J Physiol Heart Circ Physiol 2000;279:H1982-H1988.

16. Feron O, Smith TW, Michel T, Kelly RA. Dynamic targeting of the agonist-stimulated m2 muscarinic acetylcholine receptor to caveolae in cardiac myocytes. J Biol Chem 1997;272:17744-17748.

17. Feron O, Saldana F, Michel JB, Michel T. The endothelial nitric-oxide synthase-caveolin regulatory cycle. J Biol Chem 1998;273:3125-3128.

18. Hare JM, Lofthouse RA, Juang GJ, Colman L, Ricker KM, Kim B, Senzaki H, Cao S, Tunin RS, Kass DA. Contribution of caveolin protein abundance to augmented nitric oxide signaling in conscious dogs with pacing-induced heart failure. Circ Res 2000;86:1085-1092.

19. Fulton D, Gratton JP, McCabe TJ, Fontana J, Fujio Y, Walsh K, Franke TF, Papapetropoulos A, Sessa WC. Regulation of endothelium-derived nitric oxide production by the protein kinase Akt. Nature 1999;399:597-601.

20. Dimmeler S, Fleming I, Fisslthaler B, Hermann C, Busse R, Zeiher AM. Activation of nitric oxide synthase in endothelial cells by Akt-dependent phosphorylation. Nature 1999;399:601-605.

21. George WJ, Polson JB, O'Toole AG, Goldberg ND. Elevation of guanosine 3',5'-cyclic phosphate in rat heart after perfusion with acetylcholine. Proc Natl Acad Sci U S A 1970;66:398-403.

22. George WJ, Wilkerson RD, Kadowitz PJ. Influence of acetylcholine on contractile force and cyclic nucleotide levels in the isolated perfused rat heart. J Pharmacol Exp Ther 1973;184:228-235.

23. Shah AM, Lewis MJ, Henderson AH. Effects of 8-bromo-cyclic GMP on contraction and on inotropic response of ferret cardiac muscle. J Mol Cell Cardiol 1991;23:55-64.

24. Krause EG, Halle W, Wollenberger A. Effect of dibutyryl cyclic GMP on cultured beating rat heart cells. Adv Cyclic Nucleotide Res 1972;1:301-305.

25. Shah AM, Spurgeon HA, Sollott SJ, Talo A, Lakatta EG. 8-bromo-cGMP reduces the myofilament response to Ca^{2+} in intact cardiac myocytes. Circ Res 1994;74:970-978.

26. Xie YW, Shen W, Zhao G, Xu X, Wolin MS, Hintze TH. Role of endothelium-derived nitric oxide in the modulation of canine myocardial mitochondrial respiration in vitro. Implications for the development of heart failure. Circ Res 1996;79:381-387.

27. Henning RJ, Khalil IR, Levy MN. Vagal stimulation attenuates sympathetic enhancement of left ventricular function. Am J Physiol 1990;258:H1470-H1475.

28. Watanabe AM, Besch HR Jr. Interaction between cyclic adenosine monophosphate and cyclic guanosine monophosphate in guinea pig ventricular myocardium. Circ Res 1975;37:309-317.

29. Kanai AJ, Mesaros S, Finkel MS, Oddis CV, Birder LA, Malinski T. Beta-adrenergic regulation of constitutive nitric oxide synthase in cardiac myocytes. Am J Physiol 1997;273:C1371-C1377.

30. Varghese P, Harrison RW, Lofthouse RA, Georgakopoulos D, Berkowitz DE, Hare JM. Beta(3)-adrenoceptor deficiency blocks nitric oxide-dependent inhibition of myocardial contractility. J Clin Invest 2000;106:697-703.

31. Gauthier C, Leblais V, Kobzik L, Trochu JN, Khandoudi N, Bril A, Balligand JL, Le Marec H. The negative inotropic effect of beta$_3$-adrenoceptor stimulation is mediated by activation of a nitric oxide synthase pathway in human ventricle. J Clin Invest 1998;102:1377-1384.

32. Mery PF, Lohmann SM, Walter U, Fischmeister R. Ca^{2+} current is regulated by cyclic GMP-dependent protein kinase in mammalian cardiac myocytes. Proc Natl Acad Sci U S A 1991;88:1197-1201.

33. Hartzell HC, Fischmeister R. Opposite effects of cyclic GMP and cyclic AMP on Ca^{2+} current in single heart cells. Nature 1986;323:273-275.

34. Mery PF, Pavoine C, Belhassen L, Pecker F, Fischmeister R. Nitric oxide regulates cardiac Ca^{2+} current. Involvement of cGMP-inhibited and cGMP-stimulated phosphodiesterases through guanylyl cyclase activation. J Biol Chem 1993;268:26286-26295.

35. Han X, Kubota I, Feron O, Opel DJ, Arstall MA, Zhao YY, Huang P, Fishman MC, Michel T, Kelly RA. Muscarinic cholinergic regulation of cardiac myocyte ICa-L is absent in mice with targeted disruption of endothelial nitric oxide synthase. Proc Natl Acad Sci U S A 1998;95:6510-6515.

36. Han X, Shimoni Y, Giles WR. An obligatory role for nitric oxide in autonomic control of mammalian heart rate. J Physiol 1994;476:309-314.

37. Han X, Shimoni Y, Giles WR. A cellular mechanism for nitric oxide-mediated cholinergic control of mammalian heart rate. J Gen Physiol 1995;106:45-65.

38. Levi RC, Alloatti G, Penna C, Gallo MP. Guanylate-cyclase-mediated inhibition of cardiac ICa by carbachol and sodium nitroprusside. Pflugers Arch 1994;426:419-426.

39. Stamler JS, Jia L, Eu JP, McMahon TJ, Demchenko IT, Bonaventura J, Gernert K, Piantadosi CA. Blood flow regulation by S-nitrosohemoglobin in the physiological oxygen gradient. Science 1997;276:2034-2037.

40. Kojda G, Kottenberg K, Nix P, Schluter KD, Piper HM, Noack E. Low increase in cGMP induced by organic nitrates and nitrovasodilators improves contractile response of rat ventricular myocytes. Circ Res 1996;78:91-101.

41. Mohan P, Brutsaert DL, Paulus WJ, Sys SU. Myocardial contractile response to nitric oxide and cGMP. Circulation 1996;93:1223-1229.

42. Preckel B, Kojda G, Schlack W, Ebel D, Kottenberg K, Noack E, Thamer V. Inotropic effects of glyceryl trinitrate and spontaneous NO donors in the dog heart. Circulation 1997;96:2675-2682.

43. Wawrzynów A, Collins JH. Chemical modification of the Ca^{2+}-ATPase of rabbit skeletal muscle sarcoplasmic reticulum: identification of sites labeled with aryl isothiocyanates and thiol-directed conformational probes. Biochim Biophys Acta 1993;1203:60-70.

44. Eley DW, Eley JM, Korecky B, Fliss H. Impairment of cardiac contractility and sarcoplasmic reticulum Ca^{2+} ATPase activity by hypochlorous acid: reversal by dithiothreitol. Can J Physiol Pharmacol 1991;69:1677-1685.

45. Stamler JS, Hausladen A. Oxidative modifications in nitrosative stress. Nat Struct Biol 1998;5:247-249.

46. Shen W, Hintze TH, Wolin MS. Nitric oxide. An important signaling mechanism between vascular endothelium and parenchymal cells in the regulation of oxygen consumption. Circulation 1995;92:3505-3512.

47. Shen W, Wolin MS, Hintze TH. Defective endogenous nitric oxide-mediated modulation of cellular respiration in canine skeletal muscle after the development of heart failure. J Heart Lung Transplant 1997;16:1026-1034.

48. Gross WL, Bak MI, Ingwall JS, Arstall MA, Smith TW, Balligand JL, Kelly RA. Nitric oxide inhibits creatine kinase and regulates rat heart contractile reserve. Proc Natl Acad Sci U S A 1996;93:5604-5609.

49. Suto N, Mikuniya A, Okubo T, Hanada H, Shinozaki N, Okumura K. Nitric oxide modulates cardiac contractility and oxygen consumption without changing contractile efficiency. Am J Physiol 1998;275:H41-H49.

50. Recchia FA, McConnell PI, Bernstein RD, Vogel TR, Xu X, Hintze TH. Reduced nitric oxide production and altered myocardial metabolism during the decompensation of pacing-induced heart failure in the conscious dog. Circ Res 1998;83:969-979.

51. Espey MG, Miranda KM, Pluta RM, Wink DA. Nitrosative capacity of macrophages is dependent on nitric-oxide synthase induction signals. J Biol Chem 2000;275:11341-11347.

52. Chiamvimonvat N, O'Rourke B, Kamp TJ, Kallen RG, Hofmann F, Flockerzi V, Marban E. Functional consequences of sulfhydryl modification in the pore-forming subunits of cardiovascular Ca^{2+} and Na^+ channels. Circ Res 1995;76:325-334.

53. Thomas JA, Poland B, Honzatko R. Protein sulfhydryls and their role in the antioxidant function of protein S-thiolation. Arch Biochem Biophys 1995;319:1-9.

54. Takasago T, Goto Y, Kawaguchi O, Hata K, Saeki A, Nishioka T, Suga H. Ryanodine wastes oxygen consumption for Ca^{2+} handling in the dog heart. A new pathological heart model. J Clin Invest 1993;92:823-830.

55. Oyama J-I, Shimokawa H, Momii H, Cheng X-S, Fukuyama N, Arai Y, Egashira K, Nakazawa H, Takeshita A. Role of nitric oxide and peroxynitrite in the cytokine-induced sustained myocardial dysfunction in dogs in vivo. J Clin Invest 1998;101:2207-2214.

56. Ferdinandy P, Danial H, Ambrus I, Rothery RA, Schulz R. Peroxynitrite is a major contributor to cytokine-induced myocardial contractile failure. Circ Res 2000;87:241-247.

57. Ekelund UE, Harrison RW, Shokek O, Thakkar RN, Tunin RS, Senzaki H, Kass DA, Marban E, Hare JM. Intravenous allopurinol decreases myocardial oxygen consumption and increases mechanical efficiency in dogs with pacing-induced heart failure. Circ Res 1999;85:437-445.

58. Hare JM, Loh E, Creager MA, Colucci WS. Nitric oxide inhibits the positive inotropic response to beta-adrenergic stimulation in humans with left ventricular dysfunction. Circulation 1995;92:2198-2203.

59. Hare JM, Givertz MM, Creager MA, Colucci WS. Increased sensitivity to nitric oxide synthase inhibition in patients with heart failure: potentiation of beta-adrenergic inotropic responsiveness. Circulation 1998;97:161-166.

60. Barry WH. Mechanisms of immune-mediated myocyte injury. Circulation 1994;89:2421-2432.

61. Yang X, Chowdhury N, Cai B, Brett J, Marboe C, Sciacca RR, Michler RE, Cannon PJ. Induction of myocardial nitric oxide synthase by cardiac allograft rejection. J Clin Invest 1994;94:714-721.

62. Levine B, Kalman J, Mayer L, Fillit HM, Packer M. Elevated circulating levels of tumor necrosis factor in severe chronic heart failure. N Engl J Med 1990;323:236-241.

63. Torre-Amione G, Kapadia S, Benedict C, Oral H, Young JB, Mann DL. Proinflammatory cytokine levels in patients with depressed left ventricular ejection fraction: a report from the Studies of Left Ventricular Dysfunction (SOLVD). J Am Coll Cardiol 1996;27:1201-1206.

64. Torre-Amione G, Kapadia S, Lee J, Durand JB, Bies RD, Young JB, Mann DL. Tumor necrosis factor-alpha and tumor necrosis factor receptors in the failing human heart. Circulation 1996;93:704-711.

65. Nathan C. Inducible nitric oxide synthase: what difference does it make? J Clin Invest 1997;100:2417-2423.

66. Haywood GA, Tsao PS, von der Leyen HE, Mann MJ, Keeling PJ, Trindade PT, Lewis NP, Byrne CD, Rickenbacher PR, Bishopric NH, Cooke JP, McKenna WJ, Fowler MB. Expression of inducible nitric oxide synthase in human heart failure. Circulation 1996;93:1087-1094.

67. de Belder AJ, Radomski MW, Why HJ, Richardson PJ, Bucknall CA, Salas E, Martin JF, Moncada S. Nitric oxide synthase activities in human myocardium. Lancet 1993;341:84-85.

68. de Belder AJ, Radomski MW, Why HJ, Richardson PJ, Martin JF. Myocardial calcium-independent nitric oxide synthase activity is present in dilated cardiomyopathy, myocarditis, and postpartum cardiomyopathy but not in ischaemic or valvar heart disease. Br Heart J 1995;74:426-430.

69. Habib FM, Springall DR, Davies GJ, Oakley CM, Yacoub MH, Polak JM. Tumour necrosis factor and inducible nitric oxide synthase in dilated cardiomyopathy. Lancet 1996;347:1151-1155.

70. Thoenes M, Forstermann U, Tracey WR, Bleese NM, Nussler AK, Scholz H, Stein B. Expression of inducible nitric oxide synthase in failing and non-failing human heart. J Mol Cell Cardiol 1996;28:165-169.

71. Sun X, Delbridge LM, Dusting GJ. Cardiodepressant effects of interferon-gamma and endotoxin reversed by inhibition of NO synthase 2 in rat myocardium. J Mol Cell Cardiol 1998;30:989-997.

72. Bristow MR, Ginsburg R, Minobe W, Cubicciotti RS, Sageman WS, Lurie K, Billingham ME, Harrison DC, Stinson EB. Decreased catecholamine sensitivity and beta-adrenergic-receptor density in failing human hearts. N Engl J Med 1982;307:205-211.

73. Woodruff JF. Viral myocarditis. A review. Am J Pathol 1980;101:425-484.

74. Felker GM, Boehmer JP, Hruban RH, Hutchins GM, Kasper EK, Baughman KL, Hare JM. Echocardiographic findings in fulminant and acute myocarditis. J Am Coll Cardiol 2000;36:227-232.

75. McCarthy RE III, Boehmer JP, Hruban RH, Hutchins GM, Kasper EK, Hare JM, Baughman KL. Long-term outcome of fulminant myocarditis as compared with acute (nonfulminant) myocarditis. N Engl J Med 2000;342:690-695.

76. Kirchhoff LV. Chagas' disease. In: Isselbacher KJ, Braunwald E, Wilson JD, Martin JB, Fauci AS, Kasper DL, eds. Harrison's principles of internal medicine. 13th ed. Vol. 1. New York: McGraw-Hill, 1994:899-903.

77. Li BY, Qiao GF, Zhou H, Li WH, Huang ZG, Zhou LW. Cytosolic-Ca^{2+} and coxsackievirus B3-induced apoptosis in cultured cardiomyocytes of rats. Zhongguo Yao Li Xue Bao 1999;20:395-399.

78. Henke A, Launhardt H, Klement K, Stelzner A, Zell R, Munder T. Apoptosis in coxsackievirus B3-caused diseases: interaction between the capsid protein VP2 and the proapoptotic protein siva. J Virol 2000;74:4284-4290.

79. Huber SA. T cells expressing the gamma delta T cell receptor induce apoptosis in cardiac myocytes. Cardiovasc Res 2000;45:579-587.

80. Huber SA, Budd RC, Rossner K, Newell MK. Apoptosis in coxsackievirus B3-induced myocarditis and dilated cardiomyopathy. Ann N Y Acad Sci 1999;887:181-190.

81. Colston JT, Chandrasekar B, Freeman GL. Expression of apoptosis-related proteins in experimental coxsackievirus myocarditis. Cardiovasc Res 1998;38:158-168.

82. Badorff C, Lee GH, Lamphear BJ, Martone ME, Campbell KP, Rhoads RE, Knowlton KU. Enteroviral protease 2A cleaves dystrophin: evidence of cytoskeletal disruption in an acquired cardiomyopathy. Nat Med 1999;5:320-326.

83. Wessely R, Klingel K, Santana LF, Dalton N, Hongo M, Lederer WJ, Kandolf R, Knowlton KU. Transgenic expression of replication-restricted enteroviral genomes in heart muscle induces defective excitation-contraction coupling and dilated cardiomyopathy. J Clin Invest 1998;102:1444-1453.

84. Binah O. Immune effector mechanisms in myocardial pathologies. Int J Mol Med 2000;6:3-16.

85. Kawai C. From myocarditis to cardiomyopathy: mechanisms of inflammation and cell death: learning from the past for the future. Circulation 1999;99:1091-1100.

86. Gebhard JR, Perry CM, Harkins S, Lane T, Mena I, Asensio VC, Campbell IL, Whitton JL. Coxsackievirus B3-induced myocarditis: perforin exacerbates disease, but plays no detectable role in virus clearance. Am J Pathol 1998;153:417-428.

87. Felzen B, Shilkrut M, Less H, Sarapov I, Maor G, Coleman R, Robinson RB, Berke G, Binah O. Fas (CD95/Apo-1)-mediated damage to ventricular myocytes induced by cytotoxic T lymphocytes from perforin-deficient mice: a major role for inositol 1,4,5-trisphosphate. Circ Res 1998;82:438-450.

88. Seko Y, Shinkai Y, Kawasaki A, Yagita H, Okumura K, Yazaki Y. Evidence of perforin-mediated cardiac myocyte injury in acute murine myocarditis caused by coxsackie virus B3. J Pathol 1993;170:53-58.

89. Seko Y, Shinkai Y, Kawasaki A, Yagita H, Okumura K, Takaku F, Yazaki Y. Expression of perforin in infiltrating cells in murine hearts with acute myocarditis caused by coxsackievirus B3. Circulation 1991;84:788-795.

90. Young LH, Joag SV, Zheng LM, Lee CP, Lee YS, Young JD. Perforin-mediated myocardial damage in acute myocarditis. Lancet 1990;336:1019-1021.

91. Guthrie M, Lodge PA, Huber SA. Cardiac injury in myocarditis induced by coxsackievirus group B,

type 3 in Balb/c mice is mediated by Lyt 2+ cytolytic lymphocytes. Cell Immunol 1984;88:558-567.

92. Penninger JM, Bachmaier K. Review of microbial infections and the immune response to cardiac antigens. J Infect Dis 2000;181 Suppl 3:S498-S504.

93. Rose NR. Viral damage or 'molecular mimicry'—placing the blame in myocarditis. Nat Med 2000;6:631-632.

94. Gauntt CJ, Arizpe HM, Higdon AL, Wood HJ, Bowers DF, Rozek MM, Crawley R. Molecular mimicry, anti-coxsackievirus B3 neutralizing monoclonal antibodies, and myocarditis. J Immunol 1995;154:2983-2995.

95. Beisel KW, Srinivasappa J, Prabhakar BS. Identification of a putative shared epitope between coxsackie virus B4 and alpha cardiac myosin heavy chain. Clin Exp Immunol 1991;86:49-55.

96. Lanzavecchia A. How can cryptic epitopes trigger autoimmunity? J Exp Med 1995;181:1945-1948.

97. Rosas GO, Zieman SJ, Donabedian M, Vandegaer K, Hare JM. Augmented age-associated innate immune responses contribute to negative inotropic and lusitropic effects of lipopolysaccharide and interferon gamma. J Mol Cell Cardiol 2001;33:1849-1859.

98. Frantz S, Kelly RA, Bourcier T. Role of TLR-2 in the activation of nuclear factor-kappa B by oxidative stress in cardiac myocytes. J Biol Chem 2001;276:5197-5203.

99. Frantz S, Kobzik L, Kim YD, Fukazawa R, Medzhitov R, Lee RT, Kelly RA. Toll4 (TLR4) expression in cardiac myocytes in normal and failing myocardium. J Clin Invest 1999;104:271-280.

100. MacMicking J, Xie QW, Nathan C. Nitric oxide and macrophage function. Annu Rev Immunol 1997;15:323-350.

101. Hiraoka Y, Kishimoto C, Takada H, Nakamura M, Kurokawa M, Ochiai H, Shiraki K. Nitric oxide and murine coxsackievirus B3 myocarditis: aggravation of myocarditis by inhibition of nitric oxide synthase. J Am Coll Cardiol 1996;28:1610-1615.

102. Lowenstein CJ, Hill SL, Lafond-Walker A, Wu J, Allen G, Landavere M, Rose NR, Herskowitz A. Nitric oxide inhibits viral replication in murine myocarditis. J Clin Invest 1996;97:1837-1843.

103. Mikami S, Kawashima S, Kanazawa K, Hirata K, Katayama Y, Hotta H, Hayashi Y, Ito H, Yokoyama M. Expression of nitric oxide synthase in a murine model of viral myocarditis induced by coxsackievirus B3. Biochem Biophys Res Commun 1996;220:983-989.

104. Zaragoza C, Ocampo C, Saura M, Leppo M, Wi XQ, Quick R, Moncada S, Liew FY, Lowenstein CJ. The role of inducible nitric oxide synthase in the host response to coxsackievirus myocarditis. Proc Natl Acad Sci U S A 1998;95:2469-2474.

105. Zaragoza C, Ocampo CJ, Saura M, McMillan A, Lowenstein CJ. Nitric oxide inhibition of coxsackievirus replication in vitro. J Clin Invest 1997;100:1760-1767.

106. Saura M, Zaragoza C, McMillan A, Quick RA, Hohenadl C, Lowenstein JM, Lowenstein CJ. An antiviral mechanism of nitric oxide: inhibition of a viral protease. Immunity 1999;10:21-28.

107. Badorff C, Berkely N, Mehrotra S, Talhouk JW, Rhoads RE, Knowlton KU. Enteroviral protease 2A directly cleaves dystrophin and is inhibited by a dystrophin-based substrate analogue. J Biol Chem 2000;275:11191-11197.

108. Badorff C, Fichtlscherer B, Rhoads RE, Zeiher AM, Muelsch A, Dimmeler S, Knowlton KU. Nitric oxide inhibits dystrophin proteolysis by coxsackieviral protease 2A through S-nitrosylation: a protective mechanism against enteroviral cardiomyopathy. Circulation 2000;102:2276-2281.

109. Petray P, Rottenberg ME, Grinstein S, Orn A. Release of nitric oxide during the experimental infection with Trypanosoma cruzi. Parasite Immunol 1994;16:193-199.

110. Pakianathan DR, Kuhn RE. Trypanosoma cruzi affects nitric oxide production by murine peritoneal macrophages. J Parasitol 1994;80:432-437.

111. Rottenberg ME, Castanos-Velez E, de Mesquita R, Laguardia OG, Biberfeld P, Orn A. Intracellular co-localization of Trypanosoma cruzi and inducible nitric oxide synthase (iNOS): evidence for dual pathway of iNOS induction. Eur J Immunol 1996;26:3203-3213.

112. Abrahamsohn IA, Coffman RL. *Trypanosoma cruzi*: IL-10, TNF, IFN-gamma, and IL-12 regulate innate and acquired immunity to infection. Exp Parasitol 1996;84:231-244.

113. Silva JS, Vespa GN, Cardoso MA, Aliberti JC, Cunha FQ. Tumor necrosis factor alpha mediates resistance to *Trypanosoma cruzi* infection in mice by inducing nitric oxide production in infected gamma interferon-activated macrophages. Infect Immun 1995;63:4862-4867.

114. Munoz-Fernandez MA, Fernandez MA, Fresno M. Synergism between tumor necrosis factor-alpha and interferon-gamma on macrophage activation for the killing of intracellular *Trypanosoma cruzi* through a nitric oxide-dependent mechanism. Eur J Immunol 1992;22:301-307.

115. Vespa GN, Cunha FQ, Silva JS. Nitric oxide is involved in control of *Trypanosoma cruzi*-induced parasitemia and directly kills the parasite *in vitro*. Infect Immun 1994;62:5177-5182.

116. Petray P, Castanos-Velez E, Grinstein S, Orn A, Rottenberg ME. Role of nitric oxide in resistance and histopathology during experimental infection with *Trypanosoma cruzi*. Immunol Lett 1995;47:121-126.

117. Chandrasekar B, Melby PC, Troyer DA, Freeman GL. Differential regulation of nitric oxide synthase isoforms in experimental acute chagasic cardiomyopathy. Clin Exp Immunol 2000;121:112-119.

118. Huang H, Chan J, Wittner M, Jelicks LA, Morris SA, Factor SM, Weiss LM, Braunstein VL, Bacchi CJ, Yarlett N, Chandra M, Shirani J, Tanowitz HB. Expression of cardiac cytokines and inducible form of nitric oxide synthase (NOS2) in *Trypanosoma cruzi*-infected mice. J Mol Cell Cardiol 1999;31:75-88.

119. Holscher C, Kohler G, Muller U, Mossmann H, Schaub GA, Brombacher F. Defective nitric oxide effector functions lead to extreme susceptibility of *Trypanosoma cruzi*-infected mice deficient in gamma interferon receptor or inducible nitric oxide synthase. Infect Immun 1998;66:1208-1215.

120. Perez-Fuentes R, Sanchez-Guillen MC, Gonzalez-Alvarez C, Monteon VM, Reyes PA, Rosales-Encina JL. Humoral nitric oxide levels and antibody immune response of symptomatic and indeterminate Chagas' disease patients to commercial and autochthonous *Trypanosoma cruzi* antigen. Am J Trop Med Hyg 1998;58:715-720.

121. Ishiyama S, Hiroe M, Nishikawa T, Shimojo T, Hosokawa T, Ikeda I, Toyozaki T, Kasajima T, Marumo F. Inhibitory effects of vesnarinone in the progression of myocardial damage in experimental autoimmune myocarditis in rats. Cardiovasc Res 1999;43:389-397.

122. Goren N, Leiros CP, Sterin-Borda L, Borda E. Nitric oxide synthase in experimental autoimmune myocarditis dysfunction. J Mol Cell Cardiol 1998;30:2467-2474.

123. Shin T, Tanuma N, Kim S, Jin J, Moon C, Kim K, Kohyama K, Matsumoto Y, Hyun B. An inhibitor of inducible nitric oxide synthase ameliorates experimental autoimmune myocarditis in Lewis rats. J Neuroimmunol 1998;92:133-138.

124. Ishiyama S, Hiroe M, Nishikawa T, Abe S, Shimojo T, Ito H, Ozasa S, Yamakawa K, Matsuzaki M, Mohammed MU, Nakazawa H, Kasajima T, Marumo F. Nitric oxide contributes to the progression of myocardial damage in experimental autoimmune myocarditis in rats. Circulation 1997;95:489-496.

125. Hirono S, Islam MO, Nakazawa M, Yoshida Y, Kodama M, Shibata A, Izumi T, Imai S. Expression of inducible nitric oxide synthase in rat experimental autoimmune myocarditis with special reference to changes in cardiac hemodynamics. Circ Res 1997;80:11-20.

126. Bachmaier K, Neu N, Pummerer C, Duncan GS, Mak TW, Matsuyama T, Penninger JM. iNOS expression and nitrotyrosine formation in the myocardium in response to inflammation is controlled by the interferon regulatory transcription factor 1. Circulation 1997;96:585-591.

127. Olivetti G, Abbi R, Quaini F, Kajstura J, Cheng W, Nitahara JA, Quaini E, Di Loreto C, Beltrami CA, Krajewski S, Reed JC, Anversa P. Apoptosis in the failing human heart. N Engl J Med 1997;336:1131-1141.

128. Narula J, Haider N, Virmani R, DiSalvo TG, Kolodgie FD, Hajjar RJ, Schmidt U, Semigran MJ, Dec GW, Khaw BA. Apoptosis in myocytes in end-stage heart failure. N Engl J Med 1996;335:1182-1189.

129. Dimmeler S, Haendeler J, Nehls M, Zeiher AM. Suppression of apoptosis by nitric oxide via inhibition of interleukin-1 beta-converting enzyme (ICE)-like and cysteine protease protein (CPP)-32-like proteases. J Exp Med 1997;185:601-607.

130. Li J, Billiar TR, Talanian RV, Kim YM. Nitric oxide reversibly inhibits seven members of the caspase family via S-nitrosylation. Biochem Biophys Res Commun 1997;240:419-424.

131. Mohr S, Zech B, Lapetina EG, Brune B. Inhibition of caspase-3 by S-nitrosation and oxidation caused by nitric oxide. Biochem Biophys Res Commun 1997;238:387-391.

132. Mannick JB, Hausladen A, Liu L, Hess DT, Zeng M, Miao QX, Kane LS, Gow AJ, Stamler JS. Fas-induced caspase denitrosylation. Science 1999;284:651-654.

Life and Death Signaling Pathways in CVB3-Induced Myocarditis

Bobby Yanagawa, B.Sc., Mitra Esfandiarei, B.Sc., M.Sc.,
Chris Carthy, B.Sc., Paul Cheung, B.Sc., Honglin Luo, M.D.,
David Granville, B.Sc., Ph.D., Decheng Yang, Ph.D.,
Jonathan Choy, B.Sc., Amy Lui, M.Sc., Darya Dabiri,
Janet E. Wilson, B.Sc., MT (ASCP), Aikun Wang, M.D.,
Mary Zhang, M.Sc., Simon Sinn, B.Sc.,
Bruce M. McManus, M.D., Ph.D., Kevin Wei, B.Sc., M.D.,
and Ismail Laher, B.Sc., M.Sc., Ph.D.

INTRODUCTION TO SIGNALING

When Rodbell and co-workers discovered the role of cyclic adenosine monophosphate (cAMP) as a cellular second messenger, the world of life sciences moved to a new conceptual plateau.[1-5] Since then, signaling, in and out of cells, through or bypassing the genome has become a protracted and revealing focus of investigation and discovery. In 1979, the breakthrough discovery that the activity of an enzyme can be reversibly regulated through the action of phosphatases and kinases greatly enriched the concept of cellular homeostasis: how it is maintained in health and disrupted in disease states.[6] Tyrosine phosphorylation was also uncovered as a mediator of growth control,[7] and mitogen-activated protein kinase signaling was discovered by groups studying transcription factor phosphorylation and protein-serine kinases activated by receptor protein tyrosine kinases.[8] The identification of a large family of small monomeric G proteins was a giant step forward in understanding intracellular signaling.[9] Ras was the first protein found to be conserved from yeast to vertebrates, and Ras-associated signaling pathways include Sos,[10] guanosine triphosphate-guanosine diphosphate (GTP-GDP) exchange, Ras-GAP, and Raf.[11] Finally, the discovery of transcription factor NFκB was important in understanding nuclear translocation of a cytoplasmically sequestered transcription factor.[12]

Cell death has been a topic of scientific interest for more than a century. Virchow[13] suggested the importance of cell death in atheromas, and at the gross level, the process was described as degeneration, mortification, softening, and necrosis of cells. Since the acknowledgment that apoptosis is as fundamental to cellular and tissue physiology as are cell division and differentiation, apoptosis has become the focus of intense scientific inquiry. Originally, regulators of the executioner phase of apoptotic cell death were discovered in the nematode *Caenorhabditis elegans*.[14,15] The finding that *ced-3* encodes a protein that is highly homologous to the mammalian interleukin-1β-converting enzyme strongly suggests that the biochemical events governing apoptosis are highly conserved from nematodes to mammals.[14]

There are currently 14 known human homologues in the caspase family.[16] The specificity of caspases-2, -3, and -7 and CED-3 (DEXD) suggests that these enzymes may function to incapacitate essential homeostatic pathways during the effector phase of apoptosis by proteolyzing and deactivating functional proteins.[17] Conversely, the optimal substrate specificity for caspases-6, -8, and -9 and granzyme B ([I/L/V]EXD) corresponds to cleavage sites in effector caspase proenzymes, suggesting that these enzymes may activate cleavages downstream of executioner caspases, resulting in a proteolytic cascade that amplifies the death signal.[17] More than 70 caspase substrates have now been identified, which are involved in cell regulation, signaling, DNA repair, homeostasis, and survival.[16] As noted, apoptosis is now known to be involved in many physiologic and pathologic processes including viral infection.

It was once thought that infection by viruses simply involved overwhelming the cellular transcriptional and translational machinery and compromise of membrane integrity.[18] Indeed, acute infection by certain viruses can lead to oncotic death.[19,20] However, some viruses can disrupt host cell transcriptional and translational apparatus or use viroporins to alter membrane permeability to cause cell death.[21] Still other viruses take advantage of apoptotic apparatus to induce cell death.[22] In fact, many of the cellular antiapoptotic or proapoptotic proteins and genes were discovered by virologists.[23-25] The Src protein tyrosine kinase was originally discovered as v-Src, a Rous sarcoma virus oncogene product.[25] Thus, viruses can modulate host apoptotic machinery to prolong infection or kill the cell. If an "apoptotic" virus is blocked by host antiapoptotic proteins, the virus can *actively* kill the cell by necrosis. Pro-life signaling may save the cell by activation of a stress response or other antiapoptotic mechanisms.

Are pro-life and pro-death signaling occurring all of the time? It is conceivable that life signaling and death signaling are in fact occurring concomitantly and continuously throughout the life of any given cell, usually balanced in opposition to each other but in favor of life. Ultimately, such a balance may swing toward death by environmental insults (like viruses) or by telomerases.[26] Thus, loss or gain of specific signaling may lead to catastrophic one-sidedness and the occurrence of either cell death or cell survival.[27]

VIRAL MYOCARDITIS

Myocarditis, infectious and noninfectious, is a major cause of sudden unexpected death in patients younger than age 40 years, and it contributes significantly to the societal burden of heart failure.[28] There were strong suspicions of an infectious-immune cause for dilated cardiomyopathy,[29-31] and now significant evidence from animal models and clinical studies suggests that viral myocarditis is important in the etiology of dilated cardiomyopathy.[32,33] Group B coxsackieviruses (CVBs) are the most frequent cause of symptomatic viral myocarditis.[34] Molecular diagnostic approaches have confirmed that coxsackieviral RNA, plus and minus strands, is present for extended periods in the heart of experimentally infected mice and in ill humans.[28,32,35,36] Other viral agents causing myocarditis include Coxsackie A and, at times, echovirus, poliovirus, unclassified or uncharacterized enteroviruses, and adenovirus.[28] Our review focuses primarily on signaling mechanisms invoked in CVB3 infection but refers to other viral systems. In particular, we refer to the well-characterized poliovirus, as a comparator model organism to the coxsackievirus, because they are similar in their genomic organization, viral proteases, and life cycle.

Myocarditic damage related to viruses was, until the 1990s, considered predominantly an immune-mediated event.[37-39] Early immune responses and inflammatory processes are initiated by an influx of macrophages, natural killer cells, and humoral neutralizing antibody responses.[28] The next wave of immune defense to reach the myocardium includes the antigen-specific T lymphocytes and antibodies.[40,41] Often, this barrage of innate immune and antigen-specific reactions rids the heart of virus, killing virus-infected heart muscle cells. The Myocarditis Treatment Trial determined that immunosuppressive agents do not improve cardiac function in patients with myocarditis and further suggested that the inflammatory response may reduce disease severity.[42] Experience with mouse models has shown unequivocally that viral infection causes extensive cellular damage before immune cell infiltration.[43] Such findings lead readily to the studies of apoptotic and necrotic mechanisms induced by CVB3.[44]

Direct virus-induced damage has an important role in early ventricular compromise and is a major determinant of long-term sequelae. Early and widespread coagulative necrosis and contraction band necrosis resulting from CVB3 infections have no evident local inflammatory response.[45,46] Prominent cytopathic alterations colocalized to cells with viral replication, as identified by in situ hybridization of positive- and negative-strand viral RNA, reinforce the importance of direct viral-induced damage[47] (Fig. 7-1; see color plate 9). Chow et al.[45] used a severe combined immunodeficient murine model of myocarditis to illustrate extensive CVB3-induced myocarditis and high subsequent mortality. There is still debate as to whether the immune system is always beneficial or at times destructive in the development of myocarditis.[48] Whether primarily caused by direct viral damage or contributed to by activated immune cells, histologic evidence of cellular damage in myocarditic hearts is well characterized and is a major determinant of myocardial outcome and host prognosis. The definition of myocarditis should be situational, and typically it includes early myocyte death associated with direct viral infection, followed by inflammation with further damage, and later by reclamation and ultimate remodeling.

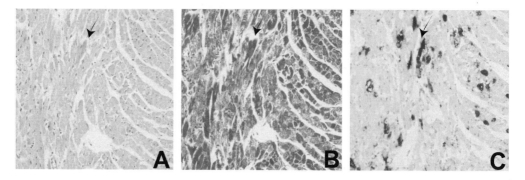

Fig. 7-1. Serial sections stained with hematoxylin and eosin (A) and Masson trichrome (B) or studied by in situ hybridization for viral RNA (C). Patchy areas of myocardial damage (arrows) are colocalized to active viral infection (arrows). (x50.) See color plate 9.

Information on coxsackieviruses and their mechanisms as human pathogens has come from human studies and cellular and animal models as well as from comparator viruses such as the closely related poliovirus. Mouse models and samples from patients have led to understanding of early infectious events. Human cervical carcinoma (HeLa) cells can be manipulated easily and thus serve as a useful model in which to study host signaling mechanisms in response to CVB3 infection. The success of cardiac myocyte isolation and culture techniques will boost investigations of cardiac diseases of infectious and noninfectious cause. Infection of cultures of cells with virus for study not only reduces the possibility of the effects of cytokine release from neighboring cells but also eliminates the contributions from systemic immune responses. The use of microarrays for analysis of myocarditis and other cardiac diseases has revealed the regulation of thousands of genes that reflect the host response to a diverse set of agonists.[49-51]

OVERVIEW OF CVB3 LIFE CYCLE

To gain an understanding of the signaling pathways invoked by CVB3, one must appreciate the complexity of the picornavirus life cycle (Fig. 7-2). CVB3 is a nonenveloped, single-strand, positive polarity, small RNA virus. The viral genome is about 7.4 kb and contains an untranslated region at the 5′ and 3′ termini.[1-4] Instead of a cap structure 7-methyl-guanosine triphosphate group, a small viral protein (Vpg) is attached to the 5′ end. The viral RNA is polyadenylated at the 3′ end.[1,5] A sine qua non of viral pathogenesis is the presence of a functional cell surface protein(s) that can facilitate viral attachment,[52-55] virus-induced host cell surface rearrangements,[56] and internalization. Coxsackieviruses appear to use the decay-accelerating factor (DAF) as a primary attachment protein (coreceptor) and the coxsackievirus and adenovirus receptor (CAR) to be internalized (a concept reminiscent of the human immunodeficiency virus [HIV]-1 receptor complex).[57-59] DAF (CD55) is a membrane glycoprotein anchored to the extracellular surface by glycosylphosphatidylinositol (GPI).[60] Notably, the GPI anchor may mediate *src* family kinase signaling through p56lck, essential for productive CVB3 infection.[61-63] These early DAF- and potentially CAR-mediated signaling modalities may influence the extent of infection and are an active area of study. There are other putative CVB3 receptors or coreceptors—for example, the 100-kDa nucleolin-like protein, also known to interact with coxsackieviruses and adenoviruses.[64,65]

After viral entry and uncoating, the genomic RNA acts as a template for translation and subsequent transcription, with initial synthesis of minus-strand RNA. This minus-strand RNA acts as an essential template for transcription of complementary viral plus-strand RNA genomes, these being finally packaged into new virions. However, minus-strand

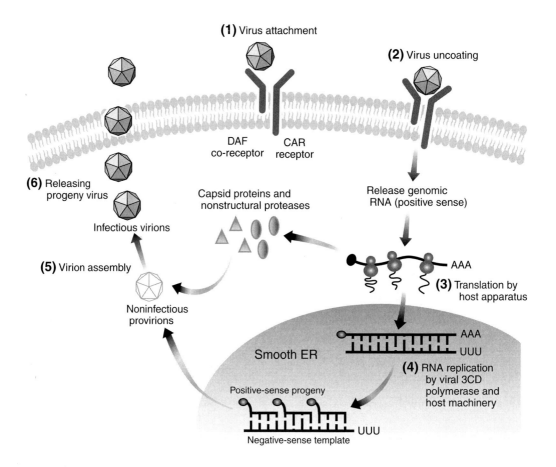

Fig. 7-2. *1 and 2,* Host cell receptor proteins (coxsackievirus and adenovirus receptor [*CAR*] and decay-accelerating factor [*DAF*]) mediate virion attachment and uncoating. *3,* The virus-positive single-strand RNA genome is released into the cytoplasm and serves as a direct template for protease translation. Viral proteases are involved in the further synthesis of capsid proteins and other nonstructural proteases that mediate pathogenesis. *4,* RNA genome replication occurs in the smooth endoplasmic reticulum (*ER*) and involves viral proteases (3CD) and other host proteins. Multiple positive-sense progeny strand synthesis occurs on the negative-sense template and they are released to be incorporated into noninfectious provirions. *5,* Final assembly of the virion and closure of the viral capsid give a potent progeny virus. *6,* Cytolysis releases the virions as infectious particles.

RNA synthesis cannot start until the viral enzymes for RNA transcription have been successfully manufactured by confiscating ribosomes and other host transcriptional machinery. The incoming plus-strand RNA directs synthesis of a polyprotein via cap-independent internal ribosome entry mechanisms.[66] This polyprotein is processed subsequently into individual structural (Vp1-Vp4) and nonstructural proteins. Cleavages of the polyprotein are made mainly by viral proteases 2A[pro], 3C[pro], and conceivably 3CD[pro]. The structural proteins formed by partial cleavage of the P1 precursor associate with positive-strand RNA molecules that retain Vpg to form progeny virions, which are released from the cell by lysis.

The mechanism by which CVB3 induces cell lysis and virion release is unclear. van Kuppeveld et al.[67] found that coxsackievirus protein 2B modifies endoplasmic and plasma membrane permeability and facilitates virus release from the host cells. However, mechanisms of cellular destabilization are also operative. The viral progeny may be released through holes in the cell membrane made by viral protein 2B. Along with viral release, proteolytically processed host proteins are released that may be targeted by autoantibodies, thereby exacerbating myocardial damage.

DEATH SIGNALING

Questions regarding the mechanisms and consequences of cell death in the heart are of interest to researchers and of importance to clinicians. Apoptosis and necrosis occur in the heart and contribute differently to developmental, adaptive, reparative, and degenerative processes. Necrosis is the equivalent of accidental cell death associated with loss of cellular homeostasis. Necrosis does not require de novo gene expression but is characterized by rupture of mitochondrial or plasma membranes leading to death. Cellular swelling due to water and electrolytes, rounding up, loss of plasma and nuclear membrane integrity, and release of contents into surrounding tissue space are classic features of oncosis.[68,69] Releasing intracellular contents induces an inflammatory response that augments this necrotic process.[69-72]

First "discovered" by Kerr, Wyllie, and Currie,[73,74] apoptosis is a tightly regulated, organized, and energy-consuming cell death process. Apoptosis is critically involved in embryogenesis and tissue homeostasis.[75] In normal tissue, apoptotic mechanisms eliminate cells that are genetically unstable or that are no longer functional.[76] The main apoptotic agents are a family of death proteases, known as caspases, which proteolyze proteins that are necessary for cell life and apoptotic signaling. The majority of caspase substrates identified thus far are involved in cell signaling, DNA repair, cellular homeostasis, and cell survival. Cleavage and subsequent inactivation or alteration of these proteins is a critical event contributing to the apoptotic phenotype.

Apoptosis can be considered in terms of morphologic consequences or biochemical mechanisms.[69,72] Morphologic changes during apoptosis include cell and nuclear shrinkage, nuclear chromatin condensation and breakdown into nucleosomal fragments, vesicle formation, budding of apoptotic bodies, and phagocytosis by neighboring macrophages and parenchymal cells.[70,71,77] Caspase targeting of structural proteins and degradation of such proteins may be responsible for the cellular morphologic changes that are observed during apoptosis. Structural proteins that are cleaved in apoptosis include actin,[78] α-fodrin,[79] lamin A,[80] lamin B,[81] nuclear mitotic-associated protein, focal adhesion kinase,[82] rabaptin-5,[83] keratin 88,[84] and gelsolin.[85]

Apoptosis can occur through receptor- and mitochondrial-mediated pathways (Fig. 7-3). Receptor-mediated pathways are induced by binding of death-inducing ligands such as Fas-L, tumor necrosis factor-α, and tumor necrosis factor-related apoptosis-inducing ligand to their respective receptors.[86] Subsequent recruitment of adapter proteins and binding of procaspase-8 forms the death-inducing signaling complex[87] and initiates activation of caspase-8, followed by activation of downstream caspases.[88] Alternatively, cellular stresses can induce apoptosis through activation of a mitochondrial-regulated pathway. Exposure to cellular insults can release cytochrome c (cyt c) from the mitochondria. Cytosolic cyt c associates with Apaf-1 and procaspase-9 and, in the presence of dATP, activates caspase-9.[89] Caspase-9 can then cleave and activate caspase-3, leading to apoptosis through downstream events similar to those that occur in receptor-mediated processes. Although the decision to use a mitochondrial or a receptor-mediated pathway often depends on the death stimulus, receptor-mediated processes can activate a mitochondrial pathway through induction of cyt c release to amplify the apoptotic signal and lead to more efficient cell death.[90]

Biochemical mechanisms of the cell death machinery consist of 3 major components: the Bcl-2 family of proteins, mitochondrial factors, and caspases. Molecular and biochemical studies have demonstrated that several Bcl-2 family proteins such as Bcl-2 and Bcl-xL can prevent apoptosis. Overexpression of the apoptotic suppressor Bcl-2 in mitochondria can block cyt c efflux and apoptosis.[91,92] Conversely, the proapoptotic members of the Bcl-2 family, including Bad, Bax, Bak, Bim, and Bid, promote cyt c release and induce apoptosis.[93,94] Bad and Bax are normally located in the cytosol and actively translocate to mitochondria during apoptosis.[95] Although it is unknown how this regulation takes place, popular theories involve regulation of the permeability transition pore. Alterations in membrane permeability release mitochondrial cyt c, apoptosis-inducing factor, second mitochondrial-derived activator, caspase-2, and caspase-9.[96] Apoptosis-inducing factor is a flavoprotein that translocates from the mitochondria to the nucleus during apoptosis[97,98] and initiates stage I DNA fragmentation,[98] and second mitochondrial-derived activator blocks the inhibitory activities of inhibitors of apoptosis proteins (IAPs).[99] Mitochondrial caspases-2 and -9 are also released into the cytosol to contribute to the activation of effector caspases.

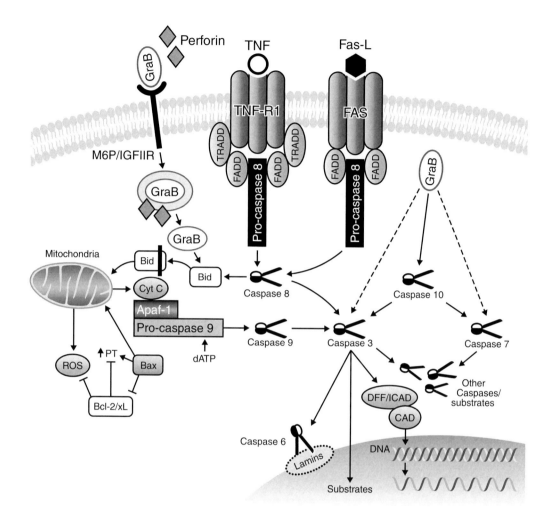

Fig. 7-3. Molecular pathways involved in Fas-L-, tumor necrosis factor (*TNF*)-, and granzyme B (*GraB*)-mediated apoptosis. Binding of TNF or Fas-L to their respective receptors results in the recruitment of adapter proteins to form a death-inducing signaling complex, thereby inducing oligomerization and activation of caspase-8, which activates downstream executioner caspases. GraB is internalized in a mannose-6-phosphate/insulin-like growth factor II receptor-dependent manner. In the presence of perforin, GraB can enter the target cell cytoplasm where it induces apoptosis in a mitochondria-dependent manner through the cleavage of Bid. However, in the absence of this pathway, GraB can induce apoptosis through the direct cleavage of several caspases. Many proapoptotic stimuli induce the mitochondria to release cytochrome c (*cyt c*) via proapoptotic Bcl-2 family proteins, such as Bid, which is blocked by Bcl-2 or Bcl-xL. Release of cyt c facilitates apoptotic protease-activating factor (*Apaf-1*)-mediated caspase-9 activation, which then cleaves caspase-3. Caspase-3 induces DNA fragmentation by cleaving DFF/ICAD, which then allows translocation of CAD into the nucleus and subsequent DNA fragmentation. Caspase-3 may also cleave other structural or repair proteins or other caspases such as caspase-6, which cleaves nuclear lamins.

A role for apoptosis in myocarditis has been doubted,[100] but mounting histologic and ultrastructural evidence and specific assays for key apoptosis markers have shown that apoptosis participates in the pathogenesis of myocarditis, although the extent of this effect is unclear.[44,101,102] Infected cells may induce apoptosis to abort the viral life cycle and prevent viral spread. This biologic response is not a surprising homeostatic check, because viruses have incorporated both apoptotic and antiapoptotic processes into their own life cycles and are able to shorten or to prolong cell viability according to need. Such proteins include adenovirus E1B (19kDa), homologous to Bcl-2, which can directly interact with and inactivate p53, a well-characterized proto-oncogene that can induce apoptosis.[103,104]

Picornaviruses have a relatively short life cycle, and prolonging survival of the host cell may be of less value to such viruses than to larger, more complex viruses that possess a longer life cycle. Although in other viral systems apoptosis is beneficial to the host in preventing viral dissemination, some literature has suggested that the opposite is true during CVB3 infection.[105] Target cell apoptosis has been found to occur in several models of picornavirus infection.[44,106-110] Induction of host cell apoptosis by CVB3 would facilitate the timely release of progeny virus, and the phagocytosis of infected cells would help evade the immune response. Rapid phagocytosis would delay the onset of inflammation and may be important in the prevention of CVB3 dissemination. Although infected cells may die by necrosis and allow for localized viral spread, immediate activation of the immune response quickly clears the viral particles. Particularly in cardiac myocytes, a cell population that cannot be replenished, virus-induced apoptosis or necrosis is especially harmful to the host. Apoptosis can be stimulated by the presence of viral antigens, by viral protease-based disruption of cellular homeostasis, and by influences on host gene transcription and protein translation.

Immediately after infection, viral proteins, particularly virus structural proteins, may contribute as a direct cause of apoptosis. For example, in HIV infections, it has frequently been observed that uninfected bystander cells undergo more extensive cell death than infected cells. Exposure to extracellular HIV coat protein gp120 alone can induce apoptosis, whereas infected cells are resistant to proapoptotic stimuli owing to the presence of virus-derived antiapoptotic proteins.[111] Similarly, the pro-apoptotic protein referred to as siva is up-regulated in CVB3-induced apoptosis and found to interact with VP2.[112] Other virus proteins such as VP3 of chicken anemia virus,[113] HIV-1 Tat and gp120,[114] and human T-cell leukemia virus-1 Tax protein[115] cause apoptosis. Furthermore, ultraviolet-inactivated, replication-incompetent viruses that attach to cellular receptors and enter the cell cause apoptosis.[106,116] It is likely that death mechanisms are triggered by either immediate and direct receptor signaling or by the presence of viral antigens.

Direct viral protease-induced cleavage of host proteins is a specific event. In addition to the viral polyprotein, a small number of cellular proteins are cleaved. Furthermore, cellular proteins have a hierarchy of susceptibility to cleavage that roughly corresponds to the time and extent of proteolysis observed postinfection.[117] Interestingly, overexpression of viral protease 2A[pro] in a cell line is sufficient to induce cell death, although the exact mechanism is unclear.[118]

2A[pro] cleaves eukaryotic initiation factor 4-gamma (eIF4γ)I and to a lesser extent eIF4γII. These proteins are necessary for host cap-dependent protein formation by bridging the RNA and ribosome (Fig. 7-4).[118-122] Decreased host protein translation results in an imbalance of protein synthesis and degradation, most likely contributing to myofibrillar disarray and an atrophic phenotype. However, the story is more complex, because there is an increasing number of cellular proteins containing an internal ribosome entry site and

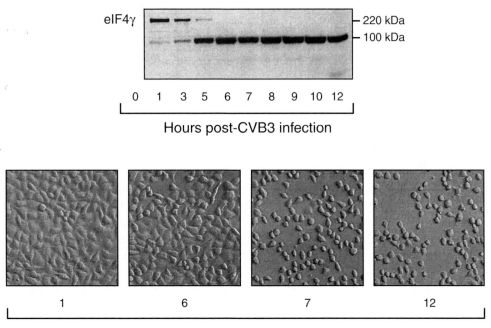

Fig. 7-4. Coxsackievirus B3 *(CVB3)* viral protease cleavage of host eukaryotic initiation factor 4-γ *(eIF4γ)*. Cell morphology changes after infection with CVB3. Cellular lysate was collected from CVB3-infected HeLa cells. Cytosolic extract was then analyzed for the presence of the 220-kDa eIF4γ component of the translation initiation complex. Phase-contrast microscopy of HeLa cells at 1, 6, 7, and 12 h postinfection was performed. Note the extensive cytopathic changes that occurred between 6 and 7 h postinfection. (From Carthy et al.[44] By permission of the American Society for Microbiology.)

undergoing translation in a cap-independent fashion.[123] Cap-independent translation of host proteins that contain an internal ribosome entry site is increased in response to blocked formation of the translation complex. To date, these proteins include VEGF,[124] c-myc,[125] apoptotic protease-activating factor-1,[126] death-associated protein 5,[127] X-linked inhibitor of apoptosis,[128] and possibly heat shock proteins[119] and eIF4γ.[129]

The story is even more complex in that genes such as c-*myc* can undergo cap-dependent translation as well as cap-independent translation whereas proteins such as apoptotic protease-activating factor-1 can be translated only in a cap-independent manner.[126] Furthermore, under restricted protein translation, among the proteins with an internal ribosome entry site, some proteins are translated more actively than others.[126] Heat shock proteins are also found to be transcriptionally up-regulated post-CVB3 infection, serving as a component of the protective response to stress.[49] eIF4γ cleavage by 2A^{pro} or by caspase-3 would cause an imbalance in host cap-dependent and cap-independent translation, of which the results are uncertain.[130] If the net effect of selective inhibition of cap-dependent translation and an increase in cap-independent translation serves to promote apoptosis,[118] it may be a component of a cell-programmed response to blocked translation, which can be life threatening for a cell, to initiate a death response.

Viral protease 2A also cleaves poly-A binding protein, which interacts with eIF4γI and eIF4γII to circularize mRNA and facilitate the reattachment of the ribosome after a round of translation.[131] Poly-A binding protein cleavage may function to arrest viral protein synthesis and to begin RNA packaging late in infection.[122,132,133] Such a cleavage event is compensated for by CVB3-induced host transcriptional up-regulation in infected cells as detected with oligonucleotide arrays.[49]

Poliovirus 3C^{pro} induces drastic morphologic alterations and apoptotic cell death by a caspase-dependent mechanism.[134] Poliovirus 3C^{pro} cleaves c-AMP response element binding protein (CREB/ATF); the transcription factors octomer-binding transcription factor (Oct-1),[135] TFIIIC, and TFIIID (the TATA-binding protein); the histone protein H3;[136,137] and the La autoantigen.[138] Oct-1 regulates the expression of host genes, including H2B and snRNA. Thus, transcription is markedly dysregulated by poliovirus 3C^{pro} and similar effects might be expected for the analogous protease of CVB3. CREB influences transcriptional regulation; nitric oxide slows coxsackieviral replication, and this may be partly explained by its inactivation of the 3C protease.[139] The 3C^{pro}-cleaved fragment of the La protein accumulates in the cytoplasm and is thought to stimulate internal initiation of picornavirus translation in the cytoplasm.[138]

There is a delicate balance between selective membrane permeability and cellular homeostasis that is disrupted during CVB3 infection. As noted earlier, the viral protein 2B can modify plasma membrane, mitochondrial, and endoplasmic reticulum permeability. Damage to the endoplasmic reticulum releases calcium into the cytosol and contributes to cellular damage.[67] Ukimura et al.[140] provided electron microscopic evidence of mitochondrial swelling and rupture in infected mouse hearts, which may involve 2B. Li et al.[141] used confocal microscopy to show increased intracellular calcium concentrations before apoptosis. The increase in calcium is either a catalyst for apoptosis or an epiphenomenon of an increase in membrane permeability. However, increased early cytosolic free calcium plays a role in triggering cardiomyocyte apoptosis.[141] Another direct outcome of the loss of mitochondrial membrane integrity is the release of death "triggers," cyt c, apoptosis-inducing factor, and caspases-2 and -9.[96,98,142] Membrane permeability and calcium release, signaling pathways through Bap31,[143] or the tremendous cellular stress from packaging an influx of viral proteins may all contribute to damage of the endoplasmic reticulum. Endoplasmic reticulum injury activates several pathways, some of which lead to cell death.[143,144]

CVB3 infection leads to 2 separate but related phenomena: cytopathic effect and apoptosis. It is plausible that cytopathic effect is caused by viral protease cleavage of host structural proteins, a subject to be discussed briefly later in this chapter. Carthy et al.[44] demonstrated caspase activation and cleavage of downstream poly-ADP ribose polymerase, a DNA repair enzyme and the inhibitor of DNA fragmentation factor (also known as ICAD) by CVB3 infection. The crucial role of the mitochondrial pathway in activating death processes that occur with CVB3 has been illustrated in work by Carthy et al. (unpublished data). We have shown clearly that cyt c release is upstream of caspase-8 cleavage, and that this release can be blocked by overexpression of Bcl-2 or Bcl-xL.

Viral infection may stimulate apoptosis by several routes, but the most significant contribution seems to come from viral protease cleavage of host structural proteins. Ultraviolet-inactivated encephalomyocarditis virus does not trigger apoptosis, suggesting that virus-mediated apoptosis may be mainly a cytoplasmic event.[109] A better understanding of virus protease cleavage of cell apoptotic, translational, and homeostatic apparatus will be a great step forward in preventing target cell death.

LIFE SIGNALING

The heart encounters a wide variety of insults and has developed mechanisms to protect itself against myocardial ischemia, anoxia, pressure overload, volume overload, viral infection, toxins, and others. Adaptive responses can protect the heart, and such often coincide in fetal gene expression, various stress responses, cytokine induction, and cytoskeletal remodeling, repair, and reclamation.[27] The inability of cardiac myocytes to replicate means that these cells must have an extensive arsenal of host protective mechanisms. Among such mechanisms are those capable of attenuating viral infection, even before the arrival of infiltrating immune cells. There is evidence that the myocytes actively use their antiviral protective mechanisms to protect the heart from CVB3 infections. The interplay between virus-induced death mechanisms and host cell protective mechanisms is a duel for survival not only of individual cells or the organ but also of the host itself. Although there are several groups of viruses that boast effective antiapoptosis proteins that benefit from maintaining host viability, picornaviruses have the opposite strategy. Because they have a short life cycle, these viruses may actually benefit from rapid host cell degradation and apoptotic cell death as opposed to necrotic death, which would bring about a fulminant immune response. We will discuss 6 major groups of protective mechanisms: proteins that target specific apoptosis-mediating molecules, specific MAPK proteins, tyrosine kinases, the phosphatidylinositol-3-kinase (PI3K) signaling pathway, the NFκB signaling pathway, and cytokine release.

Many proteins share high sequence homology to caspases but cannot be processed into active enzymes. Several host antiapoptotic proteins are able to inhibit caspase activity directly. These include the IAP and the FLICE inhibitory protein (FLIP). IAPs were first characterized in baculoviruses and can inhibit the activity of caspases-3 and -7 by binding to these proteases through baculovirus inhibitory domains present in all IAPs.[80,145,146] FLIP was originally characterized as a virally encoded protein isolated from γ-herpesviruses that can inhibit caspase-8 activation in response to death stimuli from Fas-L and tumor necrosis factor-α. Presumably, FLIP can inhibit caspase-8 recruitment to and activation at the death-inducing signaling complex.[147] Although these proteins were originally identified in viruses, many human homologues have been discovered that function in similar fashions to inhibit apoptosis and these include c-IAP-1[148] and c-IAP-2,[146] X chromosome-linked IAP,[149] neuronal apoptosis inhibitor protein,[150] survivin,[151] and c-FLIP.[152] To date, host IAP responses have not been shown to contribute to CVB3 and other enterovirus infections, but it is likely that translation of internal ribosome entry site-containing X chromosome-linked IAP is increased with virus inhibition of cap-dependent translation machinery.[128]

MAPKs are serine/threonine protein kinases that play important roles in intracellular signal transduction pathways that are activated in response to a wide variety of extracellular stimuli, including viral infection. At least 3 kinase members of the MAPK family have been identified in mammals: extracellular signal-regulated kinase (ERK),[153,154] p38 MAPK,[155-157] and c-Jun N-terminal kinase.[158,159] They are characterized by phosphorylation on threonine and tyrosine residues in a TXY motif. Each MAPK pathway consists of 3 kinase modules composed of a MAPK, an upstream MAPK kinase (MAPKK), and a farther upstream MAPKK kinase (MAPKKK). These kinase modules are differentially activated by cellular stimuli and contribute to distinct cellular functions. MAPKs regulate many cellular processes including cell proliferation, differentiation, cell death, and stress responses. This family of proteins may play an important role in viral replication by mediating host cell survival or directly interfering with the virus life cycle.

A diverse set of viruses is known to interact with host cell MAPKs, often by a viral mechanism to augment their survival or as an adaptation to host defense mechanisms. Picornaviruses and adenoviruses have been shown to induce specific MAPKs.[160] In echovirus infection, host gene expression mediated via p38 and ERK1/2 phosphorylation is thought to be an important regulator of host cell behavior.[161] In CVB3-infected HeLa cells, RasGAP cleavage, and Sam68, ERK are phosphorylated and may contribute to pathogenesis.[162] RasGAP and Sam68 mediate signals upstream of Ras and, as alluded to earlier, may be key players in the pathogenesis of CVB3 infection.

Ras is a membrane-bound guanine nucleotide binding protein that interacts with a GTP or GDP molecule to become active or nonactive, respectively.[163] Ras is involved in several important cell signaling mechanisms with an apoptotic and an antiapoptotic contribution, either through JNK or PI3K and ERK.[164-166] This pathway may be activated in response to viral infection to maintain cell viability and to prevent production of viral progeny within the cell and subsequent release into the noncellular environment. Further evidence has shown that in infected isolated non-neonatal murine cardiac myocytes, ERK and p38 are phosphorylated post CVB3 infection (unpublished data). We suspect that the host cell activates ERK to maintain cell viability and that this process initiates an antiviral response.

The significance of MAPK activation is demonstrated in HIV infection, but specific MAPK maintenance of infected cells' lives here is beneficial to the virus and detrimental to the host. Unlike picornaviruses, retroviruses have an extended life cycle, including an extended dormant stage; therefore, prolongation of host viability permits further viral progeny production and infection. ERK activation is considered to increase viral infectivity and viral replication by direct phosphorylation of viral proteins or maintenance of cell viability to allow for viral replication.[167-170] In addition, p38 activation has been shown to increase viral production, and a p38 inhibitor has significantly decreased viral replication.[171,172] Teleologically, cellular ERK stimulation may be aimed at preventing death, and the HIV virus may have adapted to take advantage of this response.

Phosphorylation of MAPKs postinfection with picornaviruses leads to the transcription of immediate early host genes. Echovirus infection induces immediate early gene transcription of *junB*, *jun*, and *fos*, all involved in cell survival, growth, and differentiation.[161] The precise signaling pathway and resultant gene induction depend on the specific agonist, but there seems to be considerable overlap (cross talk) among the different MAPK pathways. CVB3 infection also induces transcription of c-*jun*, c-*fos*, c-*myc*, Elk, and ATF3; a MAPK contribution to transcriptional activation is likely but undetermined (unpublished data). Microarray data from CVB3-infected HeLa cells have shown up-regulation of c-*fos* and MAPK phosphatase-2, suggesting that MAPKs are functionally activated in HeLa cells (unpublished data). MAPK phosphatase-2 (commonly coexpressed with MAPK phosphatase-1) can be stimulated in response to various growth stimuli via ERK and has been shown to limit MAPK-dependent gene expression in vivo.[173,174] As noted, signaling is an interplay of kinases and phosphatases, and if transient or sustained MAPK activation results in proliferation or destructive responses, MAPK phosphatase-2 may be an important determinant of cell viability resulting from MAPK activation post CVB3 infection.[175] Several cardiovascular diseases involve the MAPKs in survival and apoptotic signaling; whether these kinases are primarily responsible for disease or protection against disease is incompletely understood.

Tyrosine phosphorylation is a ubiquitous and important covalent modification in cellular signal transduction. Our group and others have found key tyrosine phosphorylation events that occur during viral infection.[62,176,177] During CVB3 infection, protein tyrosine phosphorylation of a cytosolic 48-kDa and membrane-bound 200-kDa protein occurs 4 hours postinfection.[176] Herbimycin A, a specific inhibitor of src-like tyrosine kinases, reduces tyrosine phosphorylation and the production of progeny virions.[176] It was found that p56*lck* may be necessary for CVB3 replication in T-cell lines, and mice lacking this gene were completely protected from infection.[62]

As mentioned earlier, GPI-anchored proteins, such as DAF, are localized to distinct membrane microdomains or caveolae, a proposed site for increased signal transduction and transcytosis.[178] Signal mediation may be a requirement for internalization either by DAF directly or by a CAR/DAF complex. Notably, p56lck and p59fyn are also associated with the T-cell antigen receptor on Jurkat cells, although only the latter is found to coimmunoprecipitate, implicating a regulatory role for lck.[179] DAF is associated with p56lck, p59fyn, and a yet unidentified 40- to 85-kDa protein.[61] Given that DAF is localized to the outer leaflet of the plasma membrane and tyrosine kinases exist strictly on the inner leaflet, the 85-kDa protein may be a transmembrane protein that binds the receptor-kinase complex.

Protein tyrosine kinase-viral interplay is an important characteristic of CVB3 infection in T cells. HIV-tat also interacts with p56lck, although the precise role of this interaction is incompletely understood.[180] Work by Opavsky et al.[181] has uncovered ERK as one of the downstream targets of p56lck in CVB3-infected T cells. Tyrosine kinases have also been found to induce phosphorylation of Akt during infection with Epstein-Barr virus, although cell survival was not detected.[182] Further work in this exciting area will provide insights into downstream targets of p56lck signaling and its potential role in CVB3 infections in T cells and analogous pathways in cardiac myocytes.

PI3K is activated by growth factors and hormones to deliver cell proliferation and survival signals.[183,184] One of the major downstream targets of PI3K is Akt (*PKB*), a proto-oncogene encoding a serine threonine kinase containing a pleckstrin homology domain at the amino terminal.[185] Akt is a major hypertrophic protein[186] and may exert its cardioprotective effects by phosphorylating the proapoptotic protein BAD and caspase-9, impairing proapoptotic transcription[187] and induction of NFκB transcription.[188-190] Encephalomyocarditis virus infection, in the setting of wortmannin and rapamycin (PI3K pathway inhibitors) enhanced infectivity.[191] It has been shown that the extracellular HIV-1 Tat protein can rapidly stimulate the PI3K pathway to decrease apoptosis in Jurkat cells.[192] Hepatitis B virus X protein also alleviates apoptosis through the activation of the PI3-kinase signaling pathway.[193] Thus, the PI3K pathway may contribute a similar protective function in CVB3 infections.

NFκB was first described as an activator of gene transcription in B-lymphocyte nuclei and is now known to be a ubiquitous transcriptional regulator that controls various cellular functions ranging from immune reactions to growth control.[194] The NFκB pathway is activated by several growth factors and cytokines, stress stimuli, free radicals, and viral agents. NFκB proteins all contain an N-terminal Rel-homology domain that mediates dimerization, its interaction with the inhibitor of NFκB (IκB-alpha, -beta, -epsilon, -gamma, -delta; Bcl-3),[195] nuclear translocation, and DNA binding. Activation of the NFκB pathway, in most instances, involves the phosphorylation of IκB and degradation of IκB by the 26s proteasome and subsequent NFκB nuclear translocation and gene transcription. Such genes transcribed include the apoptosis inhibitors TRAF1, TRAF2, c-IAP1, and c-IAP2.[196]

The NFκB family of transcription factors is a double-edged sword in viral infections. Although in most instances pro-life genes are up-regulated, NFκB can also facilitate death through either pro-death genes or other unknown pathways. The contrasting effects of NFκB may be partly explained by formation of different Rel/NFκB, homodimers and heterodimers, which have various affinities for different κB sites.[197] Potential proapoptotic gene products under the control of the NFκB family of transcription factors are caspase-1, Fas-L, and p53.[197] Evidence suggests early cytoprotection by NFκB, but prolonged activation appears to lead to death. Perhaps such activation provides a way to distinguish between cells that are recoverable and those that are irreversibly damaged. This balance of proapoptotic and antiapoptotic signaling of NFκB illustrates the cell's intricate system of checks and balances.

HIV-1,[198] cytomegalovirus, Simian virus 40, adenovirus, and other viruses have effects through modulation of NFκB. In HIV-1, NFκB binds the genome and allows for efficient transcription.[199] Viral induction of NFκB may serve 2 countering functions: NFκB mediates ligand-induced cell death but is well recognized as a cytoprotective protein. Numerous antiapoptotic gene products have been recognized, including the zinc finger protein A20, IAPs,[200] and members of the Bcl-2 family.[198] Bcl-2-mediated loss of IκB-alpha and subsequent NFκB translocation illustrate an interaction between these 2 pathways.[201] On the other hand, encephalomyocarditis virus, a picornavirus, requires NFκB for infection.[105]

Reovirus, a double-stranded RNA virus, uses NFκB as a proapoptotic protein, and the use of proteasome inhibitors has been shown to circumvent apoptosis.[202] Human T-cell leukemia virus Tax protein induces NFκB, which in turn promotes transcription of cellular proteins that complement human T-cell leukemia virus proteins.[203] The ability of infected cells to circumvent apoptotic processes supports an attractive hypothesis that failure to activate the death pathway results in chronic infection.[204]

Finally, in response to viral infection, cardiac myocytes release cytokines such as CT-1, interleukin-1α, and tumor necrosis factor-α, which may be considered a survival mechanism.[205] CT-1 may play an important role in infection, by regulation of other cytokines and prevention of apoptosis by gp130 and leukemia inhibitory factor signaling and possibly by a MAPK signaling pathway.[206] Infected myocytes release tumor necrosis factor-α, a multifunctional proinflammatory cytokine that can induce life or death machinery. Besides catalyzing the immune response, increased tumor necrosis factor-α has been shown to depress cardiac function and may beget skeletal muscle atrophy that occurs primarily through the NFκB pathway.[207,208] Tumor necrosis factor-α, interleukin-1α, interleukin-6, and interferon-β were increased at day 3 after experimental CVB3 infection.[209] These cytokines are also potent inducible nitric oxide synthase regulators in the myocardium and can lead to formation of nitric oxide, which has antiviral properties.[210] Nitric oxide has been shown to nitrosylate and attenuate viral protease 3C,[139] caspase-3,[211] and just recently viral protease 2A.[212] Through activation of host protective mechanisms, attenuation of viral proteases, and other yet to be determined mechanisms, cytokines may prolong the survival of target cells.

LATE PHENOTYPIC CHANGES

The determining factors for late phenotypic changes in the heart are enterovirus-mediated injury, pretranslational altered gene expression, and post-translational modifications of key myocyte and interstitial cell proteins. The interplay of life and death signaling pathways invoked by virus and host is pertinent to the discussion of what is host-beneficial and what is host-detrimental (Fig. 7-5). Structurally, cardiac hypertrophy is considered a disease of the sarcomere,[213,214] but the primary cytoskeletal disruption in other cardiomyopathies, including myocarditis and subsequent dilated cardiomyopathy (DCM) is less clear. DCM may result from cytoskeletal protein mutation, post-translational alteration, or cytoskeletal accumulation.[215]

Viral infection leads to extensive cytoskeletal alterations through actions of viral proteases; this is an important step for progeny virus release. 3C^pro cleavage of the microtubule-associated protein MAP-4 is thought to contribute to late cytoskeletal remodeling.[216] The 2A^pro-specific cleavage of dystrophin at the hinge 3 region disconnects

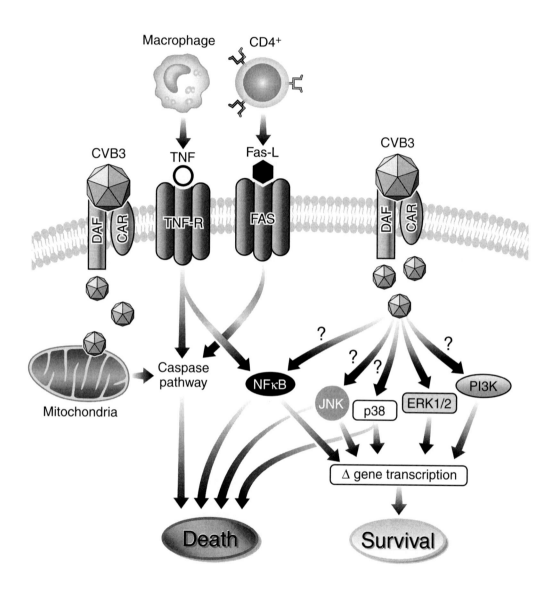

Fig. 7-5. Conceptual model for the delicate balance between intracellular pro-life and pro-death signaling, as triggered by coxsackievirus B3 (*CVB3*) infection. Viral coligation to the coxsackievirus and adenovirus receptor (*CAR*) and decay-accelerating factor (*DAF*) receptor and endocytosis activate mitochondrial-mediated death signaling. Activated macrophages and CD4+ T cells release tumor necrosis factor (*TNF*) family cytokines and Fas ligand, respectively, thereby stimulating receptor-mediated apoptotic and anti-apoptotic pathways. Specific MAPK signaling modules, NFκB, and PI3K pathways are potential host survival signaling mechanisms stimulated in response to CVB3 infection. *JNK*, c-Jun N-terminal kinase.

the cytoskeletal actin-binding site from the beta-dystroglycan extracellular matrix anchor, completely disrupting the cytoskeletal architecture.[217] Structural proteins may have scaffolding or docking functions especially important to forming carefully constructed signaling highways. Therefore, dystrophin cleavage by 2A[pro] may affect scaffolding functions of this cytoskeletal protein.[218] Host protein synthesis shutoff (mentioned earlier) during these structural cleavage events prevents replacement of cleaved proteins, augmenting the damaging effects of structural loss. The dystrophin-glycoprotein complex is the primary cause of Duchenne muscular dystrophy[213,214] and has been identified in patients with familial DCM and more recently in viral myocarditis leading to DCM.[219] The progression of myocarditis to DCM has been confirmed in experimental models and in patient populations.[220] The 2A protease has also been shown to cleave the intermediate filament family member, cytokeratin 8, which corresponds to the onset of observed cytopathic effect.[117]

Repetitive or persistent CVB3 infection, a product of restricted viral replication and gene expression, may also lead to a phenotype similar to that seen in DCM, the primary cause of which is viral myocarditis.[221-224] DCM from myocarditis is particularly devastating because dystrophin cleavage is a sudden occurrence that does not allow for any compensatory mechanisms. Dystrophin loss has been shown to result in necrosis, hypertrophy, activation of stress-activated signaling, key destructive processes leading to defective signaling, and contractile insufficiency eventually resulting in cell death.[225] Severe cytoskeletal disruption may lead to accumulation of dysfunctional cytoskeletal proteins. Cytoskeletal abnormalities are particularly devastating because they may contribute to substantial instability by dislodging mitochondria, Golgi apparatus, nuclei, and myofibrils. Architectural changes also contribute to cellular signal transduction dysfunction, especially that of membrane-nuclear signaling.

The ventricular myocardium normally consists of cardiac myocytes (20% of cells), endothelial cells (10%), and connective tissue fibroblasts (70%). The muscle is well organized, such that every myocyte is directly perfused and the contractile force generated is transmitted to the extracellular matrix. The cardiac myocyte cytoskeleton is made up of sarcomeric proteins, the cytoskeletal proteins, the membrane-associated proteins, and the proteins of the intercalated disk.[215] Introduction of a viral agonist to this highly ordered system results in a complex, multistaged potentially destructive duel between the virus and host.

Viral myocarditis results in a patchy pattern of infection, which has an important impact on resultant myocardial organization postinfection.[45] Often a myocyte will have a fulminant viral load, whereas its neighbors remain wholly unaffected. The importance of viral receptors in determining tissue tropism suggests the possibility of a "receptor-mediated pattern" in the heart; some heart tissues may be naturally more resistant to viral injury than others.[35,226,227] However, patchy distributions of infection within the same heart seems unlikely to be a result of receptor expression or function. Differences in intracellular protein interactions involved in viral transcription and translation, antiviral factors, and virus-activating proteins-host proteinases may be determining factors.

The overall results of varying viral activity and host response include heterogeneity in integrity, size, and other characteristics of the myocytes. Some cells undergo infection and overloading of the cell circuitry, leading to necrosis. Others may succumb to apoptosis by virus-induced death or "host-protective" machinery. The observed heterogeneous phenotype of the healing heart is consistent with apoptosis, wherein dying cells minimally disrupt their neighbors. Myocyte dropout by either of these processes, necrosis or apoptosis, alters the intricate organization of the myocardium that leads to inefficient force transmission, an inability to normalize chamber pressure, and mediation of the destructive process of dilation. Myocyte death, myocyte slippage, and excessive interstitial fibrosis alter the dynamics of load distribution in the myocardium, eventually leading to diastolic dysfunction. Cardiac fibrosis entails increases in matrix collagens and changes in ratio of type, cross-links, and organization. Microarray analysis revealed that extracellular matrix proteins were up-regulated early postinfection, suggestive of an active reparative process.[49]

Infected myocytes that remain alive may atrophy by ATP-dependent degradation of the cytoskeleton, viral inhibition of host structural protein translation, and a resultant mismatch in the myosin heavy chain (MHC) isoforms. Viral infection results in MHC alteration to a slow (α) isoform and reduced unloaded sarcomere shortening.[228] Failing ventricles often exhibit loss of α-MHC and concomitant up-regulation of β-MHC. The reduced enzymatic activity of β-MHC generates substantial loss in myofibrillar ATPase activity and systolic contractile function which may contribute to diastolic dysfunction.[229] Atrophic phenotypes are comparable to skeletal muscle wasting in cancer-associated cachexia[207] and to decreased load causing myocardial atrophy,[230] which target MHC and other contractile proteins.[231]

Still other myocytes may exhibit a forme fruste of all or some of the above conditions. In response to an agonist, the heart may undergo myocyte migration and slippage, rearrangement of the cytoskeleton, alterations in metabolism, or increased vascularization that adds to cardiac disorganization. Controversial evidence suggests that adult myocytes can replicate in response to stress.[232,233] Perhaps increased load due to dying myocytes forces others to replicate in a limited fashion. Finally, noninfected myocytes must take up the responsibility for contraction and hypertrophy to normalize excess wall stress. Load increases in the heart have been identified as a precursor in cardiac diseases, which suggests a vicious cycle of heterogeneity and myocardial inefficiency. Cytokines play an important role in myocarditis and it is perplexing that myocytes can coexist in a similar microenvironment yet exhibit such varying phenotypes.

FUTURE DIRECTIONS

The search for transcriptional regulatory events postinfection has led to some interesting hypotheses regarding the contribution of death-regulating proteins in viral infections. Using mRNA differential display, we have found several important regulatory and structural proteins that are up- or down-regulated postinfection.[234] Among the down-regulated proteins are Nip21, a Bcl-2 binding protein structurally similar to human Nip2.[104, 234] The Nip proteins interact with the adenovirus E1B (19-kDa protein), the Epstein-Barr virus BHRF1, and Bcl-2 but not Bax, suggesting that they promote Bcl-2-mediated cell survival in several viral systems.[104, 235] The significance of Nip21 in cell survival and death is first due to its high sequence homology (66% similarity in a 126-amino acid region) to the GTPase-activating protein, Rho-GAP,[236] which raises the possibility that Nip21 is involved in signal transduction pathways. Second, Nip21 shares high sequence similarity with human Nip2, which is capable of interacting with the apoptosis regulator Bcl-2 and a homologous protein, the adenovirus E1B (19-kDa protein).[104] Mutational analysis has indicated that human Nip2 may interact with Bcl-2 to promote cell survival. Therefore, Nip21 down-regulation by CVB3 infection in the host may promote myocyte cell death, an early feature of CVB3-induced disease.[46]

Oligonucleotide arrays, biostatistics, and bioinformatics combine as powerful tools for studying the transient up- and down-regulation of specific signaling pathways and resultant transcriptional activity.[237] Several strategies have been used to uncover the transcriptional events surrounding infection by echovirus,[238] HIV-1,[239] herpes simplex virus,[240,241] and cytomegalovirus.[242] An interesting observation coming from these studies is the similarities of the cell response to various agonists, which begs the question whether there is a stereotypic cell response to a range of pathogens.[243] DNA arrays have also shed some light on the time-dependent changes in transcriptional activity in an in vivo mouse model of CVB3-induced myocarditis.[49] Oligonucleotide or cDNA array data must include a combination of replicates and be supported by confirmatory assays such as northern blot or quantitative reverse transcription polymerase chain reaction.[237] Genomics and soon high-throughput proteomics will play an increasingly important role in developing hypotheses and identifying key signaling events.[244]

Currently, there are no clinically relevant antiviral drugs for the treatment of enterovirus infection. One promising strategy is antisense oligonucleotides targeting the viral multiplication cycle. Sequence complementation between the antisense oligonucleotides and key sites within viral RNA could effectively arrest viral transcription and translation. Additional targets are genes encoding enzymes critical for viral proliferation and other factors inducing myocyte death.

CONCLUSION

Viral infection of the heart is not a unilateral attack on the myocardium, with the tissue waiting helplessly for the systemic immune response to come to the rescue. The virus is met with strategic defensive and offensive tactics evolved to preserve the integrity of the heart, truly creating a duel between virus and host target organs. Once the virus infects its host by the use of viral protease cleavages and compromise of mitochondrial integrity, it then attempts to induce cell death. Myocyte survival mechanisms such as IAPs, the MAPK family of proteins, PI3K, and NFκB are able to block a quick death at the hands of CVB3, but pro-life mechanisms in the cell may prove detrimental for the organ and the host. Resultant apoptosis and necrosis are at an extreme end of a wide range of potential processes that lead to an altered cell phenotype. Infected myocytes express phenotypes that are reminiscent of apoptotic and necrotic processes. A pertinent question of apoptosis relevant to many diseases is whether these cells are irreversibly damaged or whether they can retain their function and contribute synergistically with the rest of the myocardium. However, prolonging survival of infected myocytes may just provide a reservoir for virus that facilitates chronic infection of the heart.[105] It is uncertain if the progression of myocarditis to DCM can be stopped or slowed by salvage of the myocytes that are on a path to apoptosis. Through elucidation of important signaling events after viral infection, we will gain insight into the complex interplay between virus and host and the dance of life and death signals.

ACKNOWLEDGMENTS

The authors thank the Heart and Stroke Foundation of British Columbia and Yukon, the Medical Research Council of Canada, the Michael Smith Foundation for Health Research, and the St. Paul's Hospital Foundation for support. The authors are also grateful to other members of the Cardiovascular Research Laboratory for their critical appraisal of this manuscript.

REFERENCES

1. Pohl SL, Birnbaumer L, Rodbell M. The glucagon-sensitive adenyl cyclase system in plasma membranes of rat liver. I. Properties. J Biol Chem 1971;246:1849-1856.
2. Rodbell M, Birnbaumer L, Phol SL, Krans HM. The glucagon-sensitive adenylcyclase system in plasma membranes of rat liver. V. An obligatory role of guanylnucleotides in glucagon action. J Biol Chem 1971;246:1877-1882.

3. Taylor SS, Buechler JA, Yonemoto W. cAMP-dependent protein kinase: framework for a diverse family of regulatory enzymes. Annu Rev Biochem 1990;59:971-1005.

4. Ross EM, Gilman AG. Resolution of some components of adenylate cyclase necessary for catalytic activity. J Biol Chem 1977;252:6966-6969.

5. Ross EM, Howlett AC, Ferguson KM, Gilman AG. Reconstitution of hormone-sensitive adenylate cyclase activity with resolved components of the enzyme. J Biol Chem 1978;253:6401-6412.

6. Krebs EG, Beavo JA. Phosphorylation-dephosphorylation of enzymes. Annu Rev Biochem 1979;48:923-959.

7. Hunter T, Cooper JA. Protein-tyrosine kinases. Annu Rev Biochem 1985;54:897-930.

8. Seger R, Krebs EG. The MAPK signaling cascade. FASEB J 1995;9:726-735.

9. Gilman AG. G proteins: transducers of receptor-generated signals. Annu Rev Biochem 1987;56:615-649.

10. Egan SE, Giddings BW, Brooks MW, Buday L, Sizeland AM, Weinberg RA. Association of Sos Ras exchange protein with Grb2 is implicated in tyrosine kinase signal transduction and transformation. Nature 1993;363:45-51.

11. Santos E, Nebreda AR. Structural and functional properties of ras proteins. FASEB J 1989;3:2151-2163.

12. Karin M, Hunter T. Transcriptional control by protein phosphorylation: signal transmission from the cell surface to the nucleus. Curr Biol 1995;5:747-757.

13. Virchow R. Cellular pathology. As based upon physiological and pathological histology. Lecture XVI—Atheromatous affection of arteries, 1858. Nutr Rev 1989;47:23-25.

14. Yuan J. Evolutionary conservation of a genetic pathway of programmed cell death. J Cell Biochem 1996;60:4-11.

15. Chinnaiyan AM, O'Rourke K, Lane BR, Dixit VM. Interaction of CED-4 with CED-3 and CED-9: a molecular framework for cell death. Science 1997;275:1122-1126.

16. Nicholson DW. Caspase structure, proteolytic substrates, and function during apoptotic cell death. Cell Death Differ 1999;6:1028-1042.

17. Thornberry NA, Rano TA, Peterson EP, Rasper DM, Timkey T, Garcia-Calvo M, Houtzager VM, Nordstrom PA, Roy S, Vaillancourt JP, Chapman KT, Nicholson DW. A combinatorial approach defines specificities of members of the caspase family and granzyme B. Functional relationships established for key mediators of apoptosis. J Biol Chem 1997;272:17907-17911.

18. Voiculescu M, Ciugarin-Brailoiu M, Dancu I, Chiotan M, Baltiev A. Enterovirus diseases with neurological determinations in adults. Clinical and virological study. Virologie 1979;30:207-216.

19. Leroy EM, Baize S, Volchkov VE, Fisher-Hoch SP, Georges-Courbot MC, Lansoud-Soukate J, Capron M, Debre P, McCormick JB, Georges AJ. Human asymptomatic Ebola infection and strong inflammatory response. Lancet 2000;355:2210-2215.

20. Berger TM, Caduff JH, Gebbers JO. Fatal varicella-zoster virus antigen-positive giant cell arteritis of the central nervous system. Pediatr Infect Dis J 2000;19:653-656.

21. Hardwick JM. Virus-induced apoptosis. Adv Pharmacol 1997;41:295-336.

22. Granville DJ, Carthy CM, Yang D, Hunt DW, McManus BM. Interaction of viral proteins with host cell death machinery. Cell Death Differ 1998;5:653-659.

23. Duckett CS, Nava VE, Gedrich RW, Clem RJ, Van Dongen JL, Gilfillan MC, Shiels H, Hardwick JM, Thompson CB. A conserved family of cellular genes related to the baculovirus iap gene and encoding apoptosis inhibitors. EMBO J 1996;15:2685-2694.

24. Rapp UR, Goldsborough MD, Mark GE, Bonner TI, Groffen J, Reynolds FH Jr, Stephenson JR. Structure and biological activity of v-raf, a unique oncogene transduced by a retrovirus. Proc Natl Acad Sci U S A 1983;80:4218-4222.

25. Stehelin D, Varmus HE, Bishop JM, Vogt PK. DNA related to the transforming gene(s) of avian sarcoma viruses is present in normal avian DNA. Nature 1976;260:170-173.

26. Urguidi V, Tarin D, Goodison S. Role of telomerase in cell senescence and oncogenesis. Annu Rev Med 2000;51:65-79.

27. Hunter JJ, Chien KR. Signaling pathways for cardiac hypertrophy and failure. N Engl J Med 1999;341:1276-1283.

28. Woodruff JF. Viral myocarditis. A review. Am J Pathol 1980;101:425-484.

29. Kawai C. Idiopathic cardiomyopathy. A study on the infectious-immune theory as a cause of the disease. Jpn Circ J 1971;35:765-770.

30. Kereiakes DJ, Parmley WW. Myocarditis and cardiomyopathy. Am Heart J 1984;108:1318-1326.

31. Kopecky SL, Gersh BJ. Dilated cardiomyopathy and myocarditis: natural history, etiology, clinical manifestations, and management. Curr Probl Cardiol 1987;12:569-647.

32. Martino TA, Liu P, Petric M, Sole MJ. Enteroviral myocarditis and dilated cardiomyopathy: a review of clinical and experimental studies. In: Rotbart H, ed. Human enterovirus infections. Washington, DC: ASM Press, 1995:291-352.

33. Sole MJ, Liu P. Viral myocarditis: a paradigm for understanding the pathogenesis and treatment of dilated cardiomyopathy. J Am Coll Cardiol 1993;22 Suppl A:99A-105A.

34. Kandolf R, Ameis D, Kirschner P, Canu A, Hofschneider PH. In situ detection of enteroviral genomes in myocardial cells by nucleic acid hybridization: an approach to the diagnosis of viral heart disease. Proc Natl Acad Sci U S A 1987;84:6272-6276.

35. Carthy CM, Yang D, Anderson DR, Wilson JE, McManus BM. Myocarditis as systemic disease: new perspectives on pathogenesis. Clin Exp Pharmacol Physiol 1997;24:997-1003.

36. Yu JZ, Wilson JE, Wood SM, Kandolf R, Klingel K, Yang D, McManus BM. Secondary heterotypic versus homotypic infection by Coxsackie B group viruses: impact on early and late histopathological lesions and virus genome prominence. Cardiovasc Pathol 1999;8:93-102.

37. Blay R, Simpson K, Leslie K, Huber S. Coxsackievirus-induced disease. CD4+ cells initiate both myocarditis and pancreatitis in DBA/2 mice. Am J Pathol 1989;135:899-907.

38. Leslie K, Blay R, Haisch C, Lodge A, Weller A, Huber S. Clinical and experimental aspects of viral myocarditis. Clin Microbiol Rev 1989;2:191-203.

39. Lodge PA, Herzum M, Olszewski J, Huber SA. Coxsackievirus B-3 myocarditis. Acute and chronic forms of the disease caused by different immunopathogenic mechanisms. Am J Pathol 1987;128:455-463.

40. Weremeichik H, Moraska A, Herzum M, Weller A, Huber SA. Naturally occurring anti-idiotypic antibodies—mechanisms for autoimmunity and immunoregulation? Eur Heart J 1991;12 Suppl D:154-157.

41. Beck MA, Chapman NM, McManus BM, Mullican JC, Tracy S. Secondary enterovirus infection in the murine model of myocarditis. Pathologic and immunologic aspects. Am J Pathol 1990;136:669-681.

42. Mason JW, O'Connell JB, Herskowitz A, Rose NR, McManus BM, Billingham ME, Moon TE. A clinical trial of immunosuppressive therapy for myocarditis. The Myocarditis Treatment Trial Investigators. N Engl J Med 1995;333:269-275.

43. Arola A, Kalimo H, Ruuskanen O, Hyypia T. Experimental myocarditis induced by two different coxsackievirus B3 variants: aspects of pathogenesis and comparison of diagnostic methods. J Med Virol 1995;47:251-259.

44. Carthy CM, Granville DJ, Watson KA, Anderson DR, Wilson JE, Yang D, Hunt DWC, McManus BM. Caspase activation and specific cleavage of substrates after coxsackievirus B3-induced cytopathic effect in HeLa cells. J Virol 1998;72:7669-7675.

45. Chow LH, Beisel KW, McManus BM. Enteroviral infection of mice with severe combined immunodeficiency. Evidence for direct viral pathogenesis of myocardial injury. Lab Invest 1992;66:24-31.

46. McManus BM, Chow LH, Wilson JE, Anderson DR, Guilizia JM, Gauntt CJ, Klingel KE, Beisel KW, Kandolf R. Direct myocardial injury by enterovirus: a central role in the evolution of murine myocarditis. Clin Immunol Immunopathol 1993;68:159-169.

47. Klingel K, Rieger P, Mall G, Selinka HC, Huber M, Kandolf R. Visualization of enteroviral replication in myocardial tissue by ultrastructural in situ hybridization: identification of target cells and cytopathic effects. Lab Invest 1998;78:1227-1237.

48. Liu P, Martino T, Opavsky MA, Penninger J. Viral myocarditis: balance between viral infection and immune response. Can J Cardiol 1996;12:935-943.

49. Taylor LA, Carthy CM, Yang D, Saad K, Wong D, Schreiner G, Stanton LW, McManus BM. Host gene regulation during coxsackievirus B3 infection in mice: assessment by microarrays. Circ Res 2000;87:328-334.

50. Stanton LW, Garrard LJ, Damm D, Garrick BL, Lam A, Kapoun AM, Zheng Q, Protter AA, Schreiner GF, White RT. Altered patterns of gene expression in response to myocardial infarction. Circ Res 2000;86:939-945.

51. Abdellatif M. Leading the way using microarray: a more comprehensive approach for discovery of gene expression patterns. Circ Res 2000;86:919-920.

52. Rossmann MG, Bella J, Kolatkar PR, He Y, Wimmer E, Kuhn RJ, Baker TS. Cell recognition and entry by rhino- and enteroviruses. Virology 2000;269:239-247.

53. Holland JJ, McLaren LC, Syverton JT. The mammalian cell-virus relationship. IV. Infection of naturally insusceptible cells with enterovirus ribonucleic acid. J Exp Med 1959;110:65-80.

54. Kuhn RJ. Identification and biology of cellular receptors for the coxsackie B viruses group. Curr Top Microbiol Immunol 1997;223:209-226.

55. White JM, Littman DR. Viral receptors of the immunoglobulin superfamily. Cell 1989;56:725-728.

56. Crowell RL, Krah DL, Mapoles J, Landau BJ. Methods for assay of cellular receptors for picornaviruses. Methods Enzymol 1983;96:443-452.

57. Krah DL, Crowell RL. A solid-phase assay of solubilized HeLa cell membrane receptors for binding group B coxsackieviruses and polioviruses. Virology 1982;118:148-156.

58. Bergelson JM, Krithivas A, Celi L, Droguett G, Horwitz MS, Wickham T, Crowell RL, Finberg RW. The murine CAR homolog is a receptor for coxsackie B viruses and adenoviruses. J Virol 1998;72:415-419.

59. Martino TA, Petric M, Weingartl H, Bergelson JM, Opavsky MA, Richardson CD, Modlin JF, Finberg RW, Kain KC, Willis N, Gauntt CJ, Liu PP. The coxsackie-adenovirus receptor (CAR) is used by reference strains and clinical isolates representing all six serotypes of coxsackievirus group B and by swine vesicular disease virus. Virology 2000;271:99-108.

60. Medof ME, Lublin DM, Holers VM, Ayers DJ, Getty RR, Leykam JF, Atkinson JP, Tykocinski ML. Cloning and characterization of cDNAs encoding the complete sequence of decay-accelerating factor of human complement. Proc Natl Acad Sci U S A 1987;84:2007-2011.

61. Shenoy-Scaria AM, Kwong J, Fujita T, Olszowy MW, Shaw AS, Lublin DM. Signal transduction through decay-accelerating factor. Interaction of glycosyl-phosphatidylinositol anchor and protein tyrosine kinases p56lck and p59fyn 1. J Immunol 1992;149:3535-3541.

62. Liu P, Aitken K, Kong YY, Opavsky MA, Martino T, Dawood F, Wen WH, Kozieradzki I, Bachmaier K, Straus D, Mak TW, Penninger JM. The tyrosine kinase p56lck is essential in coxsackievirus B3-mediated heart disease. Nat Med 2000;6:429-434.

63. Liu PP, Opavsky MA. Viral myocarditis: receptors that bridge the cardiovascular with the immune system? Circ Res 2000;86:253-254.

64. de Verdugo UR, Selinka HC, Huber M, Kramer B, Kellermann J, Hofschneider PH, Kandolf R. Characterization of a 100-kilodalton binding protein for the six serotypes of coxsackie B viruses. J Virol 1995;69:6751-6757.

65. Qiu J, Brown KE. A 110-kDa nuclear shuttle protein, nucleolin, specifically binds to adeno-associated virus type 2 (AAV-2) capsid. Virology 1999;257:373-382.

66. Yang D, Wilson JE, Anderson DR, Bohunek L, Cordeiro C, Kandolf R, McManus BM. In vitro mutational and inhibitory analysis of the cis-acting translational elements within the 5' untranslated region of coxsackievirus B3: potential targets for antiviral action of antisense oligomers. Virology 1997;228:63-73.

67. van Kuppeveld FJ, Hoenderop JG, Smeets RL, Willems PH, Dijkman HB, Galama JM, Melchers WJ. Coxsackievirus protein 2B modifies endoplasmic reticulum membrane and plasma membrane permeability and facilitates virus release. EMBO J 1997;16:3519-3532.

68. Trump BF, Berezesky IK, Chang SH, Phelps PC. The pathways of cell death: oncosis, apoptosis, and necrosis. Toxicol Pathol 1997;25:82-88.

69. Majno G, Joris I. Apoptosis, oncosis, and necrosis. An overview of cell death. Am J Pathol 1995;146:3-15.

70. Fiers W, Beyaert R, Declercq W, Vandenabeele P. More than one way to die: apoptosis, necrosis and reactive oxygen damage. Oncogene 1999;18:7719-7730.

71. Kerr JF, Winterford CM, Harmon BV. Apoptosis. Its significance in cancer and cancer therapy. Cancer 1994;73:2013-2026.

72. Saraste A, Pulkki K. Morphologic and biochemical hallmarks of apoptosis. Cardiovasc Res 2000;45:528-537.

73. Kerr JF, Wyllie AH, Currie AR. Apoptosis: a basic biological phenomenon with wide-ranging implications in tissue kinetics. Br J Cancer 1972;26:239-257.

74. Wyllie AH, Kerr JF, Currie AR. Cell death: the significance of apoptosis. Int Rev Cytol 1980;68:251-306.

75. Wyllie AH. The genetic regulation of apoptosis. Curr Opin Genet Dev 1995;5:97-104.

76. Thompson CB. Apoptosis in the pathogenesis and treatment of disease. Science 1995;267:1456-1462.

77. Thornberry NA, Lazebnik Y. Caspases: enemies within. Science 1998;281:1312-1316.

78. Kayalar C, Ord T, Testa MP, Zhong LT, Bredesen DE. Cleavage of actin by interleukin 1 beta-converting enzyme to reverse DNase I inhibition. Proc Natl Acad Sci U S A 1996;93:2234-2238.

79. Cryns VL, Bergeron L, Zhu H, Li H, Yuan J. Specific cleavage of alpha-fodrin during Fas- and tumor necrosis factor-induced apoptosis is mediated by an interleukin-1 beta-converting enzyme/Ced-3 protease distinct from the poly(ADP-ribose) polymerase protease. J Biol Chem 1996;271:31277-31282.

80. Takahashi A, Alnemri ES, Lazebnik YA, Fernandes-Alnemri T, Litwack G, Moir RD, Goldman RD, Poirier GG, Kaufmann SH, Earnshaw WC. Cleavage of lamin A by Mch2 alpha but not CPP32: multiple interleukin 1 beta-converting enzyme-related proteases with distinct substrate recognition properties are active in apoptosis. Proc Natl Acad Sci U S A 1996;93:8395-8400.

81. Neamati N, Fernandez A, Wright S, Kiefer J, McConkey DJ. Degradation of lamin B1 precedes oligonucleosomal DNA fragmentation in apoptotic thymocytes and isolated thymocyte nuclei. J Immunol 1995;154:3788-3795.

82. Wen LP, Fahrni JA, Troie S, Guan JL, Orth K, Rosen GD. Cleavage of focal adhesion kinase by caspases during apoptosis. J Biol Chem 1997;272:26056-26061.

83. Cosulich SC, Horiuchi H, Zerial M, Clarke PR, Woodman PG. Cleavage of rabaptin-5 blocks endosome fusion during apoptosis. EMBO J 1997;16:6182-6191.

84. Caulin C, Salvesen GS, Oshima RG. Caspase cleavage of keratin 18 and reorganization of intermediate filaments during epithelial cell apoptosis. J Cell Biol 1997;138:1379-1394.

85. Kothakota S, Azuma T, Reinhard C, Klippel A, Tang J, Chu K, McGarry TJ, Kirschner MW, Koths K, Kwiatkowski DJ, Williams LT. Caspase-3-generated fragment of gelsolin: effector of morphological change in apoptosis. Science 1997;278:294-298.

86. Schulze-Osthoff K, Ferrari D, Los M, Wesselborg S, Peter ME. Apoptosis signaling by death receptors. Eur J Biochem 1998;254:439-459.

87. Muzio M, Chinnaiyan AM, Kischkel FC, O'Rourke K, Shevchenko A, Ni J, Scaffidi C, Bretz JD, Zhang M, Gentz R, Mann M, Krammer PH, Peter ME, Dixit VM. FLICE, a novel FADD-homologous ICE/CED-3-like protease, is recruited to the CD95 (Fas/APO-1) death-inducing signaling complex. Cell 1996;85:817-827.

88. Muzio M, Stockwell BR, Stennicke HR, Salvesen GS, Dixit VM. An induced proximity model for caspase-8 activation. J Biol Chem 1998;273:2926-2930.

89. Li P, Nijhawan D, Budihardjo I, Srinivasula SM, Ahmad M, Alnemri ES, Wang X. Cytochrome c and dATP-dependent formation of Apaf-1/caspase-9 complex initiates an apoptotic protease cascade. Cell 1997;91:479-489.

90. Luo X, Budihardjo I, Zou H, Slaughter C, Wang X. Bid, a Bcl2 interacting protein, mediates cytochrome c release from mitochondria in response to activation of cell surface death receptors. Cell 1998;94:481-490.

91. Yang J, Liu X, Bhalla K, Kim CN, Ibrado AM, Cai J, Peng TI, Jones DP, Wang X. Prevention of apoptosis by Bcl-2: release of cytochrome c from mitochondria blocked. Science 1997;275:1129-1132.

92. Kluck RM, Bossy-Wetzel E, Green DR, Newmeyer DD. The release of cytochrome c from mito-chondria: a primary site for Bcl-2 regulation of apoptosis. Science 1997;275:1132-1136.

93. Yang E, Zha J, Jockel J, Boise LH, Thompson CB, Korsmeyer SJ. Bad, a heterodimeric partner for Bcl-XL and Bcl-2, displaces Bax and promotes cell death. Cell 1995;80:285-291.

94. Kiefer MC, Brauer MJ, Powers VC, Wu JJ, Umansky SR, Tomei LD, Barr PJ. Modulation of apop-tosis by the widely distributed Bcl-2 homologue Bak. Nature 1995;374:736-739.

95. Gajewski TF, Thompson CB. Apoptosis meets signal transduction: elimination of a BAD influence. Cell 1996;87:589-592.

96. Susin SA, Lorenzo HK, Zamzami N, Marzo I, Brenner C, Larochette N, Prevost MC, Alzari PM, Kroemer G. Mitochondrial release of caspase-2 and -9 during the apoptotic process. J Exp Med 1999;189:381-394.

97. Daugas E, Susin SA, Zamzami N, Ferri KF, Irinopoulou T, Larochette N, Prevost MC, Leber B, Andrews D, Penninger J, Kroemer G. Mitochondrio-nuclear translocation of AIF in apoptosis and necrosis. FASEB J 2000;14:729-739.

98. Susin SA, Lorenzo HK, Zamzami N, Marzo I, Snow BE, Brothers GM, Mangion J, Jacotot E, Costantini P, Loeffler M, Larochette N, Goodlett DR, Aebersold R, Siderovski DP, Penninger JM, Kroemer G. Molecular characterization of mitochondrial apoptosis-inducing factor. Nature 1999;397:441-446.

99. Du C, Fang M, Li Y, Li L, Wang X. Smac, a mitochondrial protein that promotes cytochrome c-dependent caspase activation by eliminating IAP inhibition. Cell 2000;102:33-42.

100. Anversa P, Kajstura J. Myocyte cell death in the diseased heart. Circ Res 1998;82:1231-1233.

101. Yamada T, Matsumori A, Wang WZ, Ohashi N, Shiota K, Sasayama S. Apoptosis in congestive heart failure induced by viral myocarditis in mice. Heart Vessels 1999;14:29-37.

102. Colston JT, Chandrasekar B, Freeman GL. Expression of apoptosis-related proteins in experimental coxsackievirus myocarditis. Cardiovasc Res 1998;38:158-168.

103. Yew PR, Berk AJ. Inhibition of p53 transactivation required for transformation by adenovirus early 1B protein. Nature 1992;357:82-85.

104. Boyd. Adenovirus E1B 19 kDa and Bcl-2 proteins interact with a common set of cellular proteins. Cell 1994;79:1121.

105. Schwarz EM, Badorff C, Hiura TS, Wessely R, Badorff A, Verma IM, Knowlton KU. NF-kappaB-mediated inhibition of apoptosis is required for encephalomyocarditis virus virulence: a

mechanism of resistance in p50 knockout mice. J Virol 1998;72:5654-5660.

106. Tyler KL, Squier MK, Rodgers SE, Schneider BE, Oberhaus SM, Grdina TA, Cohen JJ, Dermody TS. Differences in the capacity of reovirus strains to induce apoptosis are determined by the viral attachment protein sigma 1. J Virol 1995;69:6972-6979.

107. Ammendolia MG, Tinari A, Calcabrini A, Superti F. Poliovirus infection induces apoptosis in CaCo-2 cells. J Med Virol 1999;59:122-129.

108. Tolskaya EA, Romanova LI, Kolesnikova MS, Ivannikova TA, Smirnova EA, Raikhlin NT, Agol VI. Apoptosis-inducing and apoptosis-preventing functions of poliovirus. J Virol 1995;69:1181-1189.

109. Jelachich ML, Lipton HL. Theiler's murine encephalomyelitis virus kills restrictive but not permissive cells by apoptosis. J Virol 1996;70:6856-6861.

110. Anderson R, Harting E, Frey MS, Leibowitz JL, Miranda RC. Theiler's murine encephalomyelitis virus induces rapid necrosis and delayed apoptosis in myelinated mouse cerebellar explant cultures. Brain Res 2000;868:259-267.

111. Corasaniti MT, Bagetta G, Rotiroti D, Nistico G. The HIV envelope protein gp120 in the nervous system: interactions with nitric oxide, interleukin-1beta and nerve growth factor signalling, with pathological implications in vivo and in vitro. Biochem Pharmacol 1998;56:153-156.

112. Henke A, Launhardt H, Klement K, Stelzner A, Zell R, Munder T. Apoptosis in coxsackievirus B3-caused diseases: interaction between the capsid protein VP2 and the proapoptotic protein siva. J Virol 2000;74:4284-4290.

113. Noteborn MH, Todd D, Verschueren CA, de Gauw HW, Curran WL, Veldkamp S, Douglas AJ, McNulty MS, van der Eb AJ, Koch G. A single chicken anemia virus protein induces apoptosis. J Virol 1994;68:346-351.

114. Lu HH, Alexander L, Wimmer E. Construction and genetic analysis of dicistronic polioviruses containing open reading frames for epitopes of human immunodeficiency virus type 1 gp120. J Virol 1995;69:4797-4806.

115. Yamada T, Yamaoka S, Goto T, Nakai M, Tsujimoto Y, Hatanaka M. The human T-cell leukemia virus type I Tax protein induces apoptosis which is blocked by the Bcl-2 protein. J Virol 1994;68:3374-3379.

116. Debiasi RL, Squier MK, Pike B, Wynes M, Dermody TS, Cohen JJ, Tyler KL. Reovirus-induced apoptosis is preceded by increased cellular calpain activity and is blocked by calpain inhibitors. J Virol 1999;73:695-701.

117. Seipelt J, Liebig HD, Sommergruber W, Gerner C, Kuechler E. 2A proteinase of human rhinovirus cleaves cytokeratin 8 in infected HeLa cells. J Biol Chem 2000;275:20084-20089.

118. Goldstaub D, Gradi A, Bercovitch Z, Grosmann Z, Nophar Y, Luria S, Sonenberg N, Kahana C. Poliovirus 2A protease induces apoptotic cell death. Mol Cell Biol 2000;20:1271-1277.

119. Novoa I, Carrasco L. Cleavage of eukaryotic translation initiation factor 4G by exogenously added hybrid proteins containing poliovirus 2Apro in HeLa cells: effects on gene expression. Mol Cell Biol 1999;19:2445-2454.

120. Lamphear BJ, Kirchweger R, Skern T, Rhoads RE. Mapping of functional domains in eukaryotic protein synthesis initiation factor 4G (eIF4G) with picornaviral proteases. Implications for cap-dependent and cap-independent translational initiation. J Biol Chem 1995;270:21975-21983.

121. Urzainqui A, Carrasco L. Degradation of cellular proteins during poliovirus infection: studies by two-dimensional gel electrophoresis. J Virol 1989;63:4729-4735.

122. Belsham GJ, Sonenberg N. Picornavirus RNA translation: roles for cellular proteins. Trends Microbiol 2000;8:330-335.

123. Johannes G, Carter MS, Eisen MB, Brown PO, Sarnow P. Identification of eukaryotic mRNAs that are translated at reduced cap binding complex eIF4F concentrations using a cDNA microarray. Proc Natl Acad Sci U S A 1999;96:13118-13123.

124. Akiri G, Nahari D, Finkelstein Y, Le SY, Elroy-Stein O, Levi BZ. Regulation of vascular endothelial growth factor (VEGF) expression is mediated by internal initiation of translation and alternative initiation of transcription. Oncogene 1998;17:227-236.

125. Nanbru C, Lafon I, Audigier S, Gensac MC, Vagner S, Huez G, Prats AC. Alternative translation of the proto-oncogene c-myc by an internal ribosome entry site. J Biol Chem 1997;272:32061-32066.

126. Coldwell MJ, Mitchell SA, Stoneley M, MacFarlane M, Willis AE. Initiation of Apaf-1 translation by internal ribosome entry. Oncogene 2000;19:899-905.

127. Henis-Korenblit S, Strumpf NL, Goldstaub D, Kimchi A. A novel form of DAP5 protein accumulates in apoptotic cells as a result of caspase cleavage and internal ribosome entry site-mediated translation. Mol Cell Biol 2000;20:496-506.

128. Holcik M, Korneluk RG. Functional characterization of the X-linked inhibitor of apoptosis (XIAP) internal ribosome entry site element: role of La autoantigen in XIAP translation. Mol Cell Biol 2000;20:4648-4657.

129. Johannes G, Sarnow P. Cap-independent polysomal association of natural mRNAs encoding c-myc, BiP, and eIF4G conferred by internal ribosome entry sites. RNA 1998;4:1500-1513.

130. Marissen WE, Lloyd RE. Eukaryotic translation initiation factor 4G is targeted for proteolytic cleavage by caspase 3 during inhibition of translation in apoptotic cells. Mol Cell Biol 1998;18:7565-7574.

131. Sachs AB, Sarnow P, Hentze MW. Starting at the beginning, middle, and end: translation initiation in eukaryotes. Cell 1997;89:831-838.

132. Kerekatte V, Keiper BD, Badorff C, Cai A, Knowlton KU, Rhoads RE. Cleavage of poly(A)-binding protein by coxsackievirus 2A protease in vitro and in vivo: another mechanism for host protein synthesis shutoff? J Virol 1999;73:709-717.

133. Joachims M, Van Breugel PC, Lloyd RE. Cleavage of poly(A)-binding protein by enterovirus proteases concurrent with inhibition of translation in vitro. J Virol 1999;73:718-727.

134. Barco A, Feduchi E, Carrasco L. Poliovirus protease 3C(pro) kills cells by apoptosis. Virology 2000;266:352-360.

135. Yalamanchili P, Weidman K, Dasgupta A. Cleavage of transcriptional activator Oct-1 by poliovirus encoded protease 3Cpro. Virology 1997;239:176-185.

136. Tesar M, Marquardt O. Foot-and-mouth disease virus protease 3C inhibits cellular transcription and mediates cleavage of histone H3. Virology 1990;174:364-374.

137. Clark ME, Lieberman PM, Berk AJ, Dasgupta A. Direct cleavage of human TATA-binding protein by poliovirus protease 3C in vivo and in vitro. Mol Cell Biol 1993;13:1232-1237.

138. Shiroki K, Isoyama T, Kuge S, Ishii T, Ohmi S, Hata S, Suzuki K, Takasaki Y, Nomoto A. Intracellular redistribution of truncated La protein produced by poliovirus 3Cpro-mediated cleavage. J Virol 1999;73:2193-2200.

139. Saura M, Zaragoza C, McMillan A, Quick RA, Hohenadl C, Lowenstein JM, Lowenstein CJ. An antiviral mechanism of nitric oxide: inhibition of a viral protease. Immunity 1999;10:21-28.

140. Ukimura A, Deguchi H, Kitaura Y, Fujioka S, Hirasawa M, Kawamura K, Hirai K. Intracellular viral localization in murine coxsackievirus-B3 myocarditis. Ultrastructural study by electron microscopic in situ hybridization. Am J Pathol 1997;150:2061-2074.

141. Li BY, Qiao GF, Zhou H, Li WH, Huang ZG, Zhou LW. Cytosolic-Ca^{2+} and coxsackievirus B3-induced apoptosis in cultured cardiomyocytes of rats. Zhongguo Yao Li Xue Bao 1999;20:395-399.

142. Zamzami N, Susin SA, Marchetti P, Hirsch T, Gomez-Monterrey I, Castedo M, Kroemer G. Mitochondrial control of nuclear apoptosis. J Exp Med 1996;183:1533-1544.

143. Granville DJ, Carthy CM, Jiang H, Shore GC, McManus BM, Hunt DW. Rapid cytochrome c release, activation of caspases 3, 6, 7 and 8 followed by Bap31 cleavage in HeLa cells treated with

photodynamic therapy. FEBS Lett 1998;437:5-10.

144. Pahl HL, Baeuerle PA. The ER-overload response: activation of NF-kappa B. Trends Biochem Sci 1997;22:63-67.

145. Crook NE, Clem RJ, Miller LK. An apoptosis-inhibiting baculovirus gene with a zinc finger-like motif. J Virol 1993;67:2168-2174.

146. Roy N, Deveraux QL, Takahashi R, Salvesen GS, Reed JC. The c-IAP-1 and c-IAP-2 proteins are direct inhibitors of specific caspases. EMBO J 1997;16:6914-6925.

147. Thome M, Schneider P, Hofmann K, Fickenscher H, Meinl E, Neipel F, Mattmann C, Burns K, Bodmer JL, Schroter M, Scaffidi C, Krammer PH, Peter ME, Tschopp J. Viral FLICE-inhibitory proteins (FLIPS) prevent apoptosis induced by death receptors. Nature 1997;386:517-521.

148. Erl W, Hansson GK, de Martin R, Draude G, Weber KS, Weber C. Nuclear factor-kappa B regulates induction of apoptosis and inhibitor of apoptosis protein-1 expression in vascular smooth muscle cells. Circ Res 1999;84:668-677.

149. Rajcan-Separovic E, Liston P, Lefebvre C, Korneluk RG. Assignment of human inhibitor of apoptosis protein (IAP) genes xiap, hiap-1, and hiap-2 to chromosomes Xq25 and 11q22-q23 by fluorescence in situ hybridization. Genomics 1996;37:404-406.

150. Liston P, Roy N, Tamai K, Lefebvre C, Baird S, Cherton-Horvat G, Farahani R, McLean M, Ikeda JE, MacKenzie A, Korneluk RG. Suppression of apoptosis in mammalian cells by NAIP and a related family of IAP genes. Nature 1996;379:349-353.

151. Ambrosini G, Adida C, Altieri DC. A novel anti-apoptosis gene, survivin, expressed in cancer and lymphoma. Nat Med 1997;3:917-921.

152. Irmler M, Thome M, Hahne M, Schneider P, Hofmann K, Steiner V, Bodmer JL, Schroter M, Burns K, Mattmann C, Rimoldi D, French LE, Tschopp J. Inhibition of death receptor signals by cellular FLIP. Nature 1997;388:190-195.

153. Widmann C, Gibson S, Jarpe MD, Johnson GL. Mitogen-activated protein kinase: conservation of a three-kinase module from yeast to human. Physiol Rev 1999;79:143-180.

154. Brunet A, Pouyssegur J. Mammalian MAP kinase modules: how to transduce specific signals. Essays Biochem 1997;32:1-16.

155. Wang Y, Huang S, Sah VP, Ross J Jr, Brown JH, Han J, Chien KR. Cardiac muscle cell hypertrophy and apoptosis induced by distinct members of the p38 mitogen-activated protein kinase family. J Biol Chem 1998;273:2161-2168.

156. Sugden PH, Clerk A. "Stress-responsive" mitogen-activated protein kinases (c-Jun N-terminal kinases and p38 mitogen-activated protein kinases) in the myocardium. Circ Res 1998;83:345-352.

157. Han J, Lee JD, Bibbs L, Ulevitch RJ. A MAP kinase targeted by endotoxin and hyperosmolarity in mammalian cells. Science 1994;265:808-811.

158. Paul A, Wilson S, Belham CM, Robinson CJ, Scott PH, Gould GW, Plevin R. Stress-activated protein kinases: activation, regulation and function. Cell Signal 1997;9:403-410.

159. Force T, Pombo CM, Avruch JA, Bonventre JV, Kyriakis JM. Stress-activated protein kinases in cardiovascular disease. Circ Res 1996;78:947-953.

160. Bruder JT, Kovesdi I. Adenovirus infection stimulates the Raf/MAPK signaling pathway and induces interleukin-8 expression. J Virol 1997;71:398-404.

161. Huttunen P, Hyypia T, Vihinin P, Nissinen L, Heino J. Echovirus 1 infection induces both stress- and growth-activated mitogen-activated protein kinase pathways and regulates the transcription of cellular immediate-early genes. Virology 1998;250:85-93.

162. Huber M, Watson KA, Selinka HC, Carthy CM, Klingel K, McManus BM, Kandolf R. Cleavage of Ras GAP and phosphorylation of mitogen-activated protein kinase in the course of coxsackievirus B3 replication. J Virol 1999;73:3587-3594.

163. Lowy DR, Willumsen BM. Function and regulation of ras. Annu Rev Biochem 1993;62:851-891.

164. Vanhaesebroeck B, Alessi DR. The P13K-PDK1 connection: more than just a road to PKB. Biochem J 2000;346:561-576.

165. Toker A. Protein kinases as mediators of phosphoinositide 3-kinase signaling. Mol Pharmacol 2000;57:652-658.

166. Wymann MP, Pirola L. Structure and function of phosphoinositide 3-kinases. Biochim Biophys Acta 1998;1436:127-150.

167. Yang X, Gabuzda D. Regulation of human immunodeficiency virus type 1 infectivity by the ERK mitogen-activated protein kinase signaling pathway. J Virol 1999;73:3460-3466.

168. Yang X, Goncalves J, Gabuzda D. Phosphorylation of Vif and its role in HIV-1 replication. J Biol Chem 1996;271:10121-10129.

169. Yang X, Gabuzda D. Mitogen-activated protein kinase phosphorylates and regulates the HIV-1 Vif protein. J Biol Chem 1998;273:29879-29887.

170. Jacque JM, Mann A, Enslen H, Sharova N, Brichacek B, Davis RJ, Stevenson M. Modulation of HIV-1 infectivity by MAPK, a virion-associated kinase. EMBO J 1998;17:2607-2618.

171. Shapiro L, Heidenreich KA, Meintzer MK, Dinarello CA. Role of p38 mitogen-activated protein kinase in HIV type 1 production in vitro. Proc Natl Acad Sci U S A 1998;95:7422-7426.

172. Cohen PS, Schmidtmayerova H, Dennis J, Dubrovsky L, Sherry B, Wang H, Bukrinsky M, Tracey KJ. The critical role of p38 MAP kinase in T cell HIV-1 replication. Mol Med 1997;3:339-346.

173. Misra-Press A, Rim CS, Yao H, Roberson MS, Stork PJ. A novel mitogen-activated protein kinase phosphatase. Structure, expression, and regulation. J Biol Chem 1995;270:14587-14596.

174. Brondello JM, Brunet A, Pouyssegur J, McKenzie FR. The dual specificity mitogen-activated protein kinase phosphatase-1 and -2 are induced by the p42/p44MAPK cascade. J Biol Chem 1997;272:1368-1376.

175. Nguyen TT, Scimeca JC, Filloux C, Peraldi P, Carpentier JL, Van Obberghen E. Co-regulation of the mitogen-activated protein kinase, extracellular signal-regulated kinase 1, and the 90-kDa ribosomal S6 kinase in PC12 cells. Distinct effects of the neurotrophic factor, nerve growth factor, and the mitogenic factor, epidermal growth factor. J Biol Chem 1993;268:9803-9810.

176. Huber M, Selinka HC, Kandolf R. Tyrosine phosphorylation events during coxsackievirus B3 replication. J Virol 1997;71:595-600.

177. Cooper JA, Gould KL, Cartwright CA, Hunter T. Tyr527 is phosphorylated in pp60c-src: implications for regulation. Science 1986;231:1431-1434.

178. Wang X, Bergelson JM. Coxsackievirus and adenovirus receptor cytoplasmic and transmembrane domains are not essential for coxsackievirus and adenovirus infection. J Virol 1999;73:2559-2562.

179. Straus DB, Weiss A. Genetic evidence for the involvement of the lck tyrosine kinase in signal transduction through the T cell antigen receptor. Cell 1992;70:585-593.

180. Manna SK, Aggarwal BB. Differential requirement for p56lck in HIV-tat versus TNF-induced cellular responses: effects on NF-kappa B, activator protein-1, c-Jun N-terminal kinase, and apoptosis. J Immunol 2000;164:5156-5166.

181. Opavsky MA, Martino T, Penninger J, Trinidad C, Chen J, Butcher L, Liu P. p56[lck] protein tyrosine kinase is required for coxsackievirus B3 activation of the growth-stimulated MAPK signal transduction pathway (abstract). Can J Cardiol 2000;16 Suppl F:124F.

182. Swart R, Ruf IK, Sample J, Longnecker R. Latent membrane protein 2A-mediated effects on the phosphatidylinositol 3-kinase/Akt pathway. J Virol 2000;74:10838-10845.

183. Marte BM, Downward J. PKB/Akt: connecting phosphoinositide 3-kinase to cell survival and beyond. Trends Biochem Sci 1997;22:355-358.

184. Toker A, Cantley LC. Signalling through the lipid products of phosphoinositide-3-OH kinase. Nature 1997;387:673-676.

185. Testa JR, Bellacosa A. Membrane translocation and activation of the Akt kinase in growth

factor-stimulated hematopoietic cells. Leuk Res 1997;21:1027-1031.

186. Fujio Y, Guo K, Mano T, Mitsuuchi Y, Testa JR, Walsh K. Cell cycle withdrawal promotes myogenic induction of Akt, a positive modulator of myocyte survival. Mol Cell Biol 1999;19:5073-5082.

187. Tang ED, Nunez G, Barr FG, Guan KL. Negative regulation of the forkhead transcription factor FKHR by Akt. J Biol Chem 1999;274:16741-16746.

188. Datta SR, Dudek H, Tao X, Masters S, Fu H, Gotoh Y, Greenberg ME. Akt phosphorylation of BAD couples survival signals to the cell-intrinsic death machinery. Cell 1997;91:231-241.

189. Cardone MH, Roy N, Stennicke HR, Salvesen GS, Franke TF, Stanbridge E, Frisch S, Reed JC. Regulation of cell death protease caspase-9 by phosphorylation. Science 1998;282:1318-1321.

190. del Peso L, Gonzalez-Garcia M, Page C, Herrera R, Nunez G. Interleukin-3-induced phosphorylation of BAD through the protein kinase Akt. Science 1997;278:687-689.

191. Svitkin YV, Hahn H, Gingras AC, Palmenberg AC, Sonenberg N. Rapamycin and wortmannin enhance replication of a defective encephalomyocarditis virus. J Virol 1998;72:5811-5819.

192. Borgatti P, Zauli G, Colamussi ML, Gibellini D, Previati M, Cantley LL, Capitani S. Extracellular HIV-1 Tat protein activates phosphatidylinositol3- and Akt/PKB kinases in CD4+ T lymphoblastoid Jurkat cells. Eur J Immunol 1997;27:2805-2811.

193. Shih WL, Kuo ML, Chuang SE, Cheng AL, Doong SL. Hepatitis B virus X protein inhibits transforming growth factor-beta-induced apoptosis through the activation of phosphatidylinositol 3-kinase pathway. J Biol Chem 2000;275:25858-25864.

194. Gilmore TD. The Rel/NF-κB signal transduction pathway: introduction. Oncogene 1999;18:6842-6844.

195. Stancovski I, Baltimore D. NF-κB activation: the IκB kinase revealed? Cell 1997;91:299-302.

196. Wang CY, Mayo MW, Korneluk RG, Goeddel DV, Baldwin AS Jr. NF-κB antiapoptosis: induction of TRAF1 and TRAF2 and c-IAP1 and c-IAP2 to suppress caspase-8 activation. Science 1998;281:1680-1683.

197. Chen FE, Ghosh G. Regulation of DNA binding by Rel/NF-κB transcription factors: structural views. Oncogene 1999;18:6845-6852.

198. DeLuca C, Kwon H, Lin R, Wainberg M, Hiscott J. NF-κB activation and HIV-1 induced apoptosis. Cytokine Growth Factor Rev 1999;10:235-253.

199. Riviere Y, Blank V, Kourilsky P, Israël A. Processing of the precursor of NF-κB by the HIV-1 protease during acute infection. Nature 1991;350:625-626.

200. Chu ZL, McKinsey TA, Liu L, Gentry JJ, Malim MH, Ballard DW. Suppression of tumor necrosis factor-induced cell death by inhibitor of apoptosis c-IAP2 is under NF-κB control. Proc Natl Acad Sci U S A 1997;94:10057-10062.

201. de Moissac D, Mustapha S, Greenberg AH, Kirshenbaum LA. Bcl-2 activates the transcription factor NFκB through the degradation of the cytoplasmic inhibitor IκBα. J Biol Chem 1998;273:23946-23951.

202. Connolly JL, Rodgers SE, Clarke P, Ballard DW, Kerr LD, Tyler KL, Dermody TS. Reovirus-induced apoptosis requires activation of transcription factor NF-κB. J Virol 2000;74:2981-2989.

203. Béraud C, Greene WC. Interaction of HTLV-I Tax with the human proteasome: implications for NF-κB induction. J Acquir Immune Defic Syndr Hum Retrovirol 1996;13 Suppl 1:S76-S84.

204. Levine B, Huang Q, Isaacs JT, Reed JC, Griffin DE, Hardwick JM. Conversion of lytic to persistent alphavirus infection by the bcl-2 cellular oncogene. Nature 1993;361:739-742.

205. Okuno M, Nakagawa M, Shimada M, Saito M, Hishinuma S, Yamauchi-Takihara K. Expressional patterns of cytokines in a murine model of acute myocarditis: early expression of cardiotrophin-1. Lab Invest 2000;80:433-440.

206. Sheng Z, Knowlton K, Chen J, Hoshijima M, Brown JH, Chien KR. Cardiotrophin 1 (CT-1) inhibition of cardiac myocyte apoptosis via a mitogen-activated protein kinase-dependent pathway. Divergence from downstream CT-1 signals for myocardial cell hypertrophy. J Biol Chem 1997;272:5783-5791.

207. Li YP, Schwartz RJ, Waddell ID, Holloway BR, Reid MB. Skeletal muscle myocytes undergo protein loss and reactive oxygen-mediated NF-kappaB activation in response to tumor necrosis factor alpha. FASEB J 1998;12:871-880.

208. Matsumori A, Yamada T, Suzuki H, Matoba Y, Sasayama S. Increased circulating cytokines in patients with myocarditis and cardiomyopathy. Br Heart J 1994;72:561-566.

209. Schmidtke M, Gluck B, Merkle I, Hofmann P, Stelzner A, Gemsa D. Cytokine profiles in heart, spleen, and thymus during the acute stage of experimental coxsackievirus B3-induced chronic myocarditis. J Med Virol 2000;61:518-526.

210. Zaragoza C, Ocampo CJ, Saura M, McMillan A, Lowenstein CJ. Nitric oxide inhibition of coxsackievirus replication in vitro. J Clin Invest 1997;100:1760-1767.

211. Rossig L, Fichtlscherer B, Breitschopf K, Haendeler J, Zeiher AM, Mülsch A, Dimmeler S. Nitric oxide inhibits caspase-3 by S-nitrosation in vivo. J Biol Chem 1999;274:6823-6826.

212. Badorff C, Fichtlscherer B, Rhoads RE, Zeiher AM, Muelsch A, Dimmeler S, Knowlton KU. Nitric oxide inhibits dystrophin proteolysis by coxsackieviral protease 2A through S-nitrosylation: a protective mechanism against enteroviral cardiomyopathy. Circulation 2000;102:2276-2281.

213. Towbin JA. The role of cytoskeletal proteins in cardiomyopathies. Curr Opin Cell Biol 1998;10:131-139.

214. Towbin JA, Bowles KR, Bowles NE. Etiologies of cardiomyopathy and heart failure. Nat Med 1999;5:266-267.

215. Hein S, Kostin S, Heling A, Maeno Y, Schaper J. The role of the cytoskeleton in heart failure. Cardiovasc Res 2000;45:273-278.

216. Joachims M, Harris KS, Etchison D. Poliovirus protease 3C mediates cleavage of microtubule-associated protein 4. Virology 1995;211:451-461.

217. Badorff C, Berkely N, Mehrotra S, Talhouk JW, Rhoads RE, Knowlton KU. Enteroviral protease 2A directly cleaves dystrophin and is inhibited by a dystrophin-based substrate analogue. J Biol Chem 2000;275:11191-11197.

218. Badorff C, Lee GH, Lamphear BJ, Martone ME, Campbell KP, Rhoads RE, Knowlton KU. Enteroviral protease 2A cleaves dystrophin: evidence of cytoskeletal disruption in an acquired cardiomyopathy. Nat Med 1999;5:320-326.

219. Badorff C, Lee GH, Knowlton KU. Enteroviral cardiomyopathy: bad news for the dystrophin-glycoprotein complex. Herz 2000;25:227-232.

220. Martino TA, Liu P, Sole MJ. Viral infection and the pathogenesis of dilated cardiomyopathy. Circ Res 1994;74:182-188.

221. Nakamura H, Yamamoto T, Yamamura T, Nakao F, Umemoto S, Shintaku T, Yamaguchi K, Liu P, Matsuzaki M. Repetitive coxsackievirus infection induces cardiac dilatation in post-myocarditic mice. Jpn Circ J 1999;63:794-802.

222. Tam PE, Messner RP. Molecular mechanisms of coxsackievirus persistence in chronic inflammatory myopathy: viral RNA persists through formation of a double-stranded complex without associated genomic mutations or evolution. J Virol 1999;73:10113-10121.

223. Kandolf R, Sauter M, Aepinus C, Schnorr JJ, Selinka HC, Klingel K. Mechanisms and consequences of enterovirus persistence in cardiac myocytes and cells of the immune system. Virus Res 1999;62:149-158.

224. Abelmann WH. Myocarditis and dilated cardiomyopathy. West J Med 1989;150:458-459.

225. Megeney LA, Kablar B, Perry RL, Ying C, May L, Rudnicki MA. Severe cardiomyopathy in mice lacking dystrophin and MyoD. Proc Natl Acad Sci U S A 1999;96:220-225.

226. Chow LH, Gauntt CJ, McManus BM. Differential effects of myocarditic variants of Coxsackievirus B3 in inbred mice. A pathologic characterization of heart tissue damage. Lab Invest 1991;64:55-64.

227. Gauntt CJ, Gomez PT, Duffey PS, Grant JA, Trent DW, Witherspoon SM, Paque RE. Characterization and myocarditic capabilities of coxsackievirus B3 variants in selected mouse strains. J Virol 1984;52:598-605.

228. Hamrell BB, Huber SA, Leslie KO. Reduced unloaded sarcomere shortening velocity and a shift to a slower myosin isoform in acute murine coxsackievirus myocarditis. Circ Res 1994;75:462-472.

229. Bristow MR. Why does the myocardium fail? Insights from basic science. Lancet 1998;352 Suppl 1:S8-S14.

230. Clark WA, Rudnick SJ, LaPres JJ, Andersen LC, LaPointe MC. Regulation of hypertrophy and atrophy in cultured adult heart cells. Circ Res 1993;73:1163-1176.

231. Clark WA, Rudnick SJ, Andersen LC, LaPres JJ. Myosin heavy chain synthesis is independently regulated in hypertrophy and atrophy of isolated adult cardiac myocytes. J Biol Chem 1994;269:25562-25569.

232. Kajstura J, Pertoldi B, Leri A, Beltrami CA, Deptala A, Darzynkiewicz Z, Anversa P. Telomere shortening is an in vivo marker of myocyte replication and aging. Am J Pathol 2000;156:813-819.

233. Anversa P, Leri A, Beltrami CA, Guerra S, Kajstura J. Myocyte death and growth in the failing heart. Lab Invest 1998;78:767-786.

234. Yang D, Yu J, Luo Z, Carthy CM, Wilson JE, Liu Z, McManus BM. Viral myocarditis: identification of five differentially expressed genes in coxsackievirus B3-infected mouse heart. Circ Res 1999;84:704-712.

235. Tsujimoto Y. Prevention of neuronal cell death by Bcl-2. Results Probl Cell Differ 1998;24:137-155.

236. Barfod ET, Zheng Y, Kuang WJ, Hart MJ, Evans T, Cerione RA, Ashkenazi A. Cloning and expression of a human CDC42 GTPase-activating protein reveals a functional SH3-binding domain. J Biol Chem 1993;268:26059-26062.

237. Lee ML, Kuo FC, Whitmore GA, Sklar J. Importance of replication in microarray gene expression studies: statistical methods and evidence from repetitive cDNA hybridizations. Proc Natl Acad Sci U S A 2000;97:9834-9839.

238. Pietiainen V, Huttunen P, Hyypia T. Effects of echovirus 1 infection on cellular gene expression. Virology 2000;276:243-250.

239. Geiss GK, Bumgarner RE, An MC, Agy MB, van't Wout AB, Hammersmark E, Carter VS, Upchurch D, Mullins JI, Katze MG. Large-scale monitoring of host cell gene expression during HIV-1 infection using cDNA microarrays. Virology 2000;266:8-16.

240. Hobbs WE II, DeLuca NA. Perturbation of cell cycle progression and cellular gene expression as a function of herpes simplex virus ICP0. J Virol 1999;73:8245-8255.

241. Stingly SW, Ramirez JJ, Aguilar SA, Simmen K, Sandri-Goldin RM, Ghazal P, Wagner EK. Global analysis of herpes simplex virus type 1 transcription using an oligonucleotide-based DNA microarray. J Virol 2000;74:9916-9927.

242. Zhu H, Cong JP, Mamtora G, Gingeras T, Shenk T. Cellular gene expression altered by human cytomegalovirus: global monitoring with oligonucleotide arrays. Proc Natl Acad Sci U S A 1998;95:14470-14475.

243. Manger ID, Relman DA. How the host 'sees' pathogens: global gene expression responses to infection. Curr Opin Immunol 2000;12:215-218.

244. Pandey A, Mann M. Proteomics to study genes and genomes. Nature 2000;405:837-846.

Animal Models of Autoimmune Myocarditis

**Makoto Kodama, M.D., Yuji Okura, M.D.,
Yoshifusa Aizawa, M.D., and Tohru Izumi, M.D.**

Myocarditis is defined pathologically as an inflammation of the heart muscle. There are 2 major challenges in the field of myocarditis. One is that patients with severe forms of myocarditis die from refractory heart failure because treatment of acute myocarditis is often ineffective. The other is that some of the patients who survive the active phase develop dilated cardiomyopathy. A chronic, autoimmune-mediated myocardial injury is involved in the mechanism of dilated cardiomyopathy. To clarify the pathogenesis of myocarditis and postmyocarditis dilated cardiomyopathy, viral and autoimmune animal models have been developed. In this chapter, we review the models of experimental autoimmune myocarditis (EAM).

MYOCARDITOGENIC ANTIGENS OF EAM

Various experimental models of autoimmune myocarditis have been reported during the last 4 decades (Table 8-1). Initially, outbred animals were immunized with heart tissue homogenates. Prevalence and severity of myocarditis were inconsistent in those models. The development of organ-specific autoimmune disease varies with antigens and animal strains. Subsequently, specific antigens, such as cardiac myosin, membranous protein, and sarcoplasmic reticulum protein, which were purified from heart tissue, were challenged in inbred strains of animals. From this initial work, 2 models of EAM were established by immunizing mice or rats with cardiac myosin.[6,7] The clinical and pathologic severity of EAM in mice or rats is consistent. The models are characterized by increased cardiac size, macroscopic abnormalities, or histologic evidence of myocarditis. Rat EAM has several unique characteristics. The prevalence of histologic myocarditis is 100% in Lewis rats. Pathologically, rat EAM is characterized by its clinical severity, resemblance to human fulminant myocarditis, and appearance of multinucleated giant cells in the lesions.[12] Some rats with EAM die of congestive heart failure.

Cardiac myosin is composed of 2 heavy chains and 4 light chains. The cardiac myosin heavy chain is composed of about 2,000 amino acids. In autoimmune diseases, T cells are able to recognize 10 to 20 amino acid residues, and B cells recognize 5 to 10 amino acid peptides as antigens. Therefore, knowledge of the location and structure of myocarditogenic epitopes on cardiac myosin is important to understand the pathogenesis of autoimmune myocarditis.

Three major myocarditogenic epitopes have been identified (Fig. 8-1). By use of an antigen-reactive proliferation assay of hybridoma cells, which were derived from lymphocytes of mice with EAM,[13] the myocarditogenic epitope was localized on residues 334-352 of the murine cardiac myosin α-chain. In rat EAM, mathematical analysis of the peptide sequence which could be presented by rat major histocompatibility complex (MHC) class

Table 8-1
Experimental Autoimmune Myocarditis

Reference	Animal	Antigen	Morbidity, %	Severity
Kaplan and Craig[1]	Rabbit	Heterologous heart homogenate	10	Micro lesion
Davies et al.[2]	Rabbit	Homologous heart homogenate	About 30	Micro lesion
	Rat	Heart homogenate	- - -	Micro lesion
	Guinea pig	Heart homogenate	- - -	Micro lesion
	Hamster	Heart homogenate	- - -	Micro lesion
Wittner et al.[3]	Rabbit	Heterologous cardiac myosin	Infrequent	Micro lesion
Acosta and Santos-Buch[4]	Mouse (BALB)	Sarcoplasmic reticulum protein	78	Micro lesion
Izumi et al.[5]	Mouse (NMRI)	Cardiac membranous protein	20	Micro lesion
Neu et al.[6]	Mouse (A, A.SW)	Homologous cardiac myosin	85	Macro lesion
Kodama et al.[7]	Rat (Lewis)	Heterologous cardiac myosin	100	Macro lesion, lethal GCM
Sharaf et al.[8]	Mouse (A)	SR calcium ATPase	- - -	Myocardial degeneration
Schultheiss et al.[9]	Guinea pig	ADP-ATP carrier protein	- - -	Antibody production
Huber and Cunningham[10]	Mouse (MRL)	Streptococcal M protein	75	Micro lesion
Bachmaier et al.[11]	Mouse (BALB)	*Chlamydia* protein	86	Micro-macro lesion

GCM, giant cell myocarditis; SR, sarcoplasmic reticulum.

II molecules showed that residues 1,539-1,555 of the rat cardiac myosin α-chain would be the myocarditogenic epitope of EAM.[14] Direct subfragment analysis revealed that actually several myocarditogenic epitopes existed on cardiac myosin. The most effective epitope was present on the residues 1,070-1,165 of the porcine cardiac myosin β-chain.[15]

Initiation of autoimmune disease requires the breakdown of antigen-specific self-tolerance. Molecular mimicry of myocarditogenic epitopes to viral or foreign antigens may be one of the mechanisms for loss of self-tolerance. However, the viral or foreign antigens that initiate autoimmune myocarditis have not yet been fully determined in experimental models or in clinical cases. Reports suggested that coxsackievirus B3, streptococcal M protein, and chlamydia protein have sequence homology to cardiac myosin and that these might play a role in the initiation of autoimmune myocarditis.[10,11,16]

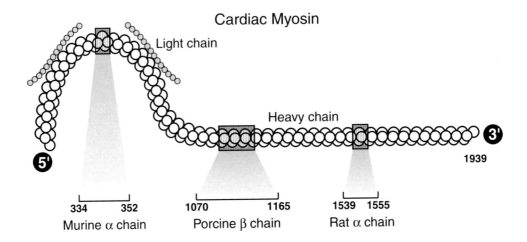

Fig. 8-1. Myocarditogenic epitopes of cardiac myosin. Three major myocarditogenic epitopes have been identified on the cardiac myosin heavy chain. The epitope of murine experimental autoimmune myocarditis (EAM) exists on residues 334-352 of murine cardiac myosin α heavy chain, and the myocarditogenic epitopes of rat EAM are present on residues 1,070-1,165 of porcine cardiac myosin β heavy chain and 1,539-1,555 of rat cardiac myosin α heavy chain.

SUSCEPTIBILITY TO EAM

Cardiac myosin-induced autoimmune myocarditis can be elicited in only certain strains of mice and rats (Table 8-2).[6,7] Susceptibility to EAM depends strongly on genetic background. It is suggested that MHC locus may control the susceptibility of mouse and human autoimmune myocarditis.[17] In the case of rat EAM, the susceptibility cannot be attributed to a single MHC haplotype.[18] The presence of cardiac myosin-reactive myocarditogenic T cells is fundamentally important. The activation and proliferation of the myocarditogenic T cells would be necessary before initiation of EAM. Genetic background, cytokines and chemokines, internal steroid hormones, and resident cells in the target organs probably regulate susceptibility to EAM.[19,20]

PATHOLOGY OF RAT EAM

Rat EAM is characterized by its high morbidity and mortality. All rats, without exception, develop a severe form of myocarditis after immunization with sufficient doses of cardiac myosin, as homologous or heterologous antigens. Pericardial effusions, cardiac enlargement, and discoloration of the cardiac surface are macroscopic findings of EAM (Fig. 8-2; see color plate 10). These macroscopic findings have been common at autopsy in patients with myocarditis but have been reported rarely in experimental models other than the

Table 8-2
Susceptibility of Animals for Cardiac Myosin-Induced Autoimmune Myocarditis

Susceptibility	Species	Strain
Susceptible		
	Mouse	A, A.SW
	Rat	Lewis
Intermediate		
	Mouse	A.CA, A.BY, B10.A, C.B-17, BALB, DBA, CAJ, C3H
	Rat	Dahl, Fisher, Wistar
Resistant		
	Mouse	C57BL, SCID
	Rat	BN, PVG, SHR
	Guinea pig	Hartley

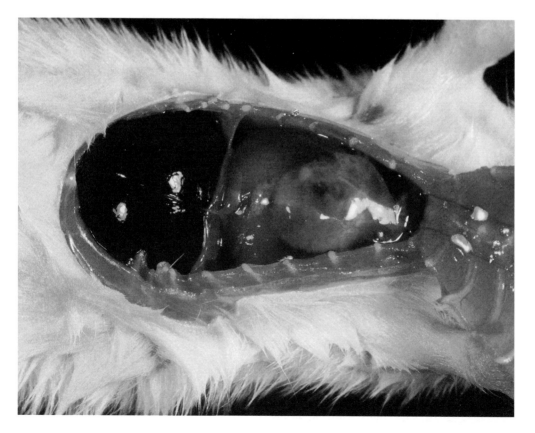

Fig. 8-2. Gross pathology of rat experimental autoimmune myocarditis. Massive pericardial effusion and discoloration of cardiac surface are evident. See color plate 10.

Lewis rat. Histologic examination reveals infiltration of inflammatory cells with myocardial degeneration and necrosis. The appearance of multinucleated giant cells in the lesions is also a characteristic and unique finding of the rat EAM (Fig. 8-3; see color plate 11). Rats with EAM become severely ill and largely immobile. Myocarditis develops about 14 days after immunization and continues for about 14 days. Then, the cellular infiltrate decreases and replacement fibrosis increases in the myocardium (Fig. 8-4). Ten to twenty percent of the rats with severe EAM die of congestive heart failure during the acute phase of the disease. This mortality rate seems to be inappropriately low for the pathologic severity. Why rats are able to survive severe congestive heart failure caused by myocarditis is unknown.

MEDIATORS OF EAM

Rat EAM is transferable into naive syngeneic animals by in vitro-activated lymphocytes.[21] Transfer experiments with sorted lymphocytes revealed that CD4-positive T cells mediated EAM.[22] Fresh sera, IgG fraction of sera, nonactivated lymphocytes, and activated CD8-positive T cells did not transfer the disease into syngeneic animals. Furthermore, the anti-$\alpha\beta$ T-cell receptor antibody was able to block the induction of EAM in Lewis rats.[23] Therefore, CD4-positive T cells bearing $\alpha\beta$ T-cell receptors are pathogenic in rat EAM. Murine EAM may be transferred into severe combined immunodeficient mice by using CD4-positive T cells but not with antimyosin antibodies.[24] Thus, rat and mouse EAM are CD4-positive, T-cell–mediated autoimmune diseases. It has remained uncertain whether CD4-positive T cells directly interact with cardiomyocytes.

Subsets of infiltrating cells have been investigated in the hearts with EAM.[25,26] The majority of infiltrating cells are composed of macrophages and CD4-positive T cells. The frequency of macrophages and of CD4-positive T cells is about 75% and 15%, respectively. CD8-positive T cells are scarce and B cells are rare in the lesions, approximately 5% and 0.5%, respectively. The dominance of macrophages and CD4-positive T cells is a constant finding among the sites of the lesions and throughout the course of the disease. The subsets of infiltrating cells in EAM differ from those of murine viral myocarditis, which are composed mainly of natural killer cells and CD8-positive T cells. Thus, myocardial T-cell subsets may differentiate viral and autoimmune myocarditis.

Infiltrating CD4-positive T cells are highly activated in the rat heart with EAM. The majority of CD4-positive T cells bear the $\alpha\beta$ T-cell receptor, lymphocyte function-associated antigen-1, and interleukin (IL)-2 receptor molecules on their cell surface.[27] T cells recognize antigenic peptides in the context of self-MHC using T-cell receptors. The repertoire of T cells corresponds to the variety of foreign antigens in the individual. T-cell repertoire depends on the highly variable region of the T-cell receptor—the complementarity deter-

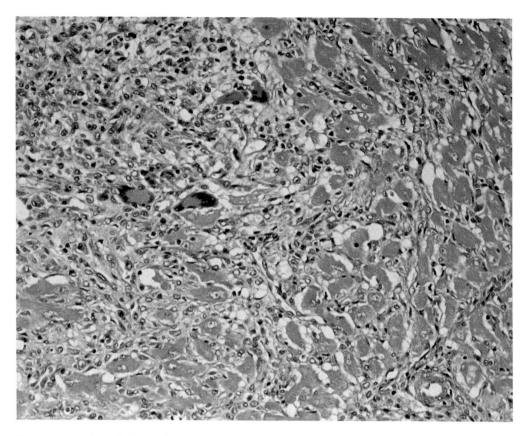

Fig. 8-3. Histologic findings of rat experimental autoimmune myocarditis. Multinucleated giant cells are observed in the lesion. (Hematoxylin and eosin; x200.) See color plate 11.

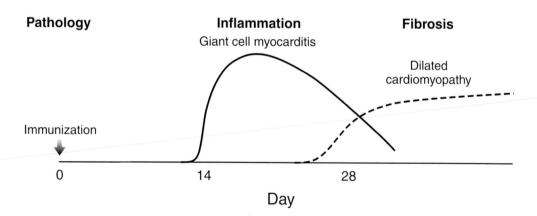

Fig. 8-4. Schema of the clinical course of rat experimental autoimmune myocarditis. Pathologic findings and possible corresponding human diseases are noted.

mining region 3 (CDR3). If inflammation is caused by specific antigens, antigen-specific T-cell clones have to exist in the lesions. In rat EAM, infiltrating T cells in the heart and pericardial space have been demonstrated to be oligoclonal, based on the analysis of CDR3 regions.[28,29] However, cardiac myosin-specific myocarditogenic T-cell clones have not been identified yet.

CYTOKINE PROFILES

Cytokines play important roles in the pathogenesis of myocarditis. When cardiac myosin-specific T cells enter the myocardium, these T cells are activated by antigen presentation from resident dendritic cells. Activated T cells secrete various cytokines and chemokines, which recruit and activate inflammatory cells in the myocardium. We investigated the myocardial cytokine expression in rat EAM (Fig. 8-5).[30] IL-2 mRNA appears in the EAM hearts at the onset of the disease. Subsequently, mRNA of IL-1β, interferon-γ (IFN-γ), and tumor necrosis factor-α increases. In the recovery phase, IL-10, a so-called Th2 cytokine, appears in the heart. The change of cytokine profile, from the Th1 to Th2 pattern, may determine the nature of the disease course, namely progression or recovery.

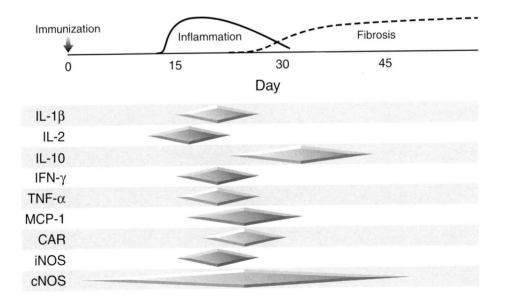

Fig. 8-5. Messenger RNA expression of inflammatory molecules in the rat hearts with experimental autoimmune myocarditis. *CAR*, coxsackievirus and adenovirus receptor; *IFN*, interferon; *IL*, interleukin; *MCP*, monocyte chemoattractant protein; *NOS*, nitric oxide synthase; *TNF*, tumor necrosis factor.

Chemokines also play important roles in the clinical course of EAM. Large numbers of inflammatory cells, including antigen-specific T cells, nonspecific macrophages, and neutrophils, infiltrate the myocardium during the course of EAM. The process may be mediated by monocyte chemoattractant protein-1 (MCP-1) or other chemokines. In rat EAM, MCP-1 mRNA is strongly expressed in the heart coincident with the onset of the disease and persists until the recovery phase. Serum concentrations of MCP-1 are also increased in rats during the acute phase of EAM.

The coxsackievirus and adenovirus receptor (CAR) is 1 of the fetal molecules of the heart. CAR belongs to the immunoglobulin superfamily and has a structure similar to that of adhesion molecules. This molecule may act on cell contact among cardiomyocytes during differentiation and development of the heart. Although the myocardium of the adult Lewis rat does not bear CARs on its cell surface, CAR is induced in the myocardium during the course of EAM.[31] Adhesion molecules, such as intercellular adhesion molecule-1 and vascular cell adhesion molecule-1, act on the inflammatory cell infiltration through the capillary wall. CAR may act on the healing process of the injured myocardium.

MYOCARDIAL INJURY IN EAM

As noted above, rat EAM is a CD4-positive, T-cell–mediated disease, and autoantibodies are not directly pathogenic. The pathogenesis of rat EAM, which is induced by active immunization with cardiac myosin, is demonstrated in Figure 8-6. Subcutaneous injection of cardiac myosin with complete adjuvant Freund leads to antigen presentation of cardiac myosin-specific T cells in the peripheral lymphatic organs. The immunoadjuvant plays an important role in the breakdown of self-tolerance by activation of antigen-presenting cells, enhancement of the expression of MHC molecules, and increases in vascular permeability.

After breakdown of self-tolerance, expansion of cardiac myosin-specific T-cell clones progresses. When cardiac myosin-specific myocarditogenic T-cell clones migrate by chance in the myocardium, resident dendritic cells, which possess cardiac myosin antigen in their MHC class II molecules, present the antigen to the T cells.[32] Subsequently, activated T cells proliferate and secrete various cytokines, such as IL-2 and IFN-γ. These cytokines activate nonspecific bystander T cells, B cells, macrophages, and neutrophils, then activated inflammatory cells secrete large amounts of various cytokines and chemokines which further promote inflammation. In the process, cytokines induce nitric oxide synthase in macrophages and cardiomyocytes.[33-35] All of these inflammatory mediators, cytokines, chemokines, nitric oxide, and leukotrienes interfere with myocardial function and may occasionally destroy the cell membrane of cardiomyocytes in a highly concentrated environment.[36-38] If cardiac myosin leaks from the injured myocardium, local antigen presentation and activation of specific T cells will be accelerated. Once the membrane of cardiomyocytes is injured, autoantibodies bind and destroy the myocardium. In the case of adoptive transfer, activation and proliferation of myocarditogenic T-cell clones in the peripheral lymphatic organs are not necessary. Accordingly, the onset of the adoptively transferred EAM is earlier than that of the actively induced EAM.

HEALING AND RECURRENCE

Although a large amount of antigen remains in the heart, active inflammation of rat EAM subsides from day 28 to day 35. The mechanisms of the healing process can be explained

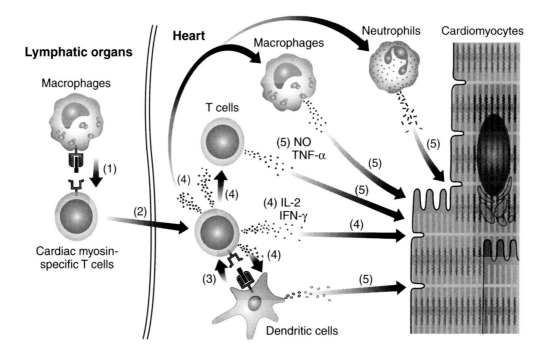

Fig. 8-6. Schema of the mechanisms of myocardial injuries in experimental autoimmune myocarditis. (1) Antigen presentation to myosin-specific myocarditogenic T cells in peripheral lymphatic organs. (2) Breakdown of self-tolerance and expansion of myocarditogenic T-cell clones. Some activated T cells migrate in the myocardium. (3) Antigen presentation and activation of migrated T cells by resident dendritic cells. (4) Activated T cells secrete various inflammatory cytokines, which act on the recruitment and activation of myosin-nonspecific T cells, macrophages, and neutrophils. (5) These activated inflammatory cells also secrete cytokines, chemokines, nitric oxide (*NO*), and leukotriene. Then tissue destructive inflammation is provoked. *IFN*, interferon; *IL*, interleukin; *TNF*, tumor necrosis factor.

by 2 steps. One is elimination of activated myosin-specific myocarditogenic T-cell clones by apoptosis,[39] and the other is changes of the cytokine profile. Th1 cytokines, such as IL-2 and IFN-γ, are predominantly expressed in the myocardium during the active phase. Then, IL-10 dominates the heart during the recovery phase. Similarly, frequency of T cells with Th1 function increases before the onset of EAM in the peripheral blood. Then, T cells with Th2 function overcome Th1 T cells during the recovery phase (Fig. 8-7). If cytokine profiles are disturbed, the natural course of EAM is modified. In vivo administration of IL-12 in rats with actively induced EAM produced persistent myocarditis.[22]

One of the unique characteristics of rat EAM is the recurrence of the disease by resensitization with the same antigen.[40] Animals cured of autoimmune disease acquire tolerance to the same antigen in other organ-specific autoimmune disease models. On the other hand, EAM may be induced in Lewis rats that were cured of actively induced EAM, at 2 months from the initial immunization. Until 2 months, rats are refractory to reinduction of EAM. The refractory period to recurrence may be explained by the Th1/Th2 balance. The mechanism of the progression from myocarditis to dilated cardiomyopathy is probably related to the above-mentioned persistent or recurrent myocarditis.

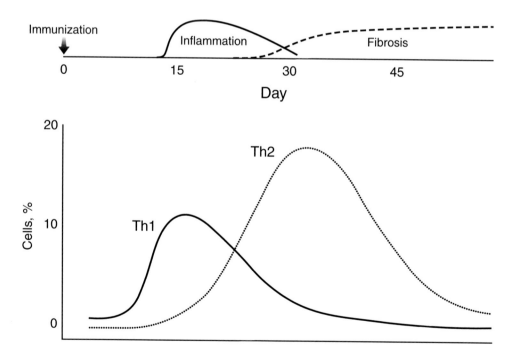

Fig. 8-7. Th1/Th2 balance of peripheral blood T cells during the course of experimental autoimmune myocarditis.

CHRONIC PHASE

Rats with EAM that survive the acute phase develop postmyocarditis dilated cardiomyopathy after 4 months or more.[40] Macroscopically, the hearts of the rats immunized with cardiac myosin are enlarged and diffusely discolored (Fig. 8-8; see color plate 12). Some rats show aneurysmal changes in the right ventricular wall. Both ventricles are dilated and heart weight increases significantly compared with normal rats. The left ventricular wall of the diseased rats is thinner than that of the normal rats. Histologically, interstitial fibrosis and replacement fibrosis spread into the entire myocardium of the hearts (Fig. 8-9; see color plate 13). Hypertrophic or atrophic myocardial fibers are observed in and around the fibrous lesions. Focal accumulations of mononuclear cells are rarely detected in the periphery of the lesions.

Collagen fibers consist of replacement fibrosis. Fibrous tissue is composed predominantly of type 1 and type 3 collagen. Expression of mRNA related to extracellular matrix components and matrix metabolism was investigated (Fig. 8-10).[41] Transforming growth factor-β is involved in the extracellular matrix production. Collagen and other extracellular matrix components play a role in protecting the left ventricle from extreme expansion after myocardial damage, but they may also interfere with left ventricular diastolic function and metabolism of residual myocardial fibers. Management of adequate replacement fibrosis may be a therapeutic strategy for postmyocarditis dilated cardiomyopathy.

RELEVANCE TO DILATED CARDIOMYOPATHY

Myocarditis is one of the important causes of dilated cardiomyopathy. How does myocarditis progress into dilated cardiomyopathy? The initial event seems to be viral infection in most cases. Organisms other than viruses, chemical substances, and disturbance of the individual immunologic environment may also be able to break self-tolerance. Infection or breakdown of self-tolerance leads to acute myocarditis. Acute myocardial injury may have 3 dominant mechanisms: direct toxic effects of viruses, an antiviral response that is valuable to the host but may be harmful for hearts lacking regeneration activity, and autoimmune myocardial injury. In viral myocarditis, all 3 pathogeneses are involved. EAM is useful to analyze autoimmune myocardial injury independent of viral effects.

Acute myocarditis shows a monophasic clinical course in human cases and in animal models. Left ventricular function improves after healing of the myocarditis. The mechanisms of how healed myocarditis progresses into dilated cardiomyopathy have been investigated extensively for a long time. Chronic myocarditis, either persistent or recurrent, is considered to be one of the mechanisms of the process (Fig. 8-11). Persistent viral infection, inappropriate antiviral immunity, and autoimmunity are proposed as the causes of

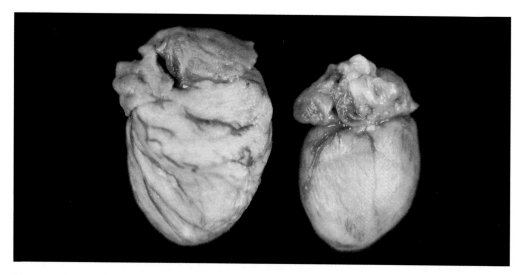

Fig. 8-8. Gross pathology of the chronic phase of experimental autoimmune myocarditis (*left*). Heart of an age-matched control rat (*right*). See color plate 12.

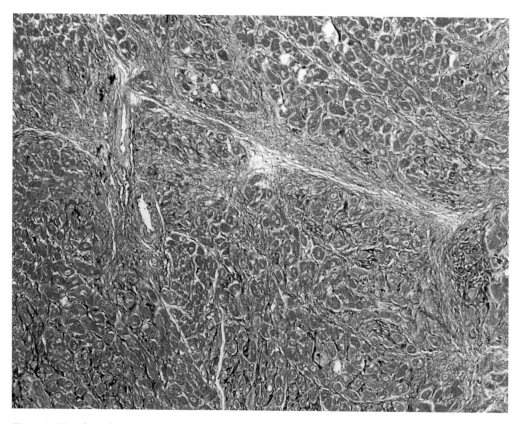

Fig. 8-9. Histologic findings of the chronic phase of experimental autoimmune myocarditis. (Azan-Mallory stain; x100.) See color plate 13.

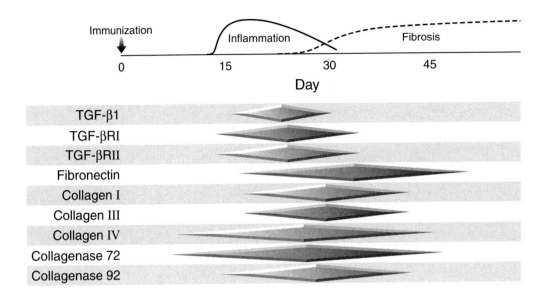

Fig. 8-10. Messenger RNA expression of extracellular matrix components during the course of experimental autoimmune myocarditis. *TGF*, transforming growth factor.

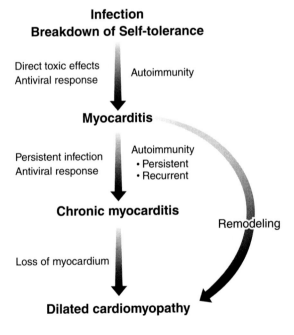

Fig. 8-11. Diagram of the pathogenesis of postmyocarditis dilated cardiomyopathy.

chronic myocarditis. The other process from myocarditis to dilated cardiomyopathy may be ventricular remodeling after myocarditis. Precise mechanisms of ventricular remodeling after inflammatory myocardial damage have not been investigated at all. Rat EAM is valuable in analyzing the process from acute myocarditis to dilated cardiomyopathy.

AN ANIMAL MODEL OF CHRONIC HEART FAILURE

Chronic heart failure is a major cardiovascular problem because of its morbidity and mortality in the population. Analysis of the pathophysiology and search for the new therapeutic strategies for chronic heart failure are required. Small animal models are useful in the basic study of chronic heart failure. Rat myocardial infarction produced by coronary ligation during open-chest surgical procedures has been used for the purpose. However, the infarction model has significant mortality due to technical problems at operation. On the other hand, rat EAM can be used as an animal model of chronic heart failure with several advantages compared to the infarction model. Rat EAM can be induced by a simple procedure: subcutaneous injection of the antigen. The morbidity is 100%. Myocardial damage is severe enough to produce chronic heart failure. Myocardial damage spreads diffusely over the entire heart. Finally, in vivo hemodynamics and left ventricular function can be measured in the chronic phase of rat EAM.[33,42,43]

Cardiac myosin-induced autoimmune myocarditis is quite useful in the study of autoimmune myocardial injuries and pathogenesis of postmyocarditis dilated cardiomyopathy. Further, rat EAM can be used as an animal model of chronic heart failure.

REFERENCES

1. Kaplan MH, Craig JM. Immunologic studies of heart tissue. VI. Cardiac lesions in rabbits associated with autoantibodies to heart induced by immunization with heterologous heart. J Immunol 1963;90:725-733.
2. Davies AM, Laufer A, Gery I, Rosemann E. Organ specificity of the heart. III. Circulating antibodies and immunopathological lesions in experimental animals. Arch Pathol 1964;78:369-376.
3. Wittner B, Maisch B, Kochsiek K. Quantification of antimyosin antibodies in experimental myocarditis by a new solid phase fluorometric assay. J Immunol Methods 1983;64:239-247.
4. Acosta AM, Santos-Buch CA. Autoimmune myocarditis induced by *Trypanosoma cruzi*. Circulation 1985;71:1255-1261.
5. Izumi T, Maisch B, Kochsiek K. Experimental murine myocarditis after immunization with cardiac membranous proteins. Eur Heart J 1987;8 Suppl J:419-424.
6. Neu N, Rose NR, Beisel KW, Herskowitz A, Gurri-Glass G, Craig SW. Cardiac myosin induces myocarditis in genetically predisposed mice. J Immunol 1987;139:3630-3636.

7. Kodama M, Matsumoto Y, Fujiwara M, Masani F, Izumi T, Shibata A. A novel experimental model of giant cell myocarditis induced in rats by immunization with cardiac myosin fraction. Clin Immunol Immunopathol 1990;57:250-262.

8. Sharaf AR, Narula J, Nicol PD, Southern JF, Khaw B-A. Cardiac sarcopic reticulum calcium ATPase, an autoimmune antigen in experimental cardiomyopathy. Circulation 1994;89: 1217-1228.

9. Schultheiss HP, Schulze K, Schauer R, Witzenbichler B, Strauer BE. Antibody-mediated imbalance of myocardial energy metabolism. A causal factor of cardiac failure? Circ Res 1995;76:64-72.

10. Huber SA, Cunningham MW. Streptococcal M protein peptide with similarity to myosin induces CD4⁺ T cell-dependent myocarditis in MRL/++ mice and induces partial tolerance against coxsackie-viral myocarditis. J Immunol 1996;156:3528-3534.

11. Bachmaier K, Neu N, de la Maza LM, Pal S, Hessel A, Penninger JM. *Chlamydia* infections and heart disease linked through antigenic mimicry. Science 1999;283:1335-1339.

12. Kodama M, Matsumoto Y, Fujiwara M, Zhang S, Hanawa H, Itoh E, Tsuda T, Izumi T, Shibata A. Characteristics of giant cells and factors related to the formation of giant cells in myocarditis. Circ Res 1991;69:1042-1050.

13. Donermeyer DL, Beisel KW, Allen PM, Smith SC. Myocarditis-inducing epitope of myosin binds constitutively and stably to I-A^k on antigen-presenting cells in the heart. J Exp Med 1995;182:1291-1300.

14. Wegmann KW, Zhao W, Griffin AC, Hickey WF. Identification of myocarditogenic peptides derived from cardiac myosin capable of inducing experimental allergic myocarditis in the Lewis rat: the utility of a class II binding motif in selecting self-reactive peptides. J Immunol 1994;153:892-900.

15. Inomata T, Hanawa H, Miyanishi T, Yajima E, Nakayama S, Maita T, Kodama M, Izumi T, Shibata A, Abo T. Localization of porcine cardiac myosin epitopes that induce experimental autoimmune myocarditis. Circ Res 1995;76:726-733.

16. Cunningham MW, Antone SN, Guilizia JM, McManus BM, Fischetti VA, Gauntt CJ. Cytotoxic and viral neutralizing antibodies crossreact with streptococcal M protein, enteroviruses, and human cardiac myosin. Proc Natl Acad Sci USA 1992;89:1320-1324.

17. Bachmaier K, Neu N, Yeung RSM, Mak TW, Liu P, Penninger JM. Generation of humanized mice susceptible to peptide-induced inflammatory heart disease. Circulation 1999;99:1885-1891.

18. Shioji K, Kishimoto C, Nakayama Y, Sasayama S. Strain difference in rats with experimental giant cell myocarditis. Jpn Circ J 2000;64:283-286.

19. Liao L, Sindhwani R, Rojkind M, Factor S, Leinwand L, Diamond B. Antibody-mediated auto-immune myocarditis depends on genetically determined target organ sensitivity. J Exp Med 1995;181:1123-1131.

20. Pummerer CL, Grässl G, Sailer M, Bachmaier KW, Penninger JM, Neu N. Cardiac myosin-induced myocarditis: target recognition by autoreactive T cells requires prior activation of cardiac interstitial cells. Lab Invest 1996;74:845-852.

21. Kodama M, Matsumoto Y, Fujiwara M. In vivo lymphocyte-mediated myocardial injuries demonstrated by adoptive transfer of experimental autoimmune myocarditis. Circulation 1992;85:1918-1926.

22. Okura Y, Takeda K, Honda S, Hanawa H, Watanabe H, Kodama M, Izumi T, Aizawa Y, Seki S, Abo T. Recombinant murine interleukin-12 facilitates induction of cardiac myosin-specific type 1 helper T cells in rats. Circ Res 1998;82:1035-1042.

23. Hanawa H, Kodama M, Inomata T, Izumi T, Shibata A, Tuchida M, Matsumoto Y, Abo T. Anti-αβ T cell receptor antibody prevents the progression of experimental autoimmune myocarditis. Clin Exp Immunol 1994;96:470-475.

24. Smith SC, Allen PM. Myosin-induced acute myocarditis is a T cell-mediated disease. J Immunol 1991;147:2141-2147.

25. Pummerer C, Berger P, Frühwirth M, Öfner C, Neu N. Cellular infiltrate, major histocompatibility antigen expression and immunopathogenic mechanisms in cardiac myosin-induced myocarditis. Lab Invest 1991;65:538-547.

26. Kodama M, Zhang S, Hanawa H, Shibata A. Immunohistochemical characterization of infiltrating mononuclear cells in the rat heart with experimental autoimmune giant cell myocarditis. Clin Exp Immunol 1992;90:330-335.

27. Hanawa H, Tsuchida M, Matsumoto Y, Watanabe H, Abo T, Sekikawa H, Kodama M, Zhang S, Izumi T, Shibata A. Characterization of T cells infiltrating the heart in rats with experimental autoimmune myocarditis: their similarity to extrathymic T cells in mice and the site of proliferation. J Immunol 1993;150:5682-5695.

28. Hanawa H, Inomata T, Sekikawa H, Abo T, Kodama M, Izumi T, Shibata A. Analysis of heart-infiltrating T-cell clonotypes in experimental autoimmune myocarditis in rats. Circ Res 1996;78:118-125.

29. Hanawa H, Inomata T, Okura Y, Hirono S, Ogawa Y, Izumi T, Kodama M, Aizawa Y. T cells with similar T-cell receptor β-chain complementarity-determining region 3 motifs infiltrate inflammatory lesions of synthetic peptides inducing rat autoimmune myocarditis. Circ Res 1998;83:133-140.

30. Okura Y, Yamamoto T, Goto S, Inomata T, Hirono S, Hanawa H, Feng L, Wilson CB, Kihara I, Izumi T, Shibata A, Aizawa Y, Seki S, Abo T. Characterization of cytokine and iNOS mRNA expression in situ during the course of experimental autoimmune myocarditis in rats. J Mol Cell Cardiol 1997;29:491-502.

31. Ito M, Kodama M, Masuko M, Yamaura M, Fuse K, Uesugi Y, Hirono S, Okura Y, Kato K, Hotta Y, Honda T, Kuwano R, Aizawa Y. Expression of coxsackievirus and adenovirus receptor in hearts of rats with experimental autoimmune myocarditis. Circ Res 2000;86:275-280.

32. Smith SC, Allen PM. Expression of myosin-class II major histocompatibility complexes in the normal myocardium occurs before induction of autoimmune myocarditis. Proc Natl Acad Sci U S A 1992;89:9131-9135.

33. Hirono S, Islam O, Nakazawa M, Yoshida Y, Kodama M, Shibata A, Izumi T, Imai S. Expression of inducible nitric oxide synthase in rat experimental autoimmune myocarditis with special reference to changes in cardiac hemodynamics. Circ Res 1997;80:11-20.

34. Ishiyama S, Hiroe M, Nishikawa T, Abe S, Shimojo T, Ito H, Ozasa S, Yamakawa K, Matsuzaki M, Mohammed MU, Nakazawa H, Kasajima T, Marumo F. Nitric oxide contributes to the progression of myocardial damage in experimental autoimmune myocarditis in rats. Circulation 1997;95:489-496.

35. Bachmaier K, Neu N, Pummerer C, Duncan GS, Mak TW, Matsuyama T, Penninger JM. iNOS expression and nitrotyrosine formation in the myocardium in response to inflammation is controlled by the interferon regulatory transcription factor 1. Circulation 1997;96:585-591.

36. Goren N, Leiros CP, Sterin-Borda L, Borda E. Nitric oxide synthase in experimental autoimmune myocarditis dysfunction. J Mol Cell Cardiol 1998;30:2467-2474.

37. Smith SC, Allen PM. Neutralization of endogenous tumor necrosis factor ameliorates the severity of myosin-induced myocarditis. Circ Res 1992;70:856-863.

38. Bachmaier K, Pummerer C, Kozieradzki I, Pfeffer K, Mak TW, Neu N, Penninger JM. Low-molecular-weight tumor necrosis factor receptor p55 controls induction of autoimmune heart disease. Circulation 1997;95:655-661.

39. Ishiyama S, Hiroe M, Nishikawa T, Shimojo T, Abe S, Fujisaki H, Ito H, Yamakawa K, Kobayashi N, Kasajima T, Marumo F. The Fas/Fas ligand system is involved in the pathogenesis of autoimmune myocarditis in rats. J Immunol 1998;161:4695-4701.

40. Kodama M, Hanawa H, Saeki M, Hosono H, Inomata T, Suzuki K, Shibata A. Rat dilated cardio-myopathy after autoimmune giant cell myocarditis. Circ Res 1994;75:278-284.

41. Tsukimata JK. Expression of TGF-β1, TGF-β receptors, extracellular matrix proteins, collagenase 72, collagenase 92 and TIMP-1 in rats with experimental autoimmune myocarditis developing into dilated cardiomyopathy. [Japanese.] Niigata Igakkai Zasshi 1997;111:509-522.

42. Koyama S, Kodama M, Izumi T, Shibata A. Experimental rat model representing both acute and chronic heart failure related to autoimmune myocarditis. Cardiovasc Drugs Ther 1995;9:701-707.

43. Watanabe K, Ohta Y, Nakazawa M, Higuchi H, Hasegawa G, Naito M, Nagatomo T, Fuse K, Ito M, Hirono S, Okura Y, Kato K, Kodama M, Aizawa Y. Effects of long-term treatment with carvedilol in rats with dilated cardiomyopathy after myocarditis. J Cardiovasc Pharmacol 1999;34 Suppl 4:S77-S80.

Progression of Myocarditis to Dilated Cardiomyopathy:

Role of the Adrenergic System and Myocardial Catecholamines

Petar M. Seferović, M.D., Ph.D.,
Arsen D. Ristić, M.D., M.Sc.,
and Ružica Maksimović, M.D., Ph.D.

INTRODUCTION

ROLE OF INOTROPIC STIMULATION IN THE PROGRESSION
OF MYOCARDITIS TO DILATED CARDIOMYOPATHY

ABNORMALITIES OF NOREPINEPHRINE UPTAKE
AND EFFECT OF β-BLOCKING AGENTS IN ACUTE
MYOCARDITIS AND DILATED CARDIOMYOPATHY

FULMINANT MYOCARDITIS:
Lessons in Pathophysiology Learned From the Assist-Device
Implantations and Percutaneous Cardiopulmonary Support

MYOCARDIAL CATECHOLAMINES:
Methodologic Aspects, Reproducibility, and Drawbacks

MYOCARDIAL CATECHOLAMINES IN ACUTE
BIOPSY-PROVEN MYOCARDITIS VERSUS IDIOPATHIC
DILATED CARDIOMYOPATHY

CONCLUSIONS

INTRODUCTION

A progression from viral myocarditis to dilated cardiomyopathy has long been hypothesized and clinically accepted, but the exact pathogenetic mechanisms remained uncertain. With developments in the molecular analyses of tissue specimens, new techniques of viral gene amplification, and biochemical analyses, this causal link became even more apparent.[1-3] Perhaps the major breakthrough in understanding this burdensome clinical issue was the demonstration of viral RNA/DNA persistence in the myocardium beyond 90 days after inoculation, confirmed by the polymerase chain reaction. Although acute viral myocarditis has various clinical presentations, only the severe cases can lead to substantial cardiac damage and development of dilated cardiomyopathy. In addition to the direct injury of the myocytes, other mechanisms are likely to be involved.[4] Several studies have revealed T-cell immune-mediated and viral-induced cardiac damage as the major pathophysiologic mechanisms.[4,5] Apoptotic cell death may provide another concept to explain the harmful clinical course of acute myocarditis.[6]

Activation of the sympathetic nervous system has been recognized recently as one of the determinants of the disease progression to dilated cardiomyopathy. Acute myocarditis is often associated with various degrees of ventricular dysfunction, which in severe cases may lead to generalized neurohumoral activation characterized by excitation of sympathetic and renin-angiotensin systems and increased synthesis of natriuretic peptides and cytokines. There is experimental and clinical evidence of detrimental effects of increased sympathetic activity in acute myocarditis.

Several investigators examined the effect of exercise on coxsackievirus B3-induced myocarditis in mice.[7-9] These studies used swimming or running on a treadmill as the exercise stressor, thus increasing the heart rate and blood pressure, effects mostly mediated through catecholamines. These experiments found more extensive heart lesions in exercised than nonexercised coxsackievirus B3-infected mice.[10] Popović et al.,[11] in an acute hemodynamic study, demonstrated the beneficial effects of metoprolol, with or without nitroglycerin, in 11 patients with left ventricular dysfunction and biopsy-proven lymphocytic myocarditis.

Therefore, this chapter reviews the current knowledge on the role of adrenergic dysfunction and myocardial catecholamines in the progression of myocarditis to dilated cardiomyopathy. In particular, the following topics are considered: the effects of inotropic stimulation in the natural history of myocarditis, the impact of β-blocking agents in acute myocarditis, studies analyzing the effect of left ventricular-assist device implantation and percutaneous cardiopulmonary support in acute myocarditis, and correlation of myocardial catecholamines and left ventricular function in acute myocarditis versus dilated cardiomyopathy. Methodologic drawbacks of catecholamine analyses in myocardial tissue are analyzed separately.

ROLE OF INOTROPIC STIMULATION IN THE PROGRESSION OF MYOCARDITIS TO DILATED CARDIOMYOPATHY

The harmful effect of catecholamines on myocardial morphology and function is well established. Deisher et al.[12] showed that epinephrine infusion resulted in myocyte hypertrophy, left ventricular fibrotic degenerative changes, diminished response to adrenergic stimuli, and enhanced left ventricular papillary contractile response to calcium. Two weeks after cessation of epinephrine infusion, left ventricular fibrotic degenerative changes were reduced, and responses to adrenergic stimuli were partially restored. However, myocyte hypertrophy and enhanced response to calcium persisted in these animals.

Exposure of adult rat ventricular myocytes to norepinephrine increases the number of apoptotic cells.[13] This effect is inhibited by propranolol, mimicked by the adenylyl cyclase stimulator forskolin, and attenuated by an inhibitor of protein kinase A, indicating that norepinephrine stimulates apoptosis via a β-adrenergic receptor–mediated increase in cyclic adenosine monophosphate (cAMP).[13] Likewise, Iwai-Kanai et al.[14] showed that β-adrenergic receptor stimulation increases apoptosis in neonatal rat cardiac myocytes by a mechanism that depends on the cAMP–protein kinase A pathway. Furthermore, Communal et al.[6] directly demonstrated that stimulation of β$_1$-adrenergic receptors increases apoptosis via a cAMP-dependent mechanism, whereas stimulation of β$_2$-adrenergic receptors inhibits apoptosis via a G(i)-protein-coupled pathway, as measured by flow cytometry. These findings support the thesis that increased sympathetic activity to the myocardium contributes to myocardial failure via β$_1$-adrenergic receptor–stimulated apoptosis of cardiac myocytes. This premise is also supported by the demonstration that mice overexpressing Gs developed dilated cardiomyopathy associated with myocyte apoptosis,[15] and mice overexpressing β$_1$-adrenergic receptors developed dilated cardiomyopathy.[16,17] In contrast, mice overexpressing β$_2$-adrenergic receptors did not develop myocardial dysfunction at ages up to 4 months.[18]

Inotropic stimulation exacerbates myocardial damage in experimental viral myocarditis.[7-9] Physical activity associated with tachycardia, increase in blood pressure, and catecholamine-mediated inotropic effect had a deleterious influence on experimental animals with viral myocarditis. Gatmaitan et al.[7] demonstrated that when coxsackievirus B3-infected mice were forced to swim in a warm pool, the virulence of the agent was significantly increased. Viral replication was augmented 530-fold over control values. Reyes et al.[8] reported that severe exercise-induced stress might be mediated by host hormonal conditions. In experiments with Swiss ICR mice infected with coxsackievirus B3, they reported that exercise is associated with the release of epinephrine and norepinephrine from the adrenal medulla. Accordingly, these neurohormones regulate the intracellular concentrations of cAMP and cyclic guanosine monophosphate (cGMP), which modulate humoral and cellular immune responses as well as inflammation, leading to the increase in susceptibility to coxsackievirus infections.[19] Altered immune function was associated with the exercised group:

increased heart-infiltrating cytotoxic T cells, decreased antibody titers, decreased interferon production, and decreased major histocompatibility complex class II expressing cells in the myocardium.[7-9]

More extensive heart damage in infected exercised animals may be caused by oxidative stress. Exercise increases the metabolic rate, which in turn leads to an increase in free-radical production.[20] Previous studies found an increase in superoxide dismutase and a decrease in glutathione peroxidase and catalase in exercised rats.[21] In this study, heart tissue in exercised animals increased free radical production, measured by the malondialdehyde reaction. Supplementation of exercised rats with vitamin E completely prevented the accumulation of malondialdehyde, suggesting that exercise-induced oxidative stress could be ameliorated with an antioxidant supplement.

Pharmacologic inotropic stimulation using digoxin also exerted adverse effects in a murine model of viral myocarditis.[22] Inbred DBA/2 mice (age 4 weeks) were inoculated intraperitoneally with encephalomyocarditis virus and treated with digoxin orally from the day of virus inoculation. The 14-day mortality tended to increase in mice treated with 1 mg/kg and was significantly increased in the group treated with 10 mg/kg per day. Myocardial necrosis and cellular infiltration on day 6 were significantly more severe in the high-dose digoxin group than in the control group. In the animals treated with 1 mg/kg digoxin, IL-1β concentration was significantly higher than in the control group. Intracardiac tumor necrosis factor (TNF)-α values also increased in a dose-dependent manner. These results suggest that in the murine model digoxin worsens viral myocarditis.

In contrast to the previous findings, Nishio et al.[23] reported the beneficial effects of denopamine, a selective β_1-adrenergic agonist, in the same murine model of congestive heart failure due to viral myocarditis. The effects of denopamine on lipopolysaccharide-induced TNF-α production were studied in murine spleen cells as well as in vivo in 4-week-old DBA/2 mice inoculated with the encephalomyocarditis virus (day 0). Denopamine (14 μmol/kg) alone, denopamine (14 μmol/kg) with a selective β_1-blocker metoprolol (42 μmol/kg), or denopamine (14 μmol/kg) with metoprolol (84 μmol/kg) was administered daily. In the in vitro study, TNF-α concentrations in treated cells were significantly lower than in controls. In the in vivo study, treatment with denopamine significantly improved the survival of the animals (56% versus 20%), attenuated myocardial lesions, and suppressed TNF-α production. There was a strong linear relationship between mortality and TNF-α values. Both in vitro and in vivo effects of denopamine were significantly inhibited by metoprolol. However, the extent of myocardial damage was not attenuated in the denopamine-treated group on day 6 or 7, despite the inhibition of TNF-α production in the heart. In contrast, denopamine did attenuate the extent of myocardial lesions and inhibited TNF-α production at day 14. Past day 7, at the stage of congestive heart failure, it exerted protective effects through its inhibitory action on TNF-α production.

Reports from several laboratories demonstrating that TNF-α exacerbates myocardial injury [24-26] contributed significantly to the understanding of the mechanisms of acute myocarditis. Increased intracellular concentration of cyclic AMP, by stimulating the β-adrenergic receptors, may accelerate the rate of cell death, and calcium overload may induce arrhythmias and myocardial injury.[27,28] Furthermore, in clinical trials an increase in mortality was associated with the long-term use of β-agonists.[29] In addition, several studies have shown an integration of neuroendocrine hormones into the immune response. Adrenergic agents, in particular, have been shown to influence cytokine production.[30-34]

ABNORMALITIES OF NOREPINEPHRINE UPTAKE AND EFFECT OF β-BLOCKING AGENTS IN ACUTE MYOCARDITIS AND DILATED CARDIOMYOPATHY

The abnormalities of norepinephrine uptake reflecting impairment of the adrenergic nerve function have been reported in several studies of acute myocarditis and dilated cardiomyopathy associated with congestive heart failure. Agostini et al.[35] demonstrated significant impairment of cardiac norepinephrine uptake in acute myocarditis by using iodine-123 M-iodobenzylguanidine (mIBG) scintigraphy. Also, a significant correlation was observed between left ventricular ejection fraction and mIBG uptake in these patients (Fig. 9-1). Reduction of myocardial mIBG uptake can most likely be explained by functional mechanisms, such as increased cardiac spillover of norepinephrine,[36] resulting in higher serum concentration and antagonistic competition for mIBG for uptake at nerve terminals. Therefore, a reduced number of sympathetic neurons with an increased amount of interstitial fibrotic tissue together with increased mIBG turnover could account for these phenomena.

Similarly, Schofer et al.[37] using identical methodology disclosed a significant positive correlation between myocardial norepinephrine concentration and left ventricular ejection fraction in 31 patients with dilated cardiomyopathy and various degrees of heart failure. Patients with diffusely reduced or no visible myocardial uptake had the lowest left ventricular ejection fraction, suggesting myocardial adrenergic disintegrity. Using a similar study design, Glowniak et al.[38] showed decreased mIBG uptake and faster mIBG washout in idiopathic dilated cardiomyopathy patients. Decreased mIBG uptake in these patients suggests sympathetic dysfunction, whereas rapid washout could reflect increased sympathetic neuron activity.

Catecholamine-induced inotropic stimulation is inhibited by β-adrenergic receptor blocking drugs. Because of this pathophysiologic background, these agents may have a beneficial effect on the natural history of myocardial inflammation. However, the experimental data are still a subject of debate. Tominaga et al.[39] reported a beneficial effect of carteolol, a nonselective β-adrenergic receptor blocker with intrinsic sympathomimetic activity,

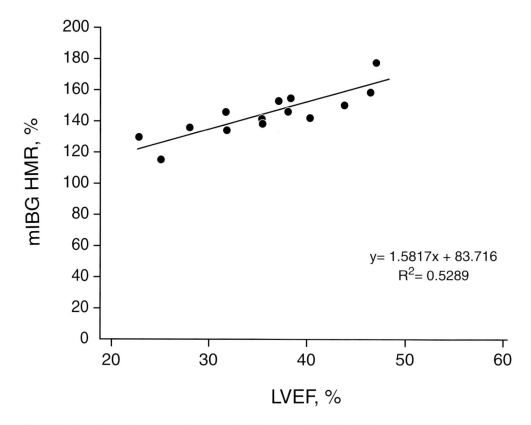

$$y = 1.5817x + 83.716$$
$$R^2 = 0.5289$$

Fig. 9-1. Correlation between cardiac meta-iodobenzylguanidine (*mIBG*) uptake expressed as heart-to-mediastinum ratio (*HMR*) and left ventricular ejection fraction (*LVEF*) with acute myocarditis. (From Agostini et al.[35] By permission of the Society of Nuclear Medicine.)

compared with metoprolol in a murine model of viral myocarditis and dilated cardiomyopathy caused by encephalomyocarditis virus. Heart weight-to-body weight ratio and histopathologic scores were significantly lower in mice given carteolol than in the infected control group. Furthermore, left ventricular dimension, wall thickness, and myocardial fiber diameter were significantly reduced in mice given carteolol compared with the control group. Metoprolol did not cause any significant changes compared with the control group.

In contrast, the β-blocking agent metoprolol exerted deleterious effects in acute coxsackievirus B3 myocarditis[40] in mice infected at the age of 3 weeks and treated with metoprolol intraperitoneally for 10 days. Mortality in the metoprolol group (*n* = 50) was 60% compared with 0% in the control group (*n* = 50) receiving isotonic saline. Whereas pathologic changes at days 3, 6, and 10 of infection were similar in the 2 groups, on day 30 of infection, inflammation, necrosis, and mineralization scores were significantly different: 1.1 ± 0.3, 2.1 ± 0.4, and 2.2 ± 0.5 for the metoprolol group versus 0.3 ± 0.1, 0.4 ± 0.3, and 0.4 ± 0.3

for the saline group, respectively. Six noninfected mice received metoprolol intraperitoneally for 10 days, and there were no deaths during 30 days of observation.

FULMINANT MYOCARDITIS:
Lessons in Pathophysiology Learned From the Assist-Device Implantations and Percutaneous Cardiopulmonary Support

Acute myocarditis complicated with severe hemodynamic compromise, requiring a left ventricular-assist device, can serve as a useful model for studying the effect of lack of the myocardial sympathetic influence. At least theoretically, the temporary use of cardiopulmonary support, offering a "resting" condition of the heart, should have a beneficial effect on recovery of the heavily diseased myocardium. However, the results of various studies in this challenging area are controversial.

Management of acute fulminant myocarditis using circulatory support systems was studied by Reiss et al.[41] who used 3 different assist devices. Two patients who initially came from another hospital died of multiorgan failure after a support time of 24 hours. The third patient, who received the Biomedicus pump, recovered after a support time of 120 hours and could be weaned. However, 2 days later, malignant arrhythmias developed and he died. The 2 remaining patients with acute fulminant viral myocarditis were supported by a biventricular-assist device (Thoratec , 111 days; Abiomed, 7 days). During the entire time of support, there were no signs of myocardial recovery.

Kato et al.[42] reported an opposite experience with percutaneous cardiopulmonary support in 9 patients with fulminant myocarditis associated with cardiogenic shock. Although 2 of the patients died, 7 improved and were able to resume social activities. Successful management of acute myocarditis with biventricular-assist devices and cardiac transplantation was also shown in the study by Starling et al.[43] In addition, a beneficial effect of percutaneous cardiopulmonary support was reported in 7 of 10 patients with acute fulminant myocarditis. Six of the 7 survivors recovered virtually normal cardiac function.

Brilakis et al.[44] compared bridging to cardiac transplantation in the giant cell myocarditis patients who received a ventricular-assist device to bridging observed in the general heart failure population. Of 9 patients with giant cell myocarditis who received ventricular-assist devices, 7 patients survived to transplantation, 4 were alive 30 days posttransplantation, and 2 survived to 1 year. The rate of successful bridging to transplantation (78%) was similar to that reported for other ventricular-assist device recipients. Posttransplantation survival of 57% at 30 days and 29% at 1 year was significantly lower compared with 93% 1-year survival of the 30 patients with giant cell myocarditis who did not receive ventricular-assist devices before transplantation.

MYOCARDIAL CATECHOLAMINES:
Methodologic Aspects, Reproducibility, and Drawbacks

Two major limitations in tissue biochemical measurements of myocardial catecholamines are the reproducibility of the method and the lack of data on myocardial catecholamine concentrations in nondiseased myocardium. Reproducibility is the inherent problem of every biopsy procedure and is more apparent if the measurement or analysis in endomyocardial biopsy samples has a higher sensitivity. The good reproducibility of measurement in endomyocardial biopsy samples is supported by the studies by Kawai et al.,[45] Regitz et al.,[46-48] and our group.[49] Kawai et al.[45] demonstrated a significant correlation between repeated measurements (n = 10) in the 2 assays for myocardial norepinephrine and epinephrine concentrations, whereas Regitz et al.[47] confirmed a high reproducibility suggested by the finding that variance between paired biopsy samples was less than 17%. More precise data on myocardial catecholamine concentration reproducibility were obtained from the examination of explanted hearts in the elegant study by De Maria et al.[50] Of 40 patients who underwent heart transplantation, the transmural myocardial samples in 27 explanted hearts (67%) gave reproducible myocardial catecholamine concentration results and were used for analysis.

In most studies using invasive methodology it is not possible to form a control group for obvious ethical reasons, and therefore the reports are scarce on values of myocardial catecholamines in nondiseased myocardium. One of the few studies addressing this issue reported myocardial catecholamine concentration values in 10 healthy controls (in pg/μg, for norepinephrine 10.3 ± 2.9, epinephrine 0.36 ± 0.51, and dopamine 0.52 ± 0.40).[11] De Maria et al.[50] also reported normal myocardial catecholamine concentration values in the explanted donor heart of a 46-year-old man.

In our institution, the measurement of myocardial catecholamine concentration is performed by a catechol O-methyltransferase (COMT) radioenzymatic method. Before analysis, the endomyocardial biopsy sample (wet weight of 2-4 mg) is divided into 2 parts: one for histology and the other for myocardial catecholamine concentration measurements. The part of the endomyocardial biopsy sample used for measurement of myocardial catecholamine concentration is immediately weighed, frozen in liquid nitrogen, and stored at -80° C. At the time of analysis, the specimens are immersed in cold (4° C) 0.1N $HClO_4$ (0.3 μg of tissue per 30 μL of 0.1N $HClO_4$). The tissue is then homogenized (10,000 rotations per minute for 15 minutes) and clear supernatant (30 μL) is used for the analysis.

We use the modified COMT radioenzymatic method of Da Prada and Zürcher,[51] Weise and Kopin,[52] and Peuler and Johnson.[53] The principle of the method is to convert the myocardial catecholamines into their corresponding O-methyl derivatives by means of purified COMT in the presence of S-adenosyl-l-([³H]methyl)-methionine. The O-methyl derivatives are extracted and oxidized into [³H]vanillin. The activity of this substance is measured by a liquid beta scintillation counter (Packard). The following substances are used: S-adenosyl-l-([^{3}H]methyl)-methionine (Amersham) and ethylenediaminetetraacetic acid (Sigma). COMT is prepared according to the method of Axelrod and Tomchick.[54] Most experts consider this method as fast, highly specific, reliable, and reproducible. Two samples from each patient are analyzed and the mean value is reported.

MYOCARDIAL CATECHOLAMINES IN ACUTE BIOPSY-PROVEN MYOCARDITIS VERSUS IDIOPATHIC DILATED CARDIOMYOPATHY

In the study by Seferović et al.,[55] myocardial catecholamine concentration was assessed in biopsy-proven myocarditis (20 patients) and idiopathic dilated cardiomyopathy (32 patients). Myocardial catecholamine concentration and left ventricular hemodynamic parameters were calculated. The diagnoses of biopsy-proven myocarditis and idiopathic dilated cardiomyopathy were established after a complete work-up that included medical history, clinical investigations, echocardiography, right-sided and left-sided heart catheterization, hemodynamic measurements, endomyocardial biopsy, and coronary arteriography. The procedure was not started before the patient had at least 1 hour in a recumbent position and 15 minutes from the latest injection of contrast material. Premedication was limited to local anesthesia.

The patients with biopsy-proven myocarditis were younger, with a higher incidence of recent viral infection, but suffered from fewer arrhythmias than the idiopathic dilated cardiomyopathy group (Table 9-1). Patients with biopsy-proven myocarditis demonstrated significantly higher mean heart rate but only a moderate decline in left ventricular function. Patients with idiopathic dilated cardiomyopathy had more severe left ventricular dysfunction.

The average myocardial norepinephrine, epinephrine, and dopamine concentrations for biopsy-proven myocarditis and idiopathic dilated cardiomyopathy are depicted in Figure 9-2. Comparison between the groups revealed significant differences for myocardial norepinephrine and epinephrine concentration ($P < 0.01$) but not for myocardial dopamine concentration. The myocardial norepinephrine and epinephrine concentrations in patients with biopsy-proven myocarditis were significantly higher than in the idiopathic dilated cardiomyopathy group. Mean myocardial dopamine concentrations were similar ($P > 0.05$).

The correlations of myocardial catecholamine concentration and the observed hemodynamic variables are shown for biopsy-proven myocarditis and idiopathic dilated cardiomyopathy groups in Tables 9-2 and 9-3, respectively. No significant correlations were found among myocardial catecholamine concentration and hemodynamic variables in patients with biopsy-proven myocarditis (Table 9-2). In patients with idiopathic dilated cardiomyopathy (Table 9-3), myocardial norepinephrine and epinephrine concentrations

Table 9-1
Clinical, Hemodynamic, and Angiographic Data of Patients
With Biopsy-Proven Myocarditis and Idiopathic Dilated Cardiomyopathy*

Characteristic	Biopsy-proven myocarditis	Idiopathic dilated cardiomyopathy
Clinical		
Patients, no.	20	32
Age, y	36.5 ± 13.3	47.3 ± 11.9
Sex, % male	80	75
Recent viral infection, % (no.)	45.0 (9)	21.8 (7)
Ventricular arrhythmias, % (no.)	35.0 (7)	56.3 (18)
Congestive heart failure, % (no.)	20.0 (4)	37.5 (12)
Hemodynamic and angiographic		
HR, beats/min	118.4 ± 8.2	82.1 ± 8.3
PCWP, mm Hg	18.2 ± 3.6	28.8 ± 2.7
LVEDP, mm Hg	19.9 ± 4.3	30.9 ± 2.7
LV max dp/dt, mm Hg x s^{-1}	1,142.3 ± 166.3	559.0 ± 151.4
LVEF, %	39.9 ± 4.7	25.1 ± 4.2
MAP, mm Hg	89.6 ± 9.3	61.1 ± 10.9

HR, heart rate; LV dp/dt max, maximal rate of change of pressure during isovolumetric contraction; LVEDP, left ventricular end-diastolic pressure; LVEF, left ventricular ejection fraction; MAP, mean arterial pressure; PCWP, pulmonary capillary wedge pressure.
*Results are shown as mean values ± SEM, unless indicated otherwise.
From Seferović et al.[55] By permission of Springer-Verlag.

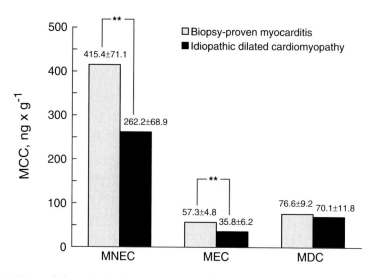

Fig. 9-2. Myocardial catecholamine concentration (*MCC*) in biopsy-proven myocarditis and idiopathic dilated cardiomyopathy. *MDC*, myocardial dopamine concentration; *MEC*, myocardial epinephrine concentration; *MNEC*, myocardial norepinephrine concentration. **$P < 0.01$.

Table 9-2
Correlation of Myocardial Catecholamine Concentration and Related Hemodynamic Variables in Biopsy-Proven Myocarditis

Hemodynamic variable	MNEC	MEC	MDC
HR, beats/min	-0.29	-0.16	-0.27
PCWP mean, mm Hg	-0.22	0.17	-0.16
LVEDP, mm Hg	-0.09	-0.13	-0.23
LV dp/dt max, mm Hg x s^{-1}	0.33	-0.18	-0.09
LVEF, %	0.34	0.08	-0.02
MAP, mm Hg	0.12	0.26	0.01

HR, heart rate; LV dp/dt max, maximal rate of change of pressure during isovolumetric contraction; LVEDP, left ventricular end-diastolic pressure; LVEF, left ventricular ejection fraction; MAP, mean arterial pressure; MDC, myocardial dopamine concentration; MEC, myocardial epinephrine concentration; MNEC, myocardial norepinephrine concentration; PCWP, pulmonary capillary wedge pressure.
From Seferović et al.[55] By permission of Springer-Verlag.

Table 9-3
Correlation of Myocardial Catecholamine Concentration and Related Hemodynamic Variables in Idiopathic Dilated Cardiomyopathy

Hemodynamic variable	MNEC	MEC	MDC
HR, beats/min	0.35	0.49	0.09
PCWP mean, mm Hg	-0.83*	-0.76*	-0.07
LVEDP, mm Hg	-0.79*	-0.75*	-0.11
LV dp/dt max, mm Hg x s^{-1}	0.87*	0.74*	0.07
LVEF, %	0.89*	0.86*	0.02
MAP, mm Hg	-0.01	0.17	-0.08

HR, heart rate; LV dp/dt max, maximal rate of change of pressure during isovolumetric contraction; LVEDP, left ventricular end-diastolic pressure; LVEF, left ventricular ejection fraction; MAP, mean arterial pressure; MDC, myocardial dopamine concentration; MEC, myocardial epinephrine concentration; MNEC, myocardial norepinephrine concentration; PCWP, pulmonary capillary wedge pressure.
*$P < 0.01$.
From Seferović et al.[55] By permission of Springer-Verlag.

demonstrated a significant positive correlation with left ventricular dp/dt max and left ventricular ejection fraction ($P < 0.01$) but a significant negative correlation with pulmonary capillary wedge pressure and left ventricular end-diastolic pressure ($P < 0.01$).

Severe cases of acute myocarditis, complicated by clinically apparent left ventricular dysfunction, can be accompanied by abnormalities in systemic and local adrenergic function. It is unclear whether the local alterations that occur in the sympathetic neuroeffector pathways are a consequence of systemic processes or whether they are under local control and may in fact contribute to the systemic abnormalities, such as increased concentration of circulating norepinephrine. At the myocardial level, several changes in the adrenergic effector systems have been described—one of the major ones being the myocardial nor-epinephrine depletion.[56] This metabolic abnormality appears to result from a profound decrease in norepinephrine reuptake. The combination of a marked decrease in neuronal uptake and, to a lesser degree, a decrease in norepinephrine release results in increased synaptic cleft/interstitial concentrations of norepinephrine and depletion in neuronal nor-epinephrine stores.[57]

In the study mentioned above, significantly higher myocardial norepinephrine and epinephrine concentrations in patients with biopsy-proven myocarditis compared with the dilated cardiomyopathy group may have pathogenetic as well as clinical implications. One can hypothesize that higher myocardial catecholamine concentrations are an inherent feature of acute myocarditis, as an initial phase of development of dilated postinflammatory heart muscle disease. However, because left ventricular ejection fraction was moderately decreased in the myocarditis group, it is unclear whether higher myocardial catecholamine values may be taken as a nonspecific marker of still maintained left ventricular function. The features of severely depressed left ventricular function, decreased myocardial norepi-nephrine and epinephrine concentrations, and their remarkable correlation demonstrated in the dilated cardiomyopathy group may reflect the severity of myocardial dysfunction and indicate the final stage of the disease. Future studies should include long-term patient follow-up and serial catecholamine measurements.

Similar findings were reported in several studies. In 72 patients who had idiopathic dilated cardiomyopathy, Schofer et al.[58] demonstrated a significant positive correlation between low myocardial norepinephrine concentration and decreased left ventricular ejection fraction, whereas myocardial norepinephrine concentration correlated negatively with myo-cyte fiber diameter. The degree of myocardial catecholamine concentration reduction in most investigations correlated with the decline of left ventricular systolic function.

Correa-Araujo et al.[59] analyzed myocardial catecholamine concentration and serotonin in apical left ventricular myocardium of 42 autopsied patients with chronic Chagas disease. A significant depletion of norepinephrine was detected in those with severe left ventricular dysfunction and manifested heart failure, whereas serotonin concentration was signifi-cantly increased. Furthermore, in heart failure patients Anderson et al.[60] revealed a positive correlation of myocardial norepinephrine and neuropeptide Y depletion, with β_1-adrenergic receptor down-regulation, whereas there was no correlation of adrenergic neurotransmitter level to β_2 receptor density. Norepinephrine, dopamine, and neuropeptide Y concentra-tions were significantly decreased in failing compared with nonfailing hearts. The mean ratio of dopamine to norepinephrine and of dopamine to neuropeptide Y in failing hearts was also significantly decreased compared with nonfailing control hearts. Thus, neuro-peptide Y depletion could be a useful marker of increased adrenergic drive in patients with congestive heart failure.

CONCLUSIONS

1. Pathogenetic mechanisms of progression from viral myocarditis to dilated cardiomyopathy are poorly understood. Circumstantial data point toward a causal role of myocardial catecholamines in the development of dilated cardiomyopathy.

2. The harmful effect of catecholamines on myocardial morphology and function in animals is well known. In acute viral myocarditis inotropic stimulation can promote myocardial damage. Inotropic stimulation using digoxin causes myocardial dysfunction in a murine model of viral myocarditis.

3. Abnormalities of norepinephrine uptake reflecting the impairment of adrenergic nerve function are associated with acute myocarditis and dilated cardiomyopathy. Catecholamine-induced inotropic stimulation is inhibited by β-adrenergic receptor blocking drugs.

4. Acute myocarditis complicated with severe hemodynamic compromise, treated with temporary left ventricular-assist support, can serve as a useful model for studying the effect of myocardial sympathetic tone. The temporary use of cardiopulmonary support, offering "resting" condition of the heart, should have a beneficial effect on recovery of the heavily diseased myocardium. However, the results of various studies are inconclusive.

5. Two major limitations in measurement of myocardial catecholamine concentration are reproducibility of the method and the lack of data on myocardial catecholamine concentration in nondiseased myocardium. The COMT radioenzymatic method is one of the most reliable methods for myocardial catecholamine concentration measurement.

6. Our study revealed significantly higher myocardial norepinephrine and epinephrine concentration in patients with biopsy-proven myocarditis than in those with idiopathic dilated cardiomyopathy. It remains unclear if this difference represents the early and the final phase of identical disease or is merely loosely associated with myocardial processes. These alterations are likely due to the impaired neuronal uptake, which could lead to further morphologic and functional consequences.

REFERENCES

1. Jin O, Sole MJ, Butany JW, Chia WK, McLaughlin PR, Liu P, Liew CC. Detection of enterovirus RNA in myocardial biopsies from patients with myocarditis and cardiomyopathy using gene amplification by polymerase chain reaction. Circulation 1990;82:8-16.

2. Weiss LM, Movahed LA, Billingham ME, Cleary ML. Detection of Coxsackievirus B3 RNA in myocardial tissues by the polymerase chain reaction. Am J Pathol 1991;138:497-503.

3. Kyu B, Matsumori A, Sato Y, Okada I, Chapman NM, Tracy S. Cardiac persistence of cardioviral RNA detected by polymerase chain reaction in a murine model of dilated cardiomyopathy. Circulation 1992;86:522-530.

4. Kawai C. From myocarditis to cardiomyopathy: mechanisms of inflammation and cell death; learning from the past for the future. Circulation 1999;99:1091-1100.

5. Kearney MT, Cotton JM, Richardson PJ, Shah AM. Viral myocarditis and dilated cardiomyopathy: mechanisms, manifestations, and management. Postgrad Med J 2001;77:4-10.

6. Communal C, Singh K, Sawyer DB, Colucci WS. Opposing effects of beta(1)- and beta(2)-adrenergic receptors on cardiac myocyte apoptosis: role of a pertussis toxin-sensitive G protein. Circulation 1999;100:2210-2212.

7. Gatmaitan BG, Chason JL, Lerner AM. Augmentation of the virulence of murine coxsackie-virus B-3 myocardiopathy by exercise. J Exp Med 1970;131:1121-1136.

8. Reyes MP, Thomas JA, Ho KL, Smith FE, Lerner AM. Elevated thymocyte norepinephrine and cyclic guanosine 3′,5′monophosphate in T-lymphocytes from exercised mice with coxsackievirus B3 myocarditis. Biochem Biophys Res Commun 1982;109:704-708.

9. Ilback NG, Fohlman J, Friman G. Exercise in coxsackie B3 myocarditis: effects on heart lymphocyte subpopulations and the inflammatory reaction. Am Heart J 1989;117:1298-1302.

10. Beck MA, Levander OA. Effects of nutritional antioxidants and other dietary constituents on coxsackievirus-induced myocarditis. Curr Top Microbiol Immunol 1997;223:81-96.

11. Popović Z, Mirić M, Vasiljević J, Sagić D, Bojić M, Popović AD. Acute hemodynamic effects of metoprolol ± nitroglycerin in patients with biopsy-proven lymphocytic myocarditis. Am J Cardiol 1998;81:801-804.

12. Deisher TA, Ginsburg R, Fowler MB, Billingham ME, Bristow MR. Spontaneous reversibility of catecholamine-induced cardiotoxicity in rats. Am J Cardiovasc Pathol 1995;5:79-88.

13. Communal C, Singh K, Pimentel DR, Colucci WS. Norepinephrine stimulates apoptosis in adult rat ventricular myocytes by activation of the beta-adrenergic pathway. Circulation 1998;98:1329-1334.

14. Iwai-Kanai E, Hasegawa K, Araki M, Kakita T, Morimoto T, Sasayama S. Alpha- and beta-adrenergic pathways differentially regulate cell type-specific apoptosis in rat cardiac myocytes. Circulation 1999;100:305-311.

15. Geng YJ, Ishikawa Y, Vatner DE, Wagner TE, Bishop SP, Vatner SF, Homcy CJ. Apoptosis of cardiac myocytes in Gs alpha transgenic mice. Circ Res 1999;84:34-42.

16. Port JD, Weinberger HD, Bisognano JD, Knudson OA, Bohlmeyer TJ, Pende A, Bristow MR. Echocardiographic and histopathological characterization of young and old transgenic mice over-expressing the human β1-adrenergic receptor (abstract). J Am Coll Cardiol 1998;31 Suppl A:177A.

17. Engelhardt S, Hein L, Wiesmann F, Lohse MJ. Progressive hypertrophy and heart failure in beta$_1$-adrenergic receptor transgenic mice. Proc Natl Acad Sci U S A 1999;96:7059-7064.

18. Rockman HA, Hamilton RA, Jones LR, Milano CA, Mao L, Lefkowitz RJ. Enhanced myocardial relaxation in vivo in transgenic mice overexpressing the beta$_2$-adrenergic receptor is associated with reduced phospholamban protein. J Clin Invest 1996;97:1618-1623.

19. Loria RM. Host conditions affecting the course of coxsackievirus infections. In: Bendinelli M, Friedman H, eds. Coxsackieviruses: a general update. New York: Plenum Press, 1988:135-157.

20. Davies RA, Laks H, Wackers FJ, Berger HJ, Williams B, Hammond GL, Geha AS, Gottschalk A, Zaret BL. Radionuclide assessment of left ventricular function in patients requiring intraoperative balloon pump assistance. Ann Thorac Surg 1982;33:123-131.

21. Kumar CT, Reddy VK, Prasad M, Thyagaraju K, Reddanna P. Dietary supplementation of vitamin E protects heart tissue from exercise-induced oxidant stress. Mol Cell Biochem 1992;111:109-115.

22. Matsumori A, Igata H, Ono K, Iwasaki A, Miyamoto T, Nishio R, Sasayama S. High doses of digitalis increase the myocardial production of proinflammatory cytokines and worsen myocardial injury in viral myocarditis: a possible mechanism of digitalis toxicity. Jpn Circ J 1999;63:934-940.

23. Nishio R, Matsumori A, Shioi T, Wang W, Yamada T, Ono K, Sasayama S. Denopamine, a beta1-adrenergic agonist, prolongs survival in a murine model of congestive heart failure induced by viral myocarditis: suppression of tumor necrosis factor-alpha production in the heart. J Am Coll Cardiol 1998;32:808-815.

24. Lane JR, Neumann DA, Lafond-Walker A, Herskowitz A, Rose NR. Interleukin 1 or tumor necrosis factor can promote Coxsackie B3-induced myocarditis in resistant B10.A mice. J Exp Med 1992;175:1123-1129.

25. Yamada T, Matsumori A, Sasayama S. Therapeutic effect of anti-tumor necrosis factor-alpha antibody on the murine model of viral myocarditis induced by encephalomyocarditis virus. Circulation 1994;89:846-851.

26. Barry WH. Mechanisms of immune-mediated myocyte injury. Circulation 1994;89:2421-2432.

27. Katz AM. Cardiomyopathy of overload. A major determinant of prognosis in congestive heart failure. N Engl J Med 1990;322:100-110.

28. Braunwald E. Mechanism of action of calcium-channel-blocking agents. N Engl J Med 1982;307:1618-1627.

29. The Xamoterol in Severe Heart Failure Study Group. Xamoterol in severe heart failure. Lancet 1990;336:1-6.

30. Talmadge J, Scott R, Castelli P, Newman-Tarr T, Lee J. Molecular pharmacology of the beta-adrenergic receptor on THP-1 cells. Int J Immunopharmacol 1993;15:219-228.

31. van der Poll T, Jansen J, Endert E, Sauerwein HP, van Deventer SJ. Noradrenaline inhibits lipopolysaccharide-induced tumor necrosis factor and interleukin 6 production in human whole blood. Infect Immun 1994;62:2046-2050.

32. Spengler RN, Allen RM, Remick DG, Strieter RM, Kunkel SL. Stimulation of alpha-adrenergic receptor augments the production of macrophage-derived tumor necrosis factor. J Immunol 1990;145:1430-1434.

33. Spengler RN, Chensue SW, Giacherio DA, Blenk N, Kunkel SL. Endogenous norepinephrine regulates tumor necrosis factor-alpha production from macrophages in vitro. J Immunol 1994;152:3024-3031.

34. Severn A, Rapson NT, Hunter CA, Liew FY. Regulation of tumor necrosis factor production by adrenaline and beta-adrenergic agonists. J Immunol 1992;148:3441-3445.

35. Agostini D, Babatasi G, Manrique A, Saloux E, Grollier G, Potier JC, Bouvard G. Impairment of cardiac neuronal function in acute myocarditis: iodine-123-MIBG scintigraphy study. J Nucl Med 1998;39:1841-1844.

36. Imamura Y, Ando H, Mitsuoka W, Egashira S, Masaki H, Ashihara T, Fukuyama T. Iodine-123 metaiodobenzylguanidine images reflect intense myocardial adrenergic nervous activity in congestive heart failure independent of underlying cause. J Am Coll Cardiol 1995;26:1594-1599.

37. Schofer J, Spielmann R, Schuchert A, Weber K, Schluter M. Iodine-123 meta-iodobenzylguanidine scintigraphy: a noninvasive method to demonstrate myocardial adrenergic nervous system disintegrity in patients with idiopathic dilated cardiomyopathy. J Am Coll Cardiol 1988;12:1252-1258.

38. Glowniak JV, Turner FE, Gray LL, Palac RT, Lagunas-Solar MC, Woodward WR. Iodine-123 metaiodobenzylguanidine imaging of the heart in idiopathic congestive cardiomyopathy and cardiac transplants. J Nucl Med 1989;30:1182-1191.

39. Tominaga M, Matsumori A, Okada I, Yamada T, Kawai C. Beta-blocker treatment of dilated cardiomyopathy. Beneficial effect of carteolol in mice. Circulation 1991;83:2021-2028.

40. Rezkalla S, Kloner RA, Khatib G, Smith FE, Khatib R. Effect of metoprolol in acute coxsackievirus B3 murine myocarditis. J Am Coll Cardiol 1988;12:412-414.

41. Reiss N, el-Banayosy A, Posival H, Morshuis M, Minami K, Korfer R. Management of acute fulminant myocarditis using circulatory support systems. Artif Organs 1996;20:964-970.

42. Kato S, Morimoto S, Hiramitsu S, Nomura M, Ito T, Hishida H. Use of percutaneous cardiopulmonary support of patients with fulminant myocarditis and cardiogenic shock for improving prognosis. Am J Cardiol 1999;83:623-625.

43. Starling RC, Galbraith TA, Baker PB, Howanitz EP, Murray KD, Binkley PF, Watson KM, Unverferth DV, Myerowitz PD. Successful management of acute myocarditis with biventricular assist devices and cardiac transplantation. Am J Cardiol 1988;62:341-343.

44. Brilakis ES, Olson LJ, Berry GJ, Daly RC, Loisance D, Zucker M, Cooper LT. Survival outcomes of patients with giant cell myocarditis bridged by ventricular assist devices. Asaio J 2000;46:569-572.

45. Kawai C, Yui Y, Hoshino T, Sasayama S, Matsumori A. Myocardial catecholamines in hypertrophic and dilated (congestive) cardiomyopathy: a biopsy study. J Am Coll Cardiol 1983;2:834-840.

46. Regitz V, Bossaller C, Strasser R, Schuler S, Hetzer R, Fleck E. Myocardial catecholamine content after heart transplantation. Circulation 1990;82:620-623.

47. Regitz V, Leuchs B, Bossaller C, Sehested J, Rappolder M, Fleck E. Myocardial catecholamine concentrations in dilated cardiomyopathy and heart failure of different origins. Eur Heart J 1991;12 Suppl D:171-174.

48. Regitz V, Fleck E. Myocardial adenine nucleotide concentrations and myocardial norepinephrine content in patients with heart failure secondary to idiopathic dilated or ischemic cardiomyopathy. Am J Cardiol 1992;69:1574-1580.

49. Seferović PM, Maksimović R, Ostojić M, Stepanović S, Nikolić J, Vasiljević JD, Kanjuh V, Seferović D, Simeunović S, Ristić A, Simić D. Myocardial catecholamines in primary heart muscle disease: fact or fancy? Eur Heart J 1995;16 Suppl O:124-127.

50. De Maria R, Accinni R, Baroldi G. Catecholamines, beta receptors and morphology in dilated cardiomyopathy: a preliminary report. In: Baroldi G, Camerini F, Goodwin JF, eds. Advances in cardiomyopathies. Berlin: Springer-Verlag, 1990:257-265.

51. Da Prada M, Zürcher G. Simultaneous radioenzymatic determination of plasma and tissue adrenaline, noradrenaline and dopamine within the femtomole range. Life Sci 1976;19:1161-1174.

52. Weise VK, Kopin IJ. Assay of catecholamines in human plasma: studies of a single isotope radioenzymatic procedure. Life Sci 1976;19:1673-1685.

53. Peuler JD, Johnson GA. Simultaneous single isotope radioenzymatic assay of plasma norepinephrine, epinephrine and dopamine. Life Sci 1977;21:625-636.

54. Axelrod J, Tomchick R. Enzymatic O-methylation of epinephrine and other catechols. J Biol Chem 1958;233:702-705.

55. Seferović PM, Maksimović R, Ristić AD, Stepanović S, Ostojić M, Kanjuh V, Seferović D, Simeunović S, Vasiljević JD. Myocardial catecholamine and inotropic response in heart muscle disease. In: Camerini F, Gavazzi A, De Maria R, eds. Advances in cardiomyopathies: Proceedings of the II Florence Meeting on Advances on Cardiomyopathies, April 24-26, 1997. Milano: Springer-Verlag, 1998:138-146.

56. Bristow MR, Minobe W, Rasmussen R, Larrabee P, Skerl L, Klein JW, Anderson FL, Murray J, Mestroni L, Karwande SV, Fowler M, Ginsburg R. Beta-adrenergic neuroeffector abnormalities in the failing human heart are produced by local rather than systemic mechanisms. J Clin Invest 1992;89:803-815.

57. Ungerer M, Weig HJ, Kubert S, Overbeck M, Bengel F, Schomig A, Schwaiger M. Regional pre- and postsynaptic sympathetic system in the failing human heart—regulation of beta ARK-1. Eur J Heart Fail 2000;2:23-31.

58. Schofer J, Tews A, Langes K, Bleifeld W, Reimitz PE, Mathey DG. Relationship between myocardial norepinephrine content and left ventricular function—an endomyocardial biopsy study. Eur Heart J 1987;8:748-753.

59. Correa-Araujo R, Oliveira JS, Ricciardi Cruz A. Cardiac levels of norepinephrine, dopamine, serotonin and histamine in Chagas' disease. Int J Cardiol 1991;31:329-336.

60. Anderson FL, Port JD, Reid BB, Larrabee P, Hanson G, Bristow MR. Myocardial catecholamine and neuropeptide Y depletion in failing ventricles of patients with idiopathic dilated cardiomyopathy. Correlation with beta-adrenergic receptor downregulation. Circulation 1992;85:46-53.

CHAPTER 10

Pathogenesis of Enteroviral Cardiomyopathy:

Interaction of Viral Proteins With Infected Myocytes

Dingding Xiong, M.D., Ph.D., Cornel Badorff, M.D., and Kirk U. Knowlton, M.D.

INTRODUCTION

Dilated cardiomyopathy, one of the leading causes of heart failure in the United States, is a multifactorial disease that includes hereditary and acquired forms.[1] Although a hereditary component of dilated cardiomyopathy is recognized in 25% to 35%[2] of cases, the majority of cases do not have a clearly defined cause. In addition, children and adults can present with an acute onset of cardiomyopathy that is often called acute myocarditis. This is usually attributed to viral infection, although limitations in our diagnostic abilities prevent precise quantitation of the incidence of viral infection in these cases.

Numerous studies have addressed the cellular immune response associated with enteroviral infection; less is known about the interaction between viral proteins and myocyte proteins that contributes to the pathogenesis of enteroviral-mediated cardiomyopathy. This chapter, therefore, focuses on the unique interaction between enteroviral proteins and the cardiac myocyte. This includes a review of murine models of viral-mediated cardiomyopathy, including transgenic mouse experiments that strengthen the evidence for a cause-effect relationship between low-level expression of enteroviral genomes in cardiac myocytes and dilated cardiomyopathy and recent evidence for a role of interferon signaling in the cardiotropic nature of coxsackievirus B3 (CVB3). In addition, evidence is reviewed that demonstrates that an enteroviral protease can directly cleave the myocyte cytoskeletal protein dystrophin, which is known to be important in hereditary dilated cardiomyopathy in humans. Furthermore, the chapter reviews the role that nitric oxide (NO) may play in inactivating this enteroviral protease.

ASSOCIATION OF ENTEROVIRAL INFECTION WITH CARDIOMYOPATHY

CLINICAL EVIDENCE OF ENTEROVIRAL INFECTION IN CARDIOMYOPATHY

Viral infection has been clearly associated with acute episodes of myocarditis in which a patient often presents with cardiomyopathy and heart failure. Many different infectious agents have been considered as the cause of viral myocarditis, including enteroviruses, adenovirus, cytomegalovirus,[3,4] hepatitis C virus,[5] and others. Among the most commonly identified infectious agents are the CVBs, members of the enterovirus genus of the picornavirus family. Reports of isolation of coxsackievirus from the heart or pericardial fluid of patients with acute myocarditis date back as far as 1965,[6,7] with numerous reports since of virus isolated from the heart or pericardial fluid or demonstrating the presence of viral antigens in diseased heart tissue.[7-14] According to World Health Organization surveys from many different countries, 34.6 per 1,000 of all CVB infections are associated with cardiovascular disease.[15]

In addition to the clear association between enteroviral infection and acute myocarditis, it has been shown that chronic, dilated cardiomyopathy can also be a sequela of viral myocarditis.[16] Attempts to isolate virus from the myocardium of patients with dilated cardiomyopathy have so far been unsuccessful. However, serologic evidence and the presence of enteroviral genomes in the heart tissue of patients with dilated cardiomyopathy have been demonstrated by molecular biologic techniques such as slot blot, in situ hybridization, and reverse transcription polymerase chain reaction. Identification of enteroviral RNA and antigen in myocardial tissue provides evidence that enteroviruses are associated with dilated cardiomyopathy. The average enterovirus detection rates from published studies that used different strategies are 10% to 30%. These studies indicate that enteroviral infection is associated with acute viral myocarditis and that it is likely to contribute to a subset of cases of chronic dilated cardiomyopathies.

MURINE MODELS OF ENTEROVIRAL CARDIOMYOPATHY

Although enteroviruses such as CVB are strongly associated with the pathogenesis of myocarditis and the evolution of dilated cardiomyopathy, the limitations of current diagnostic strategies and clinical therapies make it difficult to understand the mechanisms by which enteroviral infection causes cardiomyopathy. Fortunately, there are well-characterized murine models of CVB infection that provide a framework in which the general pathogenic mechanisms can be studied carefully. Mouse models of acute myocarditis and chronic cardiomyopathy include CVB3-infected mice and transgenic mice that express the viral genome in the cardiac myocyte.

Murine Models of Acute Coxsackieviral Myocarditis

CVB infection of many strains of mice can cause an acute myocarditis.[17] Acute viral infection causes potent activation of the cellular immune response that has been studied extensively and is reviewed elsewhere in this book. The discussion below focuses on the direct viral-mediated myocytopathic effects that occur with viral infection or expression of coxsackieviral genomes in the heart.

Viral-mediated cytotoxicity has been demonstrated in vitro and in vivo in acute viral infection. There is a large body of work that describes the direct cytopathic effect of enteroviral infection in nonmyocyte cell lines such as HeLa and Vero cells. Coxsackievirus infection can induce a direct cytopathic effect in cultured fetal human,[18] murine,[19] and rat[20] heart cells.

In vivo studies that show a direct virus-induced cytotoxicity include the presence of necrotic myofibers in the absence of an inflammatory cell infiltrate 3 days after infection;[21] extensive cardiac damage in severe combined immunodeficiency and athymic mice, where the usual inflammatory cell infiltrate is genetically reduced or absent;[22] and lack of benefit of immunosuppressive therapy in several strains of inbred mice.[23-25] These findings in combination with specific interactions between enteroviral proteins and cardiac myocytes described below provide compelling evidence that acute viral infection can have a direct effect on the cardiac myocyte independent of the cellular immune response.

Murine Models of Chronic Dilated Cardiomyopathy Caused by Coxsackievirus Infection

In addition to the acute effect of viral infection on the heart, the concept that infection of the heart could progress to a chronic dilated cardiomyopathy in mice was demonstrated as early as 1969. Wilson et al.[26] showed that experimental viral myocarditis could be associated with persistence of inflammation progressing to myocardial fibrosis. They found that acute infection with CVB3 in weanling Swiss mice was followed by marked fibrosis, dystrophic mineralization, and microscopic myocardial hypertrophy, which persisted for at least 6 months. Subsequently, they observed the natural history of the mice that were infected with CVB3 and forced to swim. Cardiomyopathy evolved after 15 months in a natural course resembling acute myocarditis that progresses to dilated cardiomyopathy in humans. Characteristics included atrial hypertrophy with thrombi and myocardial fiber disintegration with replacement by fibrous scar without mononuclear infiltration.[27]

In addition to these early experiments, evidence suggests that a viral infection and persistence of the viral genome contribute to the evolution of ongoing heart disease. The potential role of viral persistence in ongoing heart disease was demonstrated by Klingel et al.[28] in a murine model of CVB3-induced myocarditis. Murine hearts were examined by in situ hybridization for the presence of CVB3 genomic RNA. The sites where viral RNA was detected were studied further for the extent of myocardial damage and inflammatory cell infiltration.

In the first 3 days after infection, myocytes containing CVB3 RNA were distributed randomly throughout the myocardium, presumably indicating hematogenous infection during viremia. By day 6, infected myocytes were adjacent to foci of inflammatory cells. The greatest numbers of CVB3-infected myocardial cells were noted from days 6 to 9. This correlated with a significant increase in myocardial injury. From days 15 to 30 postinfection, after infectious virus could no longer be isolated from the myocardium, CVB3 genomes could still be detected in myocardial cells. These positive cells were found primarily within foci of myocardial lesions characterized by fibrosis, myocardial necrosis, and mononuclear cell infiltrates.

These observations demonstrated that CVB genomes can persist in the myocardium of infected hearts. Furthermore, the presence of viral RNA in areas that have evidence of abnormal myocardium suggests that persistence of the viral genome in CVB-infected mice may contribute to the pathogenesis of chronic myocarditis. Interestingly, there was evidence of persistent viral infection in A.CA/SnJ, A.BY/SnJ, and SWR/J mice. However, DBA/1J mice, which were capable of terminating the inflammatory processes through elimination of the virus from the heart, showed no evidence of persistent viral RNA in the myocardium.

Therefore, data obtained from murine models imply that myocardial damage in CVB3-infected mice can occur in 2 phases—an acute phase with prominent virus replication and cellular infiltration and a chronic phase characterized by progressive myocardial disease that may be associated with low-level persistence of viral genomes and progressive cardiomyopathy.

Transgenic Model of Coxsackieviral Dilated Cardiomyopathy

The data described above from the hearts of patients with dilated cardiomyopathy provide compelling evidence that there is an association between persistence of enteroviral genomes in the heart and dilated cardiomyopathy. Evidence of persistence of enteroviral genomes in the heart of mice infected with CVB3 provides additional support for this association. However, this does not prove that the presence of enteroviral genomes in the heart can cause cardiomyopathy. Acute enteroviral infection is associated with a marked inflammatory response directed against viral and some myocardial proteins. The virus is able to infect tissues in addition to the heart, including the liver, brain, pancreas, and spleen. It is, therefore, difficult to determine from these experiments whether the presence of enteroviral genomes in the myocardium in low levels, as observed in dilated cardiomyopathy, can actually cause cardiomyopathy or whether they are only remnants of a previous infection that have no significant effect on the pathogenesis of the progressive cardiomyopathy.

Persistent enteroviral infection in the murine heart and in the hearts of the patients with dilated cardiomyopathy has characteristics distinct from those observed with acute viral infection. First, in acute viral infection, there is significantly more positive- than negative-strand RNA synthesis, whereas in persistently infected mice, the amount of negative-strand RNA is approximately equivalent to the amount of positive-strand RNA, indicating restricted virus replication. Second, there is evidence of ongoing damage in the myocardium where viral RNA is detected. Third, although infectious virus is easily isolated from acute infections, infectious virus is usually not recovered from in vivo tissue samples with persistent enteroviral infection. Fourth, in persistently infected mouse hearts, viral protein expression has been difficult to detect by conventional immunohistochemistry or immunoblotting. Overall, these characteristics in persistent enteroviral infection are typical of restricted viral replication and low-level protein expression.[29]

To demonstrate that low-level expression of enteroviral genomes in the heart can cause cardiomyopathy, we generated transgenic mice that expressed replication-restricted enteroviral genomes in myocardium driven by the cardiac-specific myosin light chain-2v (MLC-2v) promoter. This allowed low-level expression of coxsackieviral genomes in the heart without formation of infectious virions, thus preventing a productive viral replication cycle. In addition, the MLC-2v promoter directs expression in the heart at day 8.5 of embryogenesis,[30] thus preventing activation of a potent immune response against viral antigens.

To accomplish this, infectious recombinant CVB3 cDNA was mutated at the autocatalytic cleavage site in the VP0 capsid protein from the amino acids asparagine and serine to lysine and alanine, thus preventing formation of infectious virus progeny.[31] In cultured neonatal ventricular myocytes transfected with the CVB3-mutated cDNA copy of the viral genome, both positive- and negative-strand viral RNAs were detected, and the levels of viral protein expression were below the limits of detection by conventional methods of protein detection, thus resembling restricted replication.[20] Nonetheless, the CVB3 mutant induced a cytopathic effect in transfected myocytes, which was demonstrated by inhibition of cotransfected MLC-2v luciferase reporter activity and an increase in release of lactate dehydrogenase from transfected cells. These results suggest that restricted replication of enteroviral genomes in myocytes in a pattern similar to that observed in hearts with persistent viral infection can induce myocytopathic effects without generation of infectious virus progeny in conditions that are independent of a cellular immune response.[20]

To determine whether a similar pathogenic effect could be observed in the intact heart, transgenic mice were generated that expressed the replication-restricted CVB3 cDNA mutant exclusively in the heart, using the cardiac myocyte-specific MLC-2v promoter. As expected, heart muscle-specific expression of the CVB3 mutant leads to the synthesis of viral plus- and minus-strand RNA without formation of infectious viral progeny. Histopathologic analysis of transgenic hearts revealed typical morphologic features of myocardial interstitial fibrosis, hypertrophy, and degeneration of myocytes, thus resembling dilated cardiomyopathy in humans (Fig. 10-1; see color plate 14). This occurred in the absence of viral neutralizing antibodies. Analysis of isolated myocytes from transgenic mice demonstrated that there is defective excitation-contraction coupling and a decrease in the magnitude of isolated cell shortening. Restricted replication of enteroviral genomes in the heart can induce cardiomyopathy with characteristics that are typical of dilated cardiomyopathy in humans.[20]

MECHANISMS OF ENTEROVIRAL INFECTION AND REPLICATION IN THE HEART

COXSACKIEVIRUS-ADENOVIRUS RECEPTORS

Significant progress has been made in understanding the mechanisms by which the virus attaches to the target cell, initiating an infectious cycle within the cell. Two receptors, the

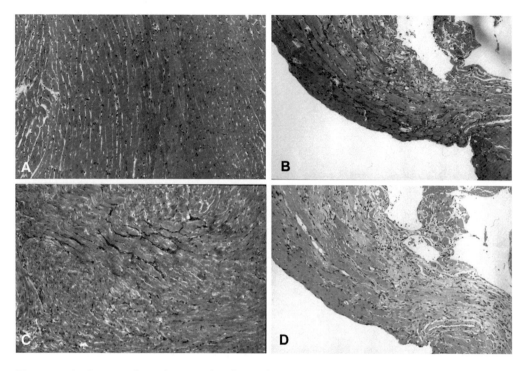

Fig. 10-1. Cardiomyopathy in the ventricles of coxsackievirus B transgenic mice. See color plate 14. (From Wessely R, Klingel K, Santana LF, Dalton N, Hongo M, Lederer WJ, Kandolf R, Knowlton KU. Transgenic expression of replication-restricted enteroviral genomes in heart muscle induces defective excitation-contraction coupling and dilated cardiomyopathy. J Clin Invest 1998;102:1444-1453. By permission of the American Society for Clinical Investigation.)

coxsackie-adenovirus receptor (CAR) and decay-accelerating factor (DAF), have been identified that play an important role in the attachment of the virus to the cell and initiation of an infectious cycle in the cells.[32,33] Either DAF or CAR can mediate viral attachment to the cell, but CAR is required for initiation of viral replication.[33] Additional details regarding viral receptor mechanisms are included in other chapters.

VIRAL REPLICATION IN THE INFECTED CELL

Enteroviral genome is an approximately 7.5-kb positive-strand RNA. It consists of a 5'-untranslated region of around 740 bp, the protein coding region, and an approximately 100-bp 3'-untranslated region. The protein coding region codes for the viral capsid proteins VP1, VP2, VP3, and VP4. The remainder of the coding region encodes nonstructural proteins that are important for viral replication. They include the viral proteases 2A and 3C that are required for cleavage of the viral polyprotein. In addition, the viral RNA-dependent RNA polymerase is a nonstructural protein that is required for replication of the viral RNA. Once the viral RNA has entered the cell, the host cell translational apparatus translates the viral RNA as a monocistronic polyprotein that is subsequently cleaved into the individual viral polyproteins by the viral proteases 2A and 3C. Viral RNA is replicated through a negative-strand RNA intermediate that serves as a template for positive-strand replication. Viral capsids assemble within the cell, encapsidating a single copy of the viral positive-strand RNA. The virus then exits the cell through mechanisms that are poorly defined.

CARDIOSELECTIVE INFECTION WITH CVB3 REQUIRES INTACT TYPE I INTERFERON SIGNALING

Infection with myocarditic variants of CVB3 causes a high virus load in the heart during acute infection compared with other tissues, and it is thought that this contributes to the ability of this virus to cause acute and chronic myocarditis.[21] The mechanisms that mediate the cardiotropic nature of CVB3 infection are not completely known. Coxsackievirus binds to the CAR that is expressed at high levels in the heart, liver, lung, and kidney of mice.[34] Although tissue-restricted expression of viral receptors is one of the mechanisms that is likely to contribute to viral tropism, other virus-host interactions, including antiviral mechanisms of the interferon system, may play an important role in determining the efficiency of viral replication in a given tissue.

Interferons of the α and β-subtypes are referred to as type I interferons and include interferon-α, -β, -ω, and -τ. Interferon-γ is the only type II interferon. Interferons exert their effect by binding to specific receptors in the cell membrane that subsequently activate intracellular signaling necessary for activation and expression of interferon-responsive genes. All type I interferons bind to the type I interferon receptors, whereas the structurally unrelated interferon-γ binds to type II interferon receptors. Genetic disruption of the type I or type II interferon receptors completely and specifically abolishes the biologic effect of type I or type II interferons, respectively.[35,36]

Previous experiments with cultured cells have suggested that both type I and type II interferons can inhibit coxsackieviral replication.[18,37] Administration of interferon-α/β can ameliorate the effect of coxsackievirus myocarditis in mice.[38-40]

Given these findings, it was anticipated that complete disruption of either type I or type II interferon receptor signaling mechanisms would markedly affect coxsackieviral replication in the heart. However, we found that CVB3 replication in type I but not type II interferon receptor-deficient mice resulted in a marked increase in viral replication in the liver. Interestingly, there was no significant increase of viral RNA in the heart of the type I interferon receptor-deficient mice. In addition to the high level of viral replication in the liver of CVB3-infected mice, there was a marked increase in mortality in CVB3-infected mice.[41]

These findings show that the presence of type I interferon receptor signaling is required to prevent high-level viral replication in the liver, but that it has no significant effect on early viral replication in the heart. In contrast, the absence of type II interferon signaling does not have a significant effect on mortality and results in only a mild increase of the viral titers in heart and liver. These results demonstrate that in addition to viral receptor-mediated viral tropism, tissue-restricted antiviral mechanisms act as important determinants of the cardioselective nature of coxsackieviral infection.[41]

VIRAL AND MYOCARDIAL PROTEIN INTERACTIONS THAT CONTRIBUTE TO ENTEROVIRAL CARDIOMYOPATHY

EFFECTS OF VIRAL PROTEASES ON INFECTED HOST CELLS

It is now clear that enteroviruses can induce a direct myocytopathic effect, and molecular mechanisms of this myocytopathic effect are being elucidated. When the enterovirus infects a cell, the positive-strand RNA genome is released from the capsid proteins. By host translational mechanisms, the viral genome is translated as a monocistronic polyprotein. This polyprotein is then cleaved into mature viral polyproteins by the viral proteases 2A and 3C. In addition to their ability to cleave the viral polyprotein, they are also able to cleave a small number of host cell proteins.

The overall folding of the enteroviral proteases resembles chymotrypsinlike serine proteases with the important distinction that there is a cysteine as the nucleophile at the catalytic active site instead of a serine.[42] Substrate recognition by the enteroviral protease 2A depends on a degenerate amino acid pattern upstream of the cleavage site. Protease 3C cleaves best at an amino acid sequence that includes an AXXQG motif with an alanine at the P4 position, a glutamate at P1, and a requirement for glycine at the P1' site. Protease 2A cleavage sites are less well defined but appear to have a higher specificity, as demonstrated by the few known proteins that can be cleaved by protease 2A. As can be seen from known CVB protease 2A cleavage sites and known CVB protease 2A cleavage sites in eukaryotic proteins shown in Table 10-1, this cleavage recognition site usually contains a T at the P2 amino acid residue and a T, I, or M at the P4 residue. In addition, a glycine residue at the P1' C-terminal side of the scissile bond of the cleavage site occurs in all known natural substrates of the enteroviral protease 2A.

Although protease 3C has been shown to cleave proteins, including some involved in TATA-dependent initiation of transcription,[43,44] protease 2A is a highly specific protease and has been shown to cleave only proteins that are important for cap-dependent initiation of translation, such as the eukaryotic initiation factor-4γ (eIF4γ) and the polyadenylate binding protein.[45-47] It can also cleave the cytoskeletal protein cytokeratin-8,[48] suggesting a potential role in release of mature virions from the infected cell.

Table 10-1
Coxsackie B Virus Protease 2A Cleavage Sites*

	P7 P4 P1	P1′
CVB1	TRSN**I**T**TT**	**G**AFGQQSG
CVB2	KRDS**LTTT**	**G**AFGQQSG
CVB3	SITT**M**T**NT**	**G**AFGQQSG
CVB4	ERAS**LITT**	**G**PYGHQSG
CVB5	EITA**M**Q**TT**	**G**VLGQQTG
MurDYS	RAPG**LSTT**	**G**ASASQTV
HumDYS	LAPG**LTTI**	**G**ASPTQTV
eIF4G-1	GRTT**LST**R	**G**PPRGGPG
HumPABP	ANTS**T**Q**T**M	**G**PRPAAAA
cytokeratin-8	KSYKVS**T**S	**G**PRAFSSR

*Shown are the protease 2A cleavage sites (represented by the space between P1 and P1′) for the coxsackie B viruses (CVB1-5) and the known cleavage sites in host-cell proteins. These include murine and human dystrophin (murDYS and humDYS) [Data from Badorff et al.[66]], eukaryotic initiation factor-4G-1 (eIF4G-1) [Data from Lamphear BJ, Rhoads RE. Biochemistry 1996;35:15726-15733], human polyadenylate binding protein (humPABP) [Data from Kerekatte et al.[47]], and cytokeratin-8 [Data from Seipelt et al.[48]].

In an attempt to identify new host cell proteins that might be cleaved by protease 2A, a computer neural network algorithm was designed from known protease 2A cleavage sites in viral and host proteins.[49] This neural network algorithm was then used to scan the Swiss human protein databank. Of all the human proteins, dystrophin was predicted to be one of the proteins most likely to be cleaved by enteroviral protease 2A.

DYSTROPHIN-GLYCOPROTEIN COMPLEX IN HEREDITARY CARDIOMYOPATHY

For coordinated contractile function of the heart, the many mechanical forces generated within the sarcomeres of individual cardiomyocytes need to be transmitted to the extracellular matrix. For this purpose, cardiomyocytes possess a highly specialized extrasarcomeric cytoskeleton[50] that includes the dystrophin-glycoprotein complex.[51] Dystrophin and the dystrophin-associated glycoproteins α-, β-, γ-, and δ-sarcoglycan; α- and β-dystroglycan; and sarcospan[52] compose a multiprotein complex that collectively connects the internal F-actin-based cytoskeleton to laminin-2 of the extracellular matrix[51] (Fig. 10-2; see color plate 15). In addition to its structural role, the dystrophin-glycoprotein complex may have signal transduction properties such as the ecto-ATPase activity that was described for α-sarcoglycan.[53] It also binds to neuronal nitric oxide synthase (NOS), localizing it to the cell membrane.

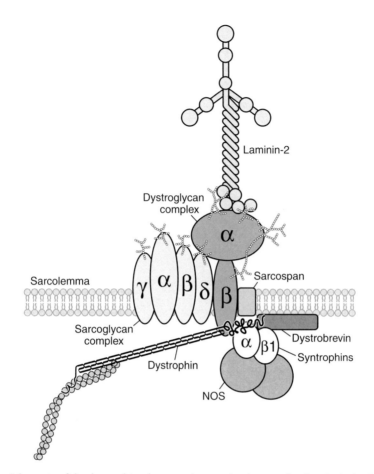

Fig. 10-2. Schematic of the dystrophin-glycoprotein complex (see text for description). See color plate 15.

Dystrophin is a 427-kDa protein with 4 major domains: an N-terminal domain, a spectrinlike repeat rod domain, a cysteine-rich domain, and a carboxy-terminal domain (Fig. 10-3). The amino-terminal domain and an epitope in the rod domain bind actin, whereas the cysteine-rich domain and carboxy-terminus contribute to binding of β-dystroglycan in the cell membrane. There are also 4 hinge regions in the rod region of dystrophin that have been shown to be accessible to proteolytic cleavage by nonviral proteases.[54]

The importance of the dystrophin-glycoprotein complex for normal cardiac function in humans and rodents is highlighted by hereditary dystrophin and sarcoglycan mutations that cause dilated cardiomyopathy. For example, dystrophin mutations in Duchenne and Becker muscular dystrophy[55] are associated with a high incidence of dilated cardiomyopathy.[56] Additionally, a mutation in dystrophin causes an X-linked dilated cardiomyopathy in patients with minimal skeletal myopathy.[57,58] Genetic defects in α-, β-, γ-, or δ-sarcoglycan are the cause of human limb-girdle muscular dystrophy types 2D, 2E, 2C, and 2F,

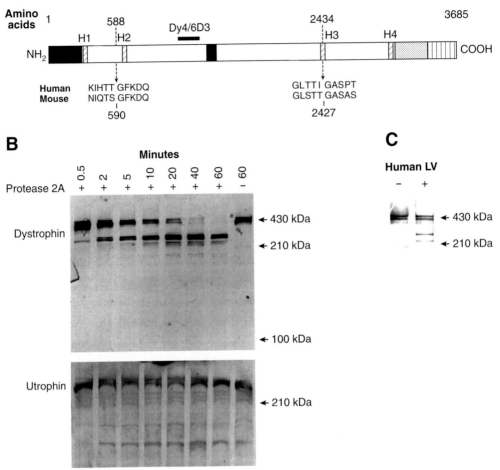

Fig. 10-3. Cleavage of dystrophin by coxsackievirus protease 2A. *Panel A,* Schematic diagram of the dystrophin molecule with known domains. Dystrophin contains actin-binding domains (black rectangles), a rod domain (open rectangles) consisting of spectrinlike repeats, a cysteine-rich domain (shaded rectangle), and a carboxy-terminal domain (vertical hatched area). Four hinge segments (H1-H4) that are accessible to proteolytic cleavage are interspersed along the rod domain (diagonal hatched areas).[40] The predicted cleavage sites in dystrophin at residues 588 and 2,434 are shown with dashed arrows. Amino acid sequences of the predicted human and mouse cleavage sites are shown below the arrows. The predicted cleavage sites in the mouse dystrophin gene are at residues 590 and 2,427. The region of dystrophin used to generate the Dy4/6D3 antibody is shown as a dark bar above dystrophin. *Panel B,* Western blot for dystrophin and utrophin in purified rat myocyte extracts after addition of purified protease 2A. Protein extract (15 μg) from cultured neonatal rat ventricular myocytes was incubated with 1 μg of purified coxsackievirus B protease 2A for the times indicated. The samples were then analyzed by sodium dodecyl sulfate polyacrylamide gel electrophoresis followed by immunoblotting for dystrophin (*Upper panel*) and utrophin (*Lower panel*). *Panel C,* Western blot for dystrophin in human heart extracts incubated with protease 2A. Protein extract (15 μg) from human left ventricle (*LV*) was incubated with 1 μg protease 2A for 60 min and analyzed as above. (From Badorff et al.[65] By permission of Nature America.)

respectively.[59] Sarcoglycan deficiency can cause dilated cardiomyopathy in these patients[60] and in the cardiomyopathic hamster in which there is a deletion in δ-sarcoglycan gene.[61] These studies and others[62,63] have led to the paradigm that familial dilated cardiomyopathy may occur secondary to defective transmission of mechanical force from the sarcomere to the extracellular matrix,[64] although the precise mechanisms by which abnormalities in the dystrophin-glycoprotein complex cause cardiomyopathy are not yet known.

CLEAVAGE OF DYSTROPHIN BY PROTEASE 2A AND DISRUPTION OF THE DYSTROPHIN-GLYCOPROTEIN COMPLEX IN VITRO AND IN CULTURED MYOCYTES

Given the importance of the dystrophin-glycoprotein complex in hereditary dilated cardio-myopathy and the role for enteroviruses in acquired cardiomyopathy, it is conceivable that disruption of the dystrophin-glycoprotein complex is also important in the pathogenesis of acquired cardiomyopathies caused by enteroviral infection.

Because of the prediction by Blom et al.[49] that dystrophin was one of the human proteins most likely to be cleaved by enteroviral protease 2A, we sought to determine experimentally whether protease 2A could cleave dystrophin. First, we applied the protease 2A cleavage site algorithm to the full dystrophin sequence and identified a second likely site for cleavage of dystrophin by protease 2A.[65] The computer-predicted protease 2A-cleavage site that we identified lies in the dystrophin hinge 3, a region that has been previously demonstrated to be accessible to proteolytic cleavage.[54] Because the hinge 3 region lies between the actin-binding sites and the β-dystroglycan anchoring motif of dystrophin,[65] cleavage at this site would disconnect the (actin-binding) N-terminal fragment from the sarcolemma (where the C-terminal fragment binds β-dystroglycan).

To determine experimentally whether enteroviral protease 2A could cleave dystrophin at the computer-predicted cleavage sites, purified protease 2A was added to neonatal rat and human myocyte extracts. Dystrophin was proteolytically cleaved by purified protease 2A whereas utrophin was not cleaved (Fig. 10-3). Dystrophin was cleaved and functionally impaired after enteroviral infection, as demonstrated by dissociation of the N-terminal rod domain fragment from the plasma membrane in cultured cardiomyocytes infected with CVB3.[65] Antibody epitope mapping of the protease 2A cleavage site in human and mouse dystrophin demonstrated that the coxsackieviral protease 2A cleaves dystrophin in the hinge 3 region.[66] By use of purified dystrophin miniproteins, it has been shown that the protease 2A-mediated cleavage in the hinge 3 region is direct and not through activation of another host-cell protease, and that cleavage occurs at the site predicted in the hinge 3 region by the neural network algorithm.[66] At the present time, it is not clear that cleavage at the second site in the spectrin repeats of dystrophin is mediated directly by protease 2A, or whether it is mediated by activation of a host-cell protease.[66] Less-efficient cleavage in spectrin repeat 3 might be explained by its triple-helical secondary structure[67] that may make that region less accessible to cleavage by protease 2A.

CVB3 infection of cultured neonatal rat ventricular myocytes confirmed that dystrophin was cleaved in infected myocytes in a pattern that was similar to that observed in vitro.[65]

PROTEASE 2A-MEDIATED DISRUPTION OF DYSTROPHIN AND THE DYSTROPHIN-GLYCOPROTEIN COMPLEX IN THE INTACT HEART

In addition to the ability of protease 2A to cleave dystrophin in vitro, dystrophin is also proteolytically cleaved and its sarcolemmal localization is disrupted in the intact heart in infected cardiac myocytes. Additionally, the sarcolemmal integrity in these cells is impaired, as determined by tracer dye uptake in a manner similar to that observed in muscular dystrophy[65] (Fig. 10-4; see color plate 16). Because genetic dystrophin deficiency leads to a loss

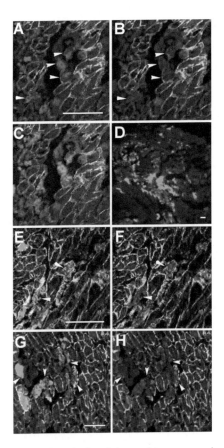

Fig. 10-4. The sarcolemmal integrity is impaired and dystrophin, α-sarcoglycan, and β-dystroglycan staining are disrupted in infected myocytes from severe combined immunodeficient mice. See color plate 16. (From Badorff et al.[65] By permission of Nature America.)

of dystrophin-associated glycoproteins,[68] we investigated whether dystrophin cleavage during CVB infection would similarly affect the sarcoglycans. The sarcoglycan complex becomes physically, morphologically, and functionally disrupted during CVB3 infection of cultured cardiomyocytes and mice, as determined by staining for the sarcoglycans (α-, β-, γ-, and δ-sarcoglycan) and β-dystroglycan (Fig. 10-4; see color plate 16).[69]

As in patients with dilated cardiomyopathy due to Duchenne muscular dystrophy, it is possible that the cleavage of dystrophin with its subsequent biochemical, morphologic, and functional disruption of the dystrophin-glycoprotein complex during CVB3 infection initiates a cascade of events that contributes to the pathogenesis of dilated cardiomyopathy.[65] Because the coxsackieviral protease 2A cleaves the human dystrophin hinge 3 region separating the actin-binding domains from the β-dystroglycan-binding domains,[66] this suggests that the dystrophin cleavage is potentially relevant for the pathogenesis of human viral heart disease (Fig. 10-5). In addition, it is also possible that cleavage of dystrophin is an important step in viral replication, facilitating viral release from the infected cell by weakening the cell membrane and allowing infection of the adjacent cardiac myocytes.

HOW COULD DYSTROPHIN CLEAVAGE LEAD TO ENTEROVIRUS-INDUCED DILATED CARDIOMYOPATHY?

Although the dystrophin cDNA was cloned more than a decade ago,[67] the exact physiologic role of the dystrophin protein is poorly defined. The current model assumes a structural role for dystrophin[51] because its N-terminus and an area in the rod domain bind F-actin,[70] whereas the cysteine-rich region near the carboxy-terminus binds the transmembrane β-dystroglycan.[71] Dystrophin, therefore, connects the internal cytoskeleton to the sarco-

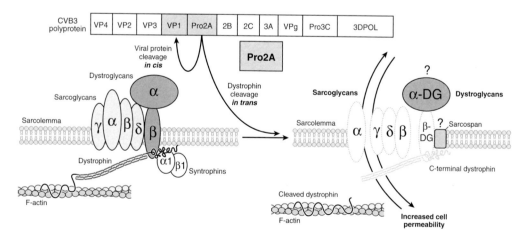

Fig. 10-5. Schematic of the effect of protease 2A on dystrophin and the dystrophin-glycoprotein complex. *CVB3,* coxsackievirus B3.

lemma via the transmembrane glycoprotein complex (Fig. 10-5). Genetic dystrophin deficiency leads to a loss of the dystrophin-glycoprotein complex, with increased myocyte permeability.[51,72] However, the downstream effectors that ultimately lead to myocyte death in Duchenne muscular dystrophy are not clear. Several potential mechanisms, including activation of reactive oxygen species[73] and lymphocyte-mediated myocyte damage,[28] have been proposed.

Our findings in enteroviral myocarditis and cardiomyopathy suggest a pathogenic link between virally induced dystrophin abnormalities and genetic dystrophin deficiency. Protease 2A cleaves dystrophin during CVB3 infection, adversely affecting myocytes by impairing transmission of mechanical force and increasing cell permeability.[65] At the organ level, myocyte dropout or dysfunction and loss of contractile force may ultimately contribute to the induction of dilated cardiomyopathy.

In addition, it is likely that cleavage of dystrophin may significantly affect viral replication in the myocyte. Previous studies with other viruses have demonstrated that viral-mediated cleavage of cytoskeletal proteins may be important for disruption of the cell membrane and release of virus from the cell. For example, the adenoviral L3 protease is able to cleave cytokeratin-18 at the junction of the globular head domain and the alpha-helical rod domain.[74] In addition, the human immunodeficiency virus (HIV) type I protease cleaves intermediate filament proteins vimentin, desmin, and glial fibrillary acidic protein.[75] It was shown that the rhinoviral protease 2A is able to cleave cytokeratin-8 late in the infection cycle in HeLa cells.[48] These studies indicate that cleavage of cytoskeletal proteins may be an important component of viral replication, perhaps facilitating efficient release of virus from infected cells, and highlight the significance of dystrophin cleavage by enteroviral protease 2A.

Important distinctions exist between virus-induced cardiomyopathy and the hereditary absence of dystrophin. In contrast to a genetic defect, enteroviral infection is focal in viral cardiomyopathy. The percentage of virally infected myocytes differs in the various stages of the disease. In the acute stage, up to 7 days after infection with CVB3, more than 10% of myocytes are infected in C3H mice (unpublished observation). This percentage may be high enough that acute cleavage of dystrophin could significantly affect overall cardiac function. A similar mechanism could occur in acute, fulminant myocarditis as is observed in children and young adults. In the chronic stage of murine infection, the percentage of cells with viral persistence appears to be much lower.[76] A similarly low percentage has been reported in human heart samples from patients with dilated cardiomyopathy.[76]

How then can enteroviruses induce dilated cardiomyopathy if the percentage of cells that express viral proteins, such as the protease 2A, is small? First, the number of infected cells in any sample indicates only the number of cells infected at the time when the tissue was harvested for analysis. Even if few cells are infected at any given time, a replicating virus can infect many cells over a prolonged time and thus cause substantial myocyte loss. The same concept has been applied to myocyte apoptosis where the percentage of apoptotic nuclei is several-fold increased in human heart failure but the absolute numbers of apoptotic cells are low.[77] Second, increased sarcolemmal permeability that occurs with cleavage of dystrophin can expose myocyte contents to immunoregulatory cells. For instance, low-level expression of coxsackieviral genomes in cultured cardiomyocytes results in release of cardiac enzymes from the cells.[20]

"Leaking" myocyte proteins from even a few infected cells could act as autoantigens and may initiate an autoreactive response. T and B lymphocytes activated in such a way may recognize diverse myocardial antigens such as myosin, the adenine-nucleotide-translocator, or the sarcolemma, all of which have been reported as autoantigens in human dilated cardiomyopathy.[78-81] This inappropriate immune response may attack and destroy many uninfected myocytes and thus cause substantial myocyte loss or dysfunction.[82] In this regard, increased lymphocytic infiltrates and enhanced expression of cytolytic mediators such as perforin and TIA-1 have been reported in endomyocardial biopsy specimens from patients with dilated cardiomyopathy.[79]

Another difference between hereditary dystrophin deficiency and cleavage of dystrophin by protease 2A is the chronic versus acute loss of dystrophin. In hereditary dystrophin deficiency, dystrophin is absent in embryonic muscle and throughout the animal's life. This allows for compensatory mechanisms such as up-regulation of the related utrophin, as has been observed in dystrophin-deficient mice.[83] However, in virally infected cells there is acute cleavage of dystrophin that is likely to occur in a cell that cannot promptly compensate for the loss of dystrophin because host cell translation mechanisms are impaired in the virally infected cells. How this would affect the cell is not known, but it may contribute to the more dramatic loss of sarcolemmal integrity that is observed in virally infected cells.[65,69]

An alternative mechanism by which disruption of the dystrophin-glycoprotein complex could cause cardiomyopathy has been proposed. In mice with genetic disruption of α-sarcoglycan, there is disruption of the typical sarcolemmal organization in the cardiac myocyte but not in the vascular smooth muscle cells; however, genetic knockout of δ- or β-sarcoglycan leads to disruption of the sarcoglycans in cardiac and vascular smooth muscle cells. Significant cardiomyopathy occurs in the mice with genetic disruption of δ- and β-sarcoglycan and disruption of the sarcoglycan complex in vascular smooth muscle cells, but the cardiomyopathy is significantly less in mice that have disruption of α-sarcoglycan with loss of the sarcoglycan complex in cardiac muscle alone. The cardiomyopathy associated with disruption of β- and δ-sarcoglycan is associated with arteriolar constriction leading to areas of apparent myocardial ischemia and cell death that are increased with exercise.[84,85] Because coxsackievirus can infect smooth muscle cells,[86] it is conceivable that enteroviral infection of smooth muscle cells can lead to disruption of the dystrophin-glycoprotein complex with focal areas of arteriolar vasospasm and cell loss through oxygen supply-demand mismatch. Arteriolar vasoconstriction has also been reported in mice that have been infected with CVB3.[87] Such a paradigm would not require that a large number of myocytes be simultaneously infected to affect a significant amount of myocardium.

The mechanisms by which disruption of the dystrophin-glycoprotein complex during coxsackieviral infection induces cardiomyopathy are still unknown. Nevertheless, cleavage of dystrophin by protease 2A is the first potential molecular mechanism that relates the pathogenesis of hereditary cardiomyopathy to events occurring in acquired cardiomyopathy. Ultimately, a complete understanding of the mechanisms by which cleavage of dystrophin by protease 2A can contribute to viral replication and cardiomyopathy depends on an improved understanding of how genetic loss of the dystrophin-glycoprotein complex causes muscular dystrophy and dilated cardiomyopathy.

INHIBITION OF PROTEASE 2A: A MECHANISM TO INHIBIT VIRAL REPLICATION

The enteroviral protease 2A is, like the HIV protease, an attractive target for antiviral drug development because both proteases are essential for viral life cycles.[88,89] Previously described inhibitors of the picornaviral protease 2A were originally designed against host enzymes such as neutrophil elastase (elastatinal and methoxysuccinyl-Ala-Ala-Pro-Val-chloromethylketone [MPCMK])[90] or identified as inhibitors of rhinoviral protease 3C (homophthalimides).[91] The enteroviral protease 2A possesses a catalytic cysteine residue, and its substrate recognition depends on the 4 to 6 amino acids upstream of the scissile bond.[92] Therefore, we hypothesized that we might be able to use the protease 2A cleavage site in dystrophin to create a protease inhibitor by using a strategy similar to that used to inhibit caspases with the peptide substrate analogue z-VAD-fmk.[93] Accordingly, we synthesized a modified tetrapeptide containing a fluoromethylketone (-fmk) group at the carboxy-terminus of the LSTT cleavage site in dystrophin (z-LSTT-fmk). The fluoromethyl ketone can form a covalent bond with the catalytic cysteine, leading to protease inactivation. A second substrate analog (z-LSTL-fmk) based on a binding peptide of the related poliovirus protease 2A was also tested.[94] The resulting components z-LSTT-fmk and z-LSTL-fmk inhibited the coxsackieviral protease 2A in vitro in a dose-dependent manner with half-maximal inhibition at 550 nM and 1,050 nM, respectively (Fig. 10-6). Preliminary evidence indicates that z-LSTL-fmk can also inhibit protease 2A in intact cells.

NITRIC OXIDE INHIBITION OF ENTEROVIRAL-MEDIATED CLEAVAGE OF DYSTROPHIN

NO, an important regulator of multiple cardiovascular responses, is synthesized from L-arginine by 3 different isoforms of NOS.[95] In human dilated cardiomyopathy, increased systemic NO production, increased myocardial NOSII mRNA, and enzymatic activity have been reported.[96-98] However, the pathophysiologic role of NO in this context remains controversial.[99] Increased cardiac NO can be myocytotoxic and reduce contractility.[22] On the other hand, Zaragoza et al.[100,101] showed that NO inhibits CVB3 replication in vitro, and targeted disruption of the NOSII gene in mice leads to aggravated myocardial damage after infection with CVB3. The mechanism(s) of the protective effect of NO in enteroviral cardiomyopathy may be related to inhibition of enteroviral proteolytic activity.

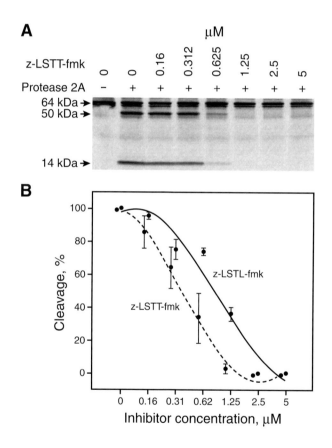

Fig. 10-6. A dystrophin-based coxsackieviral protease 2A inhibitor. *A*, A mouse dystrophin miniprotein containing the hinge 3 region was incubated with 1 μM protease 2A and the indicated concentrations of z-LSTT-fmk for 1 hour in cleavage buffer without dithiothreitol, followed by sodium dodecyl sulfate poly-acrylamide gel electrophoresis and autoradiography. Z-LSTT-fmk inhibited protease 2A in a dose-dependent manner. *B*, The cleavage inhibition by z-LSTT-fmk and z-LSTL-fmk was densitometrically calculated. Shown are the means and standard deviations from *n* = 3 independent experiments. Percentage cleavage was calculated relative to the value obtained with no inhibitor. Half-maximal inhibition of 1 μM protease 2A occurs with 550 nM z-LSTT-fmk and 1,050 nM z-LSTL-fmk, respectively.

Although NO exerts many of its physiologic functions in a cGMP-dependent fashion, it can also S-nitrosylate the sulfhydryl group of cysteine residues. This leads to enzyme inactivation in the case of cysteine protease.[102,103] Caspase-3, HIV protease, and enteroviral protease 3C are inhibited by NO through this mechanism.[104-107] Enteroviral protease 2A is not a stereotypical cysteine protease because it resembles serine-like proteases in overall folding, but it has a cysteine instead of a serine at its catalytic active site. Therefore, it is possible that protease 2A-mediated cleavage of dystrophin is inhibited by NO-mediated, S-nitrosylation of the cysteine at the catalytic active site.

Accordingly, we[108] demonstrated that NO inhibits dystrophin proteolysis by the coxsackieviral protease 2A in vitro and during CVB3 infection in cell culture. In addition, NO S-nitrosylates the active site cysteine (C110), a site that is consistent with an S-nitrosylation consensus motif, in vitro and within cells, indicating that this is a likely molecular mechanism for NO-mediated inhibition of coxsackievirus protease 2A. Because C110 is critical for protease 2A activity, nitrosylation at this site represents a molecular mechanism by which NO inactivates coxsackieviral protease 2A. Because the amino acids surrounding the active-site cysteine are conserved among all enteroviral 2A proteases known,[42] the protease 2A from all or most enteroviruses should be subject to cysteine nitrosylation.

In our experiments, protease 2A was inhibited at lower doses of NO donors than is reported for protease 3C inhibition.[107] However, because both enteroviral proteases are inactivated by S-nitrosylation, it appears that NO has a dual protective role against enteroviral infection.

CONCLUSION

Enteroviral infection of the heart plays a significant role in the pathogenesis of acute and chronic forms of cardiomyopathy. It is now clear that enteroviral infection can have a direct effect on the cardiac myocyte that contributes to viral-mediated cardiomyopathy. In addition, the viral protease 2A is able to cleave the myocyte cytoskeletal protein that has been implicated in dilated cardiomyopathy. This cleavage can be inhibited by NO-mediated nitrosylation of the catalytic active cysteine of protease 2A. Although it is highly likely that expression of the CAR in the heart contributes significantly to the cardioselective nature of coxsackievirus infection, other factors such as cleavage of dystrophin and a relative lack of effectiveness of type I interferons in the heart also contribute. Future work on viral-infected mice with a genetically manipulated dystrophin gene may shed additional insight into the mechanisms by which dystrophin deficiency and viral infection can lead to cardiomyopathy.

REFERENCES

1. Baboonian C, Davies MJ, Booth JC, McKenna WJ. Coxsackie B viruses and human heart disease. Curr Top Microbiol Immunol 1997;223:31-52.

2. Grunig E, Tasman JA, Kucherer H, Franz W, Kubler W, Katus HA. Frequency and phenotypes of familial dilated cardiomyopathy. J Am Coll Cardiol 1998;31:186-194.

3. Pauschinger M, Bowles NE, Fuentes-Garcia FJ, Pham V, Kuhl U, Schwimmbeck PL, Schultheiss HP, Towbin JA. Detection of adenoviral genome in the myocardium of adult patients with idiopathic left ventricular dysfunction. Circulation 1999;99:1348-1354.

4. Schonian U, Crombach M, Maser S, Maisch B. Cytomegalovirus-associated heart muscle disease. Eur Heart J 1995;16 Suppl O:46-49.

5. Matsumori A, Matoba Y, Sasayama S. Dilated cardiomyopathy associated with hepatitis C virus infection. Circulation 1995;92:2519-2525.

6. Cossart YE, Burgess JA, Nash PD. Fatal coxsackie B myocarditis in an adult. Med J Aust 1965;1:337-339.

7. Sun NC, Smith VM. Hepatitis associated with myocarditis. Unusual manifestation of infection with Coxsackie virus group B, type 3. N Engl J Med 1966;274:190-193.

8. Grist NR, Bell EJ. Coxsackie viruses and the heart. Am Heart J 1969;77:295-300.

9. Windorfer A, Sitzmann FC. Acute virus myocarditis in infants and children. [German.] Dtsch Med Wochenschr 1971;96:1177-1184.

10. Lerner AM, Wilson FM. Virus myocardiopathy. Prog Med Virol 1973;15:63-91.

11. Sainani GS, Dekate MP, Rao CP. Heart disease caused by Coxsackie virus B infection. Br Heart J 1975;37:819-823.

12. Sutinen S, Kalliomaki JL, Pohjonen R, Vastamaki R. Fatal generalized coxsackie B3 virus infection in an adolescent with successful isolation of the virus from pericardial fluid. Ann Clin Res 1971;3:241-246.

13. Burch GE, Sun SC, Chu KC, Sohal RS, Colcolough HL. Interstitial and coxsackievirus B myocarditis in infants and children. A comparative histologic and immunofluorescent study of 50 autopsied hearts. JAMA 1968;203:1-8.

14. Li Y, Bourlet T, Andreoletti L, Mosnier JF, Peng T, Yang Y, Archard LC, Pozzetto B, Zhang H. Enteroviral capsid protein VP1 is present in myocardial tissues from some patients with myocarditis or dilated cardiomyopathy. Circulation 2000;101:231-234.

15. Gerzen P, Granath A, Holmgren B, Zetterquist S. Acute myocarditis. A follow-up study. Br Heart J 1972;34:575-583.

16. Martino TA, Liu P, Sole MJ. Viral infection and the pathogenesis of dilated cardiomyopathy. Circ Res 1994;74:182-188.

17. Chow LH, Gauntt CJ, McManus BM. Differential effects of myocarditic variants of Coxsackievirus B3 in inbred mice. A pathologic characterization of heart tissue damage. Lab Invest 1991;64:55-64.

18. Kandolf R, Canu A, Hofschneider PH. Coxsackie B3 virus can replicate in cultured human foetal heart cells and is inhibited by interferon. J Mol Cell Cardiol 1985;17:167-181.

19. Yoneda S, Senda K, Hayashi K. Experimental study of virus myocarditis in culture. Jpn Circ J 1979;43:1048-1054.

20. Wessely R, Henke A, Zell R, Kandolf R, Knowlton KU. Low-level expression of a mutant coxsackie-viral cDNA induces a myocytopathic effect in culture: an approach to the study of enteroviral persistence in cardiac myocytes. Circulation 1998;98:450-457.

21. Mall G, Klingel K, Albrecht M, Seemann M, Rieger P, Kandolf R. Natural history of Coxsackievirus B3-induced myocarditis in ACA/Sn mice: viral persistence demonstrated by quantitative in situ hybridization histochemistry. Eur Heart J 1991;12 Suppl D:121-123.

22. Chow LH, Beisel KW, McManus BM. Enteroviral infection of mice with severe combined immunodeficiency. Evidence for direct viral pathogenesis of myocardial injury. Lab Invest 1992;66:24-31.

23. Heim A, Stille-Siegener M, Kandolf R, Kreuzer H, Figulla HR. Enterovirus-induced myocarditis: hemodynamic deterioration with immunosuppressive therapy and successful application of interferon-alpha. Clin Cardiol 1994;17:563-565.

24. Herzum M, Huber SA, Weller R, Grebe R, Maisch B. Treatment of experimental murine Coxsackie B3 myocarditis. Eur Heart J 1991;12 Suppl D:200-202.

25. Kishimoto C, Thorp KA, Abelmann WH. Immunosuppression with high doses of cyclophosphamide reduces the severity of myocarditis but increases the mortality in murine Coxsackievirus B3 myocarditis. Circulation 1990;82:982-989.

26. Wilson FM, Miranda QR, Chason JL, Lerner AM. Residual pathologic changes following murine coxsackie A and B myocarditis. Am J Pathol 1969;55:253-265.

27. Reyes MP, Ho KL, Smith F, Lerner AM. A mouse model of dilated-type cardiomyopathy due to coxsackievirus B3. J Infect Dis 1981;144:232-236.

28. Klingel K, Hohenadl C, Canu A, Albrecht M, Seemann M, Mall G, Kandolf R. Ongoing enterovirus-induced myocarditis is associated with persistent heart muscle infection: quantitative analysis of virus replication, tissue damage, and inflammation. Proc Natl Acad Sci U S A 1992;89:314-318.

29. Kandolf R, Klingel K, Mertsching H, Canu A, Hohenadl C, Zell R, Reimann BY, Heim A, McManus BM, Foulis AK, Schultheiss H-P, Erdmann E, Riecker G. Molecular studies on enteroviral heart disease: patterns of acute and persistent infections. Eur Heart J 1991;12 Suppl D:49-55.

30. O'Brien TX, Lee KJ, Chien KR. Positional specification of ventricular myosin light chain 2 expression in the primitive murine heart tube. Proc Natl Acad Sci U S A 1993;90:5157-5161.

31. Wessely R, Henke A, Kandolf R, Knowlton KU. Expression of a mutant non-infectious coxsackieviral cDNA inhibits protein expression in cardiac myocytes: a potential model of viral persistence (abstract). Circulation 1995;92 Suppl 1:527.

32. Bergelson JM, Cunningham JA, Droguett G, Kurt-Jones EA, Krithivas A, Hong JS, Horwitz MS, Crowell RL, Finberg RW. Isolation of a common receptor for Coxsackie B viruses and adenoviruses 2 and 5. Science 1997;275:1320-1323.

33. Bergelson JM, Mohanty JG, Crowell RL, St. John NF, Lublin DM, Finberg RW. Coxsackievirus B3 adapted to growth in RD cells binds to decay-accelerating factor (CD55). J Virol 1995;69:1903-1906.

34. Bergelson JM, Krithivas A, Celi L, Droguett G, Horwitz MS, Wickham T, Crowell RL, Finberg RW. The murine CAR homolog is a receptor for coxsackie B viruses and adenoviruses. J Virol 1998;72:415-419.

35. Muller U, Steinhoff U, Reis LF, Hemmi S, Pavlovic J, Zinkernagel RM, Aguet M. Functional role of type I and type II interferons in antiviral defense. Science 1994;264:1918-1921.

36. Huang S, Hendriks W, Althage A, Hemmi S, Bluethmann H, Kamijo R, Vilcek J, Zinkernagel RM, Aguet M. Immune response in mice that lack the interferon-gamma receptor. Science 1993;259:1742-1745.

37. Heim A, Canu A, Kirschner P, Simon T, Mall G, Hofschneider PH, Kandolf R. Synergistic interaction of interferon-beta and interferon-gamma in coxsackievirus B3-infected carrier cultures of human myocardial fibroblasts. J Infect Dis 1992;166:958-965.

38. Lutton CW, Gauntt CJ. Ameliorating effect of IFN-beta and anti-IFN-beta on coxsackievirus B3-induced myocarditis in mice. J Interferon Res 1985;5:137-146.

39. Sasaki O, Karaki T, Imanishi J. Protective effect of interferon on infections with hand, foot, and mouth disease virus in newborn mice. J Infect Dis 1986;153:498-502.

40. Matsumori A, Tomioka N, Kawai C. Protective effect of recombinant alpha interferon on coxsackievirus B3 myocarditis in mice. Am Heart J 1988;115:1229-1232.

41. Wessely R, Klingel K, Knowlton KU, Kandolf R. Cardioselective infection with coxsackievirus B3 requires intact type I interferon signaling: implications for mortality and early viral replication. Circulation 2001;103:756-761.

42. Petersen JF, Cherney MM, Liebig HD, Skern T, Kuechler E, James MN. The structure of the 2A proteinase from a common cold virus: a proteinase responsible for the shut-off of host-cell protein synthesis. EMBO J 1999;18:5463-5475.

43. Clark ME, Lieberman PM, Berk AJ, Dasgupta A. Direct cleavage of human TATA-binding protein by poliovirus protease 3C in vivo and in vitro. Mol Cell Biol 1993;13:1232-1237.

44. Das S, Dasgupta A. Identification of the cleavage site and determinants required for poliovirus 3CPro-catalyzed cleavage of human TATA-binding transcription factor TBP. J Virol 1993;67:3326-3331.

45. Lamphear BJ, Yan R, Yang F, Waters D, Liebig HD, Klump H, Kuechler E, Skern T, Rhoads RE. Mapping the cleavage site in protein synthesis initiation factor eIF-4 gamma of the 2A proteases from human Coxsackievirus and rhinovirus. J Biol Chem 1993;268:19200-19203.

46. Gradi A, Svitkin YV, Imataka H, Sonenberg N. Proteolysis of human eukaryotic translation initiation factor eIF4GII, but not eIF4GI, coincides with the shutoff of host protein synthesis after poliovirus infection. Proc Natl Acad Sci U S A 1998;95:11089-11094.

47. Kerekatte V, Keiper BD, Badorff C, Cai A, Knowlton KU, Rhoads RE. Cleavage of poly(A)-binding protein by coxsackievirus 2A protease in vitro and in vivo: another mechanism for host protein synthesis shutoff? J Virol 1999;73:709-717.

48. Seipelt J, Liebig HD, Sommergruber W, Gerner C, Kuechler E. 2A proteinase of human rhinovirus cleaves cytokeratin 8 in infected HeLa cells. J Biol Chem 2000;275:20085-20089.

49. Blom N, Hansen J, Blaas D, Brunak S. Cleavage site analysis in picornaviral polyproteins: discovering cellular targets by neural networks. Protein Sci 1996;5:2203-2216.

50. Chen J, Chien KR. Complexity in simplicity: monogenic disorders and complex cardiomyopathies. J Clin Invest 1999;103:1483-1485.

51. Straub V, Campbell KP. Muscular dystrophies and the dystrophin-glycoprotein complex. Curr Opin Neurol 1997;10:168-175.

52. Crosbie RH, Heighway J, Venzke DP, Lee JC, Campbell KP. Sarcospan, the 25-kDa transmembrane component of the dystrophin-glycoprotein complex. J Biol Chem 1997;272:31221-31224.

53. Betto R, Senter L, Ceoldo S, Tarricone E, Biral D, Salviati G. Ecto-ATPase activity of alpha-sarcoglycan (adhalin). J Biol Chem 1999;274:7907-7912.

54. Koenig M, Kunkel LM. Detailed analysis of the repeat domain of dystrophin reveals four potential hinge segments that may confer flexibility. J Biol Chem 1990;265:4560-4566.

55. Malhotra SB, Hart KA, Klamut HJ, Thomas NST, Bodrug SE, Burghes AHM, Bobrow M, Harper PS, Thompson MW, Ray PN, Worton RG. Frame-shift deletions in patients with Duchenne and Becker muscular dystrophy. Science 1988;242:755-759.

56. Beggs AH. Dystrophinopathy, the expanding phenotype. Dystrophin abnormalities in X-linked dilated cardiomyopathy. Circulation 1997;95:2344-2347.

57. Towbin JA, Hejtmancik JF, Brink P, Gelb B, Zhu XM, Chamberlain JS, McCabe ER, Swift M. X-linked dilated cardiomyopathy. Molecular genetic evidence of linkage to the Duchenne muscular dystrophy (dystrophin) gene at the Xp21 locus. Circulation 1993;87:1854-1865.

58. Muntoni F, Cau M, Ganau A, Congiu R, Arvedi G, Mateddu A, Marrosu MG, Cianchetti C, Realdi G, Cao A, Melis MA. Deletion of the dystrophin muscle-promoter region associated with X-linked dilated cardiomyopathy. N Engl J Med 1993;329:921-925.

59. Lim LE, Campbell KP. The sarcoglycan complex in limb-girdle muscular dystrophy. Curr Opin Neurol 1998;11:443-452.

60. van der Kooi AJ, de Voogt WG, Barth PG, Busch HF, Jennekens FG, Jongen PJ, de Visser M. The heart in limb girdle muscular dystrophy. Heart 1998;79:73-77.

61. Nigro V, Okazaki Y, Belsito A, Piluso G, Matsuda Y, Politano L, Nigro G, Ventura C, Abbondanza C, Molinari AM, Acampora D, Nishimura M, Hayashizaki Y, Puca GA. Identification of the Syrian hamster cardiomyopathy gene. Hum Mol Genet 1997;6:601-607.

62. Arber S, Hunter JJ, Ross J Jr, Hongo M, Sansig G, Borg J, Perriard JC, Chien KR, Caroni P. MLP-deficient mice exhibit a disruption of cardiac cytoarchitectural organization, dilated cardiomyopathy, and heart failure. Cell 1997;88:393-403.

63. Olson TM, Michels VV, Thibodeau SN, Tai YS, Keating MT. Actin mutations in dilated cardiomyopathy, a heritable form of heart failure. Science 1998;280:750-752.

64. Towbin JA. The role of cytoskeletal proteins in cardiomyopathies. Curr Opin Cell Biol 1998;10:131-139.

65. Badorff C, Lee G-H, Lamphear BJ, Martone ME, Campbell KP, Rhoads RE, Knowlton KU. Enteroviral protease 2A cleaves dystrophin: evidence of cytoskeletal disruption in an acquired cardiomyopathy. Nat Med 1999;5:320-326.

66. Badorff C, Berkely N, Mehrotra S, Talhouk JW, Rhoads RE, Knowlton KU. Enteroviral protease 2A directly cleaves dystrophin and is inhibited by a dystrophin-based substrate analogue. J Biol Chem 2000;275:11191-11197.

67. Koenig M, Monaco AP, Kunkel LM. The complete sequence of dystrophin predicts a rod-shaped cytoskeletal protein. Cell 1988;53:219-226.

68. Matsumura K, Tomé FMS, Ionasescu V, Ervasti JM, Anderson RD, Romero NB, Simon D, Récan D, Kaplan J-C, Fardeau M, Campbell KP. Deficiency of dystrophin-associated proteins in Duchenne muscular dystrophy patients lacking COOH-terminal domains of dystrophin. J Clin Invest 1993;92:866-871.

69. Lee G-H, Badorff C, Knowlton KU. Dissociation of sarcoglycans and the dystrophin carboxyl terminus from the sarcolemma in enteroviral cardiomyopathy. Circ Res 2000;87:489-495.

70. Rybakova IN, Ervasti JM. Dystrophin-glycoprotein complex is monomeric and stabilizes actin filaments in vitro through a lateral association. J Biol Chem 1997;272:28771-28778.

71. Roberts RG, Bobrow M. Dystrophins in vertebrates and invertebrates. Hum Mol Genet 1998;7:589-595.

72. Ervasti JM, Ohlendieck K, Kahl SD, Gaver MG, Campbell KP. Deficiency of a glycoprotein component of the dystrophin complex in dystrophic muscle. Nature 1990;345:315-319.

73. Spencer MJ, Walsh CM, Dorshkind KA, Rodriguez EM, Tidball JG. Myonuclear apoptosis in dystrophic mdx muscle occurs by perforin-mediated cytotoxicity. J Clin Invest 1997;99:2745-2751.

74. Chen PH, Ornelles DA, Shenk T. The adenovirus L3 23-kilodalton proteinase cleaves the amino-terminal head domain from cytokeratin 18 and disrupts the cytokeratin network of HeLa cells. J Virol 1993;67:3507-3514.

75. Shoeman RL, Honer B, Stoller TJ, Kesselmeier C, Miedel MC, Traub P, Graves MC. Human immunodeficiency virus type 1 protease cleaves the intermediate filament proteins vimentin, desmin, and glial fibrillary acidic protein. Proc Natl Acad Sci U S A 1990;87:6336-6340.

76. Kandolf R, Hofschneider PH. Viral heart disease. Springer Semin Immunopathol 1989;11:1-13.

77. Olivetti G, Abbi R, Quaini F, Kajstura J, Cheng W, Nitahara JA, Quaini E, Di Loreto C, Beltrami CA, Krajewski S, Reed JC, Anversa P. Apoptosis in the failing human heart. N Engl J Med 1997;336:1131-1141.

78. Maisch B, Drude L, Hengstenberg C, Herzum M, Hufnagel G, Kochsiek K, Schmaltz A, Schonian U, Schwab MD. Are antisarcolemmal (ASAs) and antimyolemmal antibodies (AMLAs) "natural" antibodies? Basic Res Cardiol 1991;86 Suppl 3:101-114.

79. Badorff C, Noutsias M, Kuhl U, Schultheiss HP. Cell-mediated cytotoxicity in hearts with dilated cardiomyopathy: correlation with interstitial fibrosis and foci of activated T lymphocytes. J Am Coll Cardiol 1997;29:429-434.

80. Lauer B, Padberg K, Schultheiss HP, Strauer BE. Autoantibodies against human ventricular myosin in sera of patients with acute and chronic myocarditis. J Am Coll Cardiol 1994;23:146-153.

81. Schulze K, Becker BF, Schultheiss HP. Antibodies to the ADP/ATP carrier, an autoantigen in myocarditis and dilated cardiomyopathy, penetrate into myocardial cells and disturb energy metabolism in vivo. Circ Res 1989;64:179-192.

82. Knowlton KU, Badorff C. The immune system in viral myocarditis: maintaining the balance. Circ Res 1999;85:559-561.

83. Grady RM, Teng H, Nichol MC, Cunningham JC, Wilkinson RS, Sanes JR. Skeletal and cardiac myopathies in mice lacking utrophin and dystrophin: a model for Duchenne muscular dystrophy. Cell 1997;90:729-738.

84. Cohn RD, Durbeej M, Moore SA, Coral-Vazquez R, Prouty S, Campbell KP. Prevention of cardiomyopathy in mouse models lacking the smooth muscle sarcoglycan-sarcospan complex. J Clin Invest 2001;107:R1-R7.

85. Coral-Vazquez R, Cohn RD, Moore SA, Hill JA, Weiss RM, Davisson RL, Straub V, Baressi R, Bansal D, Hrstka RF, Williamson R, Campbell KP. Disruption of the sarcoglycan-sarcospan complex in vascular smooth muscle: a novel mechanism for cardiomyopathy and muscular dystrophy. Cell 1999;98:465-474.

86. Godeny EK, Sprague EA, Schwartz CJ, Gauntt CJ. Coxsackievirus group B replication in cultured fetal baboon aortic smooth muscle cells. J Med Virol 1986;20:135-149.

87. Dong R, Liu P, Wee L, Butany J, Sole MJ. Verapamil ameliorates the clinical and pathological course of murine myocarditis. J Clin Invest 1992;90:2022-2030.

88. Rueckert RR. Picornaviridae: the viruses and their replication. In: Fields BN, Knipe DM, Howley PM, eds. Fundamental virology. 3rd ed. Vol. 1. New York: Lippincott-Raven, 1996:609-654.

89. Chou KC. Prediction of human immunodeficiency virus protease cleavage sites in proteins. Anal Biochem 1996;233:1-14.

90. Molla A, Hellen CU, Wimmer E. Inhibition of proteolytic activity of poliovirus and rhinovirus 2A proteinases by elastase-specific inhibitors. J Virol 1993;67:4688-4695.

91. Wang QM, Johnson RB, Jungheim LN, Cohen JD, Villarreal EC. Dual inhibition of human rhinovirus 2A and 3C proteases by homophthalimides. Antimicrob Agents Chemother 1998;42:916-920.

92. Wang QM, Johnson RB, Sommergruber W, Shepherd TA. Development of in vitro peptide substrates for human rhinovirus-14 2A protease. Arch Biochem Biophys 1998;356:12-18.

93. Nicholson DW, Thornberry NA. Caspases: killer proteases. Trends Biochem Sci 1997;22:299-306.

94. Ventoso I, Barco A, Carrasco L. Genetic selection of poliovirus 2Apro-binding peptides. J Virol 1999;73:814-818.

95. Moncada S, Higgs A. The L-arginine-nitric oxide pathway. N Engl J Med 1993;329:2002-2012.

96. Winlaw DS, Smythe GA, Keogh AM, Schyvens CG, Spratt PM, Macdonald PS. Increased nitric oxide production in heart failure. Lancet 1994;344:373-374.

97. Haywood GA, Tsao PS, von der Leyen HE, Mann MJ, Keeling PJ, Trindade PT, Lewis NP, Byrne CD, Rickenbacher PR, Bishopric NH, Cooke JP, McKenna WJ, Fowler MB. Expression of inducible nitric oxide synthase in human heart failure. Circulation 1996;93:1087-1094.

98. de Belder AJ, Radomski MW, Why HJ, Richardson PJ, Bucknall CA, Salas E, Martin JF, Moncada S. Nitric oxide synthase activities in human myocardium. Lancet 1993;341:84-85.

99. Drexler H. Nitric oxide synthases in the failing human heart: a doubled-edged sword? Circulation 1999;99:2972-2975.

100. Zaragoza C, Ocampo CJ, Saura M, McMillan A, Lowenstein CJ. Nitric oxide inhibition of coxsackievirus replication in vitro. J Clin Invest 1997;100:1760-1767.

101. Zaragoza C, Ocampo C, Saura M, Leppo M, Wei XQ, Quick R, Moncada S, Liew FY, Lowenstein CJ. The role of inducible nitric oxide synthase in the host response to Coxsackievirus myocarditis. Proc Natl Acad Sci U S A 1998;95:2469-2474.

102. Stamler JS. Redox signaling: nitrosylation and related target interactions of nitric oxide. Cell 1994;78:931-936.

103. Broillet MC. S-nitrosylation of proteins. Cell Mol Life Sci 1999;55:1036-1042.

104. Rossig L, Fichtlscherer B, Breitschopf K, Haendeler J, Zeiher AM, Mulsch A, Dimmeler S. Nitric oxide inhibits caspase-3 by S-nitrosation in vivo. J Biol Chem 1999;274:6823-6826.

105. Mannick JB, Hausladen A, Liu L, Hess DT, Zeng M, Miao QX, Kane LS, Gow AJ, Stamler JS. Fas-induced caspase denitrosylation. Science 1999;284:651-654.

106. Persichini T, Colasanti M, Lauro GM, Ascenzi P. Cysteine nitrosylation inactivates the HIV-1 protease. Biochem Biophys Res Commun 1998;250:575-576.

107. Saura M, Zaragoza C, McMillan A, Quick RA, Hohenadl C, Lowenstein JM, Lowenstein CJ. An antiviral mechanism of nitric oxide: inhibition of a viral protease. Immunity 1999;10:21-28.

108. Badorff C, Fichtlscherer B, Rhoads RE, Zeiher AM, Muelsch A, Dimmeler S, Knowlton KU. Nitric oxide inhibits dystrophin proteolysis by coxsackieviral protease 2A through S-nitrosylation: a protective mechanism against enteroviral cardiomyopathy. Circulation 2000;102:2276-2281.

Introduction to Clinical Myocarditis

G. William Dec, M.D.

HISTORICAL BACKGROUND

Myocarditis is simply defined as inflammation of the myocardium. The inflammation may involve the myocytes, interstitium, vascular elements, or pericardium. Despite its rather plain definition, the classification, diagnosis, and treatment of myocarditis continue to prompt considerable debate. The term "myocarditis" was initially used by Sobernheim[1] in 1837. The disease process was further clarified as "isolated idiopathic interstitial myocarditis" by Feidler[2] in 1899. Saphir[3] proposed one of the first classification systems for myocarditis based on disease etiology. He[3] was among the first to appreciate the disparity between pathologic findings and clinical presentation when he wrote "a gap between the abundance of anatomic changes in the myocardium and their apparent clinical insignificance." Burch and Ray,[4] in 1948, better described clinical manifestations of the disease and were the first to recognize different prognoses for acute and chronic types of myocarditis. These initial pathologic series focused on one end of the spectrum of the disease—ie, those patients who died of myocarditis. Histologic confirmation of clinical myocarditis in the living patient became possible with the advent of endomyocardial biopsy in the 1960s. The more routine use of endomyocardial biopsy has helped better define the natural history of human myocarditis and clarify clinicopathologic correlations.

Myocarditis may occur during or following a wide variety of viral, rickettsial, bacterial, and protozoal infections (Table 11-1). Infectious diseases cause myocardial injury through 3 basic mechanisms: direct invasion of the myocardium, production of a myocardial toxin (such as diphtheria), or immunologically mediated myocardial damage. Although virtually any infectious agent may produce myocardial inflammation and injury, human myocarditis is most frequently caused by viral infection.[5] The picornavirus group, which includes coxsackievirus A and B, echovirus, and poliovirus, is most frequently associated with myocardial involvement.[6] Less commonly implicated viral etiologies include orthomyxovirus (influenza A and B), paramyxovirus (rubeola, mumps), togavirus (rubella, dengue, yellow fever), herpesvirus (varicella zoster), Epstein-Barr virus, cytomegalovirus, and hepatitis virus (A, B, and C). Cardiac involvement in the acquired immunodeficiency syndrome (AIDS) may include infective or toxic forms of myocarditis. Cardiac involvement occurs in 25% to 45% of AIDS patients; however, it leads to clinically apparent heart disease in fewer than 10%.[7] Myocarditis may result from opportunistic infections of the myocardium (eg, *Pneumocystis carinii*, toxoplasmosis), viral infection (cytomegalovirus, human immunodeficiency virus), or drug toxicity (antibiotics and antiretroviral drugs). Other noninfectious causes of myocarditis include myocardial toxins, autoimmune disorders, physical agents, and hypersensitivity drug reactions (Table 11-1).

The clinical manifestations of myocarditis are highly varied and are not specific enough to establish a diagnosis with certainty. Clinicians have increasingly relied on right ventricular endomyocardial biopsy for histologic confirmation of suspected inflammatory heart

Table 11-1
Etiologies of Lymphocytic Myocarditis*

Infectious causes
    Viral agents
        Coxsackievirus (A, B), **echovirus**, **cytomegalovirus**, **adenovirus**, poliovirus, influenza, hepatitis B or **C**, encephalomyocarditis virus, Epstein-Barr virus, rubella, retrovirus, **human immunodeficiency virus**, mumps, respiratory syncytial virus, rabies, vaccinia, varicella, yellow fever
    Bacterial agents
        Endocarditis-associated myocarditis; streptococcus (rheumatic or nonrheumatic), meningococcus, salmonella, diphtheriae, brucellosis, tuberculosis, staphylococcus, hemophilus
    Chlamydial/atypical infectious agents
        Mycoplasma, psittacosis
    Rickettsial
        Q fever, Rocky Mountain spotted fever, typhus
    Fungal
        Histoplasmosis, aspergillosis, candidiasis, coccidioidomycosis, actinomycosis, cryptococcosis, blastomycosis
    Protozoal
        Trypanosoma cruzi **(Chagas disease)**, **toxoplasmosis**, *Pneumocystis carinii*, African trypanosomiasis, malaria, amebiasis
    Spirochetal
        Lyme disease, syphilis, leptospirosis, relapsing fever
    Metazoal
        Trichinosis, schistosomiasis, ascariasis, echinococcosis, cysticercosis
Autoimmune disorders
    Scleroderma, lupus erythematosus
Myocardial toxins
    Chemotherapeutic agents
        Anthracyclines, cyclophosphamide
    Antiretroviral agents
        Didanosine (ddI), **ddC (zalcitabine)**, **AZT (zidovudine)**, **ribavirin**, **interferon-α**
    Antiparasitic
        Emetine, chloroquine, antimony compounds
    Psychotropic agents
        Phenothiazine, lithium
    Metal poisoning
        Mercury, arsenic
    Animal toxins
        Snake bite, wasp sting, spider bite, scorpion sting
    Catecholamines
        Cocaine, pheochromocytoma
Physical injury
    Radiation
    Heat stroke
    Hypothermia
Hypersensitivity reaction

*Etiologies shown in **bold** are more commonly observed causes of myocarditis.

disease. Mason et al.[8] were among the first to demonstrate evidence of myocardial inflammation by using right ventricular endomyocardial biopsies in a small group of patients with presumed idiopathic dilated cardiomyopathy. Although endomyocardial biopsy has become the standard for establishing the diagnosis, the histologic criteria used for establishing the diagnosis of myocarditis have varied considerably.

In a study designed to define quantitative criteria for the diagnosis of myocarditis, Edwards et al.[9] reported that the presence of more than 5 lymphocytes/hpf was sufficient to diagnose active myocarditis. Tazelaar and Billingham,[10] however, cautioned against the use of a focal infiltrate alone in diagnosing myocarditis because isolated lymphocyte aggregations may also be seen in idiopathic dilated cardiomyopathy. To provide more uniform criteria for the pathologic diagnosis of myocarditis, a panel of cardiac pathologists developed a disease classification known as the Dallas criteria.[11] These authors define myocarditis as a process characterized by an inflammatory infiltrate of the myocardium with necrosis or degeneration of adjacent myocytes (or both), not typically seen in ischemic injury. The inflammatory infiltrate is typically lymphocytic but may also include eosinophilic, neutrophilic, granulomatous, or mixed cellularity. The amount of inflammation and its distribution may be mild, moderate, or severe and focal, confluent, or diffuse, respectively. Despite the widespread adoption of this histopathologic classification, some clinicians feel that the definition is too narrow and have proposed a clinicopathologic classification that includes histologic characteristics and clinical features (Table 11-2).[12,13] Despite its clinical appeal, this clinicopathologic approach has not been widely accepted.

Sampling error is the most critical limitation to diagnostic accuracy of endomyocardial biopsy. Hauck et al.[14] analyzed hearts from autopsies in which myocarditis was determined to have contributed directly to death. Ten biopsy specimens from the apex and septum of both ventricles were evaluated for myocarditis by the Dallas criteria. Myocarditis was correctly diagnosed from all 10 specimens in 63% of the hearts. When only the first 5 right ventricular biopsy specimens from each heart were evaluated, which is the most common clinical sampling rate, the diagnosis of myocarditis could not be established in 55% of the hearts (Fig. 11-1). In a similar postmortem study of 14 hearts, 17.2 samples per heart were required to correctly diagnose myocarditis in more than 80% of the cases.[15] Dec et al.[16] examined the results of a repeat right and left ventricular endomyocardial biopsy in patients who were strongly suspected of having myocarditis clinically but whose initial right ventricular biopsy failed to provide histologic confirmation. Repeat biopsies detected an additional 15% incidence of myocarditis. Thus, a positive endomyocardial biopsy unequivocally establishes the diagnosis; however, the absence of histologic confirmation should not exclude consideration of myocarditis in most clinical settings.

Table 11-2
Clinicopathologic Classification of Myocarditis

Characteristic	Fulminant	Acute	Chronic active	Chronic persistent
Symptom onset	Distinct	Indistinct	Indistinct	Indistinct
Presentation	Cardiogenic shock, severe LVD	CHF LVD	CHF LVD	Non-CHF symptoms, normal LV function
Biopsy findings	Multiple foci of active myocarditis	Active or borderline myocarditis	Active or borderline myocarditis	Active or borderline myocarditis
Natural history	Complete recovery or death	Partial recovery or DCM	DCM	Non-CHF symptoms, normal LV function
Histologic evolution	Complete resolution	Complete resolution	Ongoing or resolving myocarditis, fibrosis, giant cells	Ongoing or resolving myocarditis
Immunosuppression	No benefit	Sometimes beneficial	No benefit	No benefit

CHF, congestive heart failure; CM, cardiomyopathy; DCM, dilated cardiomyopathy; LV, left ventricular; LVD, left ventricular dysfunction.
From Lieberman et al.[12] By permission of the American College of Cardiology.

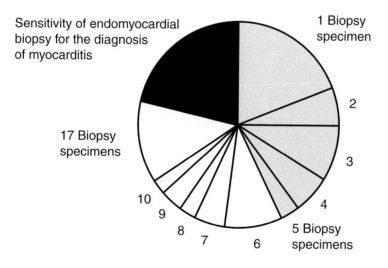

Fig. 11-1. Sensitivity of endomyocardial biopsy for detecting myocarditis in a postmortem study of 38 myocarditis hearts. Each section demonstrates the rate of detection of each additional endomyocardial biopsy specimen. One biopsy detected myocarditis in 18% of specimens. Light gray shading: 5 biopsy specimens detected myocarditis in only 43% of specimens. White: 17 biopsy specimens confirmed myocarditis in 82% of explanted hearts. Multiple biopsy specimens failed to detect known myocarditis in 18% of cases. (From Dec and Narula.[76] By permission of Edizioni Minerva Medica.)

HYPERSENSITIVITY MYOCARDITIS

Adverse effects of prescribed medications may include hypersensitivity and toxic myocarditis. Unlike toxic reactions, hypersensitivity may occur in individuals with prior uneventful exposure to the drug and is not dose related. The myocarditis is histologically characterized by a perivascular and interstitial infiltrate of the myocardium by eosinophils, leukocytes, and, rarely, multinucleated giant cells or granulomas with little or no myocyte necrosis.[17] Commonly implicated drugs are sulfonamides, penicillins, methyldopa, phenytoin, and tricyclic antidepressants (Table 11-3).[17,18] Cocaine may also rarely produce a hypersensitivity myocarditis. Unlike the hypereosinophilic syndrome, peripheral eosinophilia is typically absent.[19] Prolonged continuous infusion of dobutamine has also been associated with hypersensitivity myocarditis.[20] Hypersensitivity myocarditis is rarely recognized clinically and is often first discovered at postmortem examination. However, it may be diagnosed by endomyocardial biopsy.[17] Autopsy studies suggest that up to 50% of cases could be diagnosed by means of biopsy.[18] Like most cases of myocarditis, symptoms and physical findings do not relate to the degree of cellular infiltration. Cardiac arrhythmias or unexplained sudden death are the most common clinical presentations.[18,21] Eosinophilic myocarditis may also simulate acute myocardial infarction, with ischemic chest pain and ST-segment elevation on electrocardiography.[21] Awareness of the condition is necessary to make the correct diagnosis. Therapy includes discontinuation of the offending medication and corticosteroids, sometimes with additional immunosuppressive agents in severe cases.[17,22]

CLINICAL PRESENTATIONS OF LYMPHOCYTIC MYOCARDITIS

Clinical manifestations of lymphocytic myocarditis range from asymptomatic electrocardiographic abnormalities to severe heart failure and cardiogenic shock. Transient electrocardiographic abnormalities suggesting myocardial involvement have been reported during community viral endemics. Most patients do not have clinical manifestations of heart disease.[6,23] Typically, cardiac involvement develops 7 to 10 days after a systemic viral illness. Unrecognized myocarditis during viral infections has been supported by histologic findings obtained during routine postmortem examination.[23,24] Subepicardial myocardial involvement has been reported frequently in patients with acute myocarditis.[25] The majority of patients have no specific cardiovascular complaints. Myocarditis is often inferred from ST-segment and T-wave abnormalities noted on electrocardiogram.[6] Symptoms may include fatigue, dyspnea, palpitations, and precordial chest pain.[26] Chest pain usually reflects associated pericarditis but occasionally may suggest myocardial ischemia. Heart failure due to acute dilated cardiomyopathy is the most frequent manifestation of myocarditis that requires medical attention.[27] Myocarditis may simulate acute

Table 11-3
Common Drug Causes of Hypersensitivity Myocarditis*

Diuretics	Antituberculous	Miscellaneous
Acetazolamide	Isoniazid	**Cocaine**
Chlorthalidone	Paraminosalicylic acid	**Dobutamine**
Thiazides		**Tricyclic antidepressants**
Spironolactone	Anticonvulsants	Methyldopa
	Phenytoin	**Phenothiazines**
Antibiotics/antifungal	Carbamazepine	Sulfonylureas
Aminoglycosides		Tetanus toxoid
Penicillins	Anti-inflammatory	
Cephalosporins	Indomethacin	
Chloramphenicol	Phenylbutazone	
Sulfonamides		
Tetracyclines		
Streptomycin		
Amphotericin B		

*Etiologies shown in **bold** are more commonly observed causes of myocarditis.

myocardial infarction.[28] Ventricular arrhythmias, heart block, and sudden cardiac death are uncommon, but occasionally reported, clinical presentations.[26,29] Most patients recover from viral myocarditis within weeks, although electrocardiographic abnormalities often persist for months. Although coxsackievirus myocarditis is only occasionally fatal in adults, neonates tend to have a more malignant course.

The clinical course of myocarditis is highly variable. In the majority of patients, the disease is self-limited and there is complete resolution of myocardial inflammation without further sequelae. Myocarditis has been reported to recur in 10% to 25% of patients after apparent resolution of the initial illness.[27,30] There are no reliable predictors that identify patients likely to have a relapse, although one report indicated that pericarditis on initial presentation may be associated with a higher rate of recurrence.[31] Similar to initial presentation, recurrent myocarditis may resolve spontaneously or be associated with heart failure, arrhythmias, or death.

ACUTE DILATED CARDIOMYOPATHY

Heart failure of recent onset due to acute dilated cardiomyopathy represents one of the most dramatic and clinically relevant presentations of acute lymphocytic myocarditis.[8,32,33] Myocarditis must always be differentiated from other potentially reversible causes of acute dilated cardiomyopathy (Table 11-4). The link between clinical myocarditis and acute dilated cardiomyopathy is provided by histologic validation of acute inflammatory changes and myocyte injury. With the routine use of right ventricular endomyocardial biopsy,

Table 11-4
Reversible Causes of Acute Left Ventricular Dysfunction

Stunned myocardium following an acute ischemic insult or infarction
Sepsis-associated myocardial depression
Myocardial depression after cardiopulmonary bypass (postcardiotomy syndrome)
Acute dilated cardiomyopathies
    Peripartum cardiomyopathy
    Idiopathic
    Toxic
        Alcohol
        Cobalt (beer drinker's heart)
        Carbon monoxide
        Cocaine
    Drug-induced
        Antiretroviral agents
        Doxorubicin (acute response)
        Interferon
Myocarditis
    Lymphocytic
    Giant cell
    Eosinophilic
    Granulomatous
        Wegener granulomatosis
        Cardiac sarcoidosis

histologic evidence of active myocarditis has been reported in 1% to 67% of patients presenting with dilated cardiomyopathy (Table 11-5).[8,32,33,35,38,39,42-45]

The wide variation in reported incidence of disease has several potential explanations. Various studies have examined a heterogeneous patient mix; some series have included patients with heart failure of many years' duration whereas others have focused on those with symptoms of recent onset. In addition, the criteria for definitive diagnosis of myocarditis have varied considerably. Many series that report a biopsy incidence of myocarditis of more than 30% have used liberal definitions that included only the presence of scattered lymphocytic infiltrates. More recent series which have used the Dallas criteria have reported a substantially lower incidence of myocarditis. In the largest and most contemporary series, Mason et al.[42] reported a biopsy incidence of myocarditis of approximately 10% in the Multicenter Myocarditis Trial. Given the multifocal nature of the inflammatory infiltrate, the frequency with which myocarditis is histologically verified probably significantly underestimates its true presence. Moreover, histologic findings may be an insensitive marker of an ongoing inflammatory process, possibly inferior to histochemical and immunologic markers. The results of enteroviral genomic detection using polymerase chain reaction techniques may ultimately establish a new diagnostic standard with higher sensitivity and specificity.

Table 11-5
Incidence of Biopsy-Proven Myocarditis in Patients With Dilated Cardiomyopathy

Series	Year	Patients screened, no.	Positive biopsies*, %
Kunkel et al.[34]	1978	66	6
Mason et al.[8]	1980	400	3
Noda[35]	1980	52	0.5
Baandrup et al.[36]	1981	132	1
O'Connell et al.[37]	1981	68	7
Nippoldt et al.[38]	1982	170	5
Fenoglio et al.[39]	1983	135	25
Unverferth et al.[40]	1983	59	6
Parrillo et al.[32]	1984	74	26
Zee-Cheng et al.[33]	1984	35	63
Daly et al.[30]	1984	69	17
Bolte and Ludwig[41]	1984	91	20
Dec et al.[27]	1985	27	67
Hosenpud et al.[29]	1986	38	16
Mason et al.[42]	1995	2,233	10
		3,649	10.3

*Histologic criteria for diagnosing myocarditis varied widely among published series. The largest and most recent series from the Multicenter Myocarditis Trial[42] (n = 2,233) used the current Dallas criteria. Final mean was weighted.

It is clear that the duration of symptoms is closely related to the likelihood of detecting myocarditis on biopsy (Table 11-6). Those patients with symptoms of short duration have been found to have a higher likelihood of myocarditis or borderline myocarditis being detected.[27] Most studies have shown that the biopsy detection rate for myocarditis is less than 5% when heart failure symptoms have been present for more than 6 months.[27]

Clinical signs and symptoms of active myocarditis based on community coxsackievirus outbreaks have been described in some cases of lymphocytic myocarditis.[45-47] A viral-like illness (upper respiratory infection or gastrointestinal tract symptoms) is present in one-third of patients with coxsackievirus myocarditis but is a nonspecific finding. Pericarditis is associated with active myocarditis in 25% to 30% of patients.[27,46,47] Supportive laboratory abnormalities, including increased erythrocyte sedimentation rate, leukocytosis, or increased creatine kinase concentration, are useful when present but occur in only 10% to 20% of biopsy-proven cases.[27,48,49]

Newer laboratory markers such as serum troponin I and troponin T may be more sensitive in detecting myocardial injury and are being evaluated for diagnosis of clinical myocarditis. Thus, the classic clinical triad traditionally used to diagnose coxsackie B-induced myocarditis (ie, preceding viral illness, pericarditis, and associated laboratory abnormalities) is present in fewer than 10% of histologically proven cases.[27] Again, those patients with acute dilated cardiomyopathy of short duration are generally more likely to have a high clin-

Table 11-6
Relationship Among Duration of Illness, Clinical Features, Histopathologic Findings, and Outcome for Patients Presenting With Acute Dilated Cardiomyopathy

Onset of symptoms, wk	Patients, no.	Clinical score*	Positive[†] biopsy, %	Improved[‡], %
0-4	9	2.1	89	44
4-12	10	2.3	70	30
12-26	8	0.9	38	38

*Mean number of clinical features suggestive of myocarditis (viral syndrome by history = 1 point; pericarditis by history or examination = 1 point; supportive laboratory abnormalities [leukocytosis, increased sedimentation rate or concentration of creatine kinase] = 1 point). Score for any patient ranged from 0 to 3 points.
[†]Histologic findings confirming myocarditis or borderline myocarditis.
[‡]Improvement defined as increase in left ventricular ejection fraction > 10 units and improvement in symptoms.
Modified from Dec et al.[27] By permission of the Massachusetts Medical Society.

ical feature score (semiquantitatively defined as 0-3) than those with more long-standing symptoms (Table 11-6).[27] Therefore, a new diagnosis of acute dilated cardiomyopathy should suggest the possibility of viral myocarditis even when a prior viral illness, pericardial inflammation, or laboratory abnormalities are lacking. Conversely, the combination of one or more clinical features of coxsackie myocarditis and a subsequent substantial increase in left ventricular ejection fraction supports the clinical diagnosis of active myocarditis, even when supportive biopsy evidence is lacking.[27,50]

A patient who has acute dilated cardiomyopathy due to myocarditis generally presents in 1 of 3 ways. Typically, the patient presents with signs and symptoms of mild (New York Heart Association [NYHA] class II) heart failure of short duration. Mild cardiomegaly is noted on chest film or an increase in left ventricular end-diastolic dimension is detected on echocardiography. Systolic function is usually only mildly impaired, with left ventricular ejection fraction in the 40% to 50% range. The vast majority of these patients have spontaneous improvement in ventricular function and normalization in heart size with conservative medical management.

A second group presents more critically ill with more prominent heart failure symptoms (NYHA class III or IV). Left ventricular size is often markedly increased, with left ventricular end-diastolic dimension greater than 70 mm on echocardiography. Likewise, systolic function is more markedly impaired; left ventricular ejection fraction is almost always less than 35%. Typically, 25% of these patients have spontaneous improvement in ventricular function, 50% develop chronic left ventricular dysfunction, and the remaining 25% progress to death or need for transplantation (personal observation). Histologic findings (ie, the extent of inflammatory infiltrate, myocyte necrosis, or interstitial fibrosis) do not correlate closely with the likelihood of improvement or deterioration in ventricular function.[27,51] Among the cohort of patients who have normalization of ventricular function, biopsy-proven relapses have been noted and recurrent myocarditis should be suspected if ventricular function subsequently deteriorates.[27]

Rarely, a patient may present with fulminant myocarditis and circulatory collapse. These individuals usually have an acute onset of heart failure, severe global left ventricular function, and a minimal increase in left ventricular end-diastolic dimension.[12,52] End-organ dysfunction is frequently present with abnormalities of hepatic and renal function. Mechanical circulatory support with an intra-aortic balloon pump or unilateral or biventricular assist devices is often necessary to bridge the time to recovery of ventricular function or heart transplantation.[52-54] Despite the severity of their initial presentation, many patients exhibit partial or complete recovery of ventricular function with short- to intermediate-term inotropic or mechanical circulatory support.[52,53]

Long-term outcome with histologically verified lymphocytic myocarditis has been clarified. In a single-institution study, Grogan et al.[43] reported a 5-year survival rate of 56% for patients presenting with lymphocytic myocarditis (Fig. 11-2). Interestingly, no difference in short- or long-term survival was noted between patients with histologically verified myocarditis and those with idiopathic dilated cardiomyopathy. Similar results have been reported for patients enrolled in the Multicenter Myocarditis Trial, with a 5-year

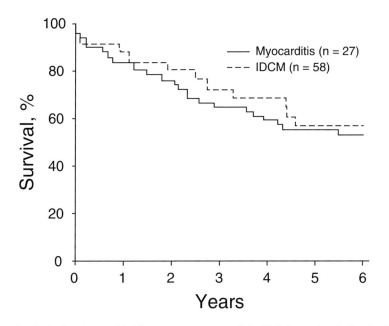

Fig. 11-2. Survival of patients with biopsy-proven myocarditis (definite or borderline by Dallas criteria) compared to that observed for patients with idiopathic dilated cardiomyopathy (*IDCM*) and negative endomyocardial biopsy findings. (From Grogan et al.[43] By permission of the American College of Cardiology.)

survival of 52% in patients treated with conventional medical therapy.[42] Some investigators have suggested that patients with borderline myocarditis may respond more favorably to immunosuppressive therapy and have a better long-term outcome, but others have been unable to confirm a better long-term outcome in this group.[51,55,56] Identification of individual patients with lymphocytic myocarditis who are at increased risk of death based on their clinical features, biopsy findings, or ventriculographic studies is not usually possible; however, the predictors of death or need for heart transplantation in two large single-center series are illustrated in Tables 11-7 and 11-8.

Table 11-7
Multivariate Predictors of Death or Transplantation in 109 Cases of Biopsy-Proven Lymphocytic Myocarditis From Massachusetts General Hospital

Variable	P	RR	CI
Syncope	0.003	8.5	2.08-34.89
BBB	0.023	2.9	1.16-7.40
EF < 40%	0.05	2.9	1.01-8.49
Borderline histologic results	0.018	0.07	0.01-0.64

BBB, bundle branch block; EF, ejection fraction.
From Goldberg LR, Suk HJ, Patton KK, Semigran MJ, Dec GW, DiSalvo TG. Predictors of adverse outcome in biopsy-proven myocarditis (abstract). J Am Coll Cardiol 1999;33 Suppl A:505A. By permission of the American College of Cardiology.

Table 11-8
Multivariate Predictors of Death or Transplantation in 147 Patients With Lymphocytic Myocarditis Diagnosed by Biopsy at Johns Hopkins Hospital

Variable*	Adjusted hazard ratio for death or transplantation (95% CI)	P value
Fulminant myocarditis at presentation	0.10 (0.01-0.88)	0.04
Increased mean pulmonary artery pressure (for each increment of 5 mm Hg)	1.50 (1.1-2.1)	0.01
Increased cardiac output (for each increment of 1 L/min)	0.75 (0.59-0.96)	0.02

*Nonsignificant predictors were age, histopathologic findings (borderline myocarditis or active myocarditis), heart rate, mean arterial pressure, mean right atrial pressure, and mean pulmonary-capillary wedge pressure. Mean pulmonary-artery pressure and cardiac output were evaluated as continuous variables. CI denotes confidence interval.
From McCarthy et al.[51] By permission of the Massachusetts Medical Society.

MYOCARDITIS MIMICKING ACUTE MYOCARDIAL INFARCTION

Myocarditis is not infrequently associated with chest pain, which is typically pleuritic in nature and related to accompanying pericardial inflammation. Patients with myocarditis may also present with angina-like chest discomfort, despite the absence of epicardial coronary artery disease. Myocarditis has been reported at autopsy in patients who presented with acute myocardial infarction, normal coronary anatomy, and documented coxsackie B viral disease.[57] Because myocarditis is associated with focal or multifocal myocardial inflammation and necrosis, it is not surprising that it may be associated with increased serum concentration of creatine kinase, electrocardiographic repolarization abnormalities, abnormal QS waves, and segmental wall motion abnormalities on left ventriculography.[57-61]

At our institution, 34 patients with clinical signs and symptoms of acute myocardial infarction underwent right ventricular endomyocardial biopsy during a 6.5-year period after angiographic identification of normal coronary anatomy.[62] Myocarditis was confirmed on biopsy in 11 of these patients (32%). Cardiogenic shock requiring transient intra-aortic balloon support developed within 6 hours of admission in 3 of these patients. Electrocardiographic abnormalities were noted, including ST-segment elevation in 2 or more contiguous leads (54%), widespread T-wave inversions (27%), ST depression (18%), and pathologic Q waves (18%) (Fig. 11-3). A clear-cut viral illness had been present in 54% of these patients. Electrocardiographic abnormalities were typically observed in the anterior precordial leads in this series; other reports confirmed abnormalities in the inferior and lateral distributions.[58-60] Left ventricular function was normal in 55% of patients at presentation and globally decreased in the remaining patients. Ejection fraction ranged from 17% to 45%. Diffuse, rather than segmental, wall motion abnormalities were present in this series. Ventricular function remained normal in all patients who presented with normal contractility; left ventricular ejection fraction normalized in 4 of the 5 patients in whom it was impaired at presentation. All patients who required transient intra-aortic balloon support survived to dismissal. One death due to progressive heart failure occurred 18 months after presentation in the only patient in the series with giant cell myocarditis on biopsy. Thus, acute myocarditis that mimics myocardial infarction is generally associated with an excellent long-term prognosis. The electrocardiographic abnormalities, including pathologic Q waves, typically resolved during the first 12 months. Likewise, reversible impairment in ventricular contractile function was evident within 3 to 6 months. Ischemic chest pain did not recur in any patient.

Clinicians should consider acute myocarditis in patients who present with ischemic chest pain syndromes when electrocardiographic abnormalities extend beyond a single vascular distribution, segmental wall motion abnormalities are lacking on echocardiography or left ventriculography in the distribution of myocardial injury, or global left ventricular hypokinesis is noted. The subsequent demonstration of normal coronary anatomy should prompt consideration of this diagnosis. Although histologic confirmation by endomyo-cardial biopsy is of theoretical interest, it is seldom clinically indicated because spontaneous improvement in electrocardiographic and ventriculographic abnormalities is quite likely. Biopsy should be considered for individuals who do not demonstrate a typical clinical course of recovery to exclude the possibility of giant cell myocarditis, which has a substantially poorer prognosis.[62-64]

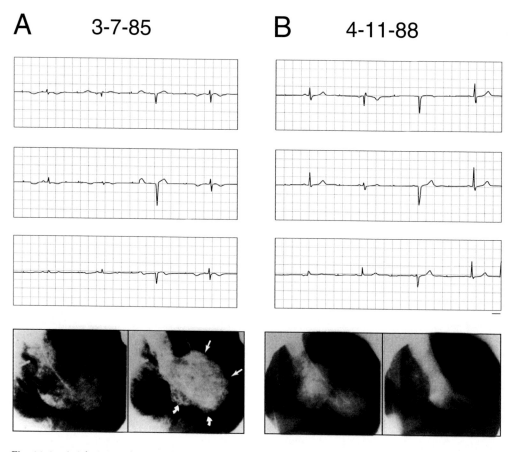

Fig. 11-3. *A,* Admission electrocardiogram (ECG) and left anterior oblique ventriculogram of a patient with biopsy-proven lymphocytic myocarditis. The ECG shows QS waves in leads V_1 and V_2 with diffuse T-wave inversions. End-diastolic (*Bottom left*) and end-systolic (*Bottom right*) frames of the ventriculogram demonstrate anteroapical and lateral akinesis (*top arrows*) and marked inferior hypokinesis (*bottom arrows*). The overall left ventricular ejection fraction was calculated at 34%. *B,* At 3-year follow-up, the ECG shows improvement in R-wave progression and resolution of the repolarization abnormalities. End-diastolic (*Bottom left*) and end-systolic (*Bottom right*) frames of the left ventriculogram demonstrate normal contractile function and an ejection fraction of 62%. Repeat right ventricular biopsy revealed healed myocarditis. (From Dec et al.[62] By permission of the American College of Cardiology.)

SUDDEN CARDIAC DEATH AND VENTRICULAR ARRHYTHMIAS

Myocarditis is a significant cause of sudden, unexpected death in adults younger than age 40 years and elite young athletes.[65,66] In these presumably healthy individuals, autopsy findings have revealed myocarditis in up to 20% of cases.[65,66] The diagnosis is now often made before death through the routine use of endomyocardial biopsy. Although heart failure, cardiomyopathy, and myocardial mimicry are more common clinical presentations, patients with myocarditis can also occasionally present with syncope or sudden cardiac death.

Several series have examined the frequency of myocarditis among patients evaluated for life-threatening ventricular arrhythmias that occurred in the absence of structural heart disease.[64,67-69] These patients tended to be young (younger than 50 years) and to have normal or near-normal left ventricular systolic function. The frequency of syncope or cardiac arrest as reported has ranged from 8% to 61%.[68,69] Biopsy evidence of myocarditis among patients without structural heart disease has ranged from 8% to 50% (Table 11-9). At our institution, granulomatous myocarditis has been associated more frequently with life-threatening ventricular arrhythmias, syncope, and high-grade atrioventricular block requiring temporary or permanent ventricular pacing than has lymphocytic myocarditis.[64]

Management of patients with ventricular arrhythmias due to lymphocytic or granulomatous myocarditis remains problematic. Electrophysiologic testing fails to provoke inducible monomorphic ventricular tachycardia or ventricular fibrillation in more than two-thirds of patients who undergo testing.[21,67,68] Many investigators use short-term immunosuppressive therapy to decrease myocardial inflammation and injury and to control ventricular tachyarrhythmias. Friedman et al.[70] reported persistent complex ventricular arrhythmias after apparent resolution of myocarditis in children and young adults. Patients with life-threatening arrhythmias generally require long-term antiarrhythmic therapy. For those with out-of-hospital cardiac arrest, an implantable defibrillator is often preferable to pharmacologic treatment. Patients with histologically documented granulomatous myocarditis and those with cardiac sarcoidosis are at particularly high risk for life-threatening

Table 11-9
Incidence of Biopsy-Proven Myocarditis in Patients
Presenting With Ventricular Arrhythmias

Series	Year	Patients, no.	Sudden death/ syncope, %	Myocarditis, %
Strain et al.[69]	1983	18	61	17
Sugrue et al.[68]	1984	12	8	8
Vignola et al.[67]	1984	12	33	50
Hosenpud et al.[29]	1986	12	33	33

ventricular tachyarrhythmias.[64,71,72] Control studies have not evaluated the success of immunosuppressive strategies, pharmacologic antiarrhythmic suppression, or implantable cardioverter-defibrillator treatment. Nonetheless, many clinicians recommend placement of an implantable cardioverter-defibrillator in such high-risk individuals.

DIAGNOSIS OF ACUTE MYOCARDITIS

CLINICAL FEATURES AND ENDOMYOCARDIAL BIOPSY

Myocarditis may be diagnosed with a moderate degree of certainty when a constellation of clinical features is present: a preceding viral illness, acute onset of symptoms, fever, pericardial inflammation, supportive laboratory abnormalities (increased erythrocyte sedimentation rate, leukocytosis, increased concentration of creatine kinase), and electrocardiographic abnormalities. As previously discussed, however, fewer than 10% of patients present with 2 or more of these supportive clinical features. Further, endomyocardial biopsy, while serving as the most appropriate way to confirm the clinically suspected diagnosis, also has substantial problems as a diagnostic tool. It is invasive, costly, and samples only a tiny portion of the myocardium. Given the focal or multifocal nature of myocarditis, it is not surprising that substantial sampling error exists. Clinicians are increasingly reluctant to recommend routine endomyocardial biopsy, even when myocarditis is clinically strongly suspected.

A noninvasive technique that possesses high sensitivity and specificity has been sought to identify those patients in whom right ventricular biopsy has a high probability of yielding a histologic diagnosis of myocarditis. Creatine kinase or its isoform is not useful as a noninvasive screening method because of low predictive value.[27,49] Recently, cardiac troponin T has been shown in a moderate-sized single center study to be useful in establishing the diagnosis. Lauer et al.[48] reported an increased serum concentration of troponin T (> 0.1 ng/mL) was associated with a sensitivity for detecting myocarditis (histologically verified by Dallas criteria, by immunohistochemical techniques, or both) of 53%; its specificity was 94%; its positive predictive value, 93%; and the negative predictive value, 56%. Additional confirmatory studies are necessary to verify the utility of this simple serologic method.

NUCLEAR IMAGING TECHNIQUES

Gallium-67 cardiac scintigraphic imaging has been used to evaluate conditions that result in myocardial inflammation. It is currently seldom performed at most centers. However, at centers with extensive experience in the technique, gallium-67 imaging has been reported to be useful as a screening tool and in predicting response to treatment.[37,73] O'Connell et al.,[73] who studied this methodology most extensively, reported a sensitivity of 36% and a specificity of 98% for histologic detection of myocarditis.

Indium-labeled monoclonal antibody fragments of antimyosin antibodies (directed against heavy chain myosin) bind to cardiac myocytes that have lost the integrity of their sarcolemma membranes and have exposed intracellular myosin to the extracellular fluid space.[74] Unlike gallium-67, which detects extent of myocardial *inflammation*, antimyosin uptake reflects the extent of myocyte *necrosis*. Because both elements are present in myocarditis, the 2 imaging modalities should provide similar or complementary information. Unfortunately, no studies have been performed that directly examine the utility of these radionuclide techniques when combined or when compared with one another. Nonetheless, published sensitivities and specificities suggest that antimyosin has a higher negative predictive value than gallium-67 scintigraphy.

Dec et al.[75] studied the utility of antimyosin imaging in 82 patients with clinically suspected myocarditis. Symptoms at presentation included congestive heart failure and cardiomyopathy (92%), chest pain mimicking myocardial infarction (6%), and life-threatening ventricular tachyarrhythmias (2%). All patients underwent planar and single photon emission computed tomographic cardiac imaging 48 hours after injection of indium-111–labeled antimyosin antibody fragments (Fig. 11-4). Right ventricular biopsy was performed within 48 hours after imaging. On the basis of right ventricular histologic

Anterior

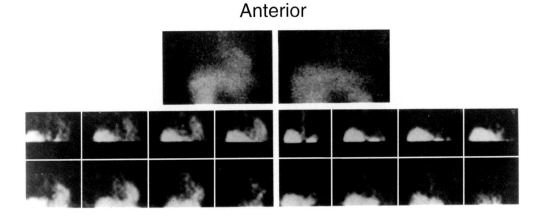

Fig. 11-4. A positive antimyosin image demonstrates diffuse tracer uptake in the cardiac region on both the anterior planar image (*Upper left*) and in all coronal tomographic reconstructions (*Bottom left*). Biopsy showed multifocal lymphocytic myocarditis. Antimyosin imaging was repeated after 6 months of immunosuppressive therapy. Biopsy showed healed myocarditis. No antimyosin uptake is visible on either the planar (*Top right*) or tomographic reconstructions (*Bottom right*). (From Dec and Narula.[76] By permission of Edizioni Minerva Medica.)

features, antimyosin was highly sensitive but moderately specific for detecting myocardial necrosis (Table 11-10).[75] The sensitivity was 83%; specificity, 53%; and predictive value of a negative scan, 92%.

Perhaps more important than the correlation between cardiac antimyosin uptake and histologic findings, improvement in left ventricular function within 6 months of treatment occurred in 54% of patients with a positive antimyosin scan but in only 18% of those with a negative scan.[75] Because spontaneous improvement in ventricular function is a well-recognized feature of acute lymphocytic myocarditis, it is suspected that several patients who were scan-positive but biopsy-negative may have, in fact, had myocarditis.[27,76] A small cohort of patients who had a negative initial antimyosin scan returned 6 to 12 months later for a second study. All showed no evidence for antimyosin uptake.[75] Repeat antimyosin imaging among 17 patients whose initial scan was positive showed persistent uptake in 9 individuals and resolution of uptake in the remaining 8 patients. No correlation could be found between ongoing myocarditis on repeat biopsy and clinical improvement.[75]

Narula et al.[61] also evaluated the role of antimyosin imaging among patients who presented with chest pain mimicking acute myocardial infarction despite normal coronary anatomy. Antimyosin uptake was global in 7 of the 8 patients with confirmed myocarditis on biopsy and equivocal in the 8th patient. Antimyosin uptake was segmental in patients with acute myocardial infarction and almost always confined to the territory of the infarct-related vessel. Thus, antimyosin uptake may be useful in differentiating unstable coronary syndromes from myocarditis.

The low specificity of cardiac antimyosin uptake results from its exquisite affinity with necrotic myocytes. Antimyosin uptake has been reported in systemic diseases that affect the heart such as Lyme disease.[77] Positive uptake has also been reported in heart transplant rejection,[78] anthracycline-induced cardiomyopathy,[79] and alcohol-related cardiomyopathy.[80] Its high sensitivity and modest specificity suggest that antimyosin scintigraphy may be useful as an initial screening tool to determine which patients should undergo biopsy. Unfortunately, this imaging agent is not currently available commercially and is restricted to research.

MAGNETIC RESONANCE IMAGING

Prior studies that demonstrated the reliability of magnetic resonance imaging (MRI) in tissue characterization of cardiac allograft rejection suggested that this technique might be useful in diagnosing acute myocarditis, which has similar histologic findings. Cardiac MRI has been shown to be effective in detecting myocardial edema. A preliminary study by Chandraratna et al.[81] detected localized myocardial edema in regions of hypokinesis or akinesis on echocardiography in 2 patients with clinically diagnosed myocarditis. After improvement in ventricular function, repeat MRI demonstrated resolution of myocardial edema.[81]

Gagliardi et al.[82] evaluated MRI and endomyocardial biopsy results in 11 consecutive children (age, 9 months to 9 years) with clinically suspected myocarditis. Tissue characterization was obtained in regions of interest of the right and left ventricles by using T1 and T2 spin-echo sequences. The myocardial/skeletal muscle signal intensity ratio was able to accurately identify all patients with histologically confirmed myocarditis (Table 11-10). While encouraging, these results were obtained in a small number of patients. Further, myocarditis in children is often associated with more prominent interstitial edema than that observed in adults. Additional MRI studies in adults are needed.

Contrast-enhanced MRI has also been evaluated.[84] Nineteen patients with clinically suspected myocarditis and the combination of electrocardiographic abnormalities, impaired left ventricular function, increased creatine kinase concentration, positive troponin T values, and positive results of antimyosin cardiac scintigraphy underwent sequential contrast-enhanced MRI. Electrocardiographic-triggered, T1-weighted images were obtained before and after administration of 0.1 mmol/kg of gadolinium. Global relative signal enhancement of the left ventricular myocardium relative to skeletal muscle was obtained and compared with measurements obtained in 18 volunteers. Global left ventricular enhancement was substantially higher in the myocarditis patients than in controls on days 2, 7, 14, and 28 after onset of acute symptoms. Although enhancement was generally focal during the initial studies, global enhancement was noted during the later times. Histologic verification of myocarditis was not obtained in any of these published studies. More importantly, the ability of this technique to differentiate viral myocarditis from other causes of acute dilated cardiomyopathy was not investigated. If additional studies confirm these findings, longitudinal follow-up of the same patient will become possible and will allow reexamination for recurrent disease or persistent myocarditis.

Table 11-10
Sensitivity, Specificity, and Predictive Value of Noninvasive Techniques for Diagnosing Myocarditis

Technique	No.	Sen, %	Spec, %	+PV, %	-PV, %	Author	Year
Troponin T	80	53	96	93	56	Lauer et al.[48]	1997
Gallium-67	71	87	86	36	98	O'Connell et al.[73]	1984
Antimyosin	82	83	53	33	92	Dec et al.[75]	1990
MRI	11	100	100	100	100	Gagliardi et al.[82]	1991
Echo	106	100	91	---	---	Leiback et al.[83]	1996

Echo, echocardiographic tissue characterization; MRI, magnetic resonance imaging; +PV, positive predictive value; -PV, negative predictive value; sen, sensitivity; spec, specificity.

ECHOCARDIOGRAPHIC TISSUE CHARACTERIZATION

Similar to MRI, echocardiography may provide precise visualization of tissue characterization and has been reported to be useful in establishing the diagnosis of myocarditis. Tissue characterization seeks to define the nature of the tissue from changes that occur in sound waves during their physical interaction with the myocardium. Quantitative approaches have used backscatter to define tissue characteristics. Backscatter is generally measured as the reflected ultrasound power at each frequency over the bandwidth of the transducer. Backscatter, like attenuation, characteristically increases with frequency. Significant increases in backscatter were described for rabbit myocardium exposed to doxorubicin.[85] Longitudinal studies of Syrian hamster cardiomyopathy revealed increasing values of backscatter as myocardial fibrosis progresses.[86] Leiback et al.[83] compared backscatter measurements among patients with persistent ($n = 12$), healed ($n = 9$), or healed myocarditis with fibrosis ($n = 17$) to measurements obtained in 35 cases of chronic dilated cardiomyopathy and 8 normal controls. Mean gray scale values were substantially higher in patients with cardiomyopathy than in normal controls. Sensitivity was 100% and specificity, 91% (Table 11-8). However, this technique was unable to differentiate myocarditis patients from those with other causes of cardiomyopathy.

CONCLUSION

Myocarditis has a wide variety of clinical presentations for the clinician to ponder. Although most cases are associated with viral pericarditis and are self-limited, the spectrum of abnormalities may include chest pain mimicking myocardial infarction, unexplained ventricular tachyarrhythmias, acute or chronic dilated cardiomyopathy, and cardiogenic shock. Awareness is necessary because characteristic clinical features (pleuritic chest pain or pericardial rub; fever; increased sedimentation rate or concentration of creatine kinase or troponin I) are lacking in the majority of patients with biopsy-proven disease. Noninvasive imaging modalities, including antimyosin cardiac scintigraphy, echocardiographic tissue characterization, and MRI, all possess sufficient sensitivity and specificity to serve as initial screening tools. Endomyocardial biopsy remains the procedure of choice for unequivocally establishing the diagnosis. It is especially useful in differentiating lymphocytic myocarditis with its more favorable prognosis from giant cell myocarditis. Clinical trials of immunosuppressive therapy or immunomodulatory therapy have failed to demonstrate a beneficial effect in this disorder. Spontaneous improvement may occur in more than 30% of patients with lymphocytic disease but is rarely, if ever, observed with granulomatous myocarditis. Effective forms of treatment are urgently needed because the 5-year mortality in patients with dilated cardiomyopathy due to myocarditis exceeds 50%. Better understanding of the cellular and immunologic abnormalities that characterize the disease process and more complete understanding of the natural history of the various subtypes of myocarditis (acute lymphocytic, fulminant, borderline) should help clinicians plan more effective therapy in the future.

REFERENCES

1. Sobernheim JF. Diagnostik der inneren Krunkheitenmit vorzuegeleicher Ruechsicht auf patholo-gische. Anatomie. Berlin: Hirschwald, 1837:1-43.
2. Feidler A. Ueber akute intestielle Myokarditis. In: Festschift des Standtkrankenhauses. Dresden: Friedrichstadt, 1899:1-10.
3. Saphir O. Myocarditis: a general review, with an analysis of two hundred and forty cases. Arch Pathol 1941;32:1000-1051; 1942;33:88-137.
4. Burch G, Ray T. Myocarditis and myocardial degeneration. Bull Tulane Med Faculty 1948;8:1-3.
5. Reyes MP, Lerner AM. Coxsackievirus myocarditis—with special reference to acute and chronic effects. Prog Cardiovasc Dis 1985;27:373-394.
6. Grist NR, Bell EJ. Coxsackie viruses and the heart (editorial). Am Heart J 1969;77:295-300.
7. Blanchard DG, Hagenhoff C, Chow LC, McCann HA, Dittrich HC. Reversibility of cardiac abnormalities in human immunodeficiency virus (HIV)-infected individuals: a serial echocardio-graphic study. J Am Coll Cardiol 1991;17:1270-1276.
8. Mason JW, Billingham ME, Ricci DR. Treatment of acute inflammatory myocarditis assisted by endomyocardial biopsy. Am J Cardiol 1980;45:1037-1044.
9. Edwards WD, Holmes DR Jr, Reeder GS. Diagnosis of active lymphocytic myocarditis by endomyo-cardial biopsy: quantitative criteria for light microscopy. Mayo Clin Proc 1982;57:419-425.
10. Tazelaar HD, Billingham ME. Leukocytic infiltrates in idiopathic dilated cardiomyopathy. A source of confusion with active myocarditis. Am J Surg Pathol 1986;10:405-412.
11. Aretz HT, Billingham ME, Edwards WD, Factor SM, Fallon JT, Fenoglio JJ Jr, Olsen EG, Schoen FJ. Myocarditis. A histopathologic definition and classification. Am J Cardiovasc Pathol 1987;1:3-14.
12. Lieberman EB, Hutchins GM, Herskowitz A, Rose NR, Baughman KL. Clinicopathologic descrip-tion of myocarditis. J Am Coll Cardiol 1991;18:1617-1626.
13. Waller BF, Slack JD, Orr CD, Adlam JH, Bournique VM. "Flaming," "smoldering" and "burned out": the fireside saga of myocarditis. J Am Coll Cardiol 1991;18:1627-1630.
14. Hauck AJ, Kearney DL, Edwards WD. Evaluation of postmortem endomyocardial biopsy specimens from 38 patients with lymphocytic myocarditis: implications for role of sampling error. Mayo Clin Proc 1989;64:1235-1245.
15. Chow LH, Radio SJ, Sears TD, McManus BM. Insensitivity of right ventricular endomyocardial biopsy in the diagnosis of myocarditis. J Am Coll Cardiol 1989;14:915-920.
16. Dec GW, Fallon JT, Southern JF, Palacios I. "Borderline" myocarditis: an indication for repeat endomyocardial biopsy. J Am Coll Cardiol 1990;15:283-289.
17. Kounis NG, Zavras GM, Soufras GD, Kitrou MP. Hypersensitivity myocarditis. Ann Allergy 1989;62:71-74.
18. Burke AP, Saenger J, Mullick F, Virmani R. Hypersensitivity myocarditis. Arch Pathol Lab Med 1991;115:764-769.
19. Isner JM, Chokshi SK. Cardiovascular complications of cocaine. Curr Probl Cardiol 1991;16:89-123.

20. Spear GS. Eosinophilic explant carditis with eosinophilia: ? hypersensitivity to dobutamine infusion. J Heart Lung Transplant 1995;14:755-760.

21. Galiuto L, Enriquez-Sarano M, Reeder GS, Tazelaar HD, Li JT, Miller FA Jr, Gleich GJ. Eosinophilic myocarditis manifesting as myocardial infarction: early diagnosis and successful treatment. Mayo Clin Proc 1997;72:603-610.

22. Taliercio CP, Olney BA, Lie JT. Myocarditis related to drug hypersensitivity. Mayo Clin Proc 1985;60:463-468.

23. Weinstein C, Fenoglio JJ. Myocarditis. Hum Pathol 1987;18:613-618.

24. Abelmann WH. Viral myocarditis and its sequelae. Annu Rev Med 1973;24:145-152.

25. Karjalainen J, Heikkila J. "Acute pericarditis": myocardial enzyme release as evidence for myocarditis. Am Heart J 1986;111:546-552.

26. Marboe CC, Fenoglio JJ Jr. Pathology and natural history of human myocarditis. Pathol Immunopathol Res 1988;7:226-239.

27. Dec GW Jr, Palacios IF, Fallon JT, Aretz HT, Mills J, Lee DC-S, Johnson RA. Active myocarditis in the spectrum of acute dilated cardiomyopathies. Clinical features, histologic correlates, and clinical outcome. N Engl J Med 1985;312:885-890.

28. Narula J, Khaw BA, Dec GW Jr, Palacios IF, Southern JF, Fallon JT, Strauss HW, Haber E, Yasuda T. Recognition of acute myocarditis masquerading as acute myocardial infarction. N Engl J Med 1993;328:100-104.

29. Hosenpud JD, McAnulty JH, Niles NR. Unexpected myocardial disease in patients with life threatening arrhythmias. Br Heart J 1986;56:55-61.

30. Daly K, Richardson PJ, Olsen EG, Morgan-Capner P, McSorley C, Jackson G, Jewitt DE. Acute myocarditis. Role of histological and virological examination in the diagnosis and assessment of immunosuppressive treatment. Br Heart J 1984;51:30-35.

31. Fowler NO, Manitsas GT. Infectious pericarditis. Prog Cardiovasc Dis 1973;16:323-336.

32. Parrillo JE, Aretz HT, Palacios I, Fallon JT, Block PC. The results of transvenous endomyocardial biopsy can frequently be used to diagnose myocardial diseases in patients with idiopathic heart failure. Endomyocardial biopsies in 100 consecutive patients revealed a substantial incidence of myocarditis. Circulation 1984;69:93-101.

33. Zee-Cheng CS, Tsai CC, Palmer DC, Codd JE, Pennington DG, Williams GA. High incidence of myocarditis by endomyocardial biopsy in patients with idiopathic congestive cardiomyopathy. J Am Coll Cardiol 1984;3:63-70.

34. Kunkel B, Lapp G, Kober G, et al. Light microscopic evaluation of myocardial biopsies. In: Kaltenbach M, Loogen F, Olsen EGJ, eds. Cardiomyopathy and myocardial biopsy. Berlin: Springer-Verlag, 1978:62-70.

35. Noda S. Histopathology of endomyocardial biopsies from patients with idiopathic cardiomyopathy; quantitative evaluation based on multivariate statistical analysis. Jpn Circ J 1980;44:95-116.

36. Baandrup U, Florio RA, Rehahn M, Richardson PJ, Olsen EGJ. Critical analysis of endomyocardial biopsies from patients suspected of having cardiomyopathy. II. Comparison of histology and clinical/haemodynamic information. Br Heart J 1981;45:487-493.

37. O'Connell JB, Robinson JA, Henkin RE, Gunnar RM. Immunosuppressive therapy in patients with congestive cardiomyopathy and myocardial uptake of gallium-67. Circulation 1981;64:780-786.

38. Nippoldt TB, Edwards WD, Holmes DR Jr, Reeder GS, Hartzler GO, Smith HC. Right ventricular endomyocardial biopsy: clinicopathologic correlates in 100 consecutive patients. Mayo Clin Proc 1982;57:407-418.

39. Fenoglio JJ Jr, Ursell PC, Kellogg CF, Drusin RE, Weiss MB. Diagnosis and classification of myocarditis by endomyocardial biopsy. N Engl J Med 1983;308:12-18.

40. Unverferth DV, Fetters JK, Unverferth BJ, Leier CV, Magorien RD, Arn AR, Baker PB. Human myocardial histologic characteristics in congestive heart failure. Circulation 1983;68:1194-1200.

41. Bolte HD, Ludwig B. Viral myocarditis: symptomatology, clinical diagnosis, and hemodynamics. In: Bolte H-D, ed. Viral heart disease. Berlin: Springer-Verlag, 1984:177-187.

42. Mason JW, O'Connell JB, Herskowitz A, Rose NR, McManus BM, Billingham ME, Moon TE, the Myocarditis Treatment Trial Investigators. A clinical trial of immunosuppressive therapy for myocarditis. N Engl J Med 1995;333:269-275.

43. Grogan M, Redfield MM, Bailey KR, Reeder GS, Gersh BJ, Edwards WD, Rodeheffer RJ. Long-term outcome of patients with biopsy-proved myocarditis: comparison with idiopathic dilated cardiomyopathy. J Am Coll Cardiol 1995;26:80-84.

44. Chow LC, Dittrich HC, Shabetai R. Endomyocardial biopsy in patients with unexplained congestive heart failure. Ann Intern Med 1988;109:535-539.

45. Smith WG. Coxsackie B myopericarditis in adults. Am Heart J 1970;80:34-46.

46. Sainani GS, Krompotic E, Slodki SJ. Adult heart disease due to the Coxsackie virus B infection. Medicine (Baltimore) 1968;47:133-147.

47. Gardiner AJ, Short D. Four faces of acute myopericarditis. Br Heart J 1973;35:433-442.

48. Lauer B, Niederau C, Kühl U, Schannwell M, Pauschinger M, Strauer B-E, Schultheiss H-P. Cardiac troponin T in patients with clinically suspected myocarditis. J Am Coll Cardiol 1997;30:1354-1359.

49. Smith SC, Ladenson JH, Mason JW, Jaffe AS. Elevations of cardiac troponin I associated with myocarditis: experimental and clinical correlates. Circulation 1997;95:163-168.

50. Narula J, Khaw BA, Dec GW, Palacios IF, Newell JB, Southern JF, Fallon JT, Strauss HW, Haber E, Yasuda T. Diagnostic accuracy of antimyosin scintigraphy in suspected myocarditis. J Nucl Cardiol 1996;3:371-381.

51. McCarthy RE III, Boehmer JP, Hruban RH, Hutchins GM, Kasper EK, Hare JM, Baughman KL. Long-term outcome of fulminant myocarditis as compared with acute (nonfulminant) myocarditis. N Engl J Med 2000;342:690-695.

52. Kesler KA, Pruitt AL, Turrentine MW, Heimansohn DA, Brown JW. Temporary left-sided mechanical cardiac support during acute myocarditis. J Heart Lung Transplant 1994;13:268-270.

53. Jett GK, Miller A, Savino D, Gonwa T. Reversal of acute fulminant lymphocytic myocarditis with combined technology of OKT3 monoclonal antibody and mechanical circulatory support. J Heart Lung Transplant 1992;11:733-738.

54. Rockman HA, Adamson RM, Dembitsky WP, Bonar JW, Jaski BE. Acute fulminant myocarditis: long-term follow-up after circulatory support with left ventricular assist device. Am Heart J 1991;121:922-926.

55. Dec GW Jr, Fallon JT, Southern JF, Palacios IF. Relation between histological findings on early repeat right ventricular biopsy and ventricular function in patients with myocarditis. Br Heart J 1988;60:332-337.

56. Jones SR, Herskowitz A, Hutchins GM, Baughman KL. Effects of immunosuppressive therapy in biopsy-proved myocarditis and borderline myocarditis on left ventricular function. Am J Cardiol 1991;68:370-376.

57. Saffitz JE, Schwartz DJ, Southworth W, Murphree S, Rodriguez ER, Ferrans VJ, Roberts WC. Coxsackie viral myocarditis causing transmural right and left ventricular infarction without coronary narrowing. Am J Cardiol 1983;52:644, 646-647.

58. Miklozek CL, Crumpacker CS, Royal HD, Come PC, Sullivan JL, Abelmann WH. Myocarditis presenting as acute myocardial infarction. Am Heart J 1988;115:768-776.

59. Costanzo-Nordin MR, O'Connell JB, Subramanian R, Robinson JA, Scanlon PJ. Myocarditis confirmed by biopsy presenting as acute myocardial infarction. Br Heart J 1985;53:25-29.

60. Desa'Neto A, Bullington JD, Bullington RH, Desser KB, Benchimol A. Coxsackie B5 heart disease. Demonstration of inferolateral wall myocardial necrosis. Am J Med 1980;68:295-298.

61. Narula J, Southern JF, Abraham S, Pieri P, Khaw BA. Myocarditis simulating myocardial infarction. J Nucl Med 1991;32:312-318.

62. Dec GW Jr, Waldman H, Southern J, Fallon JT, Hutter AM Jr, Palacios I. Viral myocarditis mimicking acute myocardial infarction. J Am Coll Cardiol 1992;20:85-89.

63. Cooper LT Jr, Berry GJ, Shabetai R, Multicenter Giant Cell Myocarditis Study Group Investigators. Idiopathic giant-cell myocarditis—natural history and treatment. N Engl J Med 1997;336:1860-1866.

64. Davidoff R, Palacios I, Southern J, Fallon JT, Newell J, Dec GW. Giant cell versus lymphocytic myocarditis. A comparison of their clinical features and long-term outcomes. Circulation 1991;83:953-961.

65. Drory Y, Turetz Y, Hiss Y, Lev B, Fisman EZ, Pines A, Kramer MR. Sudden unexpected death in persons less than 40 years of age. Am J Cardiol 1991;68:1388-1392.

66. Wesslen L, Pahlson C, Lindquist O, Hjelm E, Gnarpe J, Larsson E, Baandrup U, Eriksson L, Fohlman J, Engstrand L, Linglof T, Nystrom-Rosander C, Gnarpe H, Magnius L, Rolf C, Friman G. An increase in sudden unexpected cardiac deaths among young Swedish orienteers during 1979-1992. Eur Heart J 1996;17:902-910.

67. Vignola PA, Aonuma K, Swaye PS, Rozanski JJ, Blankstein RL, Benson J, Gosselin AJ, Lister JW. Lymphocytic myocarditis presenting as unexplained ventricular arrhythmias: diagnosis with endomyocardial biopsy and response to immunosuppression. J Am Coll Cardiol 1984;4:812-819.

68. Sugrue DD, Holmes DR Jr, Gersh BJ, Edwards WD, McLaran CJ, Wood DL, Osborn MJ, Hammill SC. Cardiac histologic findings in patients with life-threatening ventricular arrhythmias of unknown origin. J Am Coll Cardiol 1984;4:952-957.

69. Strain JE, Grose RM, Factor SM, Fisher JD. Results of endomyocardial biopsy in patients with spontaneous ventricular tachycardia but without apparent structural heart disease. Circulation 1983;68:1171-1181.

70. Friedman RA, Kearney DL, Moak JP, Fenrich AL, Perry JC. Persistence of ventricular arrhythmia after resolution of occult myocarditis in children and young adults. J Am Coll Cardiol 1994;24:780-783.

71. Sekiguchi M, Yazaki Y, Isobe M, Hiroe M. Cardiac sarcoidosis: diagnostic, prognostic, and therapeutic considerations. Cardiovasc Drugs Ther 1996;10:495-510.

72. Fleming HA, Bailey SM. Sarcoid heart disease. J R Coll Physicians Lond 1981;15:245-253.

73. O'Connell JB, Henkin RE, Robinson JA, Subramanian R, Scanlon PJ, Gunnar RM. Gallium-67 imaging in patients with dilated cardiomyopathy and biopsy-proven myocarditis. Circulation 1984;70:58-62.

74. Khaw BA, Beller GA, Haber E, Smith TW. Localization of cardiac myosin-specific antibody in myocardial infarction. J Clin Invest 1976;58:439-446.

75. Dec GW, Palacios I, Yasuda T, Fallon JT, Khaw BA, Strauss HW, Haber E. Antimyosin antibody cardiac imaging: its role in the diagnosis of myocarditis. J Am Coll Cardiol 1990;16:97-104.

76. Dec GW, Narula J. Antimyosin imaging for noninvasive recognition of myocarditis. Q J Nucl Med 1997;41 Suppl 1:128-139.

77. Casans I, Villar A, Almenar V, Blanes A. Lyme myocarditis diagnosed by indium-111-antimyosin antibody scintigraphy. Eur J Nucl Med 1989;15:330-331.

78. Ballester M, Obrador D, Carrió I, Moya C, Augè JM, Bordes R, Martí V, Bosch I, Bernà-Roqueta L, Estorch M, Pons-Lladó G, Cámara ML, Padró JM, Arís A, Caralps-Riera JM. Early postoperative reduction of monoclonal antimyosin antibody uptake is associated with absent rejection-related complications after heart transplantation. Circulation 1992;85:61-68.

79. Carrio I, Lopez-Pousa A, Estorch M, Duncker D, Berna L, Torres G, de Andres L. Detection of doxorubicin cardiotoxicity in patients with sarcomas by indium-111-antimyosin monoclonal antibody studies. J Nucl Med 1993;34:1503-1507.

80. Ballester M, Marti V, Carrio I, Obrador D, Moya C, Pons-Llado G, Berna L, Lamich R, Aymat MR, Barbanoj M, Guardia J, Carreras F, Udina C, Auge JM, Marrugat J, Permanyer G, Caralps-Riera JM. Spectrum of alcohol-induced myocardial damage detected by indium-111-labeled monoclonal antimyosin antibodies. J Am Coll Cardiol 1997;29:160-167.

81. Chandraratna PA, Bradley WG, Kortman KE, Minagoe S, Delvicario M, Rahimtoola SH. Detection of acute myocarditis using nuclear magnetic resonance imaging. Am J Med 1987;83:1144-1146.

82. Gagliardi MG, Bevilacqua M, Di Renzi P, Picardo S, Passariello R, Marcelletti C. Usefulness of magnetic resonance imaging for diagnosis of acute myocarditis in infants and children, and comparison with endomyocardial biopsy. Am J Cardiol 1991;68:1089-1091.

83. Leiback E, Hardouin I, Meyer R, Bellach J, Hetzer R. Clinical value of echocardiographic tissue characterization in the diagnosis of myocarditis. Eur Heart J 1996;17:135-142.

84. Friedrich MG, Strohm O, Schulz-Menger J, Marciniak H, Luft FC, Dietz R. Contrast media-enhanced magnetic resonance imaging visualizes myocardial changes in the course of viral myocarditis. Circulation 1998;97:1802-1809.

85. Mimbs JW, O'Donnell M, Miller JG, Sobel BE. Detection of cardiomyopathic changes induced by doxorubicin based on quantitative analysis of ultrasonic backscatter. Am J Cardiol 1981;47:1056-1060.

86. Perez JE, Barzilai B, Madaras EI, Glueck RM, Saffitz JE, Johnston P, Miller JG, Sobel BE. Applicability of ultrasonic tissue characterization for longitudinal assessment and differentiation of calcification and fibrosis in cardiomyopathy. J Am Coll Cardiol 1984;4:88-95.

Use of Cardiac Biomarkers for Detection of Myocarditis

Allan S. Jaffe, M.D.

BLOOD MARKERS OF CARDIAC INJURY

USE OF LYMPHOCYTIC IMMUNOHISTOCHEMISTRY

ANTIBODY CONCENTRATIONS

BLOOD MARKERS OF CARDIAC INJURY

Cardiac biomarkers, particularly of the older variety, have rarely assisted in the diagnosis of myocarditis[1] except for patients who present acutely.[2] In that setting, increased concentrations of creatine kinase MB (CK-MB) have been observed. Myocarditis may be confused with acute myocardial infarction because the constellation of symptoms, abnormal electrocardiograms, and increased marker protein concentrations is similar to what is seen with acute infarction. The correct diagnosis often is delineated only by demonstration of normal coronary arteries and subsequent biopsy findings.

In the more chronic setting, increased concentrations of CK-MB are unusual. In the Myocarditis Treatment Trial, mean CK-MB values were not significantly greater in patients with myocarditis than in control patients and only 5% of patients had increases.[1] The reasons for this are unclear but likely relate to 1 or several of the following.

1) **The lack of sensitivity of CK-MB**

Only 15% of the CK-MB that is depleted from the heart finds its way into the blood when ischemic heart disease is the cause of the release. Thus, the so-called release ratio for CK-MB is low. In experimental models of 2 hours of occlusion and reperfusion, this ratio doubles to 30% because release is flow limited.[3] This may be the case with myocarditis in which coronary perfusion may be normal or at least reduced to a lesser extent than with coronary occlusion. Troponin measurements are more sensitive.[4]

2) **The time window during which increased concentrations of CK-MB occur after cardiac injury is constrained**[5]

Increases usually occur early after the onset of cardiac injury (4-6 hours) and are gone within 48 to 72 hours. Thus, transitory severe injury can be missed by late presentation and the more subtle changes, because of the lack of sensitivity.

3) **Lack of specificity**

It may well be that some increases of CK-MB do occur but are ignored because of a lack of specificity of CK-MB for the heart, especially in complex medical situations.[6]

4) **Degradation in lymph**

Much of the CK and CK-MB that is released when myocytes are injured is degraded in lymph.[7] This is one of the reasons why the so-called release ratio (see above) is so low. Accordingly, a lymphocytic infiltrate associated with myocarditis might still further degrade CK-MB, further reducing its sensitivity.

The situation with troponin markers is substantially different for multiple reasons.

1) **Troponin markers are more sensitive than CK-MB**[4]

In comparative studies with troponin measurements, it is clear that the sensitivity for detection of an abnormality and the increment of change in response to a given injury are far less for CK-MB than for the troponin markers.[4,8] Some of this may be because there are constitutive levels of CK-MB in blood that are presumably from skeletal muscle that must be overcome before an abnormality can be detected. However, the cytosolic pool of CK-MB and the early releasable pool (mostly localized to the cytosol) of troponin are roughly comparable in magnitude.[8,9] The remainder of the troponin is complexed to the contractile apparatus. Overall, there is 13-fold more cardiac troponin I (cTnI)[8] and 15-fold more cardiac troponin T (cTnT) than CK-MB per gram of myocardium.[9] Furthermore, the release ratio appears to be high, approaching 100%.[10] Thus, not only are more instances of cardiac injury detected with troponin measurements but the increment of change in them is substantially greater.

2) **The time during which troponin values are increased is substantially greater**

Troponin markers frequently are increased for 10 to 14 days, depending on the specific circumstance of the cardiac injury and the assay used.[5] This is because in addition to having an early releasable pool comparable in size to the pool for CK-MB, these markers are complexed in large abundance to the contractile apparatus.[8,9] Thus, they are released early (4-6 hours) in a time course similar to that of CK-MB but also continue to be released over time from this huge complexed pool of protein as the damaged area is remodeled. Thus, the time during which cardiac injury can be detected is substantially prolonged. This allows the troponin measurements to be used similarly to lactate dehydrogenase isoenzymes for the retrospective diagnosis of acute myocardial infarction and prolongs the time during which increases can be detected.[5]

3) **Increased specificity**

Troponin markers have nearly perfect specificity for the heart. Thus, even minor increases indicate cardiac involvement.[11,12]

4) **Degradation in myocardium**

Finally, although degradation of troponin does occur, it may be (author's speculation) less extensive than with CK-MB. Such degradation also occurs at the carboxy and amino terminal ends of the molecules,[13] so that assays that use monoclonal antibodies to the central portion of the molecule are likely to be unaffected.

Nonetheless, in the Myocarditis Treatment Trial, 34% of patients had increased values of cTnI.[1] The majority of these increases were in patients whose samples were obtained within 1 month of the onset of symptoms. In the 20 early patients (within 1 month), 11 had increases compared with only 1 of 12 patients who presented later. It may well be that other increases would have been detected had the other patients been available for testing earlier or if newer more sensitive assays capable of detecting still lower values had been used. Both of these suggestions are speculative but have important potential pathophysiologic correlates.

The fact that patients who presented earlier were more likely to have increased cTnI values might be taken to suggest that the majority of damage associated with myocarditis is acute, and then subsequent damage may be due to a more indolent and thus more difficult to detect process or even "remodeling" that occurs as an acute and chronic compensation to acute cardiac injury. This speculation has potentially important therapeutic implications as well as diagnostic ones. Such an observation might fit with the impression of an improved prognosis when there is an exuberant immune response.[14] This response might lead to a greater degree of necrosis. If so, an increased troponin value could be a positive prognostic factor. Conversely, it may be that a diminished or absent immune response with less associated acute cardiac injury might mark the group most at risk for the progression of the disease. This hypothesis needs to be tested. It could be that treating patients who have troponin increases to reduce the extent of cardiac injury may require a different approach than the treatment of those with less exuberant immune responses. It may be that protocols designed to inhibit remodeling might be efficacious. In contrast, patients with a more indolent pattern in which concentrations of troponin may be low may require a totally different approach. Such a pattern might also explain why such patients are hard to diagnose biochemically because the amount of ongoing necrosis is so modest. Such a finding would also exacerbate the known difficulty with the Dallas biopsy criteria in which sampling selection can make the finding of necrosis difficult.

This synthesis suggests that troponin increases indicate irreversible injury, but this is far from proven. Experimental studies suggest that there are protein interactions that occur that could lead to the release of troponin fragments in response to reversible injury.[13] Whether this phenomenon is important pathophysiologically is unclear.

The second implication is that low levels, but ones that are above the range for normals, might be useful in this disease. The cut points used to diagnose ischemic heart disease are substantially above what we know normal values are. Thus, what has been termed this "gray area" might permit more subtle diagnoses to be made. This might be of substantial importance in those with the indolent form of myocarditis.

These speculations also have significant implications for the use of the biopsy as a diagnostic tool. It is likely that low levels of myocardial injury are difficult to detect by biopsy because of selection bias. Two experimental animal studies have documented that there is a good relationship between the histologic evidence of myocardial damage and the extent of troponin increase.[1,15] Thus, in the absence of a high-sensitivity approach (the use of abnormal values in the gray area) during a relatively indolent phase, detection of necrosis may be impossible, not only by biopsy but also by troponin measurement.

The data from Lauer and associates[16] suggest that increased troponin values should be considered a surrogate for cardiac injury. This would avoid the difficulty of selection bias as part of the cardiac biopsy. These investigators augmented the credibility of their diagnosis by looking for specific lymphocyte pools by using immunohistochemistry. They found that the cTnT value was increased in 28 of the 80 patients they found with possible myocarditis. Only 5 met biopsy criteria. However, histologic criteria using specific lymphocyte labeling revealed myocarditis in 26 of the 28 patients with increased cTnT values. They also found that 23 of the 52 patients (44%) without cTnT increases met immunohistochemical criteria. It is unclear whether including those with cTnT values in the gray area would have substantially improved sensitivity and what the cost might have been to specificity. However, at present, the use of troponin values and abnormal lymphocytes is likely adequate for the diagnosis of myocarditis. This approach will augment the diagnostic frequency of myocarditis.

The synthesis suggested is that the biopsy diagnosis of myocarditis in 6% to 10% of patients suspected of having it is a reflection of the lack of sensitivity of the Dallas criteria and specifically the criteria for necrosis.[14,16] The lymphocyte pools one might look for could vary depending on whether one is dealing with an autoimmune myocarditis, a viral etiology, a combination of both, or a better-defined entity such as giant cell myocarditis. Nonetheless, it appears likely that the difficulty with the diagnosis of myocarditis can be overcome to some extent by the use of troponin values and immunohistochemistry. With these new criteria, the diagnosis of myocarditis types is likely to increase substantially.

USE OF LYMPHOCYTIC IMMUNOHISTOCHEMISTRY

The use of lymphocytic immunohistochemistry to define abnormal lymphocytic infiltration in myocardium was developed in part because the Dallas criteria, though highly specific, lack sensitivity. This is not surprising since the reason for the development of the initial criteria was so that a consistent standard (ie, one with a high degree of specificity) could be implemented. That is why "myocyte necrosis, degeneration, or both in the absence of significant coronary artery disease *and* adjacent inflammatory infiltrate" were required for the diagnosis.[17] These criteria, however, are not sensitive enough. For example, in the Myocarditis Treatment Trial, only 10% of patients thought to have myocarditis by characteristic clinical criteria had myocarditis by biopsy criteria.[18] The reason for this is selection bias in the biopsy material because the tissue is usually obtained from only the right side of the heart, specifically from the lower septum where it is thought that the risk of perforation is minimized. Because myocarditis is a patchy process, a negative biopsy result does not exclude it. Most often, it is the lack of evidence of myocyte necrosis that makes the biopsy result negative. Thus, despite abundant and clearly abnormal lymphocytic infiltration, biopsies have to be called negative if clear evidence of necrosis is absent. False-positive biopsy results are less of a problem but can occur because inflammatory infiltrates exist in any area where there is myocardial necrosis (eg, after acute infarction).

The concept promulgated in the clinical report by Lauer et al.[16] is to use the presence of specific lymphocytes, which are usually absent in ventricular myocardium, to make the diagnosis. What Lauer and his group have in essence proposed is that a sensitive measure such as troponin be used to indicate necrosis, minimizing the problems of sampling bias. Then, the biopsy criteria require only the finding of abnormal lymphocytes. This approach might still suffer from sampling difficulties because only the right ventricle undergoes biopsy, but by eliminating the need to see histologic necrosis, it clearly enhances the frequency of the diagnosis.[16]

The substrate for the use of specific immunohistochemical pools of lymphocytes comes from many years of research starting in the 1980s. At that time, the types of lymphocytes expected to be found in normal myocardium were characterized. Subsequently, immunohistologic characterization of abnormal lymphocyte pools was reported.

The study by Linder et al.[19] originally described the number and characteristics of lymphocytes seen in normal myocardium. Fresh hearts taken at autopsy and endomyocardial biopsies were used. By use of monoclonal antibodies to T cells, B cells, and natural killer cells and of a panleukocyte marker, only small numbers of lymphocytes were found in the tissue (Table 12-1). As expected, the panleukocyte marker was the one most frequently expressed. Otherwise, there were slightly more helper T cells than others, and B cells and natural killer cells were rare. There was no correlation between the circulating lymphocyte count and the number of cells in myocardial tissue, and the number of cells defined by immunohistochemistry was similar to the number elucidated by light microscopy.

Table 12-1
Surface Marker-Positive Cells in Human Hearts*

Surface marker	Autopsy heart				RV endomyocardial biopsy specimens
	Upper RV	Mid RV	Lower RV	LVFW	
OKT-11	3.5 (1.2)	3.9 (1.2)	3.5 (1.2)	3.1 (0.9)	7.2 (2.3)
OKT-4	2.1 (0.8)	2.0 (0.8)	1.5 (0.6)	1.6 (0.5)	4.4 (0.8)
OKT-8	1.5 (0.7)	1.5 (0.7)	0.8 (0.4)	1.2 (0.6)	8.3 (2.0)
B-1	0.2 (0.1)	0.1 (0.1)	0.0	0.1 (0.0)	1.8 (1.0)
HNK-1	0.6 (0.3)	0.4 (0.2)	0.3 (0.1)	0.3 (0.1)	2.7 (1.0)
T200/CLA	15.6 (6.6)	8.0 (2.3)	6.7 (1.2)	5.3 (1.7)	13.1 (2.1)

LVFW, left ventricular free wall; RV, right ventricle.
*Measurements are means per squared millimeter; numbers in parentheses are ± standard error of the mean.
From Linder et al.[19] By permission of the American Medical Association.

In a subsequent series, the same group[20] documented an increased number of suppressor T cells in patients with histologic myocarditis but again few B cells or natural killer cells. This was in contrast to normal myocardium in which helper T cells predominated. These findings in controls have been confirmed by others with other monoclonal antibodies and even via electron microscopy.[21,22] Again, the relationship between a panleukocyte marker (ie, the number of cells) and the number of cells seen by light microscopy was close. At the time, the distribution of lymphocytes was compatible with experimental studies done with lymphocytic myocarditis.

This approach led to a considerable explosion in the use of this technique. Lauer and colleagues[16] used antibodies to CD3, CD4, and CD8 lymphocyte pools and to the expression of major histocompatibility complex I and II antigens in keeping with the experimental work on lymphocytic myocarditis to characterize the lymphocytes in their studies. Whether these lymphocyte pools exist because of molecular mimicry or develop in response to infection is unclear.

The application of this technique has already raised questions concerning the frequency of myocarditis in patients with idiopathic cardiomyopathy. Kuhl et al.[23] using this technique with increased sensitivity found 37% of patients met criteria for lymphocytic myocarditis compared with only 5% who met the Dallas criteria. Key to the proper interpretation of these findings, however, is whether the infiltrates are a cause of the cardiac abnormalities or a response to myocardial injury.

It is likely that use of this approach will increase as individual disease entities are characterized by the types of infiltrating lymphocytes. In acquired immunodeficiency syndrome myocarditis, it is $CD8^+$ lymphocytes that infiltrate myocardium.[24] With time, polymerase chain reaction techniques, which allow for viral amplification, may help to determine which cells develop as a result of direct infection and which are the result of cross-reacting epitopes. However, even if infection is present, both mechanisms could exist.

Most importantly, there is a need for more control observations in patients with both myocardial and systemic diseases. It is conceivable that the populations of cells in the myocardium may vary depending on local and systemic biologic stresses, and thus the populations of cells may reflect systemic processes and local ones. For example, natural killer cells and $CD8^+$ lymphocytes can be a sign that cell death is related to apoptosis, which occurs commonly in response to ischemic heart disease.[25] In addition, up to 40% of survivors of the syndrome of sudden cardiac death have lymphocytic infiltrates in their myocardium.[26] It is now clear that there are inflammatory mediators activated in patients with ischemic heart disease. For example, activation of nuclear factor κB and the obligatory cytokines stimulated may play an important role in patients with unstable angina[27] and may lead to abnormal lymphocytic infiltrates. In addition, there are inflammatory mediators such as the novel long chain pentraxin described in human myocardium that are released in response to injury and may help to determine which cells inhabit a given cellular infiltrate.[28] It may someday be possible to characterize the causative agent by the lymphocytes that infiltrate the myocardium.

ANTIBODY CONCENTRATIONS

Antibody studies and isolation of viral constructs from myocardium have been used to suggest that viruses may be important in the pathogenesis of idiopathic cardiomyopathy. There was the hope that such tests might be useful in identifying the cause of the disease and targeting specific therapies, such as neutralizing antibodies against a known virus. Unfortunately the viruses, and particularly the enteroviruses, that have been considered as potentially etiologic are ubiquitous. Therefore, it has been difficult to associate directly increases in the viral genome or the antibody response to the presence of disease. For example, multiple studies in the 1980s suggested there was a high frequency of coxsackievirus B immunoglobulin detected in patients with end-stage cardiomyopathy.[29-32] It was speculated that these viruses might be damaging myocardium by stimulation of conjoint antigens or via direct toxic effects.[33-35] However, in 1994 Keeling and associates[36] cast major doubt on the ability of acute and convalescent antibody titers and, for that matter, viral isolation studies to be relied on as evidence of cause. They found, as others did, that a high percentage of patients with dilated cardiomyopathy tested positive for coxsackie B-specific IgM (33%) and that this percentage was substantially greater than what was found in control subjects (5%). However, when they assessed matched community controls, they found that the relative distributions were substantially different. Of the community controls, 27% were positive. In addition, household contacts of the cardiomyopathy patients had a 28% frequency of having an IgG-specific coxsackie B response. This landmark investigation unmasked the danger of not using geographic control groups to assess the important pathophysiologic significance of specific antigens. The same group[37] used the prevalence of the enteroviral genome in myocardium by polymerase chain reaction techniques and the results were identical. The frequency of finding the enteroviral genome in myocardium was 12% in subjects with cardiomyopathy and 17% in geographic controls. Furthermore, 34% of patients with evidence of the viral genome died over 2 to 52 months compared with 33% of those without evidence of this genome but with disease. These findings have been confirmed.[38] These studies do not imply that enteroviruses cannot cause some cardiomyopathies or acute myocarditis, but they do imply that there are likely other unique determinants that must be present, some of which have been related to the different phases of myocarditis by Lieberman and co-workers.[39] Nonetheless, persistence of the viral genome (Table 12-2)[40] or the presence of the viral capsid protein may provide

Table 12-2
Predictors of Survival in Follow-up (Mean 25.2 Months) of 116 Patients
With Myocarditis or Dilated Cardiomyopathy

Variable	Significance
Detection of persisting enterovirus RNA in myocardium by molecular hybridization	<0.001
Reduced ejection fraction	<0.01
Cardiac failure	<0.05
Bundle branch block	<0.05
Arrhythmias	NS
History of viral illness and duration of symptoms	NS
Cardiothoracic ratio	NS
Left ventricular end-diastolic filling pressure	NS

NS, not significant; RNA, ribonucleic acid.
From Archard et al.[40] By permission of WB Saunders.

prognostic information.[41] The same problems exist with interpretation of studies that rely on isolation of the viral genome and those that attempt to document the importance of inflammatory markers in coronary artery disease.

In summary, present data suggest that the use of serial viral titers to attempt to identify the cause of myocarditis is no longer useful and therefore discouraged. These techniques may well make a comeback, however, as we get more specific basic science information about the pathophysiology of viral myocarditis. For now, the use of troponin concentrations combined with immunohistochemical evaluation of the lymphocytes found in myocardium has the greatest potential, especially if low levels of troponin are used. The use of values in this gray area has been advocated by some already[42] but will require further validation, similar to the data suggesting their prognostic significance in patients with cardiomyopathy[43] and improvement in the precision of the assays at these low levels.[42]

REFERENCES

1. Smith SC, Ladenson JH, Mason JW, Jaffe AS. Elevations of cardiac troponin I associated with myocarditis. Experimental and clinical correlates. Circulation 1997;95:163-168.

2. Franz WM, Remppis A, Kandolf R, Kubler W, Katus HA. Serum troponin T: diagnostic marker for acute myocarditis. Clin Chem 1996;42:340-341.

3. Vatner SF, Baig H, Manders WT, Maroko PR. Effects of coronary artery reperfusion on myocardial infarct size calculated from creatine kinase. J Clin Invest 1978;61:1048-1056.

4. Apple FS, Falahati A, Paulsen PR, Miller EA, Sharkey SW. Improved detection of minor ischemic myocardial injury with measurement of serum cardiac troponin I. Clin Chem 1997;43:2047-2051.

5. Jaffe AS, Landt Y, Parvin CA, Abendschein DR, Geltman EM, Ladenson JH. Comparative sensitivity of cardiac troponin I and lactate dehydrogenase isoenzymes for diagnosing acute myocardial infarction. Clin Chem 1996;42:1770-1776.

6. Guest TM, Ramanathan AV, Tuteur PG, Schechtman KB, Ladenson JH, Jaffe AS. Myocardial injury in critically ill patients. A frequently unrecognized complication. JAMA 1995;273:1945-1949.

7. Clark GL, Robison AK, Gnepp DR, Roberts R, Sobel BE. Effects of lymphatic transport of enzyme on plasma creatine kinase time-activity curves after myocardial infarction in dogs. Circ Res 1978;43:162-169.

8. Adams JE III, Schechtman KB, Landt Y, Ladenson JH, Jaffe AS. Comparable detection of acute myocardial infarction by creatine kinase MB isoenzyme and cardiac troponin I. Clin Chem 1994;40:1291-1295.

9. Katus HA, Remppis A, Scheffold T, Diederich KW, Kuebler W. Intracellular compartmentation of cardiac troponin T and its release kinetics in patients with reperfused and nonreperfused myocardial infarction. Am J Cardiol 1991;67:1360-1367.

10. Tanaka H, Abe S, Yamashita T, Arima S, Saigo M, Nakao S, Toda H, Nomoto K, Tahara M. Serum levels of cardiac troponin I and troponin T in estimating myocardial infarct size soon after reperfusion. Coron Artery Dis 1997;8:433-439.

11. Adams JE III, Bodor GS, Davila-Roman VG, Delmez JA, Apple FS, Ladenson JH, Jaffe AS. Cardiac troponin I. A marker with high specificity for cardiac injury. Circulation 1993;88:101-106.

12. Ricchiuti V, Voss EM, Ney A, Odland M, Anderson PA, Apple FS. Cardiac troponin T isoforms expressed in renal diseased skeletal muscle will not cause false-positive results by the second generation cardiac troponin T assay by Boehringer Mannheim. Clin Chem 1998;44:1919-1924.

13. McDonough JL, Arrell DK, Van Eyk JE. Troponin I degradation and covalent complex formation accompanies myocardial ischemia/reperfusion injury. Circ Res 1999;84:9-20.

14. Mason JW. Immunopathogenesis and treatment of myocarditis: the United States Myocarditis Treatment Trial. J Card Fail 1996;2 Suppl:S173-S177.

15. Bachmaier K, Mair J, Offner F, Pummerer C, Neu N. Serum cardiac troponin T and creatine kinase-MB elevations in murine autoimmune myocarditis. Circulation 1995;92:1927-1932.

16. Lauer B, Niederau C, Kuhl U, Schannwell M, Pauschinger M, Strauer BE, Schultheiss HP. Cardiac troponin T in patients with clinically suspected myocarditis. J Am Coll Cardiol 1997;30:1354-1359.

17. Aretz HT, Billingham ME, Edwards WD, Factor SM, Fallon JT, Fenoglio JJ Jr, Olsen EG, Schoen FJ. Myocarditis. A histopathologic definition and classification. Am J Cardiovasc Pathol 1987;1:3-14.

18. Mason JW, O'Connell JB, Herskowitz A, Rose NR, McManus BM, Billingham ME, Moon TE. A clinical trial of immunosuppressive therapy for myocarditis. The Myocarditis Treatment Trial Investigators. N Engl J Med 1995;333:269-275.

19. Linder J, Cassling RS, Rogler WC, Wilson JE, Markin RS, Sears TD, McManus BM. Immunohistochemical characterization of lymphocytes in uninflamed ventricular myocardium. Implications for myocarditis. Arch Pathol Lab Med 1985;109:917-920.

20. Cassling RS, Linder J, Sears TD, Waller BF, Rogler WC, Wilson JE, Kugler JD, Kay DH, Dillon JC, Slack JD, McManus BM. Quantitative evaluation of inflammation in biopsy specimens from idiopathically failing or irritable hearts: experience in 80 pediatric and adult patients. Am Heart J 1985;110:713-720.

21. Steenbergen C, Kolbeck PC, Wolfe JA, Anthony RM, Sanfilippo FP, Jennings RB. Detection of lymphocytes in endomyocardium using immunohistochemical techniques. Relevance to evaluation of endomyocardial biopsies in suspected cases of lymphocytic myocarditis. J Appl Cardiol 1986;1:63-73.

22. Hammond EH, Menlove RL, Anderson JL. Predictive value of immunofluorescence and electron microscopic evaluation of endomyocardial biopsies in the diagnosis and prognosis of myocarditis and idiopathic dilated cardiomyopathy. Am Heart J 1987;114:1055-1065.

23. Kuhl U, Seeberg B, Schultheiss HP, Strauer BE. Immunohistological characterization of infiltrating lymphocytes in biopsies of patients with clinically suspected dilated cardiomyopathy. Eur Heart J 1994;15 Suppl C:62-67.

24. Barbaro G, Di Lorenzo G, Grisorio B, Barbarini G, Gruppo Italiano per lo Studio Cardiologico dei Pazienti Affetti da AIDS. Incidence of dilated cardiomyopathy and detection of HIV in myocardial cells of HIV-positive patients. N Engl J Med 1998;339:1093-1099.

25. Gottlieb RA, Burleson KO, Kloner RA, Babior BM, Engler RL. Reperfusion injury induces apoptosis in rabbit cardiomyocytes. J Clin Invest 1994;94:1621-1628.

26. Frustaci A, Bellocci F, Olsen EG. Results of biventricular endomyocardial biopsy in survivors of cardiac arrest with apparently normal hearts. Am J Cardiol 1994;74:890-895.

27. Ritchie ME. Nuclear factor-kappa B is selectively and markedly activated in humans with unstable angina pectoris. Circulation 1998;98:1707-1713.

28. Peri G, Introna M, Corradi D, Iacuitti G, Signorini S, Avanzini F, Pizzetti F, Maggioni AP, Moccetti T, Metra M, Cas LD, Ghezzi P, Sipe JD, Re G, Olivetti G, Mantovani A, Latini R. PTX3, a prototypical long pentraxin, is an early indicator of acute myocardial infarction in humans. Circulation 2000;102:636-641.

29. Cambridge G, MacArthur CG, Waterson AP, Goodwin JF, Oakley CM. Antibodies to Coxsackie B viruses in congestive cardiomyopathy. Br Heart J 1979;41:692-696.

30. Kawai C. Idiopathic cardiomyopathy. A study on the infectious-immune theory as a cause of the disease. Jpn Circ J 1971;35:765-770.

31. Falase AO, Fabiyi A, Odegbo-Olukoya OO. Coxsackie B viruses and heart muscle disease in Nigerian adults. Trop Georgr Med 1979;31:237-243.

32. Lau RC. Coxsackie B virus infections in New Zealand patients with cardiac and non-cardiac diseases. J Med Virol 1983;11:131-137.

33. Matsumori A, Kawai C. An animal model of congestive (dilated) cardiomyopathy: dilatation and hypertrophy of the heart in the chronic stage in DBA/2 mice with myocarditis caused by encephalomyocarditis virus. Circulation 1982;66:355-360.

34. Neu N, Craig SW, Rose NR, Alvarez F, Beisel KW. Coxsackievirus induced myocarditis in mice: cardiac myosin autoantibodies do not cross-react with the virus. Clin Exp Immunol 1987;69:566-574.

35. Wilson FM, Miranda QR, Chason JL, Lerner AM. Residual pathologic changes following murine coxsackie A and B myocarditis. Am J Pathol 1969;55:253-265.

36. Keeling PJ, Lukaszyk A, Poloniecki J, Caforio AL, Davies MJ, Booth JC, McKenna WJ. A prospective case-control study of antibodies to coxsackie B virus in idiopathic dilated cardiomyopathy. J Am Coll Cardiol 1994;23:593-598.

37. Keeling PJ, Jeffery S, Caforio AL, Taylor R, Bottazzo GF, Davies MJ, McKenna WJ. Similar prevalence of enteroviral genome within the myocardium from patients with idiopathic dilated cardiomyopathy and controls by the polymerase chain reaction. Br Heart J 1992;68:554-559.

38. Jeffery S, Kelling PJ, Lukaszyk A, Boriskin YS, Booth JC, Hodgson J, Davies MJ, McKenna WJ. Molecular evaluation of enteroviruses in the pathogenesis of idiopathic dilated cardiomyopathy. Clin Cardiol 1997;20:857-863.

39. Lieberman EB, Hutchins GM, Herskowitz A, Rose NR, Baughman KL. Clinicopathologic description of myocarditis. J Am Coll Cardiol 1991;18:1617-1626.

40. Archard LC, Bowles NE, Cunningham L, Freeke CA, Olsen EG, Rose ML, Meany B, Why HJ, Richardson PJ. Molecular probes for detection of persisting enterovirus infection of human heart and their prognostic value. Eur Heart J 1991;12 Suppl D:56-59.

41. Li Y, Bourlet T, Andreoletti L, Mosnier JF, Peng T, Yang Y, Archard LC, Pozzetto B, Zhang H. Enteroviral capsid protein VP1 is present in myocardial tissues from some patients with myocarditis or dilated cardiomyopathy. Circulation 2000;101:231-234.

42. Jaffe AS, Ravkilde J, Roberts R, Naslund U, Apple FS, Galvani M, Katus H. It's time for a change to a troponin standard. Circulation 2000;102:1216-1220.

43. Sato Y, Yamada T, Taniguchi R, Nagai K, Makiyama T, Okada H, Kataoka K, Ito H, Matsumori A, Sasayama S, Takatsu Y. Persistently increased serum concentrations of cardiac troponin T in patients with idiopathic dilated cardiomyopathy are predictive of adverse outcomes. Circulation 2001;103:369-374.

Molecular Biologic Detection of Virus Infection in Myocarditis and Dilated Cardiomyopathy

Karin Klingel, M.D.

INTRODUCTION

Although the course of viral myocarditis in most patients is subclinical, some patients develop a severe, sometimes fatal disease.[1,2] In susceptible individuals, viral myocarditis may result in sudden death or the patient may present with cardiac failure with a clinical picture similar to that of idiopathic dilated cardiomyopathy (DCM).[3] Enteroviruses, and especially coxsackieviruses of group B (CVB), are the most common infectious agents.[2,4]

Enteroviruses of the Picornaviridae are nonenveloped icosahedral viruses that contain a single plus-strand RNA genome of about 7,500 bp. The genomic viral RNA, which is polyadenylylated at its 3′-end, serves as messenger for the translation of virus-directed structural and nonstructural proteins and as a template for transcription of a minus-strand RNA intermediate by the virus-encoded RNA-dependent RNA-polymerase $3D^{pol}$. Minus-strand RNA is transcribed again by $3D^{pol}$, providing large amounts of plus-strand RNA genomes, which are encapsidated into new virions. The acute infectious cycle is usually completed by cell lysis and release of newly synthesized virus particles.

Other viruses, such as adenoviruses,[5-9] cytomegalovirus,[5,6,9-11] herpes simplex virus,[5,6] Epstein-Barr virus,[12] human herpesvirus 6,[13] human immunodeficiency virus (HIV),[14] parvovirus B19 (PVB19),[15-17] influenza A,[18] mumps virus,[19] rubella virus,[20] and hepatitis C virus,[21,22] have also been linked with acute and chronic myocarditis. However, few data are available to establish a direct role for these viruses in the pathogenesis of the disease.

Diagnosis of viral heart disease is difficult and generally depends on clinical criteria combined with histologic findings in endomyocardial biopsy specimens. Morphologic features in heart muscle of patients thought to have viral myocarditis, however, cannot be definitely distinguished from inflammatory heart diseases of nonviral origin. Therefore, virologic diagnosis may be of great value in differentiating heart disease of viral etiology from that of other causes. For a long time, diagnosis of myocardial virus infections relied on the time-consuming virus isolation in tissue culture or on serologic tests.[23] However, attempts to isolate virus were unrewarding because patients are rarely viremic or excrete infectious virus in stool or nasopharyngeal secretions beyond the acute phase of virus infection. In addition, the conventional virologic techniques, including virus isolation and immunohistochemical staining of serotype-specific viral antigens, were successful only in cases of fulminant acute viral myocarditis owing to the low sensitivity of these methods.[24]

In the last decade, advances in molecular biology resulted in the development of more sensitive assays for the detection of viral genomes in the myocardium. The establishment of an in situ hybridization technique for the visualization of enteroviral genomes at the cellular level allowed definition of the role of enteroviruses in the induction and maintenance of myocarditis as well as study of the molecular basis of pathogenicity. By application of enterovirus group-specific in situ hybridization, it was demonstrated that enterovirus infection is detectable in a significant proportion of patients with acute and chronic myocarditis and also in patients with end-stage dilated cardiomyopathy, indicating that chronic myocardial injury may be associated with persistent enterovirus infection.[25-28] The capability of enteroviruses to persist in myocardial cells was confirmed by in situ hybridization studies in various murine models of chronic myocarditis, demonstrating that CVB3, typically a cytolytic virus, is capable of evading the immunologic surveillance in a host-dependent manner.[29-32]

In addition to in situ hybridization, the application of the polymerase chain reaction (PCR) has offered new possibilities for sensitive and rapid detection of infectious agents in viral heart disease. Primer pairs and amplification protocols have been published for the identification of RNA viruses (eg, enteroviruses) and also for DNA viruses (eg, Epstein-Barr virus and adenoviruses) in frozen as well as in paraffin-embedded heart muscle tissue.[4-10,12-22]

This chapter focuses on the currently available methods for detecting viral nucleic acids in the myocardium with special reference to the most common cause of viral heart disease—the enteroviruses. The technical principles discussed in this review, which are of general importance for the diagnosis of virus infections, comprise detection of viral nucleic acid sequences by blot hybridization, light and electron microscopic in situ hybridization, PCR, and in situ PCR.

TECHNIQUES FOR THE DETECTION OF VIRAL GENOMES IN MYOCARDITIS AND DILATED CARDIOMYOPATHY

SLOT BLOT HYBRIDIZATION IN THE DIAGNOSIS OF MYOCARDIAL VIRUS INFECTION

In the 1980s, the development of molecular probes facilitated insights into the biologic mechanism of human heart disease. Cloning of viral complementary DNA (cDNA) obtained by reverse transcription (RT) of enteroviral RNA was a major prerequisite for the detection of viral RNA in clinical specimens by RNA/cDNA hybridization.[33-36] In hybridization studies it was shown that because of the high degree of nucleic acid sequence homology shared among the numerous serotypes of the human enterovirus group, multiple enterovirus serotypes can be detected in a single hybridization assay.[37] As demonstrated by spot hybridization (Fig. 13-1), radioactively labeled cloned cDNA of CVB3 functioned as an enterovirus group-specific probe visualizing coxsackieviruses of group B,[34] coxsackieviruses of group A, echoviruses, and also poliovirus type 1.[26,33,36] The wide spectrum of enteroviruses detected by CVB3 cDNA greatly facilitates the diagnosis of viral heart disease, as from the clinical point of view, identification of single specific enterovirus serotypes is of secondary importance. In addition to cDNA probes, synthetic oligonucleotides prepared from highly conserved sequences in the 5′-noncoding region of the enterovirus genome

Slot Blot

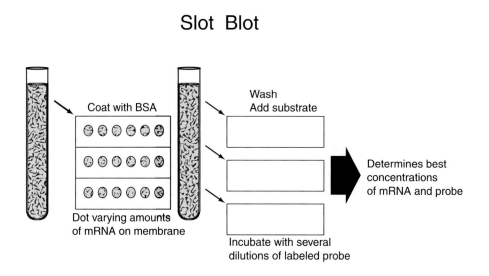

Fig. 13-1. A rapid hybridization method to partially quantify a specific RNA or DNA fragment found in a specimen without the need for a northern or Southern blot. After serially diluting DNA, it is "spotted" on a nylon or nitrocellulose membrane and then denatured with NaOH. It is then exposed to a heat-denatured DNA fragment probe that is believed to be complementary to the nucleic acid fragment whose identity is being sought. The probe is labeled with ^{32}P or ^{35}S. When the 2 strands are complementary, hybridization takes place. This is detected by autoradiography of the radiolabeled probe. Enzymatic, nonradioactive labels may also be used. *BSA*, bovine serum albumin. (From Cruse JM, Lewis RE. Illustrated dictionary of immunology. Boca Raton, FL: CRC Press, 1995:94. By permission of the publisher.)

were useful as universal probes for the detection of any enterovirus.[38] If required, type-specific identification of CVBs can also be performed by application of synthetic oligodeoxyribonucleotides determined by the nucleotide sequences of VP1 capsid protein of different coxsackieviruses.[39]

Various enterovirus-specific cDNA probes and oligodeoxynucleotides have been used in dot or slot blot hybridization studies to prove the relationship between enterovirus infection and heart diseases.[40-43] Applying radioactively labeled CVB2-derived hybridization probes in a slot blot hybridization assay, Bowles et al.[40] found enteroviral sequences in more than 50% of patients with histologic evidence of active or healing myocarditis or dilated cardiomyopathy. Despite the generally low sensitivity of this assay, the same group reported in a second study the presence of enterovirus RNA in 28 of 50 patients with myocarditis or dilated cardiomyopathy.[42] A comparison with other studies using in situ hybridization and PCR as detection methods for the presence of enteroviral RNA suggests that the number of virus-positive patients in these blot assays was overestimated. False-positive results obtained by this method might result from nonspecific cross-reactions of the radiolabeled probes with human myocardial RNA or DNA immobilized on membrane filters.

DETECTION OF VIRAL RNA IN THE HEART MUSCLE BY NORTHERN BLOT HYBRIDIZATION

Northern blot hybridization is a technically more difficult filter hybridization assay that can be used to detect viral RNA (Fig. 13-2). After isolation of total RNA from myocardial tissue and gel electrophoresis, the nucleic acids are transferred onto nylon membranes and hybridized with ^{32}P-labeled cDNA probes, RNA probes, or synthetic oligonucleotides. Because of electrophoretic resolution of nucleic acids before the hybridization procedure, nonspecific cross-reactions as observed in slot blot hybridization are usually not a problem. Whereas northern blotting was suitable for the detection of enteroviral sequences in the myocardium of mice acutely infected with CVB3[44] and encephalomyocarditis (EMC) virus,[45] no viral RNA was found in 40 samples from explanted hearts of patients with idiopathic DCM and noncardiomyopathic cardiac failure[46] using this method. Importantly, the finding that in contrast to in situ hybridization and PCR results no hybridization signals can be obtained from hearts of susceptible mice 10 days postinfection with CVB3[44] and 28 days postinfection with EMC virus[45] indicates a low sensitivity of this blotting technique.

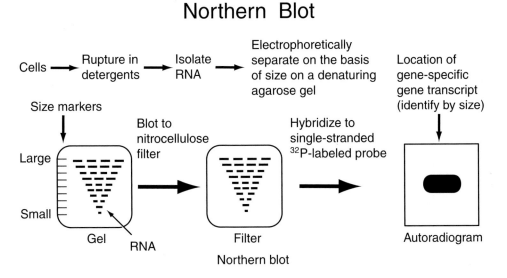

Fig. 13-2. Northern blotting is a method to identify specific mRNA molecules. Following denaturation of RNA in a particular preparation with formaldehyde to cause the molecule to unfold and become linear, the material is separated by size through gel electrophoresis and blotted onto a natural cellulose or nylon membrane. This is then exposed to a solution of labeled DNA "probe" for hybridization. This step is followed by autoradiography. Northern blotting corresponds to a similar method used for DNA fragments which is known as Southern blotting. (From Cruse JM, Lewis RE. Illustrated dictionary of immunology. Boca Raton, FL: CRC Press, 1995:219. By permission of the publisher.)

Thus, northern blotting is generally not the method of choice for diagnosis of viral heart disease, especially when small amounts of tissue probes, such as endomyocardial biopsy specimens, are investigated.

IN SITU DETECTION OF VIRAL RNA IN MURINE MODELS OF VIRAL MYOCARDITIS

A more sensitive and highly specific method for the detection of viral nucleic acids in myocardial tissue is provided by the in situ hybridization technique. In contrast to other viral detection systems, the in situ hybridization technique offers the unique possibility to localize viral RNA and DNA in single cells of frozen as well as of paraffin-embedded myocardial tissue. Because infected cells can be identified easily in hematoxylin and eosin-stained heart muscle tissue sections, the detection of viral RNA can be combined with histologic findings of myocardial injury and inflammation.

A full-length, reverse-transcribed cDNA of CVB3[35] was used to generate an entero-virus-group-specific probe, thus providing the basis for the development of a radioactive in situ hybridization assay capable of visualizing enteroviral RNA in the heart muscle.[26] In CVB3-infected mice, which are used as a model system of enteroviral heart disease, it has been shown that autoradiographic silver grains, which indicate hybridization between viral RNA and the radiolabeled CVB3 cDNA or RNA probes, are clearly localized to individual infected myocytes as visualized in consecutive heart tissue sections[26,29,47] (Fig. 13-3; see color plate 17).

With this model it has been demonstrated that radioactive in situ hybridization not only provides a powerful tool in the diagnosis of viral heart disease but also contributes to the understanding of its pathogenesis. In adult T-cell-deficient mice, it was shown by this method that myocytolysis is closely associated with virus replication. Virus-induced myocyte injury after CVB3 replication was further confirmed by in situ hybridization studies performed in T-cell-deficient athymic mice[26,48] and in severe combined immuno-deficient (SCID) mice.[49]

Furthermore, in immunocompetent mice the relevance of virus replication in the induction of myocardial damage was proven by the finding of single infected necrotic myofibers as soon as 3 days postinfection with CVB3 before the onset of the reactive cellular immune response.[29] The application of single-stranded in vitro transcribed CVB3 RNA probes in in situ hybridization of cultured cells[50] and murine hearts[29,51] revealed that during acute CVB3 infection viral genomic plus-strand RNA is synthesized in great excess compared with the synthesis of relatively low-copy numbers of the viral minus-strand RNA interme-diate. Interestingly, the extent and severity of enterovirus infection in the heart muscle depended on host-specific factors, excluding the H-2 haplotype.[29,30] The most extensive virus cell-to-cell spread was in the myocardium of permissive mouse strains (A/J, A.CA/J,

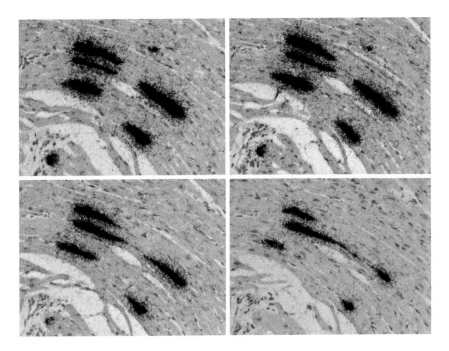

Fig. 13-3. Visualization of coxsackievirus B (CVB)3 RNA in consecutive 5-μm-thick tissue sections of a paraffin-embedded mouse heart by ^{35}S-labeled CVB3 cDNA probes. See color plate 17.

A.BY/J, A.SW/J, SWR/J), which revealed high initial virus loads in the heart muscle. In contrast to resistant mice (C57BL/6, DBA1/J), permissive animals were not capable of eliminating virus infection in the course of acute disease despite a prominent cellular immune response, thus inducing a persistent infection of the heart.[29-31] As visualized by strand-specific in situ hybridization, persistent myocardial infection was characterized by the presence of comparable amounts of viral plus- and minus-strand RNA in myocardial cells of consecutive tissue sections from permissive animals,[29] indicating that viral plus-strand RNA synthesis is restricted during viral persistence.

Tam and Messner[52] reported that coxsackieviral RNA may persist in myofibers in a double-stranded conformation. Muir and colleagues demonstrated that a much slower rate of decline in viral RNA levels occurs in persistently CVB3-infected mouse hearts than in acutely infected mouse hearts.[53] The critical role of persistent picornavirus infection in the pathogenesis of chronic myocarditis was not only proven in murine models of cox-sackievirus infection[26-32,53,54] but also in EMC virus-infected mice by PCR[55] and in situ hybridization. EMC RNA was detected in situ by ^{35}S-labeled RNA probes within the inflamed myocardium up to 3 weeks after infection.[56]

To detect virus persistence in the heart muscle a highly sensitive detection method is required. Quantification of the CVB3 genome copy number in infected cells by RNA blot analysis and comparison with results of isotopic in situ hybridization using cells from the same culture indicated that as few as 20 viral copies are detectable within 2 weeks of autoradiographic exposure.[26] Owing to the capability of isotopic in situ hybridization to detect one infected cell in a persistently infected mouse heart, this assay proved to be as sensitive as nested RT-PCR. A comparable sensitivity of these 2 methods was also reported by Muir et al.[57] with regard to the detection of enteroviral RNA in human myocardium.

A disadvantage of the radioactive in situ hybridization method is the long exposure time and the requirements of a specialized isotopic laboratory. Nonradioactive in situ hybridization techniques have been applied successfully in the detection of acute enterovirus infections of the heart muscle. With biotin-labeled CVB3 RNA probes, acute myocardial infections are easily detectable in murine paraffin-embedded heart muscle tissue by immunogold-silver labeling (Fig. 13-4 *A*; see color plate 18)[58] or via streptavidin conjugated to alkaline phosphatase-new fuchsin (Fig. 13-4 *B*; see color plate 18). However, the detection of low copy numbers of viral RNA in the myocardium by such assays usually fails. Besides biotinylated cDNA probes,[59] digoxigenin-labeled oligonucleotides[60] were suitable for the detection of enteroviral RNA in mouse hearts acutely infected with CVB3. To improve sensitivity of nonradioactive in situ hybridization, a protocol for the in situ PCR of CVB3 RNA in the heart tissue of mice has been developed by using digoxigenin-deoxyuridine triphosphate during the amplification process.[61] In situ PCR is an emerging technique that has an enormous potential in the research of viral heart disease; however, difficulties have to be overcome before this assay can be used as a reliable and a reproducible technique in our laboratories.[62] In situ PCR absolutely requires extensive control experiments to avoid false-positive results.

Also, in in situ hybridization experiments, precautions should be taken to guarantee high specificity. Appropriate measures are recommended to ensure that cross-hybridization of the oligonucleotides and cDNA or RNA probes with human myocardial RNA or DNA does not occur. Thus, the use of unrelated (vector) probes as controls is strongly suggested. The most appropriate control for specificity of hybridization results, however, is the localization of hybridization signals in the same myocardial cells of adjacent tissue sections. Because the diameter of myocardial cells is generally thicker than the 5-μm tissue sections, hybridization signals have to be detected in 2 or more consecutive sections (Fig. 13-3). The possibility of performing such specificity controls represents an enormous advantage of in situ hybridization over other hybridization techniques.

PATTERNS OF ACUTE AND PERSISTENT ENTEROVIRUS INFECTIONS IN THE HUMAN HEART

In situ hybridization as a diagnostic tool in the search for viral genomes in patients with suspected myocarditis was successfully applied in the late 1980s. After application of a

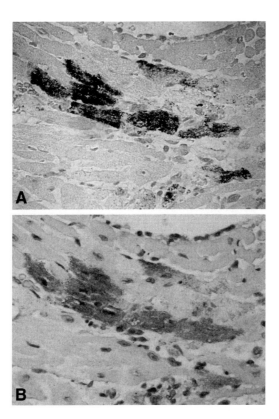

Fig. 13-4. In situ detection of coxsackievirus B (CVB)3 RNA on 2 consecutive myocardial tissue sections by different nonisotopic in situ hybridization assays. See color plate 18.

biotin-labeled 400-bp probe of CVB4 in an in situ hybridization study, 46% of patients with acute coxsackievirus infection had enteroviral RNA in the myocardium.[25] By isotopic in situ hybridization, replicating enterovirus was detected in 24% of patients with clinically suspected acute myocarditis and DCM of recent onset.[63] Tracy et al.[64] reported that 18% of patients with myocarditis were positive for enterovirus as detected by radioactively labeled CVB3 RNA probes. Furthermore, in situ hybridization studies not only have demonstrated that fulminant viral myocarditis in children is caused by enterovirus infection[65] but have pointed out that acute enterovirus myocarditis may result in chronic myocarditis and DCM.[66,67] Chronic myocarditis with cardiac dysfunction has been defined as inflammatory dilated cardiomyopathy (DCMI) by the World Health Organization/International Society and Federation of Cardiology task force.[68]

Major insights have been obtained regarding pathogenetic mechanisms in the development of myocardial enterovirus infection from in situ hybridization studies of human autopsy hearts.[69] Figure 13-5 (see color plate 19) summarizes typical patterns of acute and persistent enterovirus infections of the human heart, illustrating the development and course of myocardial organ infection. Figure 13-5 *A* reflects the establishment of myocardial infection with in situ detection of acute virus replication predominantly in myocytes, which are infected during the viremic phase. After hematogenous infection of cardiac myocytes, a characteristic feature of the developing organ infection is progression of the cardiac virus load by direct cell-to-cell spread of the virus (Figure 13-5 *B*). The increased area of infected myocardial cells is retarded by innate, early, nonadoptive antiviral mechanisms until effector cells of the adoptive immune response begin to clear the infection.

In agreement with results obtained in various murine models of coxsackievirus myocarditis,[29,30,71,72] a reactive infiltration of macrophages and T lymphocytes is the hallmark of enterovirus myocarditis. The early formation of inflammatory foci in the infected human heart is shown in Figure 13-5 *C*. The number of infected myocytes is still increasing during induction of the adoptive immune response, but it is finally controlled by lymphocyte-mediated protective processes, usually achieving elimination of the virus from the heart. Thus, most adult patients recover from acute viral myocarditis. However, acute myocarditis can result in a fulminant lethal disease, which is usually observed in young children (Fig. 13-5 *D*). In such cases, acutely infected myocytes not only are characterized by high transcription activity but also by high translation rates of viral RNA. Effective translation of viral RNA leads to the accumulation of viral structural and nonstructural proteins in myocytes and this can be detected by immunohistochemistry.[73,74] Figure 13-5 *E* is an example of the visualization of enteroviral capsid proteins VP4, VP3, and VP2 by enterovirus-specific antisera[70] in single myocytes of a fatal case of CVB4 myocarditis in a neonate. On the basis of these findings in human autopsy hearts, we are able to interpret in situ patterns of enterovirus infections in endomyocardial biopsy specimens of patients. Figure 13-5 *F* illustrates enterovirus replication in the presence of a reactive cellular immune response in a patient with clinically suspected myocarditis associated with congestive heart failure of recent onset.

As confirmed in the murine model of CVB3-myocarditis, cytolytic enteroviruses may also evade immunologic surveillance in a host-dependent fashion, thus inducing a persistent type of heart muscle infection. Figure 13-5 *G* illustrates evasion of the virus from a fully developed cellular immune response in the late phase of acute myocarditis. In agreement with animal studies, typical patterns of persistent infections of the human heart are characterized by restricted viral replication and gene expression. A relatively small number of persistently infected myocardial cells was sufficient for maintenance of chronic inflammation, as observed during the chronic phase of disease. In addition, typical patterns of persistent infections are detectable in patients with end-stage DCM (Fig. 13-5 *H*), indicating that DCM may evolve from acute and chronic enterovirus myocarditis in certain patients. Consequently, myocardial enterovirus persistence has been shown in explanted hearts of patients who underwent heart transplantation because of end-stage DCM.[63,75]

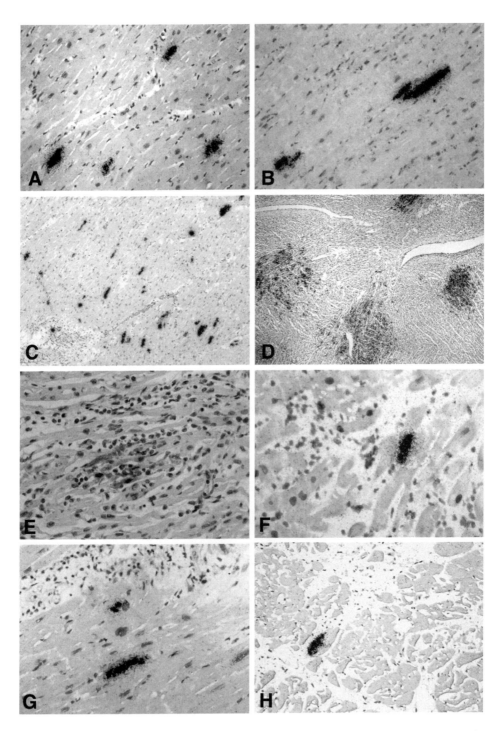

Fig. 13-5. Patterns of acute (*A, B, C, D, F*) and persistent (*G, H*) enterovirus infections of the human heart as detected by radioactive in situ hybridization. See color plate 19. (*B, C, F* from Kandolf et al.[69] By permission of Elsevier Science.)

A small single-stranded DNA virus, PVB19, was identified by PCR techniques in the myocardium of patients with myocarditis.[15-17] The association of heart muscle diseases with PVB19 has been confirmed by in situ hybridization studies demonstrating for the first time that PVB19 can infect endothelial cells of small cardiac vessels (Fig. 13-6 *A*; see color plate 20) as well as interstitial cells (Fig. 13-6 *B*; see color plate 20). Systematic evaluation of interrelationships among PVB19 infection, inflammation, and histopathologic changes of the myocardium at the cellular level is required to establish the role of PBV19 infections in the etiology of viral heart diseases.

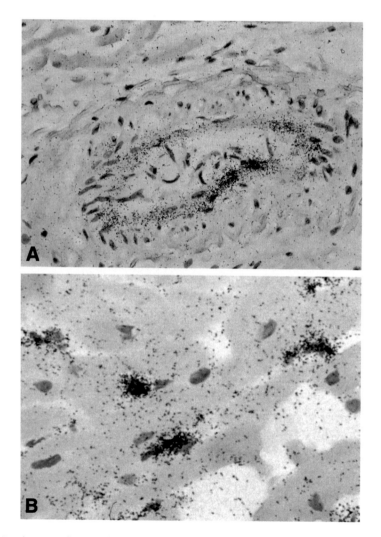

Fig. 13-6. Visualization of myocardial parvovirus B19 infection. See color plate 20.

VISUALIZATION OF VIRAL GENOMES IN THE MYOCARDIUM BY ULTRA-STRUCTURAL IN SITU HYBRIDIZATION

In humans as well as in murine models, enteroviruses have been shown to induce specific cytotoxic alterations in infected heart muscle cells. To evaluate the exact mechanisms of myocyte damage, electron microscopic studies have been performed in vitro and in vivo. Important details of direct enterovirus-induced myocytolysis were obtained in CVB3-infected cultured human myocardial cells[76] and rat myocytes.[77] By electron microscopy it has been shown that infected cultured human myocytes exhibit typical cytopathic effects with destruction of the cytoarchitecture within 20 hours postinfection. Productive infection of these cells was further indicated by the presence of crystal arrays of virus particles in association with the formation of vesicles and proliferated smooth membranes. In vivo, virus crystals have been observed in only rare cases[78,79] and isolated virus particles can usually not be identified definitely by electron microscopy because of their indistinguishability in size and density from ribosomes.[27,30]

Therefore, the in situ detection of enteroviral nucleic acids in the myocardium has been adapted to the ultrastructural level.[58,80-83] To gain insight into the interplay of virus infection and myocardial cell organelles, CVB3-infected mouse hearts were investigated by means of biotinylated enterovirus-specific cDNA or cRNA probes that are visualized with colloidal gold.[58] After the viremic phase (Fig. 13-7 A), the virus invaded the heart via endothelial cells of capillaries (Fig. 13-5 A). In myocytes early virus replication, as visualized by the detection of viral minus-strand RNA, was related to dilation of the sarcoplasmic reticulum in the perinuclear region (Fig. 13-7 B). In the course of virus replication, the majority of 5-nm gold particles, visualizing viral RNA of plus-strand polarity, were found in close vicinity to vesiculated regions (Fig. 13-7 C). In addition, acutely infected myocytes developed large autophagosome-resembling vacuoles containing organelle-like material and cellular debris (Fig. 13-7 D). In peripheral cell regions of infected myocytes an attachment of viral RNA to cytoskeletal filaments was observed in close proximity to obviously intact plasma membranes of adjacent myocytes (Fig. 13-7 E). This finding supports the concept that in addition to virus-induced cell lysis virus spread is mediated by elements of the cytoskeleton before the infected cells are disrupted. The observation of prominent cytopathic alterations in close spatial association with viral replication before the development of the reactive cellular immune response proves that the loss of host cell integrity is a direct consequence of acute viral replication.

Further progression of virus-induced cytopathologic findings in myocytes acutely infected with CVB3 is characterized by a dramatic disruption of the cardiomyocyte cytoarchitecture (Fig. 13-7 F). In the course of myocyte infection, viral RNA was found to be related to histopathologic findings typical for myocyte necrosis, revealing rupture of the plasma membrane and complete destruction of myofilaments associated with aggregated and partially calcified mitochondria. Typically, myocyte lysis results in the release of progeny viruses, which are capable of infecting healthy myocytes in the surroundings of the destroyed cell. According to our previous report,[58] persistently infected myocytes in

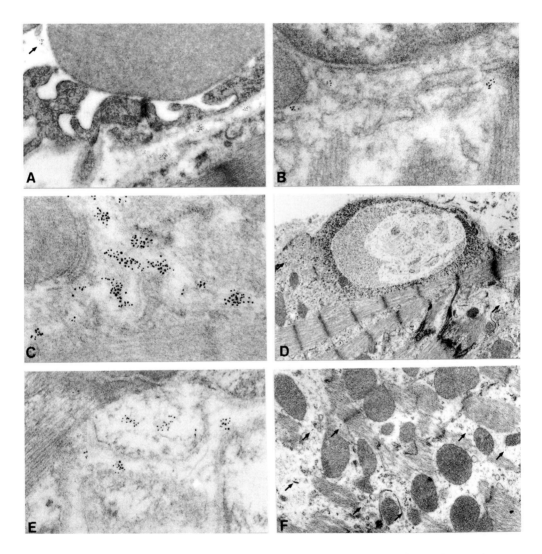

Fig. 13-7. Electron microscopic views of in situ hybridization for the detection of coxsackievirus B3 RNA in acute murine myocarditis. *A,* After viremia and infection of endothelial cells, the virus is spread to myocytes (*arrow*). In infected myocytes, viral RNA is first detected in association with dilated sarcoplasmic reticulum (*B*) and then in vesiculated regions (*C*) and near autophagosome-resembling vacuoles (*D*). *E,* The association of viral RNA with filaments of the cytoskeleton at the periphery of infected myocytes indicates cell-to-cell spread before cellular lysis occurs. *F,* In the course of infection, a complete disruption of the cardiomyocyte cytoarchitecture is noted (*arrows*). Gold particles (5 nm). (*B, C, D, E, F* from Klingel et al.[58] By permission of The United States and Canadian Academy of Pathology.)

association with chronic inflammatory lesions were also detected at the ultrastructural level during chronic myocarditis. Importantly, persistence of viral RNA within myocytes was related to morphologic changes of the myofibrils. As expected, alterations of the structural integrity in persistently infected myocytes appear to be more subtle than those observed in infected myocytes during acute disease, thus reflecting restricted virus replication.[58]

In addition to myocytes, fibroblasts and immune cells, such as B lymphocytes, were found to be infected. Productive enterovirus infection has also been reported in lymphoid cell lines with B- and T-cell characteristics[84] as well as in cultivated fibroblasts isolated from human hearts.[76,85] Enterovirus-infected myocardial cells may trigger immune cells and other myocardial cells to release specific mediators that would interfere with regulatory processes of cardiac metabolism and function.

To investigate whether low-level enteroviral gene expression can induce myocyte damage in the absence of formation of infectious virus particles, the infectious recombinant CVB3 cDNA[35,86] was mutated at the VP0 cleavage site from Asn-Ser to Lys-Ala, thus preventing the formation of infectious viral progeny. In cultured myocytes transfected with this mutated CVB3 cDNA, low-level viral gene expression similar to that observed in the heart of persistently infected mice induced cytopathic effects, which were demonstrated by inhibition of cotransfected luciferase reporter gene activity and an increase in release of lactate dehydrogenase from transfected cells.[77] From these data it can be concluded that restricted viral replication interferes with myocyte function in the presence of low-level viral protein expression and in absence of a cell-mediated immune response.

To further substantiate pathogenic consequences of persistent infection, transgenic mice were generated that express the replication-restricted CVB3 cDNA mutant exclusively in the heart, driven by the cardiac myocyte-specific myosin light chain-2v promoter.[87,88] As expected, heart muscle-specific expression of the CVB3 mutant results in the synthesis of viral plus- and minus-strand RNA without formation of infectious viral progeny, thus simulating the persistent type of heart muscle infection. Typical morphologic features of transgenic murine hearts revealing myocardial interstitial fibrosis, hypertrophy, and degeneration of myocytes were comparable to those observed in hearts of patients with DCM. Moreover, similar to pressure overload models of DCM, abnormalities were observed in the excitation-contraction coupling as well as dilation of the ventricles.[89]

Cellular injury in enterovirus-infected myocardium is mediated via expression of viral proteinases. CVB3 proteinase 2A^{pro}, which is known to cleave the eukaryotic initiation factor 4G[90] and the poly(A)-binding protein,[91] was also found to mediate cleavage of dystrophin, a large extrasarcomeric cytoskeletal protein.[92] In CVB3-infected cultured myocytes and mouse hearts, cleavage of dystrophin was closely associated with the destruction of the intracellular architecture of infected host cells.[92] In addition, our laboratory[93] demonstrated that CVB3 proteinases 3C^{pro}/3CD^{pro} are capable of inducing cleavage of the p21^ras GTPase-activating protein (RasGAP), the major down-regulator of p21^ras. As a consequence of RasGAP cleavage, p21^ras is kept in an activated state and initiates activation of the extracellular signal-regulated protein kinase ERK/MAPK pathway of mitogenic signaling in temporal correlation with the appearance of the RasGAP cleavage product.[93] In addition, there is experimental evidence that the MAP-kinase may participate in the mobilization of intracellular calcium during virus replication and may thereby contribute to morphologic and physiologic destruction of infected myocytes.

DETECTION OF VIRAL GENOMES IN THE HEART BY RT-PCR

In the last decade, another highly sensitive technique, the PCR, has become the most commonly used method for the detection of viral DNA and RNA sequences in the heart of patients with myocarditis and DCM. Primarily as a result of the identification of different viral nucleic acids in the myocardium of these patients by PCR, it is widely thought that myocarditis can develop as a result of infection with enteroviruses,[4] adenoviruses,[5,6] cytomegalovirus,[6,9] Epstein-Barr virus,[12] herpes simplex virus,[6] human herpesvirus-6,[13] HIV,[14] influenza A and influenza B virus,[18] PVB19,[15-17] or hepatitis C virus.[21,22] Martin et al.[5] reported in a PCR analysis of children with acute myocarditis that viral sequences were present in 26 of 38 myocardial samples (68%): 8 enterovirus, 15 adenovirus, 2 herpes simplex virus, and 1 cytomegalovirus. In addition, PCR analysis of endomyocardial biopsy specimens suggests that fibroelastosis is a sequela of viral myocarditis after infection with mumps virus (> 70% positive samples) and adenovirus (28% positive samples).[19]

Regarding the presence of infectious agents in the heart of patients with DCM, there are rather divergent PCR results. Whereas in patients with DCM Pankuweit et al.[9] found an incidence of cytomegalovirus DNA of 12%, adenoviral DNA of 15%, and borreliosis of 0.5%, Galama's group did not detect any nucleic acids from enteroviruses, cytomegalovirus, hepatitis B and C viruses, *Borrelia burgdorferi*, *Chlamydia* species, mycoplasmata, or *Toxoplasma gondii* in patients with end-stage DCM.[94]

PCR provides a fast and sensitive method to detect microbial nucleic acid sequences in cardiac tissue. However, a major disadvantage of the PCR technique is the failure to differentiate among infected cell types, and detection of virus in endomyocardial biopsy specimens might reflect accidental amplification of viral sequences in persistently infected blood cells. Thus, PCR results provide only circumstantial evidence for a pathogenic role of several infectious agents in suspected myocarditis. Further substantiation by in situ hybridization and exclusion of systemic infections is needed.

However, there is firm evidence for a causal link between myocarditis and DCM with acute and persistent enterovirus infection not only from findings in the murine models of enteroviral heart disease[95-98] but also from in situ hybridization studies in children and adults.[26,28,57,64,65,67,99] Unlike other infectious agents, the importance of enteroviruses in the development of heart diseases was proved by visualizing the cytotoxicity of enterovirus replication in myocytes and the consequent invasion of the reactive immune response, leading to acute and chronic myocarditis. Because the in situ hybridization technique is not available in all laboratories, the widely used PCR method was also introduced to diagnose enteroviral myocarditis.

For the identification of enteroviral sequences in clinical material, various PCR protocols have been developed. Generally, the detection of enteroviral RNA in fresh-frozen or formalin-fixed and paraffin-embedded[100-105] heart muscle tissue by RT-PCR requires several steps: 1) isolation of viral RNA from tissue, 2) reverse transcription of RNA into cDNA, 3) amplification of a specific region of the cDNA by PCR and application of enterovirus-specific primers and a heat-stable DNA polymerase, 4) confirmation of specificity by nested PCR or Southern blot hybridization, and 5) sequencing of PCR products. Most reports describe the use of enterovirus-specific primers from the well-conserved 5′ noncoding region of the enteroviral RNA, which are capable of detecting a majority of enteroviral serotypes (Fig. 13-8). Because of the high number of potentially cardiotropic serotypes, serotype-specific PCRs are usually not practical for clinical purposes. If, however, the identification of genotypes of enteroviruses is required, a PCR can be performed using primers covering the enterovirus VP2 region[106,107] in addition to single-strand conformation

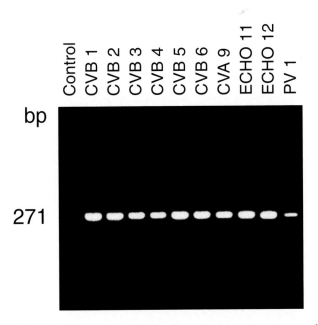

Fig. 13-8. Identification of different potentially cardiotropic enterovirus serotypes by nested reverse transcription-polymerase chain reaction. Primer sequences from highly conserved 5′-noncoding regions of the enterovirus genome are used for group-specific amplification of enteroviral RNA. *CV*, coxsackievirus; *ECHO*, echovirus; *PV*, poliovirus.

polymorphism analysis[108] or nucleotide sequencing of PCR products.[109] Several improvements in the sensitivity and specificity of enterovirus-specific RT-PCR assays have been introduced by establishing nested PCR.[97,105] Furthermore, the establishment of an antigen capture PCR,[110] a single-step PCR,[111] a commercially available assay (Amplicor, Roche Diagnostic Systems),[112] a quantitative (RT-) PCR,[113,114] and a PCR combined with a microwell capture hybridization assay[115] have been described.

A multicenter evaluation of commercial and in-house PCR methods for the identification of enteroviral RNA revealed that most PCR systems can detect enteroviral RNA derived from 0.01 $TCID_{50}$ and are generally more sensitive than cell culture for enterovirus detection in clinical samples.[116] A few laboratories experienced false-positive results from PCR contamination. The problem of PCR contamination (eg, resulting from cross-contamination during RNA extraction) might be a reason why there is a discrepancy in the literature regarding the prevalence of enteroviruses in the heart of patients with myocarditis and DCM. Some groups reported that more than 50% of patients who had DCM were positive for enteroviral RNA in the heart muscle,[117-119] whereas others did not find any evidence for the presence of enteroviruses in patients with DCM.[120-123] The failure to detect enteroviral RNA in these patients might result from limitations in RNA isolation or in the efficiency of reverse transcription or from the sampling error of endomyocardial biopsies. Because enterovirus infection is a focal infection (Fig. 13-5), it is absolutely necessary to investigate several biopsy specimens from different regions of the myocardium to get reliable results.

In 1997, a meta-analysis of 29 papers on the association of enteroviruses with myocarditis and DCM was published by Baboonian and Treasure.[4] Analysis of the data revealed that 11 of 12 studies recorded a higher number of patients (children and adults) with myocarditis who were positive for enteroviral RNA than control patients. Altogether, 23% with myocarditis and 6% of controls had enteroviral RNA in the myocardium, resulting in an odds ratio of 4.4 (95% confidence interval, 2.4 to 8.2). The review of 17 studies regarding DCM patients revealed that 23% (406 patients) of DCM patients and 7% (438 patients) of the control patients were positive for enteroviral RNA (odds ratio, 3.8; 95% confidence interval, 2.1 to 4.6).[4] Positivity in patients with DCM ranged from 0%[120-123] to 75%.[117] An overview of the studies investigating the association of enterovirus infection with myocarditis and DCM is given in Tables 13-1 and 13-2. Divergent results for the presence of enteroviruses were also reported for patients with arrhythmogenic right ventricular cardiomyopathy (ARVC). Whereas Grumbach et al.[142] detected enteroviral RNA with homology to CVBs in 37.5% (3 of 8) of ARVC patients, Calabrese et al.[143] did not find any enterovirus-specific sequences in the heart of these patients.

In addition, there is uncertainty regarding the prevalence of particular enterovirus genotypes in patients with myocarditis and DCM. Nicholson et al.[104] and Archard et al.[109]

reported that coxsackie B serotypes are most frequently involved in myocarditis and DCM, whereas other groups found that no particular type of enterovirus is present in the myocardium of patients with myocarditis.[64] It is also a matter of debate whether enterovirus infection influences the clinical outcome of DCM. Why et al.[144] and also Terasaki et al.[140] reported that the presence of enterovirus RNA in the myocardium of patients with DCM is associated with an adverse prognosis. In contrast, Figulla et al.[67] did not find this relationship. Calabrese et al.[141] reported that enterovirus infection predicts a poor prognosis in cardiac transplant patients.

Table 13-1
Prevalence of Enterovirus RNA in Cardiac Tissue of Patients With Acute Myocarditis

| Author | Year | Methods | Patients, % (no.) | |
			Positive myocarditis	Positive controls
Bowles et al.[40]	1986	Slot blot hybridization	50 (4/8)	0 (0/4)
Archard et al.[42]	1987	Slot blot hybridization	57 (12/21)	0 (0/22)
Easton and Eglin[25]	1988	In situ hybridization	46 (6/13)	0 (0/5)
Kandolf[27]	1988	In situ hybridization	25 (3/12)	0 (0/8)
Kandolf et al.[28]	1993	In situ hybridization	24 (23/95)	0 (0/53)
Jin et al.[124]	1990	RT-PCR	7 (2/28)	0 (0/9)
Tracy et al.[64]	1990	In situ hybridization	18 (3/17)	ND
Weiss et al.[125]	1991	RT-PCR	20 (1/5)	0 (0/21)
Petitjean et al.[126]	1992	RT-PCR	30 (3/10)	39 (9/23)
Koide et al.[32]	1992	RT-PCR	33 (3/9)	0 (0/9)
Hilton et al.*[65]	1993	In situ hybridization/RT-PCR	20 (2/10)	0 (0/10)
Giacca et al.[127]	1994	Nested RT-PCR	33 (1/3)	4 (1/28)
Satoh et al.[128]	1994	Nested RT-PCR	33 (12/36)	0 (0/10)
Martin et al.*[5]	1994	RT-PCR	21 (8/38)	0 (0/17)
Griffin et al.*[6]	1995	RT-PCR	21 (12/58)	0 (0/22)
Ueno et al.[129]	1995	RT-PCR	80 (4/5)	11 (3/27)
Fujioka et al.[108]	1996	PCR-SSCP	18 (5/28)	22 (5/23)
Nicholson et al.[104]	1995	RT-PCR	83 (5/6)	0 (0/8)
Pauschinger et al.[130]	1999	RT-PCR/Southern blot hybridization	40 (18/45)	0 (0/26)
Li et al.[131]	2000	Nested RT-PCR	54 (6/11)	0 (0/11)

ND, not done; RT-PCR, reverse transcription-polymerase chain reaction; SSCP, single-strand conformation polymorphism.

*The papers of Hilton, Martin, and Griffin comprise investigations of myocarditis in childhood.

Table 13-2
Prevalence of Enterovirus RNA in Cardiac Tissue of Patients With Dilated Cardiomyopathy

			Patients, % (no.)	
Author	Year	Methods	Positive DCM	Positive controls
Bowles et al.[40]	1986	Slot blot hybridization	55 (5/9)	0 (0/4)
Archard et al.[42]	1987	Slot blot hybridization	55 (16/29)	0 (0/22)
Kandolf[27]	1988	In situ hybridization	20 (3/15)	0 (0/2)
Bowles et al.[41]	1989	Slot blot hybridization	29 (6/21)	5 (1/19)
Jin et al.[124]	1990	RT-PCR	15 (3/20)	0 (0/9)
Cochrane et al.[46]	1991	Northern blot hybridization	0 (0/19)	0 (0/21)
Weiss et al.[125]	1991	RT-PCR	0 (0/11)	0 (0/21)
Weiss et al.[121]	1992	RT-PCR	45 (5/11)	38 (9/24)
Petitjean et al.[126]	1992	RT-PCR	67 (30/45)	39 (9/23)
Grasso et al.[122]	1992	RT-PCR	0 (0/21)	0 (0/60)
Chiang et al.[117]	1992	RT-PCR	75 (3/4)	0 (0/6)
Keeling et al.[132]	1992	RT-PCR	12 (6/50)	17 (13/75)
Koide et al.[32]	1992	RT-PCR	32 (8/25)	0 (0/9)
Zoll et al.[133]	1992	RT-PCR	20 (1/5)	0 (0/8)
Kandolf et al.[28]	1993	In situ hybridization	17 (8/47)	0 (0/53)
Liljeqvist et al.[123]	1993	RT-PCR	0 (0/35)	0 (0/23)
Schwaiger et al.[134]	1993	RT-PCR	32 (6/19)	0 (0/21)
Werner et al.[99]	1993	In situ hybridization	35 (6/17)	ND
Giacca et al.[127]	1994	Nested RT-PCR	8 (4/53)	4 (1/28)
Khan et al.[135]	1994	Nested RT-PCR	53 (8/15)	11 (1/9)
Satoh et al.[136]	1994	Nested RT-PCR	49 (17/35)	0 (0/10)
Figulla et al.[67]	1995	In situ hybridization	26 (20/77)	ND
Ueno et al.[129]	1995	RT-PCR	17 (7/42)	11 (3/27)
Satoh et al.[137]	1996	RT-PCR	43 (9/21)	0 (0/15)
Andreoletti et al.[119]	1996	RT-PCR/slot blot hybridization	58 (11/19)	57 (8/14)
Muir et al.[57]	1996	RT-PCR/sequencing	4 (1/24)	8 (4/51)
Muir et al.[57]	1996	In situ hybridization	20 (2/10)	41 (5/12)
Fujioka et al.[108]	1996	PCR-SSCP	19 (6/31)	22 (5/23)
Arbustini et al.[79]	1997	RT-PCR	13 (4/31)	4 (1/24)
Arola et al.[138]	1998	RT-PCR	3 (1/32)	0 (0/34)
de Leeuw et al.[120]	1998	Nested RT-PCR	0 (0/38)	0 (0/39)
Pauschinger et al.[139]	1998	RT-PCR/Southern blot hybridization	36 (27/75)	0 (0/41)
Archard et al.[109]	1998	RT-PCR/sequencing	43 (9/21)	7 (1/14)
Terasaki et al.[140]	1999	RT-PCR	15 (2/13)	ND
Calabrese et al.[141]	1999	RT-PCR	4 (1/27)	0 (0/17)
Li et al.[131]	2000	Nested RT-PCR	37 (3/8)	0 (0/11)

DCM, dilated cardiomyopathy; ND, not done; RT-PCR, reverse transcription-polymerase chain reaction; SSCP, single-strand conformation polymorphism.

CONCLUSIONS

The development of molecular biologic techniques described in this chapter not only has facilitated the diagnosis of virus infection in the heart of patients with myocarditis and DCM but also has shed light on the pathogenesis of viral heart disease. Above all, the in situ hybridization techniques for the detection of enteroviral RNA at the light and electron microscopic level and their application in diseased human hearts and animal models of myocarditis proved to be powerful tools for the elucidation of molecular and structural interrelationships in heart muscle abnormality.

Unlike in situ hybridization, the second highly sensitive detection method for viral RNA, the PCR technique, does not allow correlation of morphology with presence of viral nucleic acids, but it has proved to be a rapid and sensitive detection system suitable for routine diagnostics. The application of enterovirus group-specific PCR in numerous diagnostic studies of endomyocardial biopsies has provided strong evidence for a high prevalence of enteroviruses in patients with acute and chronic heart diseases. All methods for the detection of viral nucleic acids in cardiac tissue require invasive tissue sampling and are likely to underestimate enteroviral involvement because of sampling error resulting from the focal distribution of virus-replicating cells as visualized by in situ hybridization. On the other hand, misleading information regarding the role of enteroviruses in heart muscle diseases might result from local differences in the prevalence of enteroviruses or from small enterovirus epidemics that might artificially increase the number of virus-positive patients. Divergent results with regard to the presence of myocardial enterovirus sequences in patients with suspected myocarditis and DCM might also reflect investigation of a rather inhomogeneous population of patients owing to high variations in the clinical outcome of a myocardial virus infection.

Further improvements of existing techniques and developments of new assays are required to determine the extent and distribution and also the replicative state of the virus as well as the nature of the patient's immune response to the infection. The answers to these questions will have significant implications for the management and the successful treatment of enterovirus-infected patients with heart diseases. It is hoped that antiviral treatment with interferons may provide protection against myocardial infection.[145]

ACKNOWLEDGMENTS

The work summarized in this chapter was supported by the Federal Ministry of Education, Science, Research and Technology and the Interdisciplinary Center for Clinical Research (IZKF 01 KS9602) of the Medical Faculty at the University of Tübingen and the Dr. Karl-Kuhn Foundation. In addition, the productive collaboration with the laboratories of Bruce

McManus, University of British Columbia, Vancouver, and Kirk Knowlton, University of California, San Diego, is appreciated. The author is indebted to Reinhard Kandolf, Department of Molecular Pathology, University Hospital of Tübingen, for generous support and is grateful to Annie Canu, U.F.R. des Sciences Pharmaceutiques, Caen, and Peter Rieger, Institute for Pathology, University of Heidelberg, for contributions to the studies.

REFERENCES

1. Woodruff JF. Viral myocarditis. A review. Am J Pathol 1980;101:425-484.
2. Martino TA, Liu P, Sole MJ. Viral infection and the pathogenesis of dilated cardiomyopathy. Circ Res 1994;74:182-188.
3. Dec GW Jr, Palacios IF, Fallon JT, Aretz HT, Mills J, Lee DC, Johnson RA. Active myocarditis in the spectrum of acute dilated cardiomyopathies. Clinical features, histologic correlates, and clinical outcome. N Engl J Med 1985;312:885-890.
4. Baboonian C, Treasure T. Meta-analysis of the association of enteroviruses with human heart disease. Heart 1997;78:539-543.
5. Martin AB, Webber S, Fricker FJ, Jaffe R, Demmler G, Kearney D, Zhang Y-H, Bodurtha J, Gelb B, Ni J, Bricker JT, Towbin JA. Acute myocarditis. Rapid diagnosis by PCR in children. Circulation 1994;90:330-339.
6. Griffin LD, Kearney D, Ni J, Jaffe R, Fricker FJ, Webber S, Demmler G, Gelb BD, Towbin JA. Analysis of formalin-fixed and frozen myocardial autopsy samples for viral genome in childhood myocarditis and dilated cardiomyopathy with endocardial fibroelastosis using polymerase chain reaction (PCR). Cardiovasc Pathol 1995;4:3-11.
7. Pauschinger M, Bowles NE, Fuentes-Garcia FJ, Pham V, Kuhl U, Schwimmbeck PL, Schultheiss HP, Towbin JA. Detection of adenoviral genome in the myocardium of adult patients with idiopathic left ventricular dysfunction. Circulation 1999;99:1348-1354.
8. Grumbach IM, Heim A, Pring-Akerblom P, Vonhof S, Hein WJ, Muller G, Figulla HR. Adenoviruses and enteroviruses as pathogens in myocarditis and dilated cardiomyopathy. Acta Cardiol 1999;54:83-88.
9. Pankuweit S, Hufnagel G, Eckhardt H, Herrmann H, Uttecht S, Maisch B. Cardiotropic DNA viruses and bacteria in the pathogenesis of dilated cardiomyopathy with or without inflammation. Med Klin 1998;93:223-228.
10. Schönian U, Crombach M, Maser S, Maisch B. Cytomegalovirus-associated heart muscle disease. Eur Heart J 1995;16 Suppl O:46-49.
11. Wu TC, Pizzorno MC, Hayward GS, Willoughby S, Neumann DA, Rose NR, Ansari AA, Beschorner WE, Baughman KL, Herskowitz A. In situ detection of human cytomegalovirus immediate-early gene transcripts within cardiac myocytes of patients with HIV-associated cardiomyopathy. AIDS 1992;6:777-785.
12. Hebert MM, Yu C, Towbin JA, Rogers BB. Fatal Epstein-Barr virus myocarditis in a child with repetitive myocarditis. Pediatr Pathol Lab Med 1995;15:805-812.
13. Fukae S, Ashizawa N, Morikawa S, Yano K. A fatal case of fulminant myocarditis with human herpesvirus-6 infection. Intern Med 2000;39:632-636.
14. Herskowitz A, Wu TC, Willoughby SB, Vlahov D, Ansari AA, Beschorner WE, Baughman KL. Myocarditis and cardiotropic viral infection associated with severe left ventricular dysfunction in

late-stage infection with human immunodeficiency virus. J Am Coll Cardiol 1994;24:1025-1032.

15. Schowengerdt KO, Ni J, Denfield SW, Gajarski RJ, Bowles NE, Rosenthal G, Kearney DL, Price JK, Rogers BB, Schauer GM, Chinnock RE, Towbin JA. Association of parvovirus B19 genome in children with myocarditis and cardiac allograft rejection: diagnosis using the polymerase chain reaction. Circulation 1997;96:3549-3554.

16. Enders G, Dotsch J, Bauer J, Nutzenadel W, Hengel H, Haffner D, Schalasta G, Searle K, Brown KE. Life-threatening parvovirus B19-associated myocarditis and cardiac transplantation as possible therapy: two case reports. Clin Infect Dis 1998;26:355-358.

17. Nigro G, Bastianon V, Colloridi V, Ventriglia F, Gallo P, D'Amati G, Koch WC, Adler SP. Human parvovirus B19 infection in infancy associated with acute and chronic lymphocytic myocarditis and high cytokine levels: report of 3 cases and review. Clin Infect Dis 2000;31:65-69.

18. Ray CG, Icenogle TB, Minnich LL, Copeland JG, Grogan TM. The use of intravenous ribavirin to treat influenza virus-associated acute myocarditis. J Infect Dis 1989;159:829-836.

19. Ni J, Bowles NE, Kim YH, Demmler G, Kearney D, Bricker JT, Towbin JA. Viral infection of the myocardium in endocardial fibroelastosis. Molecular evidence for the role of mumps virus as an etiologic agent. Circulation 1997;95:133-139.

20. Thanopoulos BD, Rokas S, Frimas CA, Mantagos SP, Beratis NG. Cardiac involvement in postnatal rubella. Acta Paediatr Scand 1989;78:141-144.

21. Matsumori A, Yutani C, Ikeda Y, Kawai S, Sasayama S. Hepatitis C virus from the hearts of patients with myocarditis and cardiomyopathy. Lab Invest 2000;80:1137-1142.

22. Okabe M, Fukuda K, Arakawa K, Kikuchi M. Chronic variant of myocarditis associated with hepatitis C virus infection. Circulation 1997;96:22-24.

23. Javett SN, Heyman S, Mundel B, Pepler WJ, Lurie HI, Gear J, Maesroch V, Kirsch Z. Myocarditis in the newborn infant. J Pediatr 1956;48:1-22.

24. Grandien M, Forsgren M, Ehrnst A. Enteroviruses and reoviruses. In: Schmidt NJ, Emmons RW, eds. Diagnostic procedures for viral, rickettsial, and chlamydial infections. Washington, DC: American Public Health Association, 1989:513-569.

25. Easton AJ, Eglin RP. The detection of coxsackievirus RNA in cardiac tissue by in situ hybridization. J Gen Virol 1988;69:285-291.

26. Kandolf R, Ameis D, Kirschner P, Canu A, Hofschneider PH. In situ detection of enteroviral genomes in myocardial cells by nucleic acid hybridization: an approach to the diagnosis of viral heart disease. Proc Natl Acad Sci U S A 1987;84:6272-6276.

27. Kandolf R. The impact of recombinant DNA technology on the study of enterovirus heart disease. In: Bendinelli M, Friedman H, eds. Coxsackieviruses--a general update. New York: Plenum Press, 1988:293-318.

28. Kandolf R, Klingel K, Zell R, Selinka HC, Raab U, Schneider-Brachert W, Bültmann B. Molecular pathogenesis of enterovirus-induced myocarditis: virus persistence and chronic inflammation. Intervirology 1993;35:140-151.

29. Klingel K, Hohenadl C, Canu A, Albrecht M, Seemann M, Mall G, Kandolf R. Ongoing enterovirus-induced myocarditis is associated with persistent heart muscle infection: quantitative analysis of virus replication, tissue damage, and inflammation. Proc Natl Acad Sci U S A 1992;89:314-318.

30. Klingel K, Kandolf R. The role of enterovirus replication in the development of acute and chronic heart muscle disease in different immunocompetent mouse strains. Scand J Infect Dis Suppl 1993;88:79-85.

31. Gauntt CJ, Tracy SM, Chapman N, Wood HJ, Kolbeck PC, Karaganis AG, Winfrey CL, Cunningham MW. Coxsackievirus-induced chronic myocarditis in murine models. Eur Heart J 1995;16 Suppl O:56-58.

32. Koide H, Kitaura Y, Deguchi H, Ukimura A, Kawamura K, Hirai K. Genomic detection of enteroviruses in the myocardium--studies on animal hearts with coxsackievirus B3 myocarditis and endomyocardial biopsies from patients with myocarditis and dilated cardiomyopathy. Jpn Circ J 1992;56:1081-1093.

33. Hyypiä T, Stalhandske P, Vainionpaa R, Pettersson U. Detection of enteroviruses by spot hybridization. J Clin Microbiol 1984;19:436-438.

34. Tracy S. A comparison of genomic homologies among the coxsackievirus B group: use of fragments of the cloned coxsackievirus B3 genome as probes. J Gen Virol 1984;65:2167-2172.

35. Kandolf R, Hofschneider PH. Molecular cloning of the genome of a cardiotropic Coxsackie B3 virus: full-length reverse-transcribed recombinant cDNA generates infectious virus in mammalian cells. Proc Natl Acad Sci U S A 1985;82:4818-4822.

36. Rotbart HA, Levin MJ, Villareal LP. Factors affecting the detection of enteroviruses in cerebrospinal fluid with coxsackievirus B3 and poliovirus type 1 cDNA probes. J Clin Microbiol 1985;22:220-224.

37. Rotbart HA, Romero JR. Laboratory diagnosis of enteroviral infections. In: Rotbart HA, ed. Human enterovirus infections. Washington, DC: ASM Press, 1995:401-418.

38. Bruce C, al-Nakib W, Forsyth M, Stanway G, Almond JW. Detection of enteroviruses using cDNA and synthetic oligonucleotide probes. J Virol Methods 1989;25:233-240.

39. Alksnis M, Lindberg M, Stalhandske P, Hultberg H, Pettersson U. Use of synthetic oligodeoxyribo-nucleotides for type-specific identification of coxsackie B viruses. Mol Cell Probes 1989;3:103-108.

40. Bowles NE, Richardson PJ, Olsen EG, Archard LC. Detection of Coxsackie-B-virus-specific RNA sequences in myocardial biopsy samples from patients with myocarditis and dilated cardiomyopathy. Lancet 1986;1:1120-1123.

41. Bowles NE, Rose ML, Taylor P, Banner NR, Morgan-Capner P, Cunningham L, Archard LC, Yacoub MH. End-stage dilated cardiomyopathy. Persistence of enterovirus RNA in myocardium at cardiac transplantation and lack of immune response. Circulation 1989;80:1128-1136.

42. Archard LC, Richardson PJ, Olsen EG, Dubowitz V, Sewry C, Bowles NE. The role of Coxsackie B viruses in the pathogenesis of myocarditis, dilated cardiomyopathy and inflammatory muscle disease. Biochem Soc Symp 1987;53:51-62.

43. Wiegand V, Tracy S, Chapman N, Wucherpfennig C. Enteroviral infection in end stage dilated cardiomyopathy. Klin Wochenschr 1990;68:914-920.

44. Okada I, Matsumori A, Kawai C, Yodoi J, Tracy S. The viral genome in experimental murine Coxsackievirus B3 myocarditis: a Northern blotting analysis. J Mol Cell Cardiol 1990;22:999-1008.

45. Wee L, Liu P, Penn L, Butany JW, McLaughlin PR, Sole MJ, Liew CC. Persistence of viral genome into late stages of murine myocarditis detected by polymerase chain reaction. Circulation 1992;86:1605-1614.

46. Cochrane HR, May FE, Ashcroft T, Dark JH. Enteroviruses and idiopathic cardiomyopathy. J Pathol 1991;163:129-131.

47. Kallajoki M, Kalimo H, Wesslen L, Auvinen P, Hyypia T. In situ detection of enterovirus genomes in mouse myocardial tissue by ribonucleic acid probes. Lab Invest 1990;63:669-675.

48. Sato S, Tsutsumi R, Burke A, Carlson G, Porro V, Seko Y, Okumura K, Kawana R, Virmani R. Persistence of replicating coxsackievirus B3 in the athymic murine heart is associated with development of myocarditic lesions. J Gen Virol 1994;75:2911-2924.

49. Chow LH, Beisel KW, McManus BM. Enteroviral infection of mice with severe combined immuno-deficiency. Evidence for direct viral pathogenesis of myocardial injury. Lab Invest 1992;66:24-31.

50. Rotbart HA, Abzug MJ, Murry RS, Murphy NL, Levin MJ. Intracellular detection of sense and antisense enteroviral RNA by in situ hybridization. J Virol Methods 1988;22:295-301.

51. Hohenadl C, Klingel K, Mertsching J, Hofschneider PH, Kandolf R. Strand-specific detection of enteroviral RNA in myocardial tissue by in situ hybridization. Mol Cell Probes 1991;5:11-20.

52. Tam PE, Messner RP. Molecular mechanisms of coxsackievirus persistence in chronic inflammatory myopathy: viral RNA persists through formation of a double-stranded complex without associated genomic mutations or evolution. J Virol 1999;73:10113-10121.

53. Reetoo KN, Osman SA, Illavia SJ, Cameron-Wilson CL, Banatvala JE, Muir P. Quantitative analysis of viral RNA kinetics in coxsackievirus B3-induced murine myocarditis: biphasic pattern of clearance following acute infection, with persistence of residual viral RNA throughout and beyond the inflammatory phase of disease. J Gen Virol 2000;81:2755-2762.

54. Leipner C, Borchers M, Merkle I, Stelzner A. Coxsackievirus B3-induced myocarditis in MHC class II-deficient mice. J Hum Virol 1999;2:102-114.

55. Kyu B, Matsumori A, Sato Y, Okada I, Chapman NM, Tracy S. Cardiac persistence of cardioviral RNA detected by polymerase chain reaction in a murine model of dilated cardiomyopathy. Circulation 1992;86:522-530.

56. Cronin ME, Love LA, Miller FW, McClintock PR, Plotz PH. The natural history of encephalo-myocarditis virus-induced myositis and myocarditis in mice. Viral persistence demonstrated by in situ hybridization. J Exp Med 1988;168:1639-1648.

57. Muir P, Nicholson F, Illavia SJ, McNeil TS, Ajetunmobi JF, Dunn H, Starkey WG, Reetoo KN, Cary NR, Parameshwar J, Banatvala JE. Serological and molecular evidence of enterovirus infection in patients with end-stage dilated cardiomyopathy. Heart 1996;76:243-249.

58. Klingel K, Rieger P, Mall G, Selinka H-C, Huber M, Kandolf R. Visualization of enteroviral replication in myocardial tissue by ultrastructural in situ hybridization: identification of target cells and cytopathic effects. Lab Invest 1998;78:1227-1237.

59. Zhang HY, Yousef GE, Bowles NE, Archard LC, Mann GF, Mowbray JF. Detection of enterovirus RNA in experimentally infected mice by molecular hybridisation: specificity of subgenomic probes in quantitative slot blot and in situ hybridisation. J Med Virol 1988;26:375-386.

60. Hilton DA, Day C, Pringle JH, Fletcher A, Chambers S. Demonstration of the distribution of coxsackie virus RNA in neonatal mice by non-isotopic in situ hybridization. J Virol Methods 1992;40:155-162.

61. Berger MM, See DM, Redl B, Aymard M, Lina B. Comparison of procedures for the detection of enteroviruses in murine heart samples by in situ polymerase chain reaction. Res Virol 1997;148:409-416.

62. Teo IA, Shaunak S. Polymerase chain reaction in situ: an appraisal of an emerging technique. Histochem J 1995;27:647-659.

63. Kandolf R, Hofschneider PH. Viral heart disease. Springer Semin Immunopathol 1989;11:1-13.

64. Tracy S, Chapman NM, McManus BM, Pallansch MA, Beck MA, Carstens J. A molecular and serologic evaluation of enteroviral involvement in human myocarditis. J Mol Cell Cardiol 1990;22:403-414.

65. Hilton DA, Variend S, Pringle JH. Demonstration of Coxsackie virus RNA in formalin-fixed tissue sections from childhood myocarditis cases by in situ hybridization and the polymerase chain reaction. J Pathol 1993;170:45-51.

66. Muir P, Kandolf R. The laboratory diagnosis of enterovirus-induced heart disease. In: Banatvala JE, ed. Viral infections of the heart. London: E. Arnold, 1996:211-230.

67. Figulla HR, Stille-Siegener M, Mall G, Heim A, Kreuzer H. Myocardial enterovirus infection with left ventricular dysfunction: a benign disease compared with idiopathic dilated cardiomyopathy. J Am Coll Cardiol 1995;25:1170-1175.

68. Richardson P, McKenna W, Bristow M, Maisch B, Mautner B, O'Connell J, Olsen E, Thiene G, Goodwin J, Gyarfas I, Martin I, Nordet P. Report of the 1995 World Health Organization/International Society and Federation of Cardiology Task Force on the Definition and Classification of Cardiomyopathies. Circulation 1996;93:841-842.

69. Kandolf R, Sauter M, Aepinus C, Schnorr J-J, Selinka H-C, Klingel K. Mechanisms and consequences of enterovirus persistence in cardiac myocytes and cells of the immune system. Virus Res 1999;62:149-158.

70. Werner S, Klump WM, Schönke H, Hofschneider PH, Kandolf R. Expression of coxsackievirus B3 capsid proteins in *Escherichia coli* and generation of virus-specific antisera. DNA 1988;7:307-316.

71. Herskowitz A, Wolfgram LJ, Rose NR, Beisel KW. Coxsackievirus B3 murine myocarditis: a pathologic spectrum of myocarditis in genetically defined inbred strains. J Am Coll Cardiol 1987;9:1311-1319.

72. Craighead JE, Huber SA, Sriram S. Animal models of picornavirus-induced autoimmune disease: their possible relevance to human disease. Lab Invest 1990;63:432-446.

73. Zhang H, Li Y, Peng T, Aasa M, Zhang L, Yang Y, Archard LC. Localization of enteroviral antigen in myocardium and other tissues from patients with heart muscle disease by an improved immunohistochemical technique. J Histochem Cytochem 2000;48:579-584.

74. Foulis AK, Farquharson MA, Cameron SO, McGill M, Schönke H, Kandolf R. A search for the presence of the enteroviral capsid protein VP1 in pancreases of patients with type 1 (insulindependent) diabetes and pancreases and hearts of infants who died of coxsackieviral myocarditis. Diabetologia 1990;33:290-298.

75. Kandolf R, Klingel K, Zell R, Canu A, Fortmüller U, Hohenadl C, Albrecht M, Reimann B-Y, Franz WM, Heim A, Raab U, McPhee F. Molecular mechanisms in the pathogenesis of enteroviral heart disease: acute and persistent infections. Clin Immunol Immunopathol 1993;68:153-158.

76. Kandolf R, Canu A, Hofschneider PH. Coxsackie B3 virus can replicate in cultured human foetal heart cells and is inhibited by interferon. J Mol Cell Cardiol 1985;17:167-181.

77. Wessely R, Henke A, Zell R, Kandolf R, Knowlton KU. Low-level expression of a mutant coxsackieviral cDNA induces a myocytopathic effect in culture: an approach to the study of enteroviral persistence in cardiac myocytes. Circulation 1998;98:450-457.

78. Arbustini E, Porcu E, Bellini O, Grasso M, Pilotto A, Dal Bello B, Morbini P, Diegoli M, Gavazzi A, Specchia G, Tavazzi L. Enteroviral infection causing fatal myocarditis and subclinical myopathy. Heart 2000;83:86-90.

79. Arbustini E, Grasso M, Porcu E, Bellini O, Diegoli M, Fasani R, Banchieri N, Pilotto A, Morbini P, Dal Bello B, Campana C, Gavazzi A, Vigano M. Enteroviral RNA and virus-like particles in the skeletal muscle of patients with idiopathic dilated cardiomyopathy. Am J Cardiol 1997;80:1188-1193.

80. Hofschneider PH, Klingel K, Kandolf R. Toward understanding the pathogenesis of enterovirus-induced cardiomyopathy: molecular and ultrastructural approaches. J Struct Biol 1990;104:32-37.

81. Klingel K, Kandolf R. Molecular in situ localization techniques in diagnosis and pathogenecity studies of enteroviral heart disease. Clin Diagn Virol 1996;5:157-166.

82. Ukimura A, Deguchi H, Kitaura Y, Fujioka S, Hirasawa M, Kawamura K, Hirai K. Intracellular viral localization in murine coxsackievirus-B3 myocarditis. Ultrastructural study by electron microscopic in situ hybridization. Am J Pathol 1997;150:2061-2074.

83. Klingel K, Selinka HC, Huber M, Sauter M, Leube M, Kandolf R. Molecular pathology and structural features of enteroviral replication. Toward understanding the pathogenesis of viral heart disease. Herz 2000;25:216-220.

84. Vuorinen T, Vainionpää R, Kettinen H, Hyypiä T. Coxsackievirus B3 infection in human leukocytes and lymphoid cell lines. Blood 1994;84:823-829.

85. Heim A, Brehm C, Stille-Siegener M, Müller G, Hake S, Kandolf R, Figulla HR. Cultured human myocardial fibroblasts of pediatric origin: natural human interferon-alpha is more effective than recombinant interferon-alpha 2a in carrier-state coxsackievirus B3 replication. J Mol Cell Cardiol 1995;27:2199-2208.

86. Klump WM, Bergmann I, Müller BC, Ameis D, Kandolf R. Complete nucleotide sequence of infectious Coxsackievirus B3 cDNA: two initial 5' uridine residues are regained during plus-strand RNA synthesis. J Virol 1990;64:1573-1583.

87. Franz WM, Breves D, Klingel K, Brem G, Hofschneider PH, Kandolf R. Heart-specific targeting of firefly luciferase by the myosin light chain-2 promoter and developmental regulation in transgenic mice. Circ Res 1993;73:629-638.

88. Franz WM, Brem G, Katus HA, Klingel K, Hofschneider PH, Kandolf R. Characterization of a cardiac-selective and developmentally upregulated promoter in transgenic mice. Cardioscience 1994;5:235-243.

89. Wessely R, Klingel K, Santana LF, Dalton N, Hongo M, Lederer WJ, Kandolf R, Knowlton KU. Transgenic expression of replication-restricted enteroviral genomes in heart muscle induces defective excitation-contraction coupling and dilated cardiomyopathy. J Clin Invest 1998;102:1444-1453.

90. Lamphear BJ, Yan R, Yang F, Waters D, Liebig HD, Klump H, Kuechler E, Skern T, Rhoads RE. Mapping the cleavage site in protein synthesis initiation factor eIF-4 gamma of the 2A proteases from human Coxsackievirus and rhinovirus. J Biol Chem 1993;268:19200-19203.

91. Joachims M, Van Breugel PC, Lloyd RE. Cleavage of poly(A)-binding protein by enterovirus proteases concurrent with inhibition of translation in vitro. J Virol 1999;73:718-727.

92. Badorff C, Lee GH, Lamphear BJ, Martone ME, Campbell KP, Rhoads RE, Knowlton KU. Enteroviral protease 2A cleaves dystrophin: evidence of cytoskeletal disruption in an acquired cardiomyopathy. Nat Med 1999;5:320-326.

93. Huber M, Watson KA, Selinka HC, Carthy CM, Klingel K, McManus BM, Kandolf R. Cleavage of RasGAP and phosphorylation of mitogen-activated protein kinase in the course of coxsackievirus B3 replication. J Virol 1999;73:3587-3594.

94. de Leeuw N, Melchers WJ, Balk AH, de Jonge N, Galama JM. Study on microbial persistence in end-stage idiopathic dilated cardiomyopathy. Clin Infect Dis 1999;29:522-525.

95. Okada I, Matsumori A, Kyu B. Detection of viral RNA in experimental coxsackievirus B3 myocarditis of mice using the polymerase chain reaction. Int J Exp Pathol 1992;73:721-731.

96. Leparc I, Fuchs F, Kopecka H, Aymard M. Use of the polymerase chain reaction with a murine model of picornavirus-induced myocarditis. J Clin Microbiol 1993;31:2890-2894.

97. Klingel K, Stephan S, Sauter M, Zell R, McManus BM, Bültmann B, Kandolf R. Pathogenesis of murine enterovirus myocarditis: virus dissemination and immune cell targets. J Virol 1996;70:8888-8895.

98. Andreoletti L, Hober D, Becquart P, Belaich S, Copin MC, Lambert V, Wattre P. Experimental CVB3-induced chronic myocarditis in two murine strains: evidence of interrelationships between virus replication and myocardial damage in persistent cardiac infection. J Med Virol 1997;52:206-214.

99. Werner GS, Figulla HR, Munz DL, Klingel K, Kandolf R, Emrich D, Kreuzer H. Myocardial indium-111 antimyosin uptake in patients with idiopathic dilated cardiomyopathy: its relation to haemodynamics, histomorphometry, myocardial enteroviral infection, and clinical course. Eur Heart J 1993;14:175-184.

100. Rotbart HA. Enzymatic RNA amplification of the enteroviruses. J Clin Microbiol 1990;28:438-442.

101. Chapman NM, Tracy S, Gauntt CJ, Fortmüller U. Molecular detection and identification of enteroviruses using enzymatic amplification and nucleic acid hybridization. J Clin Microbiol 1990;28:843-850.

102. Redline RW, Genest DR, Tycko B. Detection of enteroviral infection in paraffin-embedded tissue by the RNA polymerase chain reaction technique. Am J Clin Pathol 1991;96:568-571.

103. Shimizu H, Schnurr DP, Burns JC. Comparison of methods to detect enteroviral genome in frozen and fixed myocardium by polymerase chain reaction. Lab Invest 1994;71:612-616.

104. Nicholson F, Ajetunmobi JF, Li M, Shackleton EA, Starkey WG, Illavia SJ, Muir P, Banatvala JE. Molecular detection and serotypic analysis of enterovirus RNA in archival specimens from patients with acute myocarditis. Br Heart J 1995;74:522-527.

105. Nicholson F, Meetoo G, Aiyar S, Banatvala JE, Muir P. Detection of enterovirus RNA in clinical samples by nested polymerase chain reaction for rapid diagnosis of enterovirus infection. J Virol Methods 1994;48:155-166.

106. Arola A, Santti J, Ruuskanen O, Halonen P, Hyypiä T. Identification of enteroviruses in clinical specimens by competitive PCR followed by genetic typing using sequence analysis. J Clin Microbiol 1996;34:313-318.

107. Santti J, Vainionpää R, Hyypiä T. Molecular detection and typing of human picornaviruses. Virus Res 1999;62:177-183.

108. Fujioka S, Koide H, Kitaura Y, Deguchi H, Kawamura K, Hirai K. Molecular detection and differentiation of enteroviruses in endomyocardial biopsies and pericardial effusions from dilated cardiomyopathy and myocarditis. Am Heart J 1996;131:760-765.

109. Archard LC, Khan MA, Soteriou BA, Zhang H, Why HJ, Robinson NM, Richardson PJ. Characterization of Coxsackie B virus RNA in myocardium from patients with dilated cardiomyopathy by nucleotide sequencing of reverse transcription-nested polymerase chain reaction products. Hum Pathol 1998;29:578-584.

110. Shen S, Desselberger U, McKee TA. The development of an antigen capture polymerase chain reaction assay to detect and type human enteroviruses. J Virol Methods 1997;65:139-144.

111. Quiros E, Piedrola G, Maroto MC. Detection of enteroviral RNA by a new single-step PCR. Scand J Clin Lab Invest 1997;57:415-419.

112. Bourlet T, Omar S, Grattard F, Pozzetto B. Detection of coxsackievirus B3 in intestinal tissue of orally-infected mice by a standardized RT-PCR assay. Clin Diagn Virol 1997;8:143-150.

113. Reetoo KN, Osman SA, Illavia SJ, Banatvala JE, Muir P. Development and evaluation of quantitative-competitive PCR for quantitation of coxsackievirus B3 RNA in experimentally infected murine tissues. J Virol Methods 1999;82:145-156.

114. Monpoeho S, Dehee A, Mignotte B, Schwartzbrod L, Marechal V, Nicolas JC, Billaudel S, Ferre V. Quantification of enterovirus RNA in sludge samples using single tube real-time RT-PCR. Biotechniques 2000;29:88-93.

115. Andreoletti L, Hober D, Belaich S, Lobert PE, Dewilde A, Wattre P. Rapid detection of enterovirus in clinical specimens using PCR and microwell capture hybridization assay. J Virol Methods 1996;62:1-10.

116. Muir P, Ras A, Klapper PE, Cleator GM, Korn K, Aepinus C, Fomsgaard A, Palmer P, Samuelsson A, Tenorio A, Weissbrich B, van Loon AM. Multicenter quality assessment of PCR methods for detection of enteroviruses. J Clin Microbiol 1999;37:1409-1414.

117. Chiang FT, Lin LI, Tseng YZ, Tseng CD, Hsu KL, Wu TL, Ho SW. Detection of enterovirus RNA in patients with idiopathic dilated cardiomyopathy by polymerase chain reaction. J Formos Med Assoc 1992;91:569-574.

118. Petitjean J, Kopecka H, Freymuth F, Langlard JM, Scanu P, Galateau F, Bouhour JB, Ferrière M, Charbonneau P, Komajda M. Detection of enteroviruses in endomyocardial biopsy by molecular approach. J Med Virol 1993;41:260.

119. Andreoletti L, Hober D, Decoene C, Copin MC, Lobert PE, Dewilde A, Stankowiac C, Wattre P. Detection of enteroviral RNA by polymerase chain reaction in endomyocardial tissue of patients with chronic cardiac diseases. J Med Virol 1996;48:53-59.

120. de Leeuw N, Melchers WJ, Balk AH, de Jonge N, Galama JM. No evidence for persistent enterovirus infection in patients with end-stage idiopathic dilated cardiomyopathy. J Infect Dis 1998;178:256-259.

121. Weiss LM, Liu XF, Chang KL, Billingham ME. Detection of enteroviral RNA in idiopathic dilated cardiomyopathy and other human cardiac tissues. J Clin Invest 1992;90:156-159.

122. Grasso M, Arbustini E, Silini E, Diegoli M, Percivalle E, Ratti G, Bramerio M, Gavazzi A, Vigano M, Milanesi G. Search for Coxsackievirus B3 RNA in idiopathic dilated cardiomyopathy using gene amplification by polymerase chain reaction. Am J Cardiol 1992;69:658-664.

123. Liljeqvist JA, Bergstrom T, Holmstrom S, Samuelson A, Yousef GE, Waagstein F, Jeansson S. Failure to demonstrate enterovirus aetiology in Swedish patients with dilated cardiomyopathy. J Med Virol 1993;39:6-10.

124. Jin O, Sole MJ, Butany JW, Chia WK, McLaughlin PR, Liu P, Liew CC. Detection of enterovirus RNA in myocardial biopsies from patients with myocarditis and cardiomyopathy using gene amplification by polymerase chain reaction. Circulation 1990;82:8-16.

125. Weiss LM, Movahed LA, Billingham ME, Cleary ML. Detection of Coxsackievirus B3 RNA in myocardial tissues by the polymerase chain reaction. Am J Pathol 1991;138:497-503.

126. Petitjean J, Kopecka H, Freymuth F, Langlard JM, Scanu P, Galateau F, Bouhour JB, Ferrière M, Charbonneau P, Komajda M. Detection of enteroviruses in endomyocardial biopsy by molecular approach. J Med Virol 1992;37:76-82.

127. Giacca M, Severini GM, Mestroni L, Salvi A, Lardieri G, Falaschi A, Camerini F. Low frequency of detection by nested polymerase chain reaction of enterovirus ribonucleic acid in endomyocardial tissue of patients with idiopathic dilated cardiomyopathy. J Am Coll Cardiol 1994;24:1033-1040.

128. Satoh M, Tamura G, Segawa I. Enteroviral RNA in endomyocardial biopsy tissues of myocarditis and dilated cardiomyopathy. Pathol Int 1994;44:345-351.

129. Ueno H, Yokota Y, Shiotani H, Yokoyama M, Itoh H, Ishido S, Maeda S, Katayama Y, Hotta H. Significance of detection of enterovirus RNA in myocardial tissues by reverse transcription-polymerase chain reaction. Int J Cardiol 1995;51:157-164.

130. Pauschinger M, Dörner A, Kühl U, Schwimmbeck PL, Poller W, Kandolf R, Schultheiss HP. Enteroviral RNA replication in the myocardium of patients with left ventricular dysfunction and clinically suspected myocarditis. Circulation 1999;99:889-895.

131. Li Y, Bourlet T, Andreoletti L, Mosnier JF, Peng T, Yang Y, Archard LC, Pozzetto B, Zhang H. Enteroviral capsid protein VP1 is present in myocardial tissues from some patients with myocarditis or dilated cardiomyopathy. Circulation 2000;101:231-234.

132. Keeling PJ, Jeffery S, Caforio AL, Taylor R, Bottazzo GF, Davies MJ, McKenna WJ. Similar prevalence of enteroviral genome within the myocardium from patients with idiopathic dilated cardiomyopathy and controls by the polymerase chain reaction. Br Heart J 1992;68:554-559.

133. Zoll GJ, Melchers WJ, Kopecka H, Jambroes G, van der Poel HJ, Galama JM. General primer-mediated polymerase chain reaction for detection of enteroviruses: application for diagnostic routine and persistent infections. J Clin Microbiol 1992;30:160-165.

134. Schwaiger A, Umlauft F, Weyrer K, Larcher C, Lyons J, Mühlberger V, Dietze O, Grunewald K. Detection of enteroviral ribonucleic acid in myocardial biopsies from patients with idiopathic dilated cardiomyopathy by polymerase chain reaction. Am Heart J 1993;126:406-410.

135. Khan M, Why H, Richardson P, Archard L. Nucleotide sequencing of PCR products shows the presence of Coxsackie-B3 virus in endomyocardial biopsies from patients with myocarditis or dilated cardiomyopathy. Biochem Soc Trans 1994;22:176S.

136. Satoh M, Tamura G, Segawa I, Hiramori K, Satodate R. Enteroviral RNA in dilated cardiomyopathy. Eur Heart J 1994;15:934-939.

137. Satoh M, Tamura G, Segawa I, Tashiro A, Hiramori K, Satodate R. Expression of cytokine genes and presence of enteroviral genomic RNA in endomyocardial biopsy tissues of myocarditis and dilated cardiomyopathy. Virchows Arch 1996;427:503-509.

138. Arola A, Kallajoki M, Ruuskanen O, Hyypiä T. Detection of enteroviral RNA in end-stage dilated cardiomyopathy in children and adolescents. J Med Virol 1998;56:364-371.

139. Pauschinger M, Kühl U, Dörner A, Schieferecke K, Petschauer S, Rauch U, Schwimmbeck PL, Kandolf R, Schultheiss HP. Detection of enteroviral RNA in endomyocardial biopsies in inflammatory cardiomyopathy and idiopathic dilated cardiomyopathy. Z Kardiol 1998;87:443-452.

140. Terasaki F, Okabe M, Hayashi T, Fujioka S, Suwa M, Hirota Y, Kitaura Y, Kawamura K, Isomura T, Suma H. Myocardial inflammatory cell infiltrates in cases of dilated cardiomyopathy: light microscopic, immunohistochemical, and virological analyses of myocardium specimens obtained by partial left ventriculectomy. J Card Surg 1999;14:141-146.

141. Calabrese F, Valente M, Thiene G, Angelini A, Testolin L, Biasolo MA, Soteriou B, Livi U, Palu G. Enteroviral genome in native hearts may influence outcome of patients who undergo cardiac transplantation. Diagn Mol Pathol 1999;8:39-46.

142. Grumbach IM, Heim A, Vonhof S, Stille-Siegener M, Mall G, Gonska BD, Kreuzer H, Andreas S, Figulla HR. Coxsackievirus genome in myocardium of patients with arrhythmogenic right ventricular dysplasia/cardiomyopathy. Cardiology 1998;89:241-245.

143. Calabrese F, Angelini A, Thiene G, Basso C, Nava A, Valente M. No detection of enteroviral genome in the myocardium of patients with arrhythmogenic right ventricular cardiomyopathy. J Clin Pathol 2000;53:382-387.

144. Why HJ, Meany BT, Richardson PJ, Olsen EG, Bowles NE, Cunningham L, Freeke CA, Archard LC. Clinical and prognostic significance of detection of enteroviral RNA in the myocardium of patients with myocarditis or dilated cardiomyopathy. Circulation 1994;89:2582-2589.

145. Schmaltz AA, Demel KP, Kallenberg R, Neudorf U, Kandolf R, Klingel K, Bültmann B. Immunosuppressive therapy of chronic myocarditis in children: three cases and the design of a randomized prospective trial of therapy. Pediatr Cardiol 1998;19:235-239.

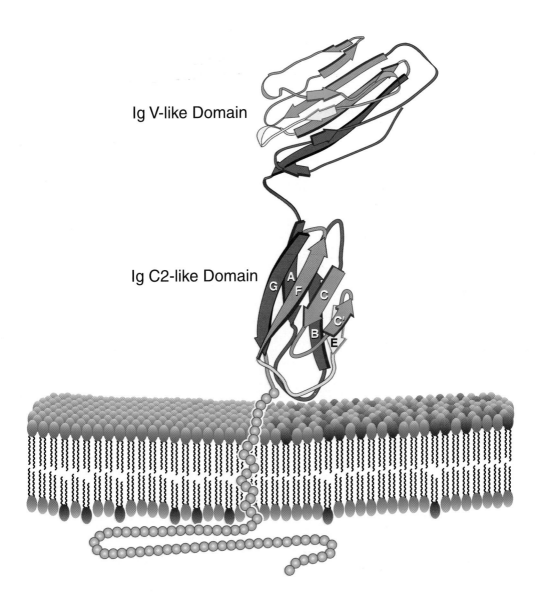

Plate 1, Fig. 2-1. A schematic representation of a feasible structure for the human coxsackievirus and adeno-virus receptor protein is depicted that is derived from the crystal structure of the Ig V-like domain[41] and a prototypical Ig C2-like domain.[42] The V-like and C2-like domains are occasionally referred to as D1 and D2, respectively. The C2-like domain is followed by a predicted single membrane-spanning sequence and a cytoplasmic domain of unknown structure (shown in green). *Flat arrows* are beta-pleated sheets. (p. 27.)

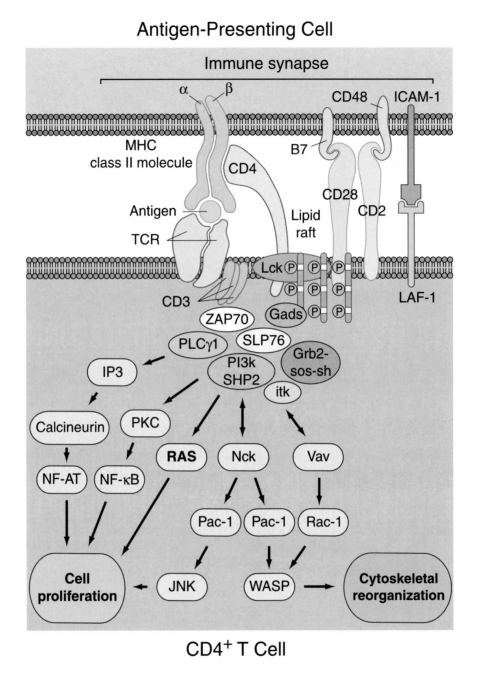

Antigen-Presenting Cell

CD4⁺ T Cell

Plate 2, Fig. 3-3. Signaling pathways in T cells after T-cell receptor (*TCR*) engagement lead to cell proliferation and cytoskeleton reorganization. Adhesion molecules in outer ring of the immune synapse stabilize connection between antigen-presenting cell and T cell. CD28 engagement amplifies signaling, especially in naïve T cells. First T-cell proliferative cycle requires 20 hours of sustained signaling between APC and T cell. Subsequent cell cycles require 6 hours. *MHC*, major histocompatibility complex; *ICAM*, intracellular adhesion molecule; *JNK*, Jun-N-terminal kinase; *NF-AT*, nuclear factor of activated T cells. (Modified from Lanzavecchia and Sallusto.[29] By permission of Excerpta Medica.) (p. 61.)

Plate 3, Fig. 3-4. Activation of virus-specific and autoimmune T cells during myocarditis. Virus infection of the heart should result in direct virus-induced lysis of some cardiocytes with release of sequestered antigens. Viral and self-antigens are taken up by immature dendritic cells (*iDC*), which subsequently are induced to mature by viral dsRNA and proinflammatory cytokines (tumor necrosis factor-α [*TNFα*] and interleukin-1 [*IL-1*]), and migrate out of the heart to draining lymphoid tissues. Before leaving the heart, DCs release chemokines (macrophage inflammatory protein [*MIP*], IL-8, monocyte chemotactic protein [*MCP*]) which stimulate additional monocyte infiltration using chemokine receptors (*CCR-1, CCR-2, CCR-5,* and *CXCR-1*) and differentiation into new DCs. Antigen-loaded mature DCs (*mDC*) enter the lymph node and stimulate both virus-specific and autoreactive T- and B-cell clones. Activated T cells stimulate mDC to higher antigen-presenting cell activity using TRANCE and CD40L. T cells leaving the lymph node migrate to the heart where they directly lyse infected or normal

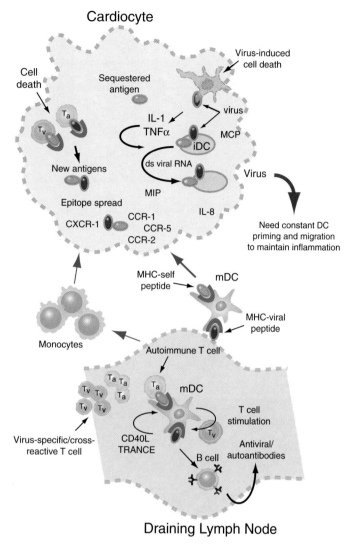

cardiocytes via major histocompatibility complex (*MHC*)-peptide-T-cell receptor interactions and release or induce cytokines, which also can cause significant cardiac dysfunction. Continuous cycles of antigen release, presentation, and lymphocyte stimulation amplify the reaction, resulting in accumulation of cardiac damage. The initial immune response may be primarily directed toward virus epitopes and viral epitopes cross-reactive to self-molecules (antigenic mimicry). However, with increased cardiocyte lysis, release and processing of sequestered self-antigens could stimulate additional autoreactive T-cell clones (epitope spreading). Remission of the initial autoimmune response may be imposed through immune regulation with virus clearing as autoantigen release is diminished without virus-specific immunity and direct viral lysis of cardiocytes. Effector lymphocytes undergo apoptosis when antigen stimulation and growth factors are removed.[99] However, reinfection of the heart with unrelated viruses[100] may trigger memory autoimmune activation as sequestered antigens are released again during the new virus infection. Whether persistent virus infections[101] could maintain chronic inflammatory responses in the heart depends on whether and how much virus antigen is produced or whether and how much self-antigen is released by ongoing autoimmunity. Sufficient antigen must be available and taken up by iDC to continually produce new effector lymphocytes. (Modified from Lanzavecchia and Sallusto.[29] By permission of Excerpta Medica.) (p. 68.)

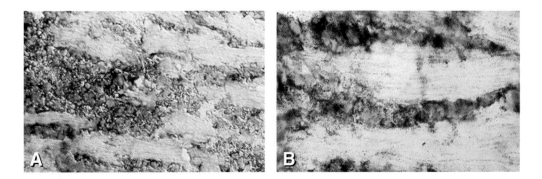

Plate 4, Fig. 4-1. Cryostat sections demonstrate CD4-positive lymphocytes in chronic myocarditis by using monoclonal antibodies to CD4 (Becton Dickinson, NJ, USA). *A*, Low magnification (x80). *B*, High magnification (x400). (From Maisch et al.[5] By permission of Urban & Vogel. (p. 79.)

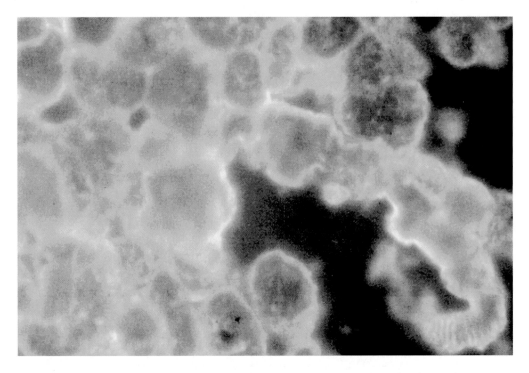

Plate 5, Fig. 4-4. Demonstration of IgG binding (fluorescein isothiocyanate-labeled F[ab]2 antihuman IgG) in dilated cardiomyopathy with inflammation. (From Maisch et al.[5] By permission of Urban & Vogel.) (p. 94.)

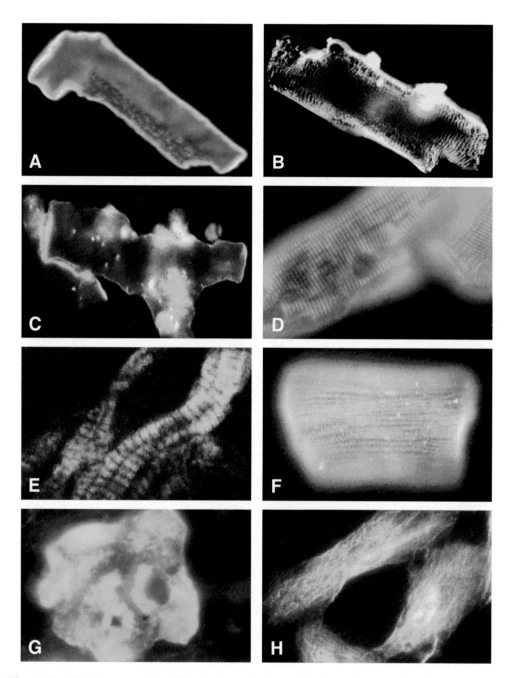

Plate 6, Fig. 4-2. Demonstration of circulating antibodies to the *A*, sarcolemma and myolemma with isolated rat cardiocytes; *B*, laminin with isolated rat cardiocytes; *C*, specific positive staining of the sarcolemma with isolated Purkinje (dog) fibers; *D*, myosin with isolated rat cardiocytes; *E*, actin with isolated rat cardiocytes; *F*, anti-interfibrillary staining (eg, antimitochondrial or anticytoplasmic antibodies against isolated rat cardiomyocytes; *G*, intracellular staining of Purkinje fibers in bovine false tendon; and *H*, antiendothelial staining on Hep2 cells. (Magnification x400.) (2 *A* and *C-H* from Maisch et al.[5] By permission of Urban & Vogel. 2 *B* from Maisch.[9] By permission of Springer-Verlag.) (p. 86.)

Sarcolemma

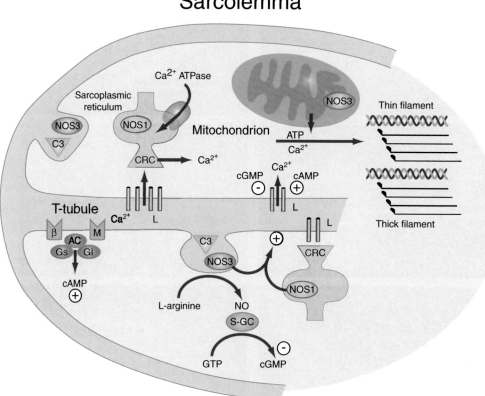

Plate 7, Fig. 6-1. Location and action of nitric oxide synthase (*NOS*) isoforms in the cardiac myocyte. The action potential initiated in the sinoatrial node opens a sarcolemmal Ca^{2+} pore (L-type channel). Ca^{2+} entering the myocyte (I_{Ca}) binds to the sarcoplasmic reticulum (SR) calcium release channel (*CRC*) and triggers a large release of Ca^{2+}, which in turn initiates myofilament contraction (excitation-contraction coupling). Systole (contraction phase) terminates when Ca^{2+} is actively pumped back into the SR by the calcium reuptake pump (Ca^{2+}-ATPase). Cyclic AMP (*cAMP*) stimulates contraction, partly by activation of the L-type Ca^{2+} channel. Increases in cAMP are produced by β-adrenergic coupling to adenylyl cyclase via a stimulatory G protein. cAMP effects are offset by inhibitory G proteins and cGMP, which is produced by particulate and soluble guanylyl cyclases, sensitive to natriuretic peptides and nitric oxide (*NO*), respectively. NO or related molecules also activate the L-type Ca^{2+} channel and CRC and inhibit the Ca^{2+}-ATPase by S-nitrosylation, thiol oxidation, or both. Alternative isoforms of NOS subserve different functions by virtue of their subcellular localization: NOS1 localizes to the SR (with the Ca^{2+}-ATPase and the CRC)[5] and NOS3 to the sarcolemma/T-tubule network (in proximity to the L-type channel)[6] and to mitochondria (ie, with the respiratory complexes).[7] *AC,* adenylyl cyclase; *β,* β-adrenergic receptor; *C3,* caveolin-3; *G$_i$,* inhibitory G protein; *G$_s$,* stimulatory G protein; *L,* L-type Ca^{2+} channel; *M,* muscarinic receptor; *S-GC,* soluble guanylyl cyclase. (From Hare JM, Stamler JS. NOS: modulator, not mediator of cardiac performance. Nat Med 1999;5:273-274. By permission of Nature America.) (p. 138.)

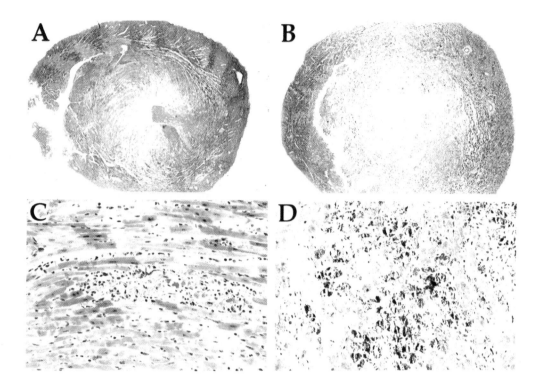

Plate 8, Fig. 6-3. Myocarditis in wild-type and NOS2 null mice. Wild-type mice (*A* and *C*) and NOS2 null mice (*B* and *D*) were infected with 107 pfu CVB3. Hearts were harvested and tissue sections were stained. (Hematoxylin and eosin; *A* and *B*, x40; *C* and *D*, x240.) (p. 149.)

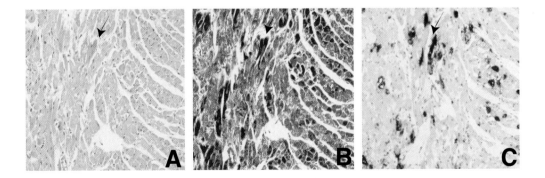

Plate 9, Fig. 7-1. Serial sections stained with hematoxylin and eosin (*A*) and Masson trichrome (*B*) or studied by in situ hybridization for viral RNA (*C*). Patchy areas of myocardial damage (*arrows*) are colocalized to active viral infection (*arrows*). (x50.) (p. 164.)

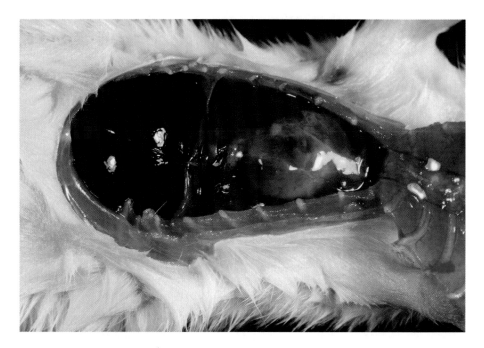

Plate 10, Fig. 8-2. Gross pathology of rat experimental autoimmune myocarditis. Massive pericardial effusion and discoloration of cardiac surface are evident. (p. 201.)

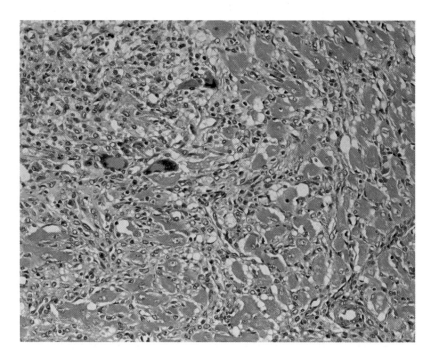

Plate 11, Fig. 8-3. Histologic findings of rat experimental autoimmune myocarditis. Multinucleated giant cells are observed in the lesion. (Hematoxylin and eosin; x200.) (p. 203.)

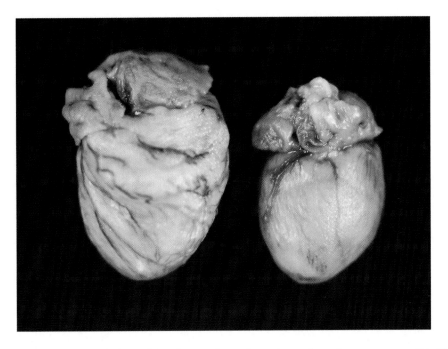

Plate 12, Fig. 8-8. Gross pathology of the chronic phase of experimental autoimmune myocarditis (*left*). Heart of an age-matched control rat (*right*). (p. 209.)

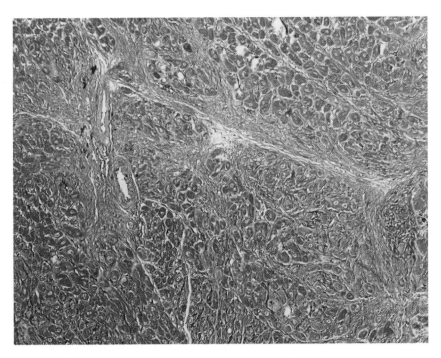

Plate 13, Fig. 8-9. Histologic findings of the chronic phase of experimental autoimmune myocarditis. (Azan-Mallory stain; x100.) (p. 209.)

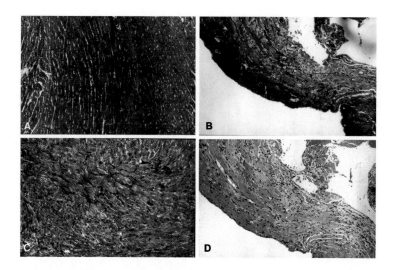

Plate 14, Fig. 10-1. Cardiomyopathy in the ventricles of coxsackievirus B (CVB) transgenic mice. Ventricular histologic findings in nontransgenic (*A*) and CVB transgenic (*B-D*) mice were analyzed with trichrome stain (*A-C*) and hematoxylin and eosin stain (*D*). There is mild (*B*) to extensive (*C* and *D*) interstitial fibrosis in the ventricles. (*A* and *C*, x200; *B* and *D*, x40.) (From Wessely R, Klingel K, Santana LF, Dalton N, Hongo M, Lederer WJ, Kandolf R, Knowlton KU. Transgenic expression of replication-restricted enteroviral genomes in heart muscle induces defective excitation-contraction coupling and dilated cardiomyopathy. J Clin Invest 1998;102:1444-1453. By permission of the American Society for Clinical Investigation.) (p. 237.)

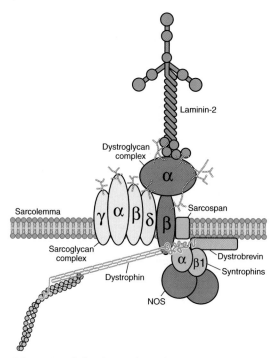

Plate 15, Fig. 10-2. Schematic of the dystrophin-glycoprotein complex (see text for description). *NOS*, nitric oxide synthase. (p. 241.)

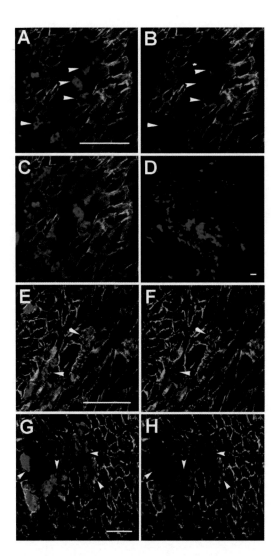

Plate 16, Fig. 10-4. The sarcolemmal integrity is impaired and dystrophin, α-sarcoglycan, and β-dystroglycan staining are disrupted in infected myocytes from severe combined immunodeficient (SCID) mice. *A-D*, SCID mouse heart infected with coxsackievirus B3 and injected with Evans blue dye 7 d later. *A-C*, Confocal images of the same high-power field. *A*, Dual stain using an antibody against coxsackievirus B3 (blue fluorescence) and an antibody against dystrophin (green fluorescence). *B*, Dystrophin immunostain only. The dystrophin staining pattern is disrupted in the virally infected myocytes (*arrowheads, A and B*). *C*, Superimposed triple fluorescence with Evans blue dye (red) uptake specifically in the virally infected cells. *D*, Lower-magnification, nonconfocal image shows many cells with Evans dye uptake (bright red) in an infected mouse heart; surrounding uninfected myocytes have a faint background fluorescence. *E-H*, Hearts from coxsackievirus B3-infected SCID mice collected 7 d after infection and dual-stained with an antibody against coxsackievirus B3 (red fluorescence, *E* and *G*) and an antibody against α-sarcoglycan (green fluorescence, *E* and *F*) or an antibody against β-dystroglycan (green fluorescence, *G* and *H*). *E* and *G*, Superimposed red and green fluorescence. *F* and *H*, Only the stain for α-sarcoglycan (*F*) or β-dystroglycan (*H*). The α-sarcoglycan and β-dystroglycan staining patterns are disrupted in virally infected cells (*arrowheads, E-H*). Scale bars represent 50 μm. (From Badorff et al.[65] By permission of Nature America.) (p. 244.)

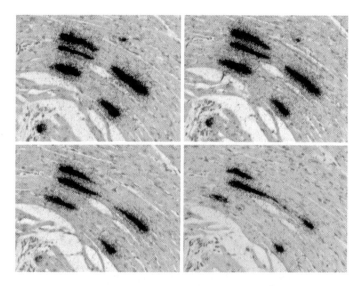

Plate 17, Fig. 13-3. Visualization of coxsackievirus B (CVB)3 RNA in 5-μm-thick tissue sections of a paraffin-embedded mouse heart by ^{35}S-labeled CVB3 cDNA probes. By radioactive in situ hybridization, the identical infected myocyte can usually be detected in more than 2 consecutive heart muscle sections. (x130.) (p. 301.)

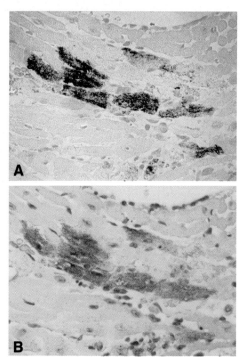

Plate 18, Fig. 13-4. In situ detection of coxsackievirus B (CVB)3 RNA on 2 consecutive myocardial tissue sections by different nonisotopic in situ hybridization assays. *A*, The visualization of biotin-labeled CVB3 cDNA probes by immunogold-silver staining. *B*, Streptavidin-alkaline phosphatase-new fuchsin in the same myocytes reflects the comparable sensitivity of both nonradioactive detection methods. (x300.) (p. 303.)

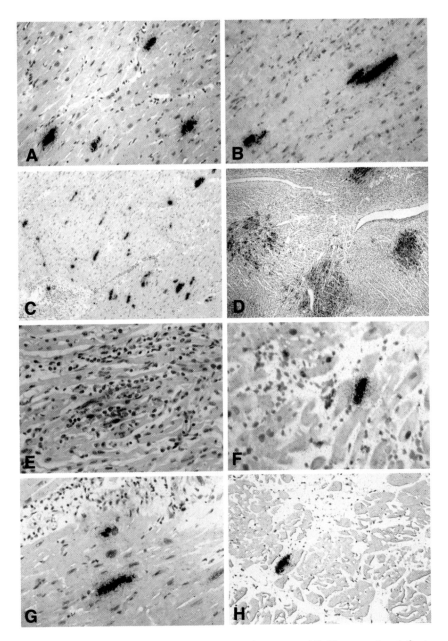

Plate 19, Fig. 13-5. Patterns of acute (*A, B, C, D, F*) and persistent (*G, H*) enterovirus infections of the human heart as detected by radioactive in situ hybridization. Evasion of the virus from the immune response induces a persistent infection as detected in the late phase of acute myocarditis (*G*) and DCM (*H*). The autoradiographic silver grains, indicating hybridization between viral RNA and an ^{35}S-labeled enterovirus-specific hybridization probe, are clearly localized to distinct infected myocardial cells, thus providing an unequivocal diagnosis of myocardial enterovirus infection. Because of high translation rates of viral RNA in acutely infected cells, enteroviral proteins[70] may be detected by immunohistochemistry in single myocytes of patients with fulminant enterovirus myocarditis (*E*). (*A, B, H*, x160; *C*, x25; *D*, x6; *E* and *F*, x200; *G*, x180.) (*B, C, F* from Kandolf et al.[69] By permission of Elsevier Science.) (p. 305.)

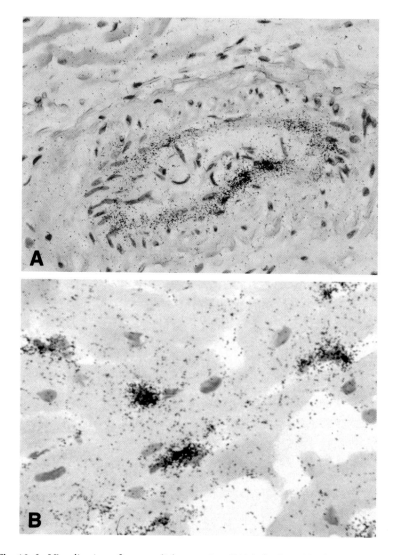

Plate 20, Fig. 13-6. Visualization of myocardial parvovirus B19 infection. Viral DNA can be detected by radioactive in situ hybridization in endothelial cells of small intramural vessels (*A*) as well as in interstitial cells (*B*) of heart from patients who have acute myocarditis. (*A*, x200; *B*, x500.) (p. 306.)

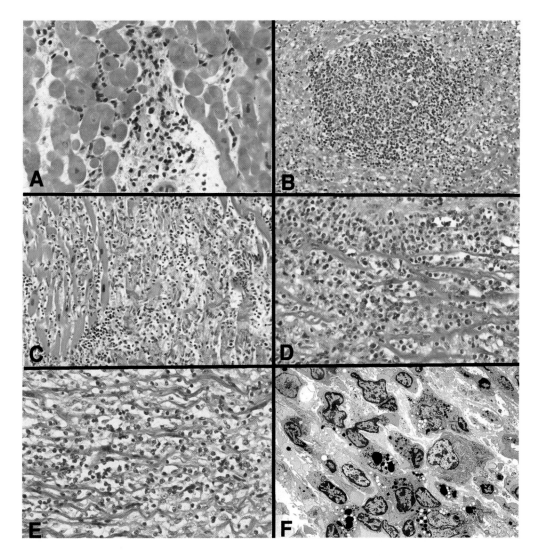

Plate 21, Fig. 14-1. Idiopathic lymphocytic myocarditis. *A*, Borderline myocarditis with sparse perivascular lymphocytic infiltrate but no myocyte damage. (x400.) *B*, Focal active lymphocytic myocarditis composed of a circumscribed nodule of mononuclear cells resulting in architectural distortion and myocyte damage. (x200.) *C*, Diffuse lymphocytic myocarditis shows interstitial inflammatory infiltrates and damage. (x300.) *D*, High-power magnification of myocyte damage and inflammation. (x400.) *E*, Diffuse lymphocytic myocarditis in a 4-month-old infant after viral-like infection. (x400.) *F*, Transmission electron photomicrograph shows numerous lymphocytes replacing myocardial tissue. (x3,400.) (*A* through *E*, hematoxylin and eosin.) (p. 334.)

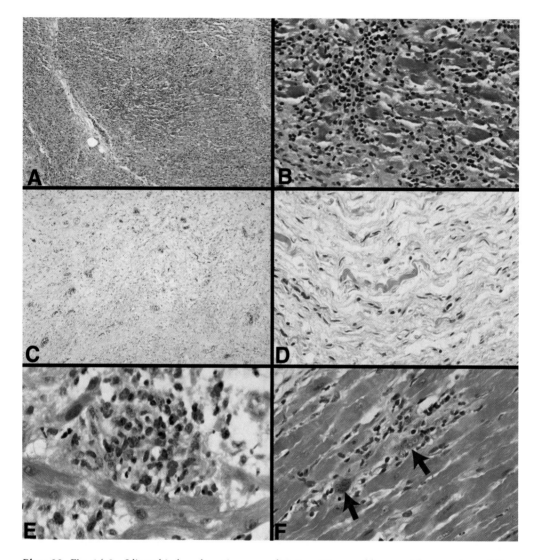

Plate 22, Fig. 14-2. Idiopathic lymphocytic myocarditis in a 28-year-old man with severe heart failure after upper respiratory tract infection. *A,* The right ventricular endomyocardial biopsy specimen and left apical specimen obtained at placement of a left ventricular assist device show florid lymphocytic myocarditis. (x100.) *B,* High-power magnification shows dense interstitial inflammation and abundant myocyte necrosis. (x400.) *C,* Postmortem left ventricular section 3 months after initial biopsy. The ventricle revealed complete replacement by dense scar tissue. (x100.) *D,* High-power magnification of isolated myocyte fibers surrounded by fibroblasts and scar tissue. (x400.) *E,* An example of lymphocytic myocarditis containing scattered eosinophils. (x400.) *F,* A case of lymphocytic myocarditis with a giant cell of myogenic origin (*arrows*). (x400.) (*A* through *F,* hematoxylin and eosin. (p. 335.)

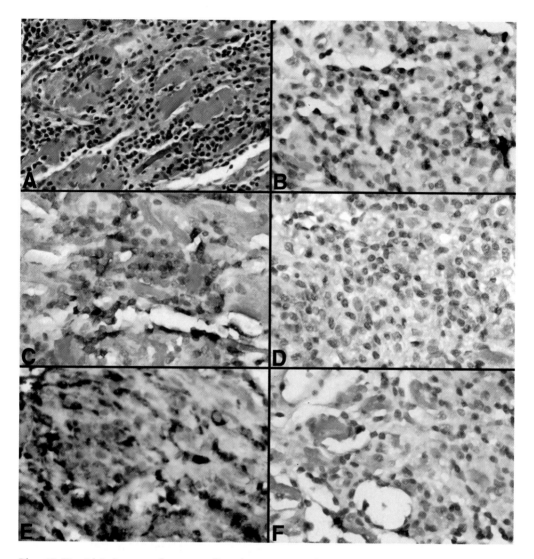

Plate 23, Fig. 14-3. Immunophenotype of lymphocytic myocarditis. *A,* High-power magnification demonstrates myocyte damage and inflammatory cell infiltrate. (Hematoxylin and eosin.) *B,* CD3⁺ staining of numerous T cells within infiltrate. *C,* CD8⁺ cytotoxic cells predominate in the infiltrate. *D,* Scattered CD4⁺ helper T cells are seen. *E,* Variable numbers of CD68⁺ macrophages within the infiltrate. *F,* Absence of CD20⁺ B cells in lymphocytic myocarditis. (*A* through *F,* x400.) (p. 337.)

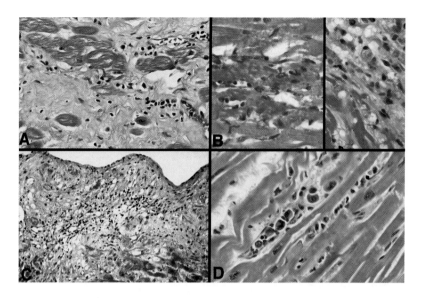

Plate 24, Fig. 14-4. Differential diagnosis of lymphocytic myocarditis. *A*, Scattered lymphocytes within scar tissue in dilated cardiomyopathy. *B, Left panel*: Focus of pressor injury with rare inflammatory cells and conspicuous focal myocyte damage. *Right panel*: Edge of ischemic necrosis containing granulation tissue. *C*, Prior biopsy-site changes with lymphocytes admixed with granulation tissue and early fibrosis. *D*, Metastatic malignant melanoma with interstitial neoplastic infiltrates. (Hematoxylin and eosin; *A*, *B*, and *D*, x400; *C*, x250.) (p. 339.)

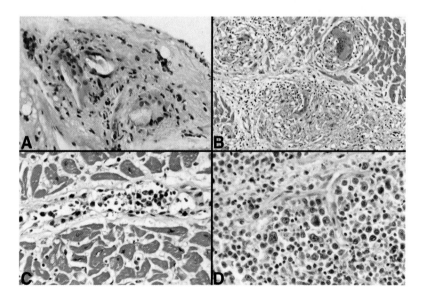

Plate 25, Fig. 14-5. Differential diagnosis of idiopathic giant cell myocarditis. *A*, Multinucleated giant cells centered on foreign material in endomyocardial biopsy specimen from right ventricle. *B*, Cardiac sarcoidosis composed of well-formed granulomas. *C*, Angiotrophic large B-cell lymphoma. *D*, Pleomorphic large B-cell lymphoma with atypical large lymphoid cells replacing myocardial tissue. (Hematoxylin and eosin; *A*, *C*, and *D*, x400; *B*, x200.) (p. 340.)

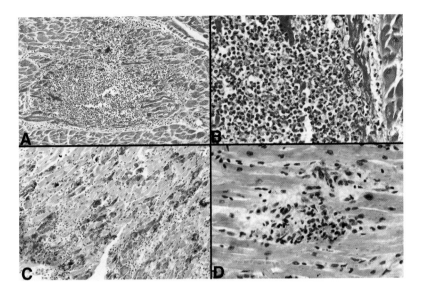

Plate 26, Fig. 14-6. Bacterial myocarditis. *A,* Intermediate magnification shows focal inflammation and myocyte damage in suppurative myocarditis. *B,* Sheets of neutrophils replace the myocardium. *C,* Diphtheritic myocarditis shows streaky myocardial degeneration and infiltrates. *D,* Mononuclear cell infiltrates composed of lymphocytes and histiocytes. (Hematoxylin and eosin; *A* and *C,* x200; *B* and *D,* x400.) (p. 342.)

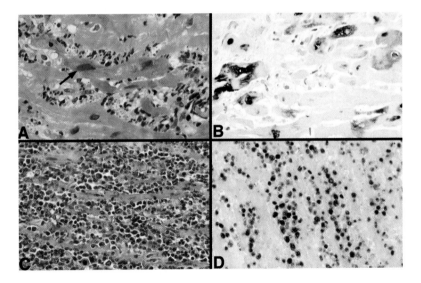

Plate 27, Fig. 14-7. Cytomegalovirus (CMV) myocarditis. *A,* CMV myocarditis shows a mixed inflammatory cell infiltrate and CMV nuclear inclusion within myocyte (*arrow*). *B,* In situ hybridization demonstrates numerous infected myocytes. *C,* Post-transplant lymphoproliferative disorder shows diffuse interstitial infiltrates of atypical large lymphoid cells. *D,* In situ hybridization for *EBER*-1 gene demonstrates the presence of Epstein-Barr virus nuclear sequences in post-transplant lymphoproliferative disorder. (*A* and *C,* hematoxylin and eosin; *A* through *D,* x400.) (p. 345.)

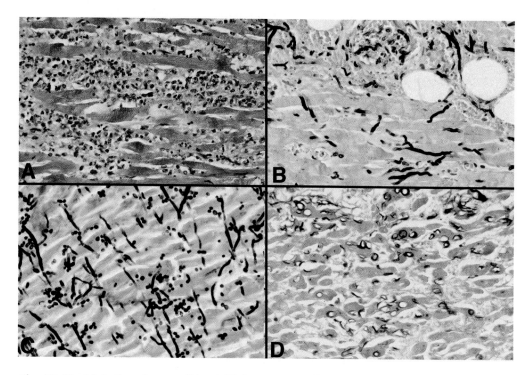

Plate 28, Fig. 14-8. Fungal myocarditis. *A,* High-power magnification shows a mixed inflammatory infiltrate with abundant neutrophils and pyknotic debris. *B,* Aspergillus myocarditis composed of septate dichotomously branching hyphae. *C, Candida* myocarditis shows oval budding yeasts and pseudohyphae. *D,* Mucormycosis myocarditis shows broad, thin-walled hyphae with random branching patterns. (*A,* hematoxylin and eosin; *B* through *D,* Gomori-methenamine-silver; *A* through *D,* x400.) (p. 347.)

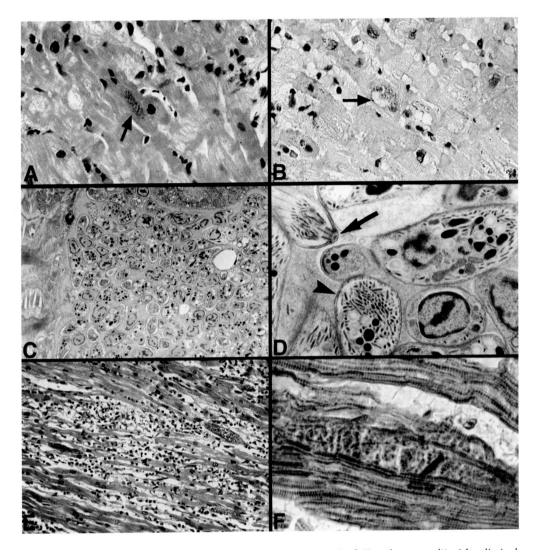

Plate 29, Fig. 14-9. Parasitic myocarditis. *A*, Bradyzoite (*arrow*) of *Toxoplasma gondii* with a limited inflammatory response. (x400.) *B*, Immunohistochemical staining for toxoplasmic cyst (*arrow*). (x400.) *C*, Transmission electron photomicrograph of encysted bradyzoite within a myocyte. (x13,000.) *D*, High-power magnification shows intracystic oval-shaped organisms with double-layered pellicle (*arrowhead*) and conoid (*arrow*). (x42,000.) *E*, Acute Chagas myocarditis shows marked inflammation and pseudocysts. (x200.) *F*, High-power magnification of pseudocyst of *Trypanosoma cruzi*. (x600.) (*A*, *E*, and *F*, hematoxylin and eosin.) (p. 349.)

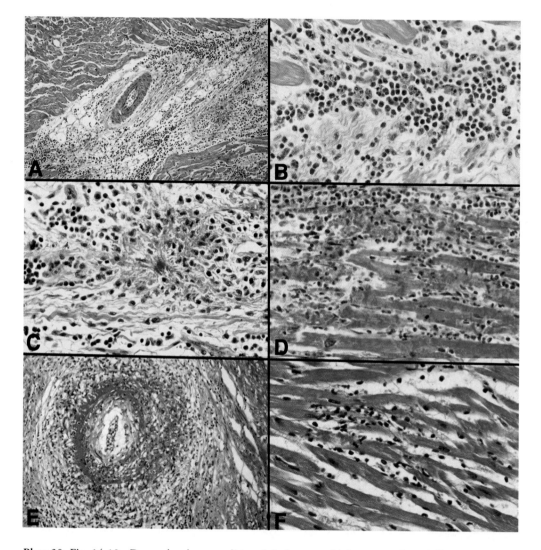

Plate 30, Fig. 14-10. Drug-related myocarditis. *A,* In hypersensitivity myocarditis, diffuse eosinophilic infiltrates are located around perivascular structures. *B,* High-power magnification shows predominance of eosinophils admixed with histiocytes. *C,* Poorly formed granulomas centered on degenerated collagen bundles. *D,* Diffuse eosinophilic myocarditis shows marked myocyte necrosis with numerous interstitial eosinophils. *E,* In toxic myocarditis, necrotizing vasculitis with surrounding mixed inflammatory infiltrate in patient receiving cyclophosphamide. *F,* Acute anthracycline cardiotoxicity shows focal myocarditis. (Hematoxylin and eosin; *A,* x150; *B* through *F,* x400.) (p. 352.)

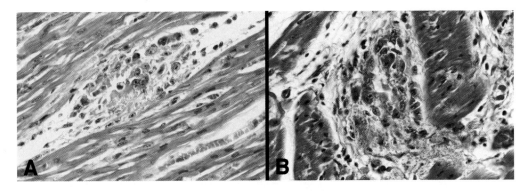

Plate 31, Fig. 14-11. Acute rheumatic myocarditis. *A,* Aschoff nodule composed of circumscribed collection of mononuclear cells distributed along the interstitial tissue planes and perivascular spaces. (x300.) *B,* High-power magnification shows histiocytes and small multinucleated giant cells (Aschoff cells). (x400.) (*A* and *B,* hematoxylin and eosin.) (p. 354.)

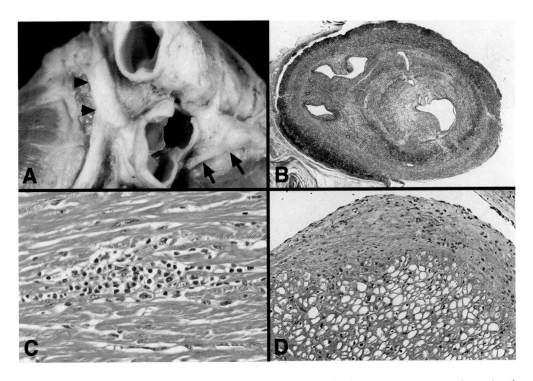

Plate 32, Fig. 14-12. Kawasaki disease. *A,* Aneurysmal dilatation of right main coronary artery (*arrows*) and proximal left anterior descending artery (*arrowheads*) in 18-month-old boy undergoing heart transplantation. *B,* Mid right coronary artery shows recanalization of lumen, disruption of internal elastic membrane, and marked fibrointimal occlusion. (x50.) *C,* Focal lymphocytic myocarditis found as an incidental lesion. (x400.) *D,* Diffuse subendocardial ischemic vacuolar myocyte degeneration. (x300.) (*B,* Elastic van Gieson; *C* and *D,* hematoxylin and eosin.) (p. 355.)

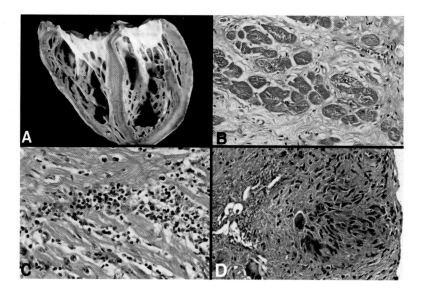

Plate 33, Fig. 14-13. Patterns in cardiac sarcoidosis. *A*, Dilated cardiomyopathy at orthotopic heart transplantation. *B*, Microscopic features of dilated cardiomyopathy, including myocyte hypertrophy and interstitial fibrosis. *C*, Lymphocytic myocarditis. *D*, Noncaseating granulomatous myocarditis contains epithelioid histiocytes, multinucleated giant cells, and scattered lymphocytes surrounded by dense collagen. (*B* and *C*, hematoxylin and eosin; *D*, trichrome; *B* through *D*, x400.) (p. 357.)

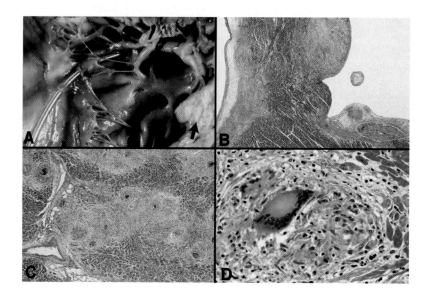

Plate 34, Fig. 14-14. Cardiac sarcoidosis. *A*, Nodular mass-like lesions (*arrows*) within myocardium. *B*, Multiple granulomas within region of atrioventricular node in young man with third degree heart block followed by sudden death. (x100.) *C*, Coalescing noncaseating granulomas within the interventricular septum. (x200.) *D*, Classic noncaseating granuloma of sarcoidosis. (x400.) (*B* through *D*, hematoxylin and eosin.) (p. 357.)

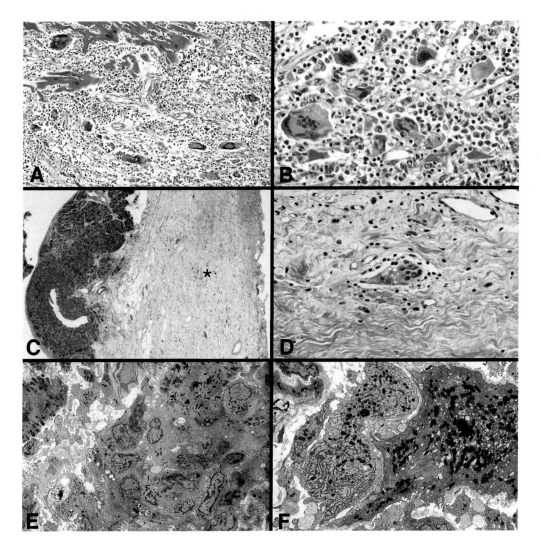

Plate 35, Fig. 14-15. Idiopathic giant cell myocarditis (IGCM). *A*, Scanning magnification shows abundant necrosis, dense infiltrates, and numerous giant cells. (x200.) *B*, Multinucleated giant cells admixed with lymphocytes, eosinophils, plasma cells, histiocytes, and necrotic myocytes. (x400.) *C*, Diffuse fibrous scarring of outer half of myocardium within region of asterisk 3 months after presentation with IGCM. (x100.) *D*, Scattered giant cells, mononuclear cells, and dense collagen bundles. (x400.) *E*, Transmission electron photomicrograph of IGCM shows histiocytes and multinucleated giant cells. (x3,400.) *F*, Histiocytic cell along damaged sarcolemmal membrane. (x27,000.) (*A*, *B*, and *D*, hematoxylin and eosin; *C*, trichrome.) (p. 359.)

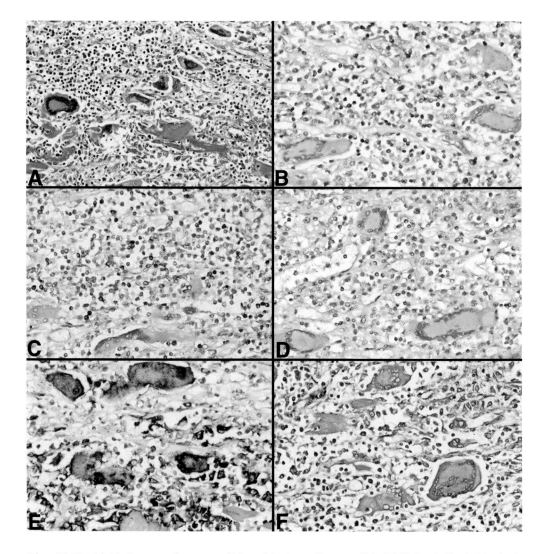

Plate 36, Fig. 14-16. Immunophenotype of idiopathic giant cell myocarditis (IGCM). *A*, Classic histologic features of IGCM. *B*, Numerous CD3$^+$ T cells within infiltrate. *C*, Predominance of CD8$^+$ cytotoxic cells. *D*, Rare CD4$^+$ cells within infiltrate. *E*, CD68$^+$ histiocytes and multinucleated giant cells. *F*, Actin staining of blood vessels but not giant cells. (*A*, Hematoxylin and eosin; *A* through *F*, x400.) (p. 361.)

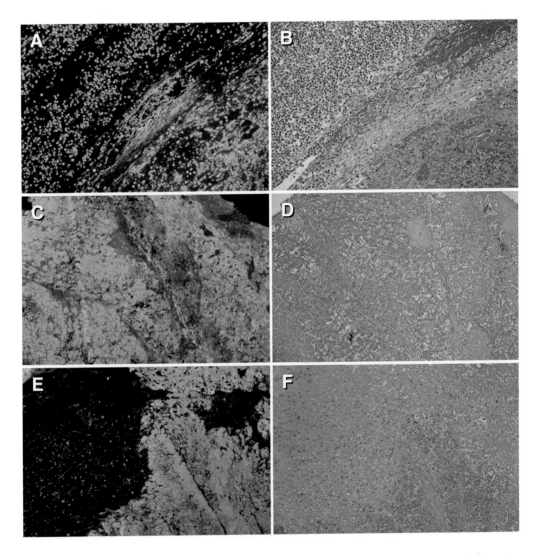

Plate 37, Fig. 19-1. Immunofluorescent localization of eosinophil granule major basic protein in heart tissue. *A* and *B*, Sections of myocardium from a patient with acute necrotizing myocarditis. This case was originally reported by deMello et al.[128] *A*, Section stained with antibody to major basic protein (*MBP*). Note the intracellular MBP staining of numerous eosinophils and the localization of extracellular MBP around myocardial fibers and sarcolemmal membranes. *B*, Section serial to *A* stained with hematoxylin and eosin. Large numbers of intact eosinophils and degenerating myofibers are evident. *C* through *F*, Sections of ventricular thrombus from a patient with eosinophilic endomyocardial disease. This case was originally reported by Wright et al.[129] *C* and *E*, Sections stained with antibody to MBP. Note the extensive, diffuse localization of MBP in *C* and the focal localization in *E*. *D* and *F*, Sections serial to *C* and *E*, respectively, stained with hematoxylin and eosin. Adjacent sections (not shown) to *A*, *C*, and *E* stained with protein A-purified normal rabbit IgG were negative. (Original magnification, x160.) (p. 444.)

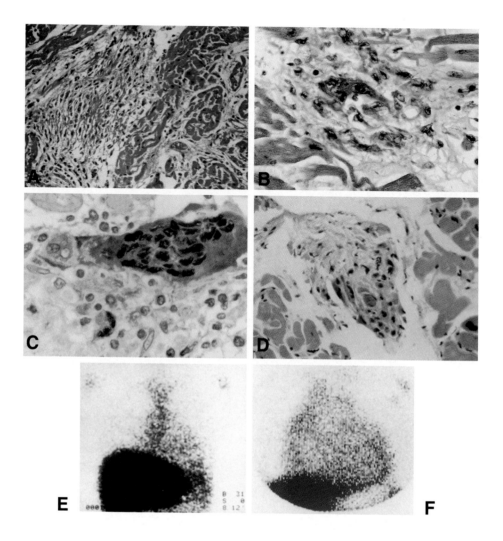

Plate 38, Fig. 21-1. Myocardial involvement in rheumatic fever (RF). Aschoff nodules are the pathologic hallmark of RF. An Aschoff nodule is present in ventricular and atrial endomyocardium and comprises perivascular fibrinoid necrosis-associated mononuclear and histiocytic cellular infiltration. Histiocytic infiltration is intermixed with giant cells or Aschoff cells, which have abundant cytoplasm and characteristic one or multiple nuclei. *A*, Perivascular interstitial Aschoff nodule at low magnification (x10), as observed in the left ventricular myocardium of a boy who died of acute RF at age 11 years. *B*, Higher magnification (x40) of the same lesion demonstrates Aschoff giant cells; the centrally located Aschoff cells are multinucleated. *C*, The giant cells are of monocyte-macrophage origin as revealed by immunostaining with α-chemotrypsin (x40). Objective evidence of rheumatic myocarditis in life has been obtained by endomyocardial biopsy and gamma imaging techniques. *D*, Presence of Aschoff nodule in biopsy specimen is pathognomonic or diagnostic of rheumatic carditis (x40). *E*, Gallium-67 nuclear imaging allows the detection of myocardial inflammation noninvasively. *F*, Nuclear imaging with antimyosin antibody, which identifies myocyte necrosis, is less sensitive and suggests that rheumatic myocarditis is a more infiltrative than degenerative disorder. (*A*, *B*, *D*, Hematoxylin and eosin.) (*C* and *F* from Massell and Narula.[2] By permission of the publisher. *E* was a gift from Jose Calegaro, M.D., Brasilia, Brazil.) (p. 510.)

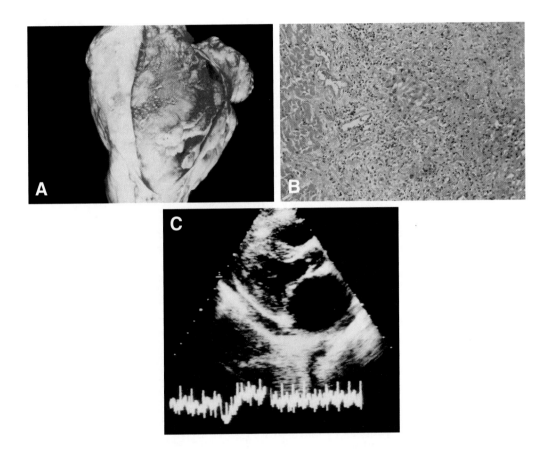

Plate 39, Fig. 21-2. Pericardial involvement in rheumatic fever. Pericarditis is typically fibrinous, and removal of the parietal pericardial layer imparts an appearance as if bread slices have been pulled apart in a buttered sandwich (*A*). Apart from fibrinous exudates, lymphomononuclear cells are seen on microscopic examination with the rare presence of Aschoff nodules, as seen in the center of the photomicrograph (*B*). Clinical presence of pericardial rub indicates the pericardial involvement in rheumatic fever. (Hematoxylin and eosin; x40.) Echocardiographically, pericardial effusion may be associated (*C*). Occasionally, a rub masks the underlying regurgitant murmurs and the echocardiogram becomes a useful diagnostic aid. (*A* and *C* from Massell and Narula.[2] By permission of the publisher.) (p. 512.)

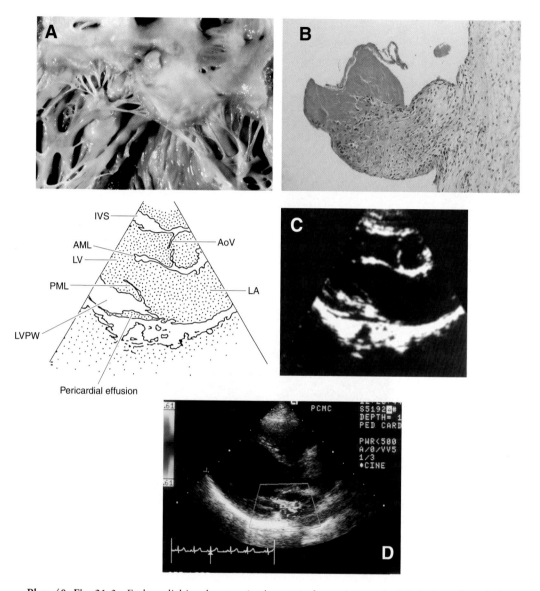

Plate 40, Fig. 21-3. Endocardial involvement in rheumatic fever. Acute valvulitis is the only pathologic abnormality that leads to permanent damage. Endocardial involvement results in development of tiny vegetations on the valve surfaces, which are noninfective and nonfragile. The vegetations comprise fibrinous material on the surface and reveal pallisading mononuclear cellular infiltration at the base of the vegetation. *A,* Gross macroscopic appearance of rheumatic vegetations on the atrial side of the mitral valve. *B,* Microscopic section through one of the vegetations; Aschoff cells are occasionally observed in the infiltrate. Noninvasive diagnosis of endocardial involvement is made currently by echocardiographic examination. (Hematoxylin and eosin; x10.) *C,* Presence of small nodular vegetations on the valve surfaces is proposed as ultrasonic counterpart of pathologic nodules. *D,* Consequent valvular regurgitation can be appreciated best by Doppler studies (eg, mitral regurgitation shown here). Regurgitation has also been described as evidence of subclinical carditis in rheumatic fever patients with no evidence of clinical carditis. (*C* from Vasan et al.[59] By permission of the American Heart Association. *D* from Massell and Narula.[2] By permission of the publisher.) (p. 513.)

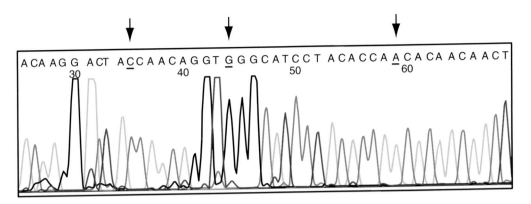

ACA AG G ACT A<u>C</u>C A A C A G GT <u>G</u> G G C A T C C T A C A C C A <u>A</u> C A C A A C A A C T
     30   40   50   60

Plate 41, Fig. 23-2. DNA sequence analysis of an adenovirus-specific polymerase chain reaction product. The region shown is highly divergent between adenovirus serotypes, allowing rapid identification of the virus amplified—in this case adenovirus type 5. Analysis of the 3 nucleotides indicated is sufficient to differentiate all adenovirus serotypes sequenced to date. (p. 563.)

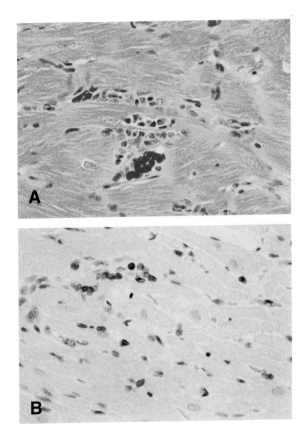

Plate 42, Fig. 23-4. Myocarditis in the cotton rat heart. *A*, Hematoxylin-eosin staining shows a discrete cluster of lymphocytes and macrophages adjacent to a degenerating myocyte. There is also focal loss of myocytes with early fibrous scarring. *B*, T-cell immunostain demonstrates a cluster of cells surrounding myocytes. (x132.) (p. 570.)

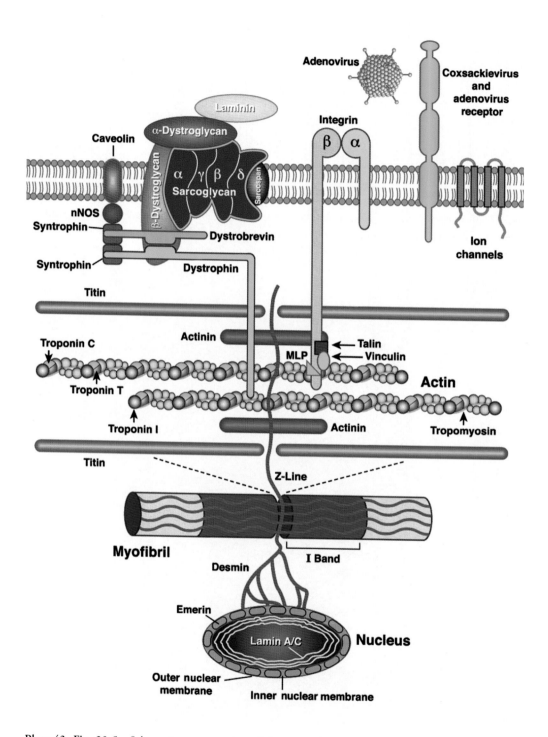

Plate 43, Fig. 23-5. Schematic representation of the cytoarchitecture of the cardiomyocyte, including components of the cytoskeleton, intermediate filaments, nuclear envelope, and dystrophin-associated glycoprotein complex. *MLP*, muscle LIM protein; *nNOS*, neuronal nitric oxide synthase. (p. 575.)

Pathology of Human Myocarditis

Gerald J. Berry, M.D., and Kristen A. Atkins, M.D.

INTRODUCTION

In spite of the remarkable advances in our understanding, diagnosis, and treatment of myocarditis in the last 150 years, it remains a diagnostic dilemma for many practicing pathologists. In a detailed review of the subject in 1941, Saphir[1] noted that the "incidence of the diagnosis of myocarditis has undergone more changes than perhaps the incidence of any other diagnosis." Much of the confusion can be traced to shifting diagnostic criteria, complex classifications, and changing patterns of infectious disease. The term was initially used by Sobernheim[2] in 1837 and popularized by Virchow[3] in 1858. After the recognition of distinct morphologic features of ischemic myocardial necrosis by Herrick[4] in 1912, the incidence of myocarditis diminished. The introduction of the transvenous endomyocardial biopsy in 1962 by Sakakibara and Konno[5] led to a renewed interest in the pathobiology, etiology, and treatment of myocarditis in antemortem specimens.

In 1984 a group of 8 cardiac pathologists met in Dallas, Texas, as an adjunct to the American College of Cardiology to develop a consensus definition and classification of morphologic criteria for the diagnosis and reporting of myocarditis in endomyocardial biopsy samples now known as the "Dallas criteria."[6] The primary goal was to provide reproducible criteria that allowed the discrimination of myocarditis from ischemic necrosis and other histopathologic mimics rather than to provide another complex temporal or etiologic grading scheme like classifications of Boikan,[7] Gore and Saphir,[8] Burch and Ray,[9] or Kline and Saphir.[10] The Dallas criteria were subsequently used for the multicenter National Institutes of Health myocarditis treatment trial and remain the standard for surgical pathologists.

ROLE OF THE SURGICAL PATHOLOGIST

Before the routine use of the endomyocardial biopsy in clinical cardiology practice, the diagnosis of myocarditis was often suspected but seldom proven before postmortem examination. Now, the surgical pathologist plays a pivotal role in the multidisciplinary team approach to the diagnosis and management of these patients.[11] Critical functions that the surgical pathologist performs in this endeavor can be summarized as: 1) to establish a histopathologic diagnosis of myocarditis using the Dallas criteria; 2) to exclude other morphologic and clinical mimics of inflammatory myocardial disease; 3) to classify the specific type of myocarditis for treatment and prognostic purposes (eg, lymphocytic, giant cell, hypersensitivity, toxic, infectious, sarcoidosis); 4) to monitor the effects of therapy (eg, antivirals, antibiotics, corticosteroids, and other immunosuppressive agents); 5) to evaluate for histopathologic evidence of progression to cardiomyopathy; and 6) to preserve tissue for research purposes (eg, microbiologic, immunohistochemical, molecular). Each of these functions is predicated on the evaluation of histologic sections prepared from adequate endomyocardial biopsy samples.

In our opinion, the diagnosis of myocarditis should not be rendered before adequate clinical information has been obtained. Direct communication between clinician and pathologist promotes clinical-pathologic correlation. The information should include the clinical history, age and sex of patient, onset and duration of symptoms, ventricular function, cardiac enzyme studies, status of coronary arteries (ideally by angiographic analysis), drug history (eg, vasopressive agents, illicit drugs, cardiotoxic or hypersensitivity-provoking agents, immunosuppressive drugs), studies for infectious etiologies, systemic illnesses such as vasculitis, and results of prior endomyocardial biopsies when available.[12]

TISSUE HANDLING AND PROCESSING

Proper tissue procurement and handling is a prerequisite for optimal microscopic examination. Biopsy specimens should be extracted gently from the bioptome with a needle to prevent crush artifact. The tissue should be placed immediately in a standard fixative such as 10% neutral buffered formalin. Frozen-section immunohistochemistry and immunofluorescence are investigative studies and are not essential to establish the diagnosis. For research purposes, the specimen should be received in saline and then snap frozen in a plastic Beem capsule containing an embedding medium. Transmission electron microscopy is also considered an optional study; an appropriate tissue fixative is required such as glutaraldehyde. Any tissue set aside for research purposes should always be examined by light microscopy before a final diagnosis is rendered because of the focal nature of many types of myocarditis.

For routine diagnostic evaluation, overnight processing and paraffin embedding are sufficient. For emergent cases, a 90-minute rapid (ultra) processing cycle is preferred, and microscopic slides are available within 2 to 3 hours. All the biopsy pieces should be embedded in the same block. At least 3 slides are prepared, each sectioned at 4- to 5-micron thickness from various depths within the block, with multiple fragments or ribbons placed on each slide. Thicker sections often result in biopsy samples appearing cellular, particularly in the interstitial regions, which can be mistaken for myocarditis. This approach also diminishes the risk of missing a focal process within the myocardium. We routinely stain with hematoxylin and eosin and a connective tissue stain such as Masson trichrome to evaluate for myocyte degeneration or damage in problematic cases. Immunohistochemical and molecular studies are performed for specific indications. In some centers, frozen-section analysis on fresh, unfixed tissue by cryomicrotome sectioning is performed for emergent circumstances. Interpretation of these cases is more problematic because of additional artifacts and requires an experienced pathologist (Table 14-1).

Table 14-1
Biopsy Requirements for the Evaluation of Myocarditis

1) Adequate biopsy samples (4-5 pieces preferred)
2) Sections prepared at 4- to 5-micron thickness in ribbons and at 3-step levels
3) Optimal staining with hematoxylin and eosin and a connective tissue stain such as Masson trichrome
4) Clinical history including symptom onset, physical findings, drug history, and status of coronary arteries
5) Biopsy specimen should be obtained during acute illness

BIOPSY LIMITATIONS AND TISSUE ARTIFACTS

Myocarditis is often a focal process, and sampling error remains a major consideration in the clinical management of patients. From the cardiac transplant literature, statistical analysis has shown an expected false-negative rate of 5% with 3 pieces and 2% with 4 pieces obtained by a 9F bioptome.[13] The reported false-negative rate in myocarditis is higher than in acute cardiac rejection. A Mayo Clinic study of endomyocardial samples obtained post mortem from hearts of patients who died of myocarditis reported a false-negative rate of 37% for the right ventricle.[14] Rather than negating the role of the endomyocardial biopsy for the diagnosis of clinically suspected myocarditis, as has been proposed by some investigators,[15-17] we think it remains the standard for this purpose. Recognition of the diminished sensitivity of the biopsy, careful patient selection, adequate biopsy sampling, and liberal use of leveled sections improve the diagnostic yield. For these reasons, a minimum of 4 to 5 pieces is recommended to minimize sampling error. Samples obtained by smaller bioptomes may require at least 5 or 6 pieces.

Various artifacts occur in endomyocardial biopsy specimens, which may mimic pathologic processes, and the surgical pathologist must be aware of these patterns. These have been reviewed in detail[18] and only selected topics are reviewed here. The most common biopsy artifact is the presence of contraction bands within myocytes. They are identical to the bands observed in acute ischemic necrosis and catecholamine (pressor) effect. These changes are induced by the biopsy procedure and can be diminished by using fixatives at room temperature. In ischemic injury, the nuclei of surrounding myocytes are usually pyknotic, whereas in artifactually induced contraction bands, the nuclei appear normal.

Another frequent artifact is intussusception or telescoping of small arteries that mimics luminal occlusion by thrombus. Connective tissue stains such as Masson trichrome or elastic van Gieson highlight the internal elastic membranes of both vessel segments. Intramyocardial accumulations of mature adipose tissue can simulate epicardial tissue, especially if associated with vessels of relatively large caliber. Both can be found in the right ventricular apical region, and adipose tissue is found not uncommonly in women and elderly patients. This should not be confused with arrhythmogenic right ventricular dysplasia or ventricular perforation; the latter is identified by the presence of mesothelial cells.

Accumulations of fresh platelet, fibrin-rich thrombus may be identified along the endocardial surface of biopsy fragments. These form by repeated placement of the bioptome along the endocardium and do not indicate chronic mural thrombi. Crush artifactual distortion of cellular components can be mistaken for inflammatory cell infiltrates. This can be reduced by gently extracting the specimen from the bioptome with a needle. Finally, artifactual widening of the interstitium may be caused by tissue procurement and processing and does not imply interstitial edema. We require the presence of interstitial, eosinophilic proteinaceous material as a minimum criterion for edema.

THE DALLAS CRITERIA

As mentioned previously, a consensus definition and classification of myocarditis were produced by a panel of cardiac pathologists at the American College of Cardiology meetings in Dallas in March 1984. The goals for the original group are enumerated in Table 14-2. Myocarditis was defined as a myocardial process characterized by the presence of an inflammatory infiltrate and myocyte damage or necrosis that is not typical of the myocardial damage of ischemic heart disease. Two distinct schemes were proposed to describe the endomyocardial biopsy findings from the timing of the biopsy procedure (Table 14-3).

The First Diagnostic Biopsy

Three diagnostic categories are possible for the initial diagnostic biopsy.[6]

Active Myocarditis — Reflecting the definitional features described above, the unequivocal diagnosis of myocarditis requires the presence of **both** inflammatory cell infiltrates and myocyte damage. The composition of the infiltrate should be described and can include predominantly lymphocytic, eosinophilic, neutrophilic, giant cell, granulomatous, or mixed cell types. The distribution and amount of inflammatory infiltrate should be assessed by patterns such as focal, confluent, or diffuse and mild, moderate, and severe degrees, respectively.

Table 14-2
Goals of the Dallas Criteria

1) To provide a morphologic definition for the diagnosis of myocarditis
2) To develop a simple, reproducible working formulation for reporting myocarditis
3) To enumerate diagnostic mimics of myocarditis
4) To assess the applicability and reproducibility of the classification

Modified from Aretz et al.[6] By permission of Field and Wood.

Table 14-3
Dallas Classification of Myocarditis

First biopsy
 I) Unequivocal myocarditis
 II) Borderline myocarditis
 III) No evidence of myocarditis

Subsequent biopsies
 I) Ongoing (persistent) myocarditis
 II) Resolving (healing) myocarditis
 III) Resolved (healed) myocarditis

Data from Billingham.[11]

A more difficult challenge is the determination of myocyte damage in the biopsy specimen. In our experience, florid myocytolysis and necrosis are not common biopsy patterns. We recognize myocyte damage by the presence of mononuclear cells that cause encroachment or scalloping of the sarcolemmal membrane of myocytes, fragmentation of myocytes with remnants of cytoplasm or bare nuclei, architectural displacement or distortion of myocytes by inflammatory cells, or partial replacement of myocytes by inflammatory cells. In equivocal cases the liberal use of leveled sections and Masson trichrome are helpful because damaged myocytes display a basophilic tinctorial quality.

Finally, the presence or absence of fibrosis should be noted for reference to changes in subsequent biopsies and the potential development of dilated cardiomyopathy. Interstitial, perivascular, and endocardial patterns can be seen. We do not attempt to quantitate the severity of fibrous replacement because it is subjective and poorly reproducible in our experience.

Borderline Myocarditis — This term is applied to biopsy samples in which the inflammatory cell infiltrate is limited and myocyte damage is not demonstrated. In some cases, unequivocal diagnostic features can be demonstrated in additional leveled sections. In others, repeat biopsies may be required.[19]

No Evidence of Myocarditis — This implies that neither diagnostic feature is present in the sample. Deeper sectioning of the paraffin blocks should be considered before this diagnosis is made because the inflammatory process may be patchy in distribution. If myocarditis is absent, attention should be focused on the presence of other myocardial disorders such as myocyte hypertrophy and interstitial fibrosis in the setting of dilated cardiomyopathy. We routinely perform histochemical stains for amyloidosis and hemochromatosis in this setting.

Follow-up Biopsy

It is not uncommon for patients with biopsy-proven myocarditis to undergo additional biopsies. In some cases, these are done after therapeutic interventions with immuno-suppressive drugs to monitor the response to drug therapy. In other patients, it is used to detect disease recurrence or progression. Three categories are used that resemble the diagnostic scheme of acute cellular rejection in cardiac allograft recipients.

Ongoing or Persistent Myocarditis — This term is applied when the degree of myocarditis is unchanged or worse than the original biopsy specimen.

Resolving or Healing Myocarditis — This category implies that the degree of inflammation or damage (or both) is diminished. Reparative changes are usually evident in the form of interstitial fibroblastic or myofibroblastic cellular infiltrates, granulation tissue, and immature collagen deposition.

Resolved or Healed Myocarditis — This term is restricted to biopsy specimens lacking either cellular infiltrates or damage. Mature collagenous scar tissue may be found in some cases, whereas others are entirely normal. The distribution of cicatricial scar tissue and the compensatory myocyte hypertrophy should be noted when present. Scattered mononuclear cells can be found within scar tissue and do not imply a recurrence or exacerbation of the disease.

We have observed cases of recurrent myocarditis after tapering of immunosuppressive therapy and previous biopsy specimens showing healed myocarditis. According to the Dallas criteria, if unequivocal or borderline myocarditis recurs, the new biopsy should be interpreted as a first biopsy.[6]

SPECIFIC TYPES OF HUMAN MYOCARDITIS

The definition and diagnostic criteria described in the preceding section illustrate a crucial point for the reporting of myocarditis by the surgical pathologist. The term is primarily a descriptive one and therefore requires a qualifier to provide the clinician with important etiologic, therapeutic, and prognostic information. The remainder of the discussion focuses on specific patterns and types of myocarditis. The composition and distribution of the inflammatory cell infiltrate and the pattern and type of injury observed in the endomyocardial biopsy specimen generally offer etiologic clues. For example, infiltrates composed predominantly of polymorphonuclear cells suggest a bacterial infection; eosinophils may be found in parasitic infestations or allergic drug reactions; giant cells can be seen in mycobacterial or fungal infections, sarcoidosis, or idiopathic giant cell myocarditis; and predominantly lymphocytic infiltrates are the typical response in myocarditis associated with systemic diseases and idiopathic (postviral), viral, rickettsial, or spirochetal infections.

IDIOPATHIC (POSTVIRAL) MYOCARDITIS

In most developed countries viral agents are thought to be the primary cause of most cases of myocarditis. Historical, clinical, and experimental evidence has identified members of the genus *Enterovirus*. These include coxsackievirus A and B, echovirus, and poliovirus. The pathogenesis of these viruses is incompletely understood and is discussed in other chapters in this book. Possible mechanisms include direct viral destruction of cardiac myocytes, T-cell-mediated autoimmune injury, and viral-mediated endothelial injury with intimal proliferation and ischemic sequelae. In many clinical cases, however, a direct causative link is not established, and these cases are classified as idiopathic myocarditis. Other terms that have been used include "acute myocarditis" to reflect the clinical onset of symptoms and absence of fibrosis in the biopsy specimen or "rapidly progressive myocarditis" in cases of multifocal damage and extensive fibrosis.[20] We prefer the term "lymphocytic" or "idiopathic myocarditis" and use the criteria in the Dallas classification. We discourage the use of the term "chronic myocarditis," because these cases usually represent dilated cardiomyopathy in our experience.

The incidence and natural history of idiopathic myocarditis remain largely undetermined. Discrepancies between clinically suspected cases and endomyocardial biopsy findings are well recognized. In a previous study from Stanford University, 30% of patients presenting with unexplained heart failure of short duration had biopsy evidence of lymphocytic myocarditis.[21] Other published series reporting the prevalence of myocarditis by using the endomyocardial biopsy as the standard are presented in Table 14-4.[22-30] The low incidence is thought to relate to the focal nature of the inflammatory cell infiltrates in both pediatric and adult cases.[31,32]

Table 14-4
Prevalence of Myocarditis in the Published Literature

Reference	Year published	Positive biopsy results	
		%	Number/total number
22	1985	67	18/27
23	1989	37	38/102
24	1990	78	14/18
25	1994	51	20/39
26	1995	10	214/2,233
27	1999	9	1/11
28	1999	16	10/62
29	2000	14	252/1,757

Modified from Feldman and McNamara.[30] By permission of the Massachusetts Medical Society.

Macroscopic Findings in Idiopathic Myocarditis

In general, examination of the heart specimen at transplantation or post mortem demonstrates 4-chamber dilatation and cardiac enlargement. Patients who die of ventricular arrhythmias or florid myocarditis, however, may have normal cardiac configurations. The papillary muscles and trabeculae carneae are often flattened, and the myocardium appears pale and flabby. Thrombi are uncommon within atrial appendages or along ventricular endocardial surfaces. The cut surface of the myocardium is usually pale, and foci of hemorrhage or hemorrhagic necrosis are found. Many cases are also associated with a fibrinous pericarditis and exudative effusions.[33]

Microscopic Findings in Idiopathic Myocarditis

The resemblance of this type of myocarditis and acute cellular rejection of the cardiac allograft was described[34] (Gopal S, Achalu R, Day JD, Huang M, Narasimhan U, Day MT, Kasper EK, Trichon BH, Chen CL, Cina SJ, Berry GJ, Robertson AL, Hruban RH, unpublished data). The cardinal features of acute allograft rejection are the presence of inflammatory cells and presence or absence of myocyte damage. The category of borderline myocarditis reflects the presence of inflammatory cells without concomitant myocyte damage and resembles the categories of focal or diffuse mild acute rejection. Typically, the infiltrates are sparse and are predominantly lymphocytic in nature. Occasional neutrophils or eosinophils may be found admixed within the infiltrate. They are more commonly distributed in the perivascular tissue spaces (Fig. 14-1 A; see color plate 21). In more advanced or severe cases of myocarditis, myocyte damage or necrosis is conspicuous. The architectural patterns include focal (Fig. 14-1 B; see color plate 21), multifocal, or diffuse interstitial infiltrates (Fig. 14-1 C; see color plate 21). Interstitial widening by tissue edema and inflammation is seen, and interstitial hemorrhage may be either punctate or diffuse. The patterns of confluent myocyte damage and necrosis are similar in the biopsy specimens of adult (Fig. 14-1 D; see color plate 21) and pediatric (Fig. 14-1 E; see color plate 21) patients. The composition of the infiltrates in the advanced stages of both groups is often polymorphous, with a predominance of mononuclear cells but variable numbers of eosinophils and neutrophils (Fig. 14-2 E; see color plate 22). Scattered multinucleated giant cells of either myogenic or macrophagic origin may also be found (Fig. 14-2 F; see color plate 22).

The treatment of idiopathic myocarditis remains controversial and is not discussed in detail here. At Stanford University, immunosuppressive agents are used routinely for biopsy-proven cases, often with dramatic clinical and morphologic responses. The progression from florid myocarditis on the initial diagnostic biopsy (Fig. 14-2 A and 2 B; see color plate 22) to healing or healed myocarditis (Fig. 14-2 C and 2 D; see color plate 22) on subsequent biopsies is well documented. The intensity of the infiltrate is diminished or absent. Reparative changes within the interstitium range from loose granulation tissue with minimal alteration of the myocardial architecture to replacement by collagenous scar tissue. Increased vascularity suggesting angiogenesis may also be seen, along with compensatory hypertrophy of residual myocytes. The findings on the follow-up biopsies should be graded as persistent, healing (resolving), or healed (resolved) myocarditis according to the Dallas criteria. The progression to dilated cardiomyopathy should also be recorded.

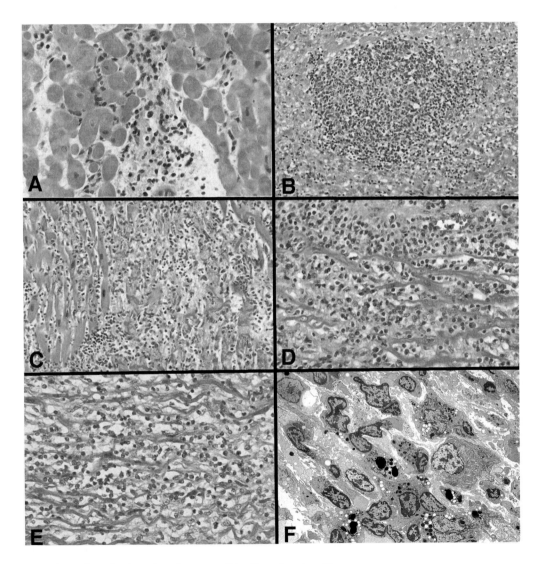

Fig. 14-1. Idiopathic lymphocytic myocarditis. See color plate 21.

Ultrastructural, Immunohistochemical, and Molecular Findings

The utility of transmission electron microscopy in the diagnosis of myocarditis is limited to research studies. Interstitial expansion by mononuclear cells dispersed among normal myocytes is observed (Fig. 14-1 *F*, see color plate 21). On occasion, myocyte necrosis characterized by lymphocytes adherent to disrupted sarcolemmal membranes, damage of the microvascular elements, and fragmented collagen bundles within the interstitium may be seen.[35] We and others have not observed viral components or immune complex deposition with these techniques.

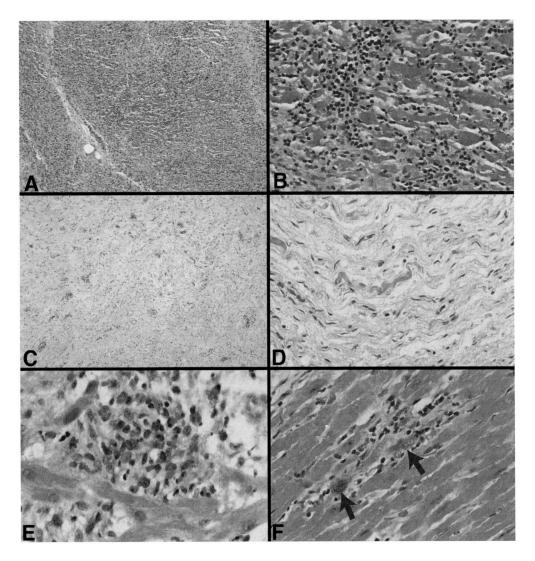

Fig. 14-2. Idiopathic lymphocytic myocarditis. See color plate 22.

Immunologic studies have expanded our understanding of the pathogenesis of this disease process. Immunofluorescence studies of cases of active myocarditis showed the presence of the third component of complement (C3) in 50% of cases; this diminished with resolution of the inflammatory lesions.[36] Indirect immunofluorescence studies also identified increased staining for antibodies directed against sarcolemmal antigens and myofibrillar components in biopsy samples showing resolving myocarditis. Different investigators reported immunophenotypic profiles of the infiltrating cells[37,38] (Gopal S, Achalu R, Day JD, Huang M, Narasimhan U, Day MT, Kasper EK, Trichon BH, Chen CL, Cina SJ, Berry GJ, Robertson AL, Hruban RH, unpublished data). The majority of lymphocytes are CD3[+] T cells with helper and suppressor subtypes. Macrophages and natural killer cells are also present, but B cells are infrequent or absent (Fig. 14-3; see color plate 23). Up to 25% of lymphocytes stain for Bcl-2, and 27% of the myocytes express p53.

Programmed cell death (apoptosis) is detectable by in situ hybridization end labeling. Early myocyte necrosis is shown by myosin light chain staining in most cases of lymphocytic myocarditis (Gopal S, Achalu R, Day JD, Huang M, Narasimhan U, Day MT, Kasper EK, Trichon BH, Chen CL, Cina SJ, Berry GJ, Robertson AL, Hruban RH, unpublished data). Other markers of immunologically mediated cell injury include the persistent expression of intercellular adhesion molecule 1 and vascular cell adhesion molecule 1 in myocardial biopsy samples.[39] Increased numbers of interstitial dendritic cells have been shown in active myocarditis, suggesting an important pathogenetic role.[40]

The role of viral infection in human myocarditis was strengthened by the identification of enterovirus genome by in situ hybridization, polymerase chain reaction (PCR), and PCR–single-strand conformation polymorphism techniques in the heart samples of patients with myocarditis and dilated cardiomyopathy.[41-44] Interestingly, enteroviral RNA sequences have been found by PCR methodologies in other conditions not related to myocarditis or dilated cardiomyopathy. These include coronary artery disease, cardiac allograft rejection, normal donor heart tissue, and cardiac fibroelastosis.[45]

Morphologic Mimics of Idiopathic Myocarditis

The common histopathologic lesions that can be mistaken for idiopathic myocarditis are presented in Table 14-5. The issue of how many lymphocytes are normally within the myocardium has been addressed. This is particularly important in assessing the possibility of lymphocytic myocarditis. Edwards et al.[46] determined that the mean number of lymphocytes within normal myocardial tissue is fewer than 5.0 per high-power field. This figure was derived from 170 endomyocardial biopsies of patients with clinical evidence of heart disease. Tazelaar and Billingham[47] examined endomyocardial biopsy specimens from 86 young disease-free cardiac transplant donors at the time of transplantation. Foci composed of at least 5 mononuclear inflammatory cells were found in 9.3% of cases.

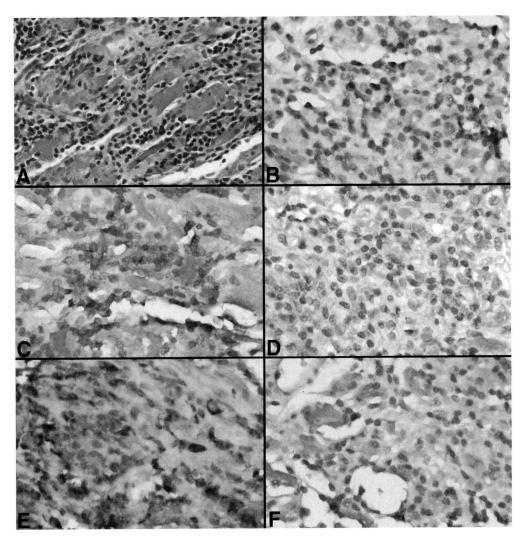

Fig. 14-3. Immunophenotype of lymphocytic myocarditis. See color plate 23.

Table 14-5
Morphologic Mimics of Idiopathic (Lymphocytic) Myocarditis

1) Lymphocytes and interstitial cells in normal myocardium
2) Lymphocytes in dilated cardiomyopathy
3) Ischemic necrosis and pressor or catecholamine effects
4) Biopsy-site changes
5) Hematolymphoid and nonhematolymphoid malignancies
6) Other types of myocarditis (eg, infectious, toxic, giant cell types)
7) Extramedullary hematopoiesis in myocardial scars

Other types of interstitial cells found within the normal myocardium that can be confused with inflammatory cells include endothelial cells, smooth muscle cells, pericytes, fibroblasts, and mast cells. Hill and Swanson[48] reported the presence of extramedullary hematopoietic cells, including immature erythroid and myeloid precursors within healing infarcts of ischemic and cardiomyopathic hearts, and areas of fibrosis in congenital defects. Interestingly, they also included 1 case of viral myocarditis within this study.

The issue of chronic myocarditis and idiopathic dilated cardiomyopathy has been mentioned. This remains a continuing source of confusion for pathologists. Our practice is to avoid the term "chronic myocarditis." Mononuclear leukocytic infiltrates are commonly found in dilated cardiomyopathy. Tazelaar and Billingham[49] examined random myocardial samples from 108 recipient hearts with end-stage idiopathic dilated cardiomyopathy and found inflammatory cells in 87% of cases. These were localized to the interstitial tissues and within fine or coarse interstitial fibrosis (Fig. 14-4 *A*; see color plate 24). The presence of myocyte hypertrophy characterized by large, irregular, hyperchromatic, and often bizarre-shaped nuclei and collagenous eosinophilic interstitial fibrosis are cardinal features of idiopathic dilated cardiomyopathy.[50] Distinguishing features are summarized in Table 14-6.

Another morphologic mimic of myocarditis is vasopressor or catecholamine effect and ischemic necrosis. Large doses of vasopressive agents may be required to support the patient hemodynamically. These can produce direct myocyte toxicity or "microinfarcts" by constriction of small "end vessels." The affected myocytes appear fragmented and hypereosinophilic and are surrounded by a minimal mixed inflammatory cell infiltrate (Fig. 14-4 *B*; see color plate 24). The distribution of the lesions near or around small intramyocardial arteries and the mixed nature of the infiltrate prevent confusion with acute myocarditis. The trichrome stain highlights the necrotic myocytes by their blue-gray tinctorial appearance. The damaged myocytes may undergo punctate calcification and mimic infectious myocarditis such as toxoplasmosis.

Ischemic necrosis can occur because of prolonged hypotension, particularly in patients with underlying coronary heart disease. Patterns include discrete subendocardial foci of necrosis characterized by hypereosinophilic myocytes with pyknotic smudged nuclei and loss of cytoplasmic striations and fine detail. This zonal injury pattern is sharply delineated by Masson trichrome stain. The normal red-orange myocytes are easily distinguished from the gray-blue necrotic fibers. In the setting of ischemia with reperfusion injury, fragmented myocytes may be found associated with foci of interstitial hemorrhage. These are caused by endothelial injury progressing to rupture of the microvasculature. In healing ischemic lesions, granulation tissue replaces the necrotic region, and histiocytes and pigment-laden macrophages are evident (Fig. 14-4 *B*). Over weeks to months, this lesion is infiltrated by mature scar tissue.

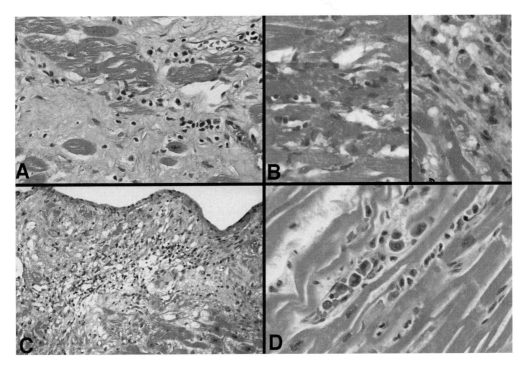

Fig. 14-4. Differential diagnosis of lymphocytic myocarditis. See color plate 24.

Table 14-6
Histopathologic Features of Lymphocytic Myocarditis (LM) and Idiopathic Dilated Cardiomyopathy (IDCM)

Finding	LM	IDCM
Focal/diffuse/cellular infiltrates	+	+
Polymorphous cell infiltrates	+	−
Endocarditis/pericarditis	+	−
Vasculitis	+	−
Global myocyte hypertrophy	−	+
Bizarre nuclear morphology	−	+
Myofibrillar loss	−	+
Myocyte damage/necrosis	+	−
Interstitial fibrosis		
Focal	+	+
Diffuse	−	+
Mature eosinophilic collagen	−	+

On occasion, we have observed changes related to previous biopsy sampling in follow-up biopsies. Two patterns are seen in biopsy-site changes. Within the first 2 weeks an endothelial-lined craterlike lesion is observed in the subendocardial tissues. Surrounding aggregates of fibrin are variable amounts of granulation tissue admixed with scattered acute and chronic inflammatory cells. Coagulative necrosis of adjacent myocytes can be seen. Progressive organization leads to replacement by cicatricial collagenous tissue with distortion of adjacent myocytes in a disarray pattern. It is not uncommon to find collections of lymphocytes and occasional hemosiderin-laden macrophages within the hyalinized tissue, including cases of dense cellular aggregates (Fig. 14-4 *C*; see color plate 24). The latter can be confused with myocarditis, but the presence of fibrous scar tissue is the key discriminator. A trichrome stain is useful in these cases. We have also seen cases of foreign material with an associated giant cell reaction in previous biopsy sites (Fig. 14-5 *A*; see color plate 25).

Neoplastic infiltrates are uncommon findings on endomyocardial biopsies. Hematolymphoid malignancies such as leukemias and lymphomas are characterized by their atypical cytologic features and the absence of necrosis and fibrosis (Fig. 14-5 *C* and 5 *D*; see color plate 25). Immunophenotypic and molecular studies are helpful to confirm the clonality of these processes and to distinguish them from myocarditis. We observed a case of

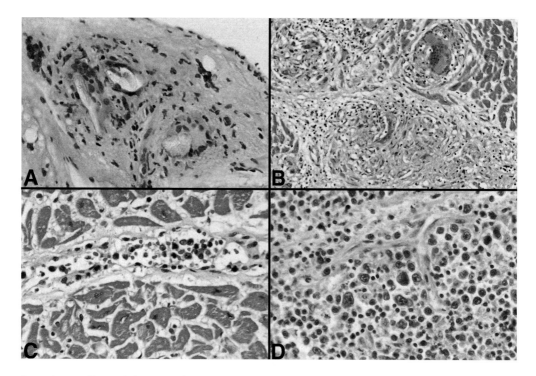

Fig. 14-5. Differential diagnosis of idiopathic giant cell myocarditis. See color plate 25.

metastatic malignant melanoma presenting as diffuse interstitial infiltrates within the myocardium in association with sparse myocyte damage (Fig. 14-4 D; see color plate 24).

INFECTIOUS MYOCARDITIS

In developed countries infectious causes of heart muscle inflammation are uncommon in immunocompetent individuals. Patients with acquired immunodeficiency syndrome (AIDS), transplant-associated immunosuppression to prevent allograft rejection, and advanced stages of malignancy are susceptible to bacterial, viral, fungal, protozoan, and rickettsial infections. In many developing countries these remain a significant cause of morbidity and mortality, and cardiac involvement is observed frequently. Some specific forms of infectious myocarditis are discussed.

Bacterial Myocarditis

The causes of bacterial myocarditis are listed in Table 14-7. Four basic morphologic patterns can be enumerated: 1) suppurative, 2) toxin-related, 3) granulomatous, and 4) nonspecific lymphocytic myocarditis. Suppurative or pyogenic myocarditis is the most common type and is usually caused by staphylococcal, streptococcal, pneumococcal, or meningococcal infections. The classic mechanisms of myocardial dissemination include septicemia or localized infection from a contiguous source such as infected lung. Infective endocarditis is the most common pattern underlying septic myocarditis in our experience.[51,52] Bacterial infections complicating myocardial infarction and coronary stent placement have been reported.[53,54]

The morphologic findings range from focal neutrophilic collections within the myocardium to microabscess formation (Fig. 14-6 *A* and 6 *B*; see color plate 26). In some

Table 14-7
Bacterial and Spirochetal Causes of Myocarditis

Bacterial	Actinomycosis	Mycoplasma
	Brucellosis	Pneumococcal
	Cholera	Salmonellosis
	Diphtheria	Staphylococcal
	Gonococcal	Streptococcal
	Haemophilus	Tularemia
	Meningococcal	Whipple disease
	Mycobacterial	
Spirochetal	Leptospirosis	Relapsing fever
	Lyme disease	Syphilis

Modified from Feldman and McNamara.[30] By permission of the Massachusetts Medical Society.

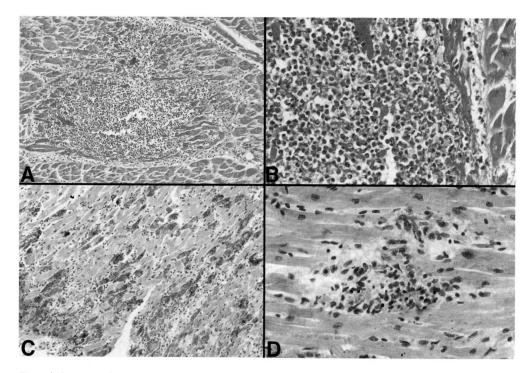

Fig. 14-6. Bacterial myocarditis. See color plate 26.

cases the collections of microorganisms are readily found on sections stained with hematoxylin and eosin, but we routinely prepare sections with Gram stain for confirmation.

Conduction abnormalities have been reported in cases of brucellosis,[55] *Mycoplasma* infection,[56] and *Legionella* infection.[57] Rare causes of bacterial myocarditis include human granulocytic ehrlichiosis,[58] psittacosis,[59] and salmonella.[60-62]

Diphtheric myocarditis occurs in up to a quarter of patients with diphtheria and remains the most frequent cause of death in patients with this disease. Myocardial dysfunction is affected by a potent exotoxin liberated by *Corynebacterium diphtheriae* that interferes with protein synthesis. Until recently, diphtheria was rare in western countries, but outbreaks have been reported in Scandinavia and the Baltic countries, particularly in alcoholics.[63] Romberg[64] described the pathologic features in the classic monograph in 1891. At postmortem examination the hearts are flabby and dilated and the myocardium exhibits a streaky appearance. Microscopic features include patchy hyaline and granular degeneration of myocytes associated with collections of mononuclear inflammation (Fig. 14-6 *C* and 6 *D*; see color plate 26). In the late or chronic stages of the disease, myocardial scarring is found. The conduction system is preferentially involved in this disease, and the development of complete atrioventricular block is regarded as a poor prognostic sign.

Tuberculosis is a rare but classic example of granulomatous bacterial myocarditis. Although uncommon in most western countries, it remains a differential diagnostic consideration in cases of myocarditis associated with giant cells. Routes of myocardial involvement include hematogenous, lymphatic, and direct contiguity. Morphologic patterns that have been described include nodular masses (tuberculoma), miliary nodules, and diffuse cellular infiltrates.[65-67] Caseating and noncaseating granulomas are found, and histochemical stains and bacteriologic studies are essential for establishing the diagnosis. Granulomatous bacterial infections have been reported in cases of Whipple disease, but the more common pattern is collections of foamy macrophages containing periodic acid-Schiff-positive granules.[68] Lymphohistiocytic infiltrates with multinucleated giant cells and liquefactive necrosis (gummatous lesions) are the hallmarks of syphilitic myocarditis in adults.[69,70] Predilection for the upper portions of the interventricular septum can result in conduction defects. In the congenital form of this disease, the histopathologic findings are mononuclear cell infiltrates without gummatous lesions.

Direct bacterial toxicity with or without a coexisting immune-mediated dysfunction is a suspected mechanism in Lyme carditis. Between 1% and 8% of patients infected by the tick-borne spirochete *Borrelia burgdorferi* develop cardiac involvement usually characterized by variable degrees of atrioventricular or interventricular block. Endomyocardial biopsy samples resemble idiopathic lymphocytic myocarditis, and in rare cases spirochetal organisms are identified by modified silver stains.[71-73] Cardiac involvement in leptospirosis (Weil syndrome) is also characterized by cellular infiltrates composed predominantly of mononuclear cells with sparse neutrophils and focal necrosis.

Viral Myocarditis

The role of viral agents in the pathogenesis of idiopathic myocarditis has been mentioned previously, and other chapters examine postviral autoimmunity mechanisms, direct viral cytopathic injury, and induction of viral-specific immune response through mediators such as interleukin -1, -2, and -6; tumor necrosis factor; interferon; and nitrous oxide.[74] In addition to the enteroviruses and echoviruses, numerous RNA and DNA viruses are linked to myocarditis (Table 14-8). Many of these viruses produce nonspecific lymphocytic myocarditis seen on histopathologic examination.[75-85] Others such as cytomegalovirus (CMV) and varicella have intranuclear inclusions that aid diagnosis.[86] The following discussion is limited to CMV myocarditis, EBV-associated lymphoproliferative disorders, and human immunodeficiency virus (HIV)-related myocardial lesions.

Cytomegalovirus Myocarditis — Human CMV is a ubiquitous virus belonging to the herpesvirus family that infects 50% to 90% of adults. Serious morbidity and mortality are limited to infections occurring in fetal development, in immunosuppressed patients receiving chemotherapy, transplant recipients, and AIDS patients.[87-91] Hepatitis, infectious

Table 14-8
Viral Causes of Myocarditis

Adenovirus	Junin virus
Arbovirus	Lymphocytic choriomeningitis
Arenavirus (Lassa fever)	Measles
Coxsackievirus	Mumps
Cytomegalovirus	Parvovirus
Dengue virus	Poliovirus
Echovirus	Rabies virus
Encephalomyocarditis virus	Respiratory syncytial virus
Epstein-Barr virus	Rubella
Hepatitis virus (A and C)	Rubeola
Herpes simplex virus	Vaccinia virus
Herpes zoster	Varicella virus
Human immunodeficiency virus	Variola virus
Influenza virus (A and B)	Yellow fever virus

Modified from Feldman and McNamara.[30] By permission of the Massachusetts Medical Society.

mononucleosis-like syndrome, pneumonitis, myocarditis, gastroenteritis, and retinitis have been described in the setting of acute infections.[92] Chronic infection plays a significant role in the development of transplant-accelerated arteriosclerosis.[93]

The diagnosis of CMV myocarditis requires the demonstration of nuclear inclusions composed of large central basophilic nuclei surrounded by a pale artifactual halo within myocytes, fibroblasts, or endothelial cells (Fig. 14-7 *A*; see color plate 27). Less frequently, cytoplasmic inclusions arranged as eosinophilic globules may be found. The density and distribution of the inflammatory response vary, and the response may be sparse or absent in the region of the inclusions. The composition of the infiltrate is generally polymorphous, with lymphocytes, histiocytes, eosinophils, and neutrophils. The presence of pyknotic debris and the mixed cell types or numerous eosinophils should heighten suspicion for infection. Immunohistochemical and molecular studies are useful in cases where the findings are equivocal[94-96] (Fig. 14-7 *B*; see color plate 27). After initiation of antiviral therapy, the inclusions appear more eosinophilic, inhomogeneous, and globular.[97] The introduction of prophylactic or preemptive strategies for CMV has resulted in a dramatic reduction in cases of CMV myocarditis at our institution.

Epstein-Barr Virus-Associated Lymphoproliferative Disorders — EBV infection involving the heart is uncommon. Nonspecific electrocardiographic alterations in patients with infectious mononucleosis have been reported. There is 1 published report of lymphocytic myocarditis on endomyocardial biopsy in a young woman with a clinical presentation simulating myocardial infarction with cardiogenic shock.[98] Immunocompromised patients

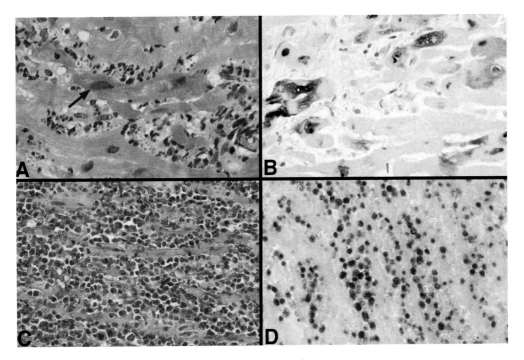

Fig. 14-7. Cytomegalovirus (CMV) myocarditis. See color plate 27.

such as transplant recipients and AIDS patients can develop EBV-driven lymphoid proliferations within the myocardium ranging from mononucleosis-like lesions to malignant lymphoma. We have encountered only 2 cases of post-transplant lymphoproliferative disease involving the allograft in endomyocardial biopsy samples. Useful morphologic clues include the presence of atypical lymphoid or lymphoplasmacytoid cells, atypical immunoblasts, brisk mitotic activity, and cellular necrosis (Fig. 14-7 C; see color plate 27). Polymorphic infiltrates may be difficult to distinguish from myocarditis and immunohistochemical and molecular studies are helpful (Fig. 14-7 D; see color plate 27). The majority of post-transplant lymphoproliferative disorders involve B cells and are EBV-associated in contrast to T-cell-mediated lesions of idiopathic myocarditis.

AIDS-Related Myocardial Lesions — Patients infected with HIV are at risk of development of various cardiac lesions (Table 14-9). These include endocardial valvular disease caused by marantic or infective endocarditis, pericardial effusions (sterile or infective), fibrinous or constrictive pericarditis, and myocardial lesions such as infectious myocarditis, neoplastic infiltration by Kaposi sarcoma or lymphoma, right ventricular hypertrophy with pulmonary hypertension, and drug toxicity.[99] Cases of dilated cardiomyopathy and non-infectious myocardial inflammation have also been reported. The changes range from borderline to active myocarditis according to the Dallas criteria and are reported in 11 of 16 HIV+ patients (69%) undergoing endomyocardial biopsy for myocardial dysfunction.[100]

Table 14-9
Cardiac Lesions in AIDS Patients

I. Endocardial disorders
    Marantic endocarditis
    Infective endocarditis (bacterial, fungal)

II. Myocardial disorders
    Opportunistic infections
        Bacterial (tuberculosis, mycobacterium avium intracellulare)
        Fungal (cryptococcosis, aspergillosis, candidiasis, histoplasmosis, coccidioidomycosis)
        Protozoan (toxoplasmosis)
        Viral (cytomegalovirus, herpes simplex, human immunodeficiency virus)
    Noninfectious myocardial necrosis
        Catecholamine effect
        Drug toxicity
        Vascular spasm
    Pulmonary hypertension with right ventricular hypertrophy
    Neoplastic processes
        Kaposi sarcoma
        Malignant lymphoma

III. Pericardial disorders
    Infectious pericarditis (opportunistic infections)
    Neoplastic infiltration (Kaposi sarcoma, non-Hodgkin lymphoma)
    Uremic/noninfectious pericarditis

Modified from Kaul et al.[99] By permission of Mosby-Year Book.

These are mediated by CD3$^+$ T cells with a suppressor/cytotoxic CD8$^+$ phenotype.[101] Possible etiologies include direct HIV viropathic effect, coinfection with another cardiotrophic virus, postviral autoimmune mechanism, and drug toxicity. In our experience, the diagnosis of HIV-associated myocarditis and cardiomyopathy is one of exclusion, and common infectious causes such as toxoplasmosis, CMV, and mycobacterial and fungal infections should be sought by histochemical, immunohistochemical, molecular, and bacteriologic methods.

Fungal Myocarditis

Fungal myocarditis is another type of opportunistic infection that occurs in iatrogenically immunosuppressed patients, AIDS patients, intravenous drug abusers, and rarely after open heart surgery.[102-104] The fungal organisms that are reported are listed in Table 14-10. In our experience, most cases occur in the setting of advanced disseminated infections. The histopathologic findings include zonal myocardial infarcts because of hematogenous spread within intramyocardial vessels. Neutrophilic microabscesses and abundant tissue necrosis are seen and warrant appropriate histochemical stains (Fig. 14-8; see color plate 28). Granulomatous formation and the presence of multinucleated giant cells are uncommon in our experience with solid organ and bone marrow transplant recipients. The presence of mixed infiltrates predominated by neutrophils and abundant pyknotic cellular debris are important clues to distinguish fungal myocarditis from idiopathic myocarditis. The number of fungal infections after thoracic transplantation at Stanford University has diminished since the introduction of aerosolized antifungal prophylaxis.[105]

Table 14-10
Fungal Causes of Myocarditis

Aspergillosis	Cryptococcosis
Blastomycosis	Histoplasmosis
Candidiasis	Mucormycosis
Coccidioidomycosis	

Modified from Feldman and McNamara.[30] By permission of the Massachusetts Medical Society.

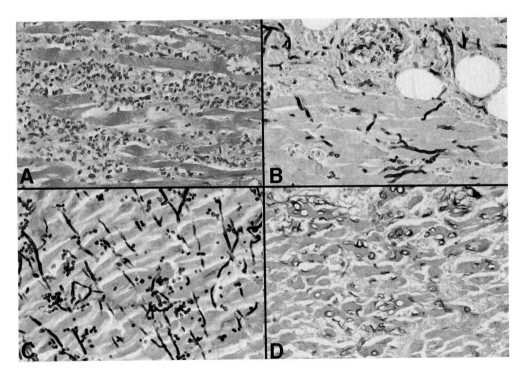

Fig. 14-8. Fungal myocarditis. See color plate 28.

Protozoan/Helminthic Myocarditis

Parasites that can cause myocarditis in humans are listed in Table 14-11. Of the protozoan causes, toxoplasmic myocarditis and Chagas disease are the most common. The helminthic infections represent tapeworm, flat-worm, and round-worm infestations and are rarely encountered in the United States. Trichinosis is the sole exception in this group, and infestation occurs after the consumption of raw or uncooked animal meat containing larval cysts.[106] Nonencysted larvae incite a brisk lymphohistiocytic response within the myocardium, and myocardial damage may be conspicuous in the early stages of the illness. Eosinophils may also be present within the inflammatory cell infiltrates.

Toxoplasmic Myocarditis — Infections by the obligate intracellular parasite, *Toxoplasma gondii*, occur clinically in congenital or acquired forms. Myocarditis is uncommon in immunocompetent adults, although rare cases are reported.[107] Three patterns of disease are recognized: acute or miliary infectious form, glandular form involving lymph nodes, and a localized form involving 1 or 2 organ systems.

We have observed cases of acquired cardiac toxoplasmosis in AIDS patients and in cardiac allograft recipients. In transplant patients, toxoplasmic myocarditis is now infrequently encountered in endomyocardial biopsy specimens because antibiotic prophylaxis is given to seronegative recipients receiving grafts from seropositive donors.[108] Like CMV, the inflammatory response may be variable and may resemble lymphocytic myocarditis or cardiac rejection. Lymphocytes and histiocytes often admixed with eosinophils are centered on necrotic, pyknotic myocytes. In some cases, toxoplasmic cysts may have sparse inflammation (Fig. 14-9 *A*; see color plate 29). Trophozoites may be difficult to identify in the biopsy samples, and immunohistochemical or molecular studies may be helpful[109] (Fig. 14-9 *B*; see color plate 29). At the ultrastructural level, encysted bradyzoites are found within myocytes. The organism is ovoid, measuring 4- to 6-microns long and 2- to 3-microns wide. The double-layered pellicle and anteriorly placed conoid are characteristic (Fig. 14-9 *C* and 9 *D*). An important diagnostic distinction must be made between bradyzoites of toxoplasmosis and the fine dystrophic calcifications within individual myocytes.[110,111] These represent encrustation of mitochondria and are usually seen in the setting of ischemic injury.

Chagas Disease — Myocarditis caused by the hemoflagellate, *Trypanosoma cruzi*, is the most common form of inflammatory heart muscle disease in Central and South America. Clinically, it is characterized by an acute phase followed by a latent phase and then the chronic phase. The acute phase develops after a short incubation period, and infection of myocytes by organisms occurs. Myocarditis occurs in a third of patients; most recover within 3 to 4 months. Death due to cardiac or neurologic complications is reported in 5% to 10% of cases, and at postmortem study the heart is enlarged, flabby, and mottled.[112] Microscopic sections reveal intact pseudocysts and a dense mixed inflammatory infiltrate of

Table 14-11
Protozoan/Helminthic Causes of Myocarditis

Toxoplasmosis	Paragonimiasis
Sarcocystosis	Trichinosis
Trypanosomiasis	Visceral larva migrans
Ascariasis	Echinococcosis
Cysticercosis	Filariasis
Schistosomiasis	

Modified from Feldman and McNamara.[30] By permission of the Massachusetts Medical Society.

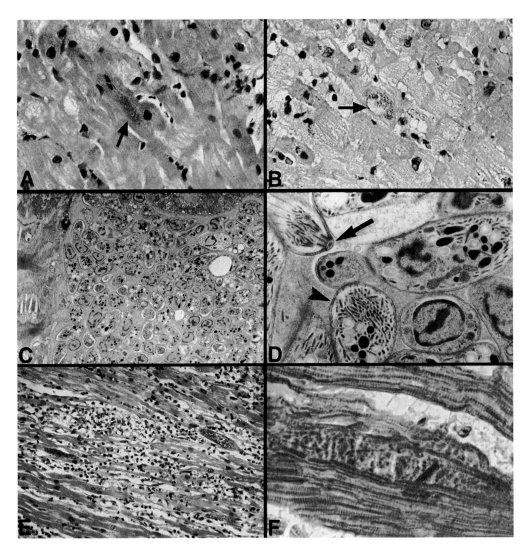

Fig. 14-9. Parasitic myocarditis. See color plate 29.

lymphocytes, plasma cells, histiocytes, and polymorphonuclear leukocytes associated with myocyte necrosis (Fig. 14-9 *E* and 9 *F*; see color plate 29). Both cell-mediated and antibody-mediated mechanisms are thought to be involved in the pathogenesis of the lesions in response to antigens released by infected cells becoming adsorbed onto surfaces of infected and noninfected host cells.[113]

The chronic phase of Chagas disease occurs years to decades after the acute infection. The morphologic findings consist of dilated cardiomyopathy. Patients can present with arrhythmias, congestive heart failure, or thromboembolic lesions.[114] Identification of parasites within the myocardium is uncommon at this time, but foci of residual myocarditis and fibrosis are reported. The role of postinfectious immunity and autoimmune-mediated myocardial disease in Chagas disease remains unresolved.

Rickettsial Myocarditis

Cardiac involvement in the rickettsial diseases is usually subclinical and consists of abnormalities in the electrocardiogram. The 3 causes–Rocky Mountain spotted fever, scrub typhus, and Q fever–are each characterized by nonsuppurative vasculitic lesions of small vessels, including capillaries, venules and arterioles, and small arteries. Endothelial and medial smooth muscle cell invasion by microorganisms results in endothelial cell injury, thrombus formation, and necrosis. An accompanying lymphocytic myocarditis is seen more frequently in Rocky Mountain spotted fever than in scrub typhus.[115-117] Organisms can be identified in tissue sections by a modified Giemsa stain. Immunofluorescence stains are also available. Endocarditis is the most common lesion in Q fever, but venous thrombosis and small vein vasculitis can occur.

DRUG-RELATED MYOCARDITIS

Drug-induced myocardial dysfunction remains a significant clinical problem and the list of drugs implicated continues to grow. Five patterns are recognized: 1) hypersensitivity myocarditis, 2) toxic myocarditis, 3) endocardial fibrosis (eg, ergotamine tartrate, methysergide, or phentermine or fenfluramine), 4) drug-induced cardiomyopathy (eg, anthracycline or chloroquine), and 5) giant cell myocarditis.[118,119] A partial list of the drugs associated with hypersensitivity and toxic myocarditis is presented in Table 14-12.

Hypersensitivity Myocarditis

Hypersensitivity myocarditis is the most common form of acute drug-related myocardial injury. More than 2 dozen drugs have been identified that cause hypersensitivity myocarditis, but the majority of cases are caused by sulfonamides, methyldopa, and penicillin and its derivatives.[120-122] It is also observed in patients undergoing cardiac transplantation and may be related to prolonged dobutamine infusion.[123-125] Clinical presentation can include rash,

Table 14-12
Drug-Induced Myocarditis

Hypersensitivity myocarditis		
Penicillin	Isoniazid	Tetanus toxoid
Sulfonamides	Amphotericin B	Indomethacin
Tetracycline	Ampicillin	Ephedra
Streptomycin	Chloramphenicol	Cefaclor
Phenylbutazone	Methyldopa	Diphtheria toxin
		Clozapine
Toxic myocarditis		
Anthracycline	Cocaine	
Cyclophosphamide	Catecholamines	
Arsenicals	Theophylline	
Fluorouracil	Quinidine	
Lithium	Barbiturates	
Amphetamines	Paraquat	

Data from Billingham,[118] La Grenade L, Graham D, Trontell A. Myocarditis and cardiomyopathy associated with clozapine use in the United States (letter to the editor). N Engl J Med 2001;345:224-225, and Kilian JG, Kerr K, Lawrence C, Celermajer DS. Myocarditis and cardiomyopathy associated with clozapine. Lancet 1999;354:1841-1845.

fever, peripheral eosinophilia, and occasionally arrhythmias, sudden death, and congestive heart failure. It is not dose-dependent and can occur at any time during drug administration.

The histopathologic features include temporally uniform lesions distributed in the subendocardial, perivascular, and interstitial tissues (Fig. 14-10 *A*; see color plate 30). The predominant inflammatory cells are eosinophils, but variable numbers of histiocytes and lymphocytes are also found (Fig. 14-10 *B*; see color plate 30). Myocyte necrosis is absent or focal and limited. Necrotizing vasculitis is not found, but infiltration of vessel walls by inflammatory cells is common.[126] Collections of histiocytes often centered on degenerated collagen bundles form ill-defined granulomas in up to 25% of cases, but fibrinoid necrosis, well-formed aggregates of epithelioid histiocytes ("hard granulomas"), multinucleated giant cells, interstitial fibrosis, and hemorrhage are absent in our experience (Fig. 14-10 *C*; see color plate 30). Immunohistochemical studies showed T-cell phenotypes of infiltrating lymphocytes and sparse or absent B cells.[126] Myocyte apoptosis was reported in 6 of 6 cases studied using in situ end-labeling techniques (Gopal S, Achalu R, Day JD, Huang M, Narasimhan U, Day MT, Kasper EK, Trichon BH, Chen CL, Cina SJ, Berry GJ, Robertson AL, Hruban RH, unpublished data). The absence of diffuse myocardial necrosis and giant cells distinguishes hypersensitivity myocarditis from drug-induced giant cell myocarditis.[119] Acute necrotizing eosinophilic myocarditis differs from hypersensitivity myocarditis by the presence of extensive necrosis and absence of systemic allergic symptoms (Fig. 14-10 *D*; see color plate 30).[127,128]

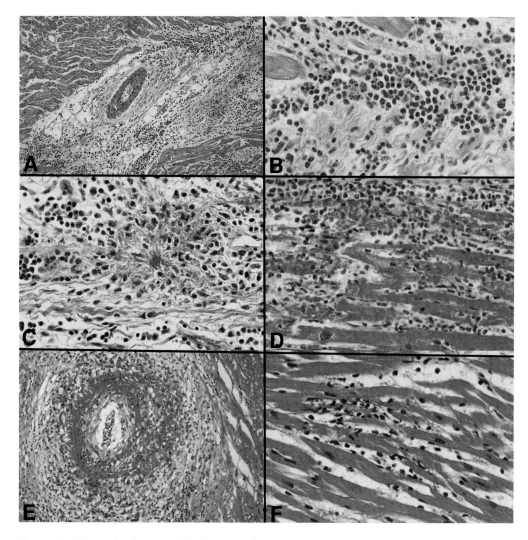

Fig. 14-10. Drug-related myocarditis. See color plate 30.

Toxic Myocarditis

Toxic myocarditis is an uncommon form of myocarditis and is characterized by direct myocyte cytotoxicity. Causative agents include antineoplastic agents such as cyclophosphamide and anthracyclines, catecholamines, cocaine, arsenicals, fluorouracil, lithium compounds, and antihypertensives. In contrast to hypersensitivity myocarditis, it is usually dose-dependent and the lesions may persist or progress after the cessation of the drug. The pathologic features reflect the cellular response to myocytopathic damage. The lesions are focal and temporally heterogeneous, reflecting the episodic or cumulative mechanism of injury. Some lesions in the biopsy sample may be acute, whereas others may be in the reparative phases. Fibrosis is not uncommon. The inflammatory infiltrates are polymorphous (lymphocytes, plasma cells, and neutrophils), but eosinophils are rare or absent. Vasculitis with associated hemorrhage has been reported in cyclophosphamide cardiotoxicity (Fig. 14-10 E; see color plate 30). Bristow and colleagues[129] reported 4 cases of early anthracycline cardiotoxicity occurring within a few days or weeks after drug administration. These were characterized by acute pericarditis-myocarditis. The myocardial lesions were typical of toxic myocarditis (Fig. 14-10 F; see color plate 30).

MYOCARDITIS ASSOCIATED WITH SYSTEMIC PROCESSES

Myocarditis has been reported in nondisease processes such as peripartum myocarditis and systemic illnesses such as thrombotic thrombocytopenic purpura. Many of these are examples of immune-mediated myocarditis.

Collagen Vascular Diseases

Myocarditis is reported in many of the connective tissue diseases, including systemic lupus erythematosus (SLE), systemic sclerosis, polyarteritis nodosa, rheumatoid arthritis, polymyositis/dermatomyositis (PM/DM), thrombotic thrombocytopenic purpura, Wegener granulomatosis, and, rarely, in ankylosing spondylitis and mixed connective tissue disease.[130-135] SLE, rheumatoid arthritis, and PM/DM are most commonly associated with myocarditis. The morphologic features on endomyocardial biopsy or in postmortem material are nonspecific myocarditis similar to the idiopathic (postviral) type of myocarditis. This emphasizes the importance of adequate clinical information in the evaluation of these cases. In SLE, fibrinoid type of vasculitis may also be observed in the small intramyocardial arteries in the biopsy specimen. Immunofluorescence studies may demonstrate immunoglobulin, complement, and fibrinogen deposition suggesting a humorally mediated form of myocarditis.

Immunosuppressive therapy remains the mainstay of treatment. Drug-related toxic myocarditis should be considered in the differential diagnosis, particularly in SLE patients receiving quinidine-based therapy.

Acute Rheumatic Fever

Rheumatic fever remains a significant cause of cardiac morbidity and mortality in underdeveloped countries.[136] It is a sequela to group A streptococcal pharyngitis and arises as an autoimmune response to extracellular or somatic bacterial antigens that share similar epitopes in human tissues. Cardiac involvement occurs in up to 55% of patients and is characterized by a pancarditis (ie, inflammation of epicardial, myocardial, and pericardial tissues). The diagnosis of rheumatic myocarditis has been made at endomyocardial biopsy, at transplantation, and at autopsy.[137,138]

The myocardial lesions consist of nonspecific lymphocytic myocarditis and Aschoff nodules. The latter may be found within the endocardium, myocardium, pericardium, and conduction system and are pathognomonic of acute rheumatic fever. They represent oval collections of histiocytes, lymphocytes, plasma cells, and giant cells (Aschoff cells) located within the interstitium adjacent to small blood vessels (Fig. 14-11; see color plate 31). This "granulomatous stage" of Aschoff nodules arises 1 to 2 months after the onset of clinical symptoms and develops within or near foci of fibrinoid necrosis. They are eventually replaced by collagenous scar tissue.

Kawasaki Disease

Kawasaki disease (mucocutaneous lymph node syndrome) is currently the most frequent cause of acquired heart disease in children in the United States.[139,140] Coronary abnormalities develop in up to 20% of patients; other cardiac manifestations include pericardial effusion, valvular insufficiency, and nonspecific lymphocytic myocarditis. Four pathologic stages are observed. Stage I occurs between days 0 and 9 and is characterized by acute perivasculitis and vasculitis of arterioles, capillaries, venules, and small arteries. An endothelitis composed of mixed inflammatory cell types is found in the major epicardial coronary arteries. Myocarditis, pericarditis, and involvement of the conduction system may occur. In stage II (12-25 days), panarteritis with thrombosis of the epicardial arteries is present. A reparative phase is seen in stage III (28-31 days) and consists of organization of thrombi and intimal proliferation. The final stage (40 days to 4 years) shows recanalization of lumens, coronary aneurysms, and myocardial ischemic injury (Fig. 14-12 *A*, 12 *B*, and 12 *D*; see color plate 32). Residual foci of lymphocytic myocarditis may be found (Fig. 14-12 C; see color plate 32). The mainstay of therapy consists of supportive care, antiplatelet drugs, and immunoglobulin given intravenously.

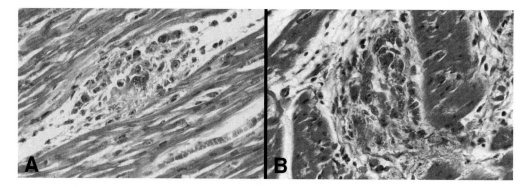

Fig. 14-11. Acute rheumatic myocarditis. See color plate 31.

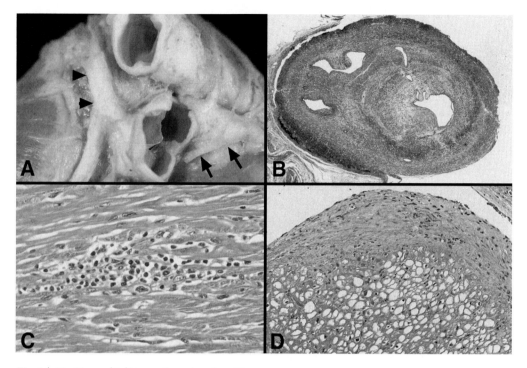

Fig. 14-12. Kawasaki disease. See color plate 32.

Peripartum Myocarditis

Peripartum myocarditis/cardiomyopathy is defined as myocardial dysfunction occurring during the third trimester of pregnancy or in the first 6 months postpartum.[141] Possible causes include viral infection, nutritional deficiencies, small vessel coronary disease, and immunologic interactions with fetal and myometrial antigens. Lymphocytic myocarditis is reported in 5% to 30% of cases. Rizeq and colleagues[141] reported an incidence of myocarditis of 8.8%, with all their cases occurring 1 to 8 weeks after onset of symptoms. All cases showed focal lymphocytic myocarditis according to the Dallas criteria. One of 3 cases had an associated cardiomyopathy. Whether postpartum myocarditis/cardiomyopathy is an entity distinct from idiopathic dilated cardiomyopathy remains unknown.

SARCOIDOSIS

Cardiac involvement in sarcoidosis occurs in 25% to 60% of patients but remains clinically silent in the vast majority of cases; isolated cardiac involvement in the absence of systemic disease is found in a minority of cases. Between 5% and 10% of patients present with cardiac dysfunction that includes: 1) arrhythmias, particularly ventricular types; 2) conduction disturbances, such as high degrees of atrioventricular block and complete bundle branch block; 3) sudden death; 4) congestive heart failure; 5) papillary muscle dysfunction; 6) acute myocardial infarction-like syndrome; 7) ventricular aneurysm; and 8) recurring pericardial effusions.[142] In a study of cardiac sarcoidosis, left-sided heart failure and syncope were the most common symptoms at hospital presentation. Atrioventricular block and ventricular tachycardia accounted for more than 75% of arrhythmias, but sudden death occurred in 2% of cases (Okura Y, Dec GW, Hare JM, Kodama M, Berry GJ, Tazelaar HD, Bailey KR, Cooper LT, unpublished data). The sensitivity of the right ventricular endomyocardial biopsy ranges from 20% to 50% because of the patchy nature of the granulomatous lesions and preferential distribution in the cephalad portion of the interventricular septum, left ventricular free wall, and papillary muscles. A negative biopsy result does not exclude the diagnosis and some have advocated institution of immunosuppressive therapy even with a negative biopsy result.[143-146] Corticosteroid therapy is effective in many cases, and cardiac transplantation remains a therapeutic option for patients who fail to respond.[147,148] Recurrence in the allograft has been reported but is uncommon; augmented immunosuppressive therapy is efficacious.[149]

Macroscopic and Histopathologic Features

Various histopathologic patterns can be observed on endomyocardial biopsy specimens from patients with cardiac sarcoidosis. These include the classic noncaseating granulomatous inflammation, lymphocytic myocarditis, dilated cardiomyopathy, and in some cases normal myocardium (Fig. 14-13; see color plate 33). Diffuse myocardial involvement progresses to myocyte hypertrophy and interstitial fibrosis resembling dilated cardiomyopathy; in a minority of cases a restrictive profile is observed. The classic granulomatous pattern is characterized by firm white nodules forming discrete masses within the interventricular septum, left ventricular free wall, or papillary muscle (Fig. 14-14 A; see color plate 34). These may be confused with metastatic deposits or fibrous tumors. The histopathologic features are similar to extracardiac lesions and consist of noncaseating, well-formed (so-called hard) granulomas composed of epithelioid histiocytes and multinucleated giant cells arranged in round or oval aggregates. These can be found as isolated lesions or may coalesce to form larger zones within the myocardium. Endocardial and pericardial involvement are observed in some cases. Scattered around and within the granulomas are mature lymphocytes, but eosinophils are absent or sparse. Mature collagenous fibrosis is present and surrounds the granulomas (Fig. 14-13 D), but active myocyte necrosis is uncommon.

Ultrastructural, Immunohistochemical, and Molecular Findings

Transmission electron microscopy shows epithelioid histiocytes containing numerous cytoplasmic dense bodies and multilobulated nuclei. Multinucleated giant cells display convoluted cytoplasmic membranes with complex interdigitating folds, multiple nuclei, and moderate

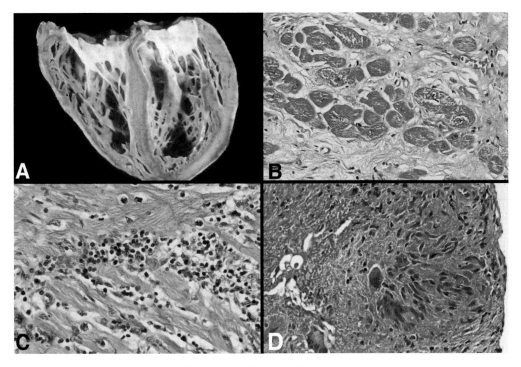

Fig. 14-13. Patterns in cardiac sarcoidosis. See color plate 33.

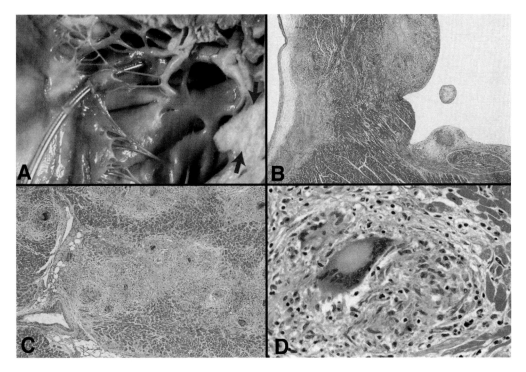

Fig. 14-14. Cardiac sarcoidosis. See color plate 34.

numbers of dense bodies, mitochondria, and endoplasmic reticulin.[142] The epithelioid histiocytes express CD68 and the infiltrating lymphocytes are almost exclusively CD3[+] T cells with a predominance of CD4[+] cells; B cells are rare.[150] Apoptotic nuclear changes and myocyte necrosis by reactivity for alpha-myosin are less intense than in lymphocytic and giant cell myocarditis (Gopal S, Achalu R, Day JD, Huang M, Narasimhan U, Day MT, Kasper EK, Trichon BH, Chen CL, Cina SJ, Berry GJ, Robertson AL, Hruban RH, unpublished data).

Differential Diagnosis in Cardiac Sarcoidosis

The differential diagnosis includes granulomatous and giant cell lesions of the heart. Granulomatous infections are uncommon in immunocompetent patients, but we routinely perform histochemical stains for fungal and mycobacterial microorganisms. In general, necrotizing granulomas are found in infectious lesions. Giant cell myocarditis is characterized by the presence of giant cells but, by definition, granulomas are absent. In hypersensitivity myocarditis, the histiocytic lesions are poorly formed and are centered on collagen fibers. Eosinophils are numerous, but multinucleated giant cells and fibrosis are not found. The granuloma-like lesions of acute rheumatic fever are poorly formed, and the giant cells are generally smaller and do not resemble Langerhans type. Foreign body-type giant cells surrounding catheter sheath fragments can be found in biopsy specimens of patients undergoing repeated biopsy procedures (Fig. 14-5 A). The edge of healing ischemic infarcts can contain giant cells of myogenic origin; lymphocytes and hemosiderin-laden macrophages are seen within the scar tissue. Granulomas are also reported in metabolic disorders such as lipogranulomatosis (Farber disease), oxalosis, and gout; in collagen vascular diseases such as rheumatoid nodules, Wegener granulomatosis, and Churg-Strauss syndrome; and in chronic granulomatous disease of childhood.[151]

IDIOPATHIC GIANT CELL MYOCARDITIS

Idiopathic giant cell myocarditis (IGCM) is a rare but frequently fatal form of myocarditis.[152] It often occurs in previously healthy young adults who present with the abrupt onset of heart failure or arrhythmias or both. Death occurs within weeks or months of onset of symptoms unless aggressive immunosuppression and cardiac transplantation are implemented.[153] Twenty percent of patients have an associated autoimmune disorder such as ulcerative colitis, cryofibrinogenemia, rheumatoid arthritis, myasthenia gravis, hyperthyroidism, or hypothyroidism. Other associations include drug hypersensitivity, Wegener granulomatosis, thymoma, sarcoidosis, and infections.[119,154] Patients receiving combination therapies such as corticosteroids plus cyclosporine or azathioprine survived for an average of 12 months compared with an average of 3 months for patients not receiving any immunosuppressive therapy.[153] In rare instances, after treatment some patients have prolonged survival before requiring cardiac transplantation.[155]

Morphologic Findings in IGCM

At postmortem examination or at transplantation, confluent or multifocal areas of necrosis are easily observed in the heart. The weight of the heart is usually normal or slightly increased. The 4 chambers of the heart are uniformly involved in most cases. In the late or healed stages of the disease, the ventricular wall may appear thin, but this reflects diffuse scarring and not aneurysmal changes because islands of myocytes are found within the collagenous scar tissue (Fig. 14-15 *C* and 15 *D*; see color plate 35). Endocardial and pericardial involvement have been described but the process is primarily centered on the myocardium.

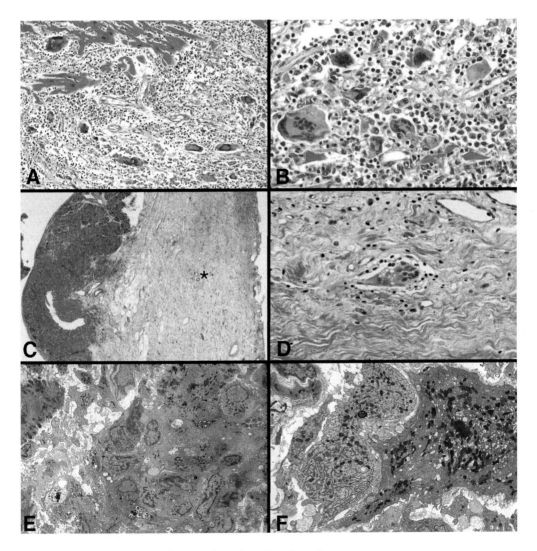

Fig. 14-15. Idiopathic giant cell myocarditis. See color plate 35.

The morphologic findings have been described.[150,153,156,157] These consist of regions of diffuse serpiginous necrosis containing multinucleated giant cells, lymphocytes, histiocytes, and eosinophils in the absence of sarcoidlike granulomas. The giant cells are distributed throughout the inflammatory infiltrates and in apposition to the sarcolemmal membranes of necrotic myocytes. They measure up to 90 x 20 microns and contain up to 20 nuclei in each cell (Fig. 14-15 *A* and 15 *B*; see color plate 35). The necrotic myocardium is replaced by edematous granulation tissue, and the border between viable and necrotic myocardium is not well delineated.

Litovsky and colleagues[150] proposed classification of IGCM into acute, healing, and healed phases. The acute or active phase is described above and is distinguished by the abundant inflammatory response, loose connective tissue stroma, and numerous giant cells of macrophage origin. In the healing or resolving stage, granulation tissue and immature fibrosis replace the myocardium, and the number of giant cells and inflammatory cells is diminished. In the healed or resolved phase, mature fibrosis is noted, with rare or absent giant cells and sparse inflammatory cells. Myocytes are found as islands of single cells or small clusters surrounded by scar tissue (Fig. 14-15 *C* and 15 *D*).

The distinction between active and resolving IGCM on endomyocardial biopsy specimen can be problematic in our experience, because the giant cells are not evenly distributed within the necrotic zones in either stage. Connective tissue stains such as Masson trichrome are helpful in identifying the quality and distribution of collagen. In explanted or postmortem heart specimens, some degree of overlap between the different stages is recognized, suggesting the temporal heterogeneity of this disease. This is an important caveat when examining endomyocardial biopsy specimens for the purpose of grading the response to immunosuppressive therapy.

Ultrastructural, Immunohistochemical, and Molecular Findings in IGCM

Until recently, the origin of the multinucleated giant cells in IGCM has been the subject of controversy. Derivation from myogenic and macrophagic cells was considered.[158,159] At the ultrastructural level, they contain large numbers of cytoplasmic vacuoles but not myofibrils, supporting macrophagic origin. Immunohistochemical studies provide further support because the giant cells stain strongly with the antibody KP1 that is raised to the macrophage-associated antigen CD68 and do not stain with muscle markers, actin, desmin, or myoglobin[150,160,161] (Fig. 14-16 *E* and 16 *F*; see color plate 36).

CD3+ T cells are the predominant inflammatory cell type; B cells are rare or absent (Fig. 14-16 *A*; see color plate 36). In the active phase, CD8 cytotoxic or suppressor cells far outnumber CD4 cells (Fig. 14-16 *C* and 16 *D*; see color plate 36). In the healing stages, occasional actin-positive myogenic-type giant cells are found at the edge of inflamed and viable myocytes, suggesting the sequela of inflammatory injury to myocytes. CD68+ giant

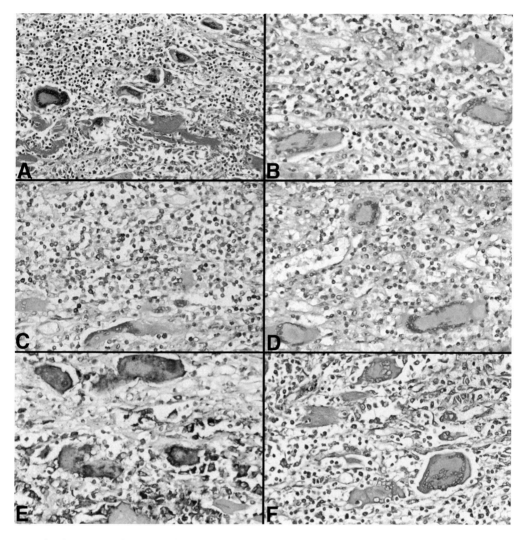

Fig. 14-16. Immunophenotype of idiopathic giant cell myocarditis. See color plate 36.

cells of macrophagic origin are more common than myogenic giant cells, but there are fewer of them than in the active phase. In one case, CD4 cells predominated over CD8 cells.[150] Apoptosis and necrosis are conspicuous by molecular techniques (Gopal S, Achalu R, Day JD, Huang M, Narasimhan U, Day MT, Kasper EK, Trichon BH, Chen CL, Cina SJ, Berry GJ, Robertson AL, Hruban RH, unpublished data).

Differential Diagnosis in IGCM

The diagnostic considerations are similar to those enumerated in the discussion of sarcoidosis. Foreign body granulomas are seen in biopsy samples of patients undergoing repetitive sampling (Fig. 14-5 *A*). The clinical and morphologic distinction between cardiac sarcoidosis and idiopathic giant cell myocarditis can be problematic. Previously, some have claimed IGCM as a type of cardiac sarcoidosis. In our experience, some degree of overlap can exist, particularly on small endomyocardial biopsy samples. In general, however, close attention to the presence or absence of granulomas is the key discriminating feature. In addition, sarcoidosis has significantly more fibrosis and few or no eosinophils within the inflammatory infiltrate. Myocyte necrosis, particularly the broad zonal distribution, is a feature of IGCM, whereas the mass-like effect is seen in sarcoidosis (Okura Y, Dec GW, Hare JM, Kodama M, Berry GJ, Tazelaar HD, Bailey KR, Cooper LT, unpublished data). Hematolymphoid malignancies can be associated with architectural distortion and myocyte necrosis (Fig. 14-5 *C* and 5 *D*). In some cases, polymorphous cell infiltrates may be present, including eosinophils. Cytologic atypia of the neoplastic cells is the cardinal feature of these lesions. Immunohistochemical and molecular studies are useful, because the majority of these lesions are B cell. Histochemical stains and bacteriologic studies are required to distinguish infectious granulomatous lesions in the heart from IGCM. Eosinophils can be found in hypersensitivity myocarditis and in IGCM. The number of eosinophils is significantly more in hypersensitivity myocarditis, and myocyte necrosis is usually absent.

CONCLUSIONS

The diagnosis and classification of myocarditis are challenging. Use of the endomyocardial biopsy for the evaluation of patients with new-onset congestive heart failure or arrhythmias places the surgical pathologist in a critical role in the diagnosis and management of myocarditis. Direct and open communication with clinicians is essential for accurate clinical-pathologic assessment. Recognition of the architectural alterations in the myocardium and the predominant inflammatory cell type narrow the diagnostic possibilities. Lymphocytic infiltrates are found in lymphocytic myocarditis, some viral types, toxic myocarditis, sarcoidosis, hematopoietic malignancies, myocarditis associated with collagen vascular diseases, and postpartum myocarditis. Infiltrates composed predominantly of neutrophils suggest suppurative myocarditis, pressor effect, ischemic necrosis, and early viral and idiopathic myocarditis (particularly in children). Eosinophils may be a minor component of idiopathic and giant cell myocarditis but are predominant in hypersensitivity and parasitic myocarditis and in hypereosinophilic syndrome. Giant cells are seen in IGCM, sarcoidosis, rheumatic fever, and granulomatous infections and occasionally in idiopathic myocarditis (often of myogenic origin).[12] The treatment and prognosis for many of these types of myocarditis differ significantly, and therefore accurate classification is important.

The relationship of idiopathic myocarditis to the subsequent development of idiopathic dilated cardiomyopathy remains controversial. The application of molecular techniques has broadened our concepts about the pathogenesis of both disease processes. These clues should lead to therapeutic strategies for their treatment and prevention. The surgical pathologist will continue to play a central role in these efforts.

REFERENCES

1. Saphir O. Myocarditis: a general review, with an analysis of two hundred and forty cases. Arch Pathol 1941;32:1000-1051.
2. Sobernheim JF. Praktische diagnostik der inneren Krankheitenvorzuglicher Rucksicht auf pathologische anatomie. Berlin: Hirschwald, 1837:118-120.
3. Virchow R. Die Cellularpathologie in ihrer Begründung auf physiologische und pathologische Gewebelehre. Berlin: August Hirschwald, 1858.
4. Herrick JB. Clinical features of sudden obstruction of the coronary arteries. JAMA 1912;59:2015-2020.
5. Sakakibara S, Konno S. Endomyocardial biopsy. Jpn Heart J 1962;3:537-543.
6. Aretz HT, Billingham ME, Edwards WD, Factor SM, Fallon JT, Fenoglio JJ Jr, Olsen EGJ, Schoen FJ. Myocarditis. A histopathologic definition and classification. Am J Cardiovasc Pathol 1986;1:3-14.
7. Boikan WS. Myocarditis perniciosa. Virchows Arch Path Anat 1931;282:46-66.
8. Gore I, Saphir O. Myocarditis: a classification of 1402 cases. Am Heart J 1947;34:827-830.
9. Burch GE, Ray CT. Myocarditis and myocardial degeneration. Bull Tulane Med Fac 1948;8:1-13.
10. Kline IK, Saphir O. Chronic pernicious myocarditis. Am Heart J 1960;59:681-697.
11. Billingham M. Acute myocarditis: a diagnostic dilemma. Br Heart J 1987;58:6-8.
12. Aretz HT. Myocarditis: the Dallas criteria. Hum Pathol 1987;18:619-624.
13. Spiegelhalter DJ, Stovin PG. An analysis of repeated biopsies following cardiac transplantation. Stat Med 1983;2:33-40.
14. Hauck AJ, Kearney DL, Edwards WD. Evaluation of postmortem endomyocardial biopsy specimens from 38 patients with lymphocytic myocarditis: implications for role of sampling error. Mayo Clin Proc 1989;64:1235-1245.
15. Lie JT. Myocarditis and endomyocardial biopsy in unexplained heart failure: a diagnosis in search of a disease. Ann Intern Med 1988;109:525-528.
16. Chow LH, Radio SJ, Sears TD, McManus BM. Insensitivity of right ventricular endomyocardial biopsy in the diagnosis of myocarditis. J Am Coll Cardiol 1989;14:915-920.
17. Davies MJ, Ward DE. How can myocarditis be diagnosed and should it be treated? Br Heart J 1992;68:346-347.
18. Hauck AJ, Edwards WD. Histopathologic examination of tissues obtained by endomyocardial biopsy. In: Fowles RE, ed. Cardiac biopsy. Mount Kisco, NY: Futura Publishing, 1992:95-153.
19. Dec GW, Fallon JT, Southern JF, Palacios I. "Borderline" myocarditis: an indication for repeat endomyocardial biopsy. J Am Coll Cardiol 1990;15:283-289.
20. Fenoglio JJ Jr, Ursell PC, Kellogg CF, Drusin RE, Weiss MB. Diagnosis and classification of myocarditis by endomyocardial biopsy. N Engl J Med 1983;308:12-18.
21. Billingham ME. The diagnostic criteria of myocarditis by endomyocardial biopsy. Heart Vessels Suppl 1985;1:133-137.

22. Dec GW Jr, Palacios IF, Fallon JT, Aretz HT, Mills J, Lee DC, Johnson RA. Active myocarditis in the spectrum of acute dilated cardiomyopathies. Clinical features, histologic correlates, and clinical outcome. N Engl J Med 1985;312:885-890.

23. Parillo JE, Cunnion RE, Epstein SE, Parker MM, Suffredini AF, Brenner M, Schaer GL, Palmeri ST, Cannon RO III, Alling D, Wittes JT, Ferrans VJ, Rodriguez ER, Fauci AS. A prospective, randomized, controlled trial of prednisone for dilated cardiomyopathy. N Engl J Med 1989;321:1061-1068.

24. Midei MG, DeMent SH, Feldman AM, Hutchins GM, Baughman KL. Peripartum myocarditis and cardiomyopathy. Circulation 1990;81:922-928.

25. Drucker NA, Colan SD, Lewis AB, Beiser AS, Wessel DL, Takahashi M, Baker AL, Perez-Atayde AR, Newburger JW. Gamma-globulin treatment of acute myocarditis in the pediatric population. Circulation 1994;89:252-257.

26. Mason JW, O'Connell JB, Herskowitz A, Rose NR, McManus BM, Billingham ME, Moon TE. A clinical trial of immunosuppressive therapy for myocarditis. The Myocarditis Treatment Trial Investigators. N Engl J Med 1995;333:269-275.

27. Bozkurt B, Villanueva FS, Holubkov R, Tokarczyk T, Alvarez RJ Jr, MacGowan GA, Murali S, Rosenblum WD, Feldman AM, McNamara DM. Intravenous immune globulin in the therapy of peripartum cardiomyopathy. J Am Coll Cardiol 1999;34:177-180.

28. McNamara DM, Starling RC, Dec GW, Loh E, Torre-Amione G, Gass A, Janosko KM, Tokarczyk T, Holubkov R, Feldman AM. Intervention in myocarditis and acute cardiomyopathy with immune globulin: results from the randomized placebo controlled IMAC trial. Circulation 1999;100 Suppl 1:I-21.

29. McCarthy RE III, Boehmer JP, Hruban RH, Hutchins GM, Kasper EK, Hare JM, Baughman KL. Long-term outcome of fulminant myocarditis as compared with acute (nonfulminant) myocarditis. N Engl J Med 2000;342:690-695.

30. Feldman AM, McNamara D. Myocarditis. N Engl J Med 2000;343:1388-1398.

31. Leatherbury L, Chandra RS, Shapiro SR, Perry LW. Value of endomyocardial biopsy in infants, children and adolescents with dilated or hypertrophic cardiomyopathy and myocarditis. J Am Coll Cardiol 1988;12:1547-1554.

32. Billingham ME. Acute myocarditis: is sampling error a contraindication for diagnostic biopsies? J Am Coll Cardiol 1989;14:921-922.

33. Billingham ME. The histopathological diagnosis and morphological features of acute myocarditis. In: Banatvala JE, ed. Viral infections of the heart. London: Edward Arnold, 1993:32-58.

34. Billingham ME. Is acute cardiac rejection a model of myocarditis in humans? Eur Heart J 1987;8 Suppl J:19-23.

35. Milin J, Stojsic D, Vuckovic D, Benc D, Hadzic M, Stojsic A, Zivkov-Saponja D. Ultrastructural aspect of myocarditis: its relevance for the diagnosis. Ultrastruct Pathol 1995;19:463-467.

36. Aretz HT, Southern JF, Palacios IF, Dec GW, Howard CA, Fallon JT. Morphological and immunological findings in heart biopsies of patients with suspected or treated myocarditis. Eur Heart J 1987;8 Suppl J:187-190.

37. Kurnick JT, Leary C, Palacios IF, Fallon JT. Culture and characterization of lymphocytic infiltrates from endomyocardial biopsies of patients with idiopathic myocarditis. Eur Heart J 1987;8 Suppl J:135-139.

38. Chow LH, Ye Y, Linder J, McManus BM. Phenotypic analysis of infiltrating cells in human myocarditis. An immunohistochemical study in paraffin-embedded tissue. Arch Pathol Lab Med 1989;113:1357-1362.

39. Ino T, Kishiro M, Okubo M, Akimoto K, Nishimoto K, Yabuta K, Okada R. Late persistent expressions of ICAM-1 and VCAM-1 on myocardial tissue in children with lymphocytic myocarditis. Cardiovasc Res 1997;34:323-328.

40. Yokoyama H, Kuwao S, Kohno K, Suzuki K, Kameya T, Izumi T. Cardiac dendritic cells and acute myocarditis in the human heart. Jpn Circ J 2000;64:57-64.

41. Bowles NE, Richardson PJ, Olsen EG, Archard LC. Detection of Coxsackie-B-virus-specific RNA sequences in myocardial biopsy samples from patients with myocarditis and dilated cardiomyopathy. Lancet 1986;1:1120-1123.

42. Kandolf R, Ameis D, Kirschner P, Canu A, Hofschneider PH. In situ detection of enteroviral genomes in myocardial cells by nucleic acid hybridization: an approach to the diagnosis of viral heart disease. Proc Natl Acad Sci U S A 1987;84:6272-6276.

43. Weiss LM, Movahed LA, Billingham ME, Cleary ML. Detection of Coxsackievirus B3 RNA in myocardial tissues by the polymerase chain reaction. Am J Pathol 1991;138:497-503.

44. Schwaiger A, Umlauft F, Weyrer K, Larcher C, Lyons J, Muhlberger V, Dietze O, Grunewald K. Detection of enteroviral ribonucleic acid in myocardial biopsies from patients with idiopathic dilated cardiomyopathy by polymerase chain reaction. Am Heart J 1993;126:406-410.

45. Weiss LM, Liu XF, Chang KL, Billingham ME. Detection of enteroviral RNA in idiopathic dilated cardiomyopathy and other human cardiac tissues. J Clin Invest 1992;90:156-159.

46. Edwards WD, Holmes DR Jr, Reeder GS. Diagnosis of active lymphocytic myocarditis by endomyocardial biopsy: quantitative criteria for light microscopy. Mayo Clin Proc 1982;57:419-425.

47. Tazelaar HD, Billingham ME. Myocardial lymphocytes. Fact, fancy, or myocarditis? Am J Cardiovasc Pathol 1987;1:47-50.

48. Hill DA, Swanson PE. Myocardial extramedullary hematopoiesis: a clinicopathologic study. Mod Pathol 2000;13:779-787.

49. Tazelaar HD, Billingham ME. Leukocytic infiltrates in idiopathic dilated cardiomyopathy. A source of confusion with active myocarditis. Am J Surg Pathol 1986;10:405-412.

50. Billingham ME. Morphology of dilated cardiomyopathy: histopathological diagnosis of acute myocarditis and dilated cardiomyopathy. In Baroldi G, Carmerini F, Goodwin JF, eds. Advances in cardiomyopathies. Berlin: Springer-Verlag, 1990:266-273.

51. Loire R. Cardiac lesions in bacterial endocarditis: from findings of pathology to possibilities and limits of surgery. [French.] Arch Mal Coeur Vaiss 1993;86 Suppl:1811-1818.

52. Hager WD, Speck EL, Mathew PK, Boger JN, Wallace WA. Endocarditis with myocardial abscesses and pericarditis in an adult: group G streptococcus as a cause. Arch Intern Med 1977;137:1725-1728.

53. McCue MJ, Moore EE. Myocarditis with microabscess formation caused by *Listeria monocytogenes* associated with myocardial infarct. Hum Pathol 1979;10:469-472.

54. Grewe PH, Machraoui A, Deneke T, Muller KM. Suppurative pancarditis: a lethal complication of coronary stent implantation. Heart 1999;81:559.

55. Jubber AS, Gunawardana DR, Lulu AR. Acute pulmonary edema in Brucella myocarditis and interstitial pneumonitis. Chest 1990;97:1008-1009.

56. Agarwala BN, Ruschhaupt DG. Complete heart block from *Mycoplasma pneumoniae* infection. Pediatr Cardiol 1991;12:233-236.

57. Armengol S, Domingo C, Mesalles E. Myocarditis: a rare complication during Legionella infection. Int J Cardiol 1992;37:418-420.

58. Jahangir A, Kolbert C, Edwards W, Mitchell P, Dumler JS, Persing DH. Fatal pancarditis associated with human granulocytic Ehrlichiosis in a 44-year-old man. Clin Infect Dis 1998;27:1424-1427.

59. Odeh M, Oliven A. Chlamydial infections of the heart. Eur J Clin Microbiol Infect Dis 1992;11:885-893.

60. Shilkin KB. *Salmonella typhimurium* pancarditis. Postgrad Med J 1969;45:40-53.

61. Burt CR, Proudfoot JC, Roberts M, Horowitz RH. Fatal myocarditis secondary to Salmonella septicemia in a young adult. J Emerg Med 1990;8:295-297.

62. Wander GS, Khurana SB, Puri S. Salmonella myopericarditis presenting with acute pulmonary oedema. Indian Heart J 1992;44:55-56.

63. Friman G, Wesslen L, Fohlman J, Karjalainen J, Rolf C. The epidemiology of infectious myocarditis, lymphocytic myocarditis and dilated cardiomyopathy. Eur Heart J 1995;16 Suppl O:36-41.

64. Romberg E. Ueber die Erkrankungen des Herz muskels bei Typhus abdominalis, Scharlach und Diphtherie. Dtsch Arch Klin Med 1891;48:369-413.

65. Horn H, Saphir O. Involvement of myocardium in tuberculosis: review of literature and report of 3 cases. Am Rev Tuberc 1935;32:492-506.

66. Chan AC, Dickens P. Tuberculous myocarditis presenting as sudden cardiac death. Forensic Sci Int 1992;57:45-50.

67. Darwish Y, Mushannen B, Hussain KM, Nititham K, Dadkhah S, Atkinson J, Zar F, Kogan A. Pancardiac tuberculosis—a case report. Angiology 1998;49:151-156.

68. Mooney EE, Kenan DJ, Sweeney EC, Gaede JT. Myocarditis in Whipple's disease: an unsuspected cause of symptoms and sudden death. Mod Pathol 1997;10:524-529.

69. Saphir O. Myocarditis: a general review, with an analysis of two hundred and forty cases. Arch Pathol 1942;33:88-137.

70. Jackman JD Jr, Radolf JD. Cardiovascular syphilis. Am J Med 1989;87:425-433.

71. McAlister HF, Klementowicz PT, Andrews C, Fisher JD, Feld M, Furman S. Lyme carditis: an important cause of reversible heart block. Ann Intern Med 1989;110:339-345.

72. Stanek G, Klein J, Bittner R, Glogar D. Isolation of *Borrelia burgdorferi* from the myocardium of a patient with longstanding cardiomyopathy. N Engl J Med 1990;322:249-252.

73. Cox J, Krajden M. Cardiovascular manifestations of Lyme disease. Am Heart J 1991;122:1449-1455.

74. Mason JW. Myocarditis. Adv Intern Med 1999;44:293-310.

75. Burk M. Viral myocarditis. Histopathology 1990;17:193-200.

76. Chaudary S, Jaski BE. Fulminant mumps myocarditis. Ann Intern Med 1989;110:569-570.

77. Ozkutlu S, Soylemezoglu O, Calikoglu AS, Kale G, Karaaslan E. Fatal mumps myocarditis. Jpn Heart J 1989;30:109-114.

78. Kabakus N, Aydinoglu H, Yekeler H, Arslan IN. Fatal mumps nephritis and myocarditis. J Trop Pediatr 1999;45:358-360.

79. Frustaci A, Abdulla AK, Caldarulo M, Buffon A. Fatal measles myocarditis. Cardiologia 1990;35:347-349.

80. Grumbach IM, Heim A, Pring-Akerblom P, Vonhof S, Hein WJ, Muller G, Figulla HR. Adenoviruses and enteroviruses as pathogens in myocarditis and dilated cardiomyopathy. Acta Cardiol 1999;54:83-88.

81. Chia JK, Jackson B. Myopericarditis due to parvovirus B19 in an adult. Clin Infect Dis 1996;23:200-201.

82. McCormick JB, King IJ, Webb PA, Johnson KM, O'Sullivan R, Smith ES, Trippel S, Tong TC. A case-control study of the clinical diagnosis and course of Lassa fever. J Infect Dis 1987;155:445-455.

83. Vilchez RA, Fung JJ, Kusne S. Influenza A myocarditis developing in an adult liver transplant recipient despite vaccination: a case report and review of the literature. Transplantation 2000;70:543-545.

84. Ursell PC, Habib A, Sharma P, Mesa-Tejada R, Lefkowitch JH, Fenoglio JJ Jr. Hepatitis B virus and myocarditis. Hum Pathol 1984;15:481-484.

85. Finlay-Jones LR. Fatal myocarditis after vaccination against smallpox. N Engl J Med 1964;270:41-42.

86. Tsintsof A, Delprado WJ, Keogh AM. Varicella zoster myocarditis progressing to cardiomyopathy and cardiac transplantation. Br Heart J 1993;70:93-95.

87. Schonian U, Crombach M, Maser S, Maisch B. Cytomegalovirus-associated heart muscle disease. Eur Heart J 1995;16 Suppl O:46-49.

88. Pucci A, Ghisetti V, Donegani E, Barbui A, David E, Fortunato M, Papandrea C, Pansini S, Zattera G, di Summa M, Marchiaro G, Mollo F. Histologic and molecular diagnosis of myocardial human cytomegalovirus infection after heart transplantation. J Heart Lung Transplant 1994;13:1072-1080.

89. Arbustini E, Grasso M, Diegoli M, Percivalle E, Grossi P, Bramerio M, Campana C, Goggi C, Gavazzi A, Vigano M. Histopathologic and molecular profile of human cytomegalovirus infections in patients with heart transplants. Am J Clin Pathol 1992;98:205-213.

90. Partanen J, Nieminen MS, Krogerus L, Lautenschlager I, Geagea A, Aarnio P, Mattila S. Cytomegalovirus myocarditis in transplanted heart verified by endomyocardial biopsy. Clin Cardiol 1991;14:847-849.

91. Adachi N, Kiwaki K, Tsuchiya H, Migita M, Yoshimoto T, Matsuda I. Fatal cytomegalovirus myocarditis in a seronegative ALL patient. Acta Paediatr Jpn 1995;37:211-216.

92. Maisch B, Schonian U, Crombach M, Wendl I, Bethge C, Herzum M, Klein HH. Cytomegalovirus associated inflammatory heart muscle disease. Scand J Infect Dis Suppl 1993;88:135-148.

93. Grattan MT, Moreno-Cabral CE, Starnes VA, Oyer PE, Stinson EB, Shumway NE. Cytomegalovirus infection is associated with cardiac allograft rejection and atherosclerosis. JAMA 1989;261:3561-3566.

94. Unger ER, Budgeon LR, Myerson D, Brigati DJ. Viral diagnosis by in situ hybridization. Description of a rapid simplified colorimetric method. Am J Surg Pathol 1986;10:1-8.

95. Weiss LM, Movahed LA, Berry GJ, Billingham ME. In situ hybridization studies for viral nucleic acids in heart and lung allograft biopsies. Am J Clin Pathol 1990;93:675-679.

96. Kemnitz J, Haverich A, Gubernatis G, Cohnert TR. Rapid identification of viral infections in liver, heart, and kidney allograft biopsies by in situ hybridization. Am J Surg Pathol 1989;13:80-82.

97. Hruban Z, Kuzo R, Heimann P, Weisenberg E, Hruban RH. Globular changes in cytomegaloviral inclusions after ganciclovir treatment. Arch Virol 1989;108:287-293.

98. Tyson AA Jr, Hackshaw BT, Kutcher MA. Acute Epstein-Barr virus myocarditis simulating myocardial infarction with cardiogenic shock. South Med J 1989;82:1184-1187.

99. Kaul S, Fishbein MC, Siegel RJ. Cardiac manifestations of acquired immune deficiency syndrome: a 1991 update. Am Heart J 1991;122:535-544.

100. Beschomer WE, Baughman K, Turnicky RP, Hutchins GM, Rowe SA, Kavanaugh-McHugh AL, Suresch DL, Herskowitz A. HIV-associated myocarditis. Pathology and immunopathology. Am J Pathol 1990;137:1365-1371.

101. Parravicini C, Baroldi G, Gaiera G, Lazzarin A. Phenotype of intramyocardial leukocytic infiltrates in acquired immunodeficiency syndrome (AIDS): a postmortem immunohistochemical study in 34 consecutive cases. Mod Pathol 1991;4:559-565.

102. Walsh TJ, Hutchins GM, Bulkley BH, Mendelsohn G. Fungal infections of the heart: analysis of 51 autopsy cases. Am J Cardiol 1980;45:357-366.

103. Atkinson JB, Connor DH, Robinowitz M, McAllister HA, Virmani R. Cardiac fungal infections: review of autopsy findings in 60 patients. Hum Pathol 1984;15:935-942.

104. Hofman P, Gari-Toussaint M, Bernard E, Michiels JF, Gibelin P, Le Fichoux Y, Morand P, Loubiere R. Fungal myocarditis in acquired immunodeficiency syndrome. [French.] Arch Mal Coeur Vaiss 1992;85:203-208.

105. Reichenspurner H, Gamberg P, Nitschke M, Valantine H, Hunt S, Oyer PE, Reitz BA. Significant reduction in the number of fungal infections after lung-, heart-lung, and heart transplantation using aerosolized amphotericin B prophylaxis. Transplant Proc 1997;29:627-628.

106. Compton SJ, Celum CL, Lee C, Thompson D, Sumi SM, Fritsche TR, Coombs RW. Trichinosis with ventilatory failure and persistent myocarditis. Clin Infect Dis 1993;16:500-504.

107. Montoya JG, Jordan R, Lingamneni S, Berry GJ, Remington JS. Toxoplasmic myocarditis and polymyositis in patients with acute acquired toxoplasmosis diagnosed during life. Clin Infect Dis 1997;24:676-683.

108. Wreghitt TG, McNeil K, Roth C, Wallwork J, McKee T, Parameshwar J. Antibiotic prophylaxis for the prevention of donor-acquired *Toxoplasma gondii* infection in transplant patients. J Infect 1995;31:253-254.

109. Holliman R, Johnson J, Savva D, Cary N, Wreghitt T. Diagnosis of toxoplasma infection in cardiac transplant recipients using the polymerase chain reaction. J Clin Pathol 1992;45:931-932.

110. Pardo-Mindan FJ, Herreros J, Marigil MA, Arcas R, Diez J. Myocardial calcification following heart transplantation. J Heart Transplant 1986;5:332-335.

111. Cohnert TR, Kemnitz J, Haverich A, Dralle H. Myocardial calcification after orthotopic heart transplantation. J Heart Transplant 1988;7:304-308.

112. Parada H, Carrasco HA, Anez N, Fuenmayor C, Inglessis I. Cardiac involvement is a constant finding in acute Chagas' disease: a clinical, parasitological and histopathological study. Int J Cardiol 1997;60:49-54.

113. Sadigursky M, von Kreuter BF, Ling PY, Santos-Buch CA. Association of elevated anti-sarcolemma, anti-idiotype antibody levels with the clinical and pathologic expression of chronic Chagas myocarditis. Circulation 1989;80:1269-1276.

114. Hagar JM, Rahimtoola SH. Chagas' heart disease in the United States. N Engl J Med 1991;325:763-768.

115. Marin-Garcia J. Left ventricular dysfunction in Rocky Mountain spotted fever. Clin Cardiol 1983;6:501-506.

116. Walker DH, Parks FM, Betz TG, Taylor JP, Muehberger JW. Histopathology and immunohisto-logic demonstration of the distribution of *Rickettsia typhi* in fatal murine typhus. Am J Clin Pathol 1989;91:720-724.

117. Woodward TE, Togo Y, Lee YC, Hornick RB. Specific microbial infections of the myocardium and pericardium. A study of 82 patients. Arch Intern Med 1967;120:270-279.

118. Billingham M. Pharmacotoxic myocardial disease: an endomyocardial study. In: Sekiguchi M, Olsen EGJ, Goodwin JF, eds. Myocarditis and related disorders: proceedings of the International Symposium on Cardiomyopathy and Myocarditis. Tokyo: Springer-Verlag, 1985:278-282.

119. Daniels PR, Berry GJ, Tazelaar HD, Cooper LT. Giant cell myocarditis as a manifestation of drug hypersensitivity. Cardiovasc Pathol 2000;9:287-291.

120. Mullick FG, McAllister HA. Myocarditis associated with methyldopa therapy. JAMA 1977;237:1699-1701.

121. Beghetti M, Wilson GJ, Bohn D, Benson L. Hypersensitivity myocarditis caused by an allergic reaction to cefaclor. J Pediatr 1998;132:172-173.

122. Zaacks SM, Klein L, Tan CD, Rodriguez ER, Leikin JB. Hypersensitivity myocarditis associated with ephedra use. J Toxicol Clin Toxicol 1999;37:485-489.

123. Gravanis MB, Hertzler GL, Franch RH, Stacy LD, Ansari AA, Kanter KR, Tazelaar HD, Rodeheffer R, McGregor C. Hypersensitivity myocarditis in heart transplant candidates. J Heart Lung Transplant 1991;10:688-697.

124. Hawkins ET, Levine TB, Goss SJ, Moosvi A, Levine AB. Hypersensitivity myocarditis in the explanted hearts of transplant recipients. Reappraisal of pathologic criteria and their clinical impli-cations. Pathol Annu 1995;30:287-304.

125. Spear GS. Eosinophilic explant carditis with eosinophilia: ? Hypersensitivity to dobutamine infusion. J Heart Lung Transplant 1995;14:755-760.

126. Burke AP, Saenger J, Mullick F, Virmani R. Hypersensitivity myocarditis. Arch Pathol Lab Med 1991;115:764-769.

127. Herzog CA, Snover DC, Staley NA. Acute necrotising eosinophilic myocarditis. Br Heart J 1984;52:343-348.

128. Getz MA, Subramanian R, Logemann T, Ballantyne F. Acute necrotizing eosinophilic myocarditis as a manifestation of severe hypersensitivity myocarditis. Antemortem diagnosis and successful treatment. Ann Intern Med 1991;115:201-202.

129. Bristow MR, Thompson PD, Martin RP, Mason JW, Billingham ME, Harrison DC. Early anthracycline cardiotoxicity. Am J Med 1978;65:823-832.

130. Ferrans VJ, Rodriguez ER. Cardiovascular lesions in collagen-vascular diseases. Heart Vessels Suppl 1985;1:256-261.

131. Kerr LD, Spiera H. Myocarditis as a complication in scleroderma patients with myositis. Clin Cardiol 1993;16:895-899.

132. Clemson BS, Miller WR, Luck JC, Feriss JA. Acute myocarditis in fulminant systemic sclerosis. Chest 1992;101:872-874.

133. Dickens P, Nicholls J, Lau CP. Acute hemorrhagic myocarditis in systemic lupus erythematosus. Heart Vessels 1992;7:104-106.

134. Scully RE, Mark EJ, McNeely WF, McNeely BU. Case records of the Massachusetts General Hospital: weekly clinicopathological exercises. Case 24-1995. N Engl J Med 1995;333:369-377.

135. Podolsky SH, Zembowicz A, Schoen FJ, Benjamin RJ, Sonna LA. Massive myocardial necrosis in thrombotic thrombocytopenic purpura: a case report and review of the literature. Arch Pathol Lab Med 1999;123:937-940.

136. Hutchison SJ. Acute rheumatic fever. J Infect 1998;36:249-253.

137. Ursell PC, Albala A, Fenoglio JJ Jr. Diagnosis of acute rheumatic carditis by endomyocardial biopsy. Hum Pathol 1982;13:677-679.

138. Silva LM, Mansur AJ, Bocchi EA, Stolf NA, Bellotti G. Unsuspected rheumatic fever carditis ending in heart transplantation. Thorac Cardiovasc Surg 1994;42:191-193.

139. Rowley AH, Shulman ST. Kawasaki syndrome. Clin Microbiol Rev 1998;11:405-414.

140. Takahashi M. Kawasaki disease. Curr Opin Pediatr 1997;9:523-529.

141. Rizeq MN, Rickenbacher PR, Fowler MB, Billingham ME. Incidence of myocarditis in peripartum cardiomyopathy. Am J Cardiol 1994;74:474-477.

142. Roberts WC, McAllister HA Jr, Ferrans VJ. Sarcoidosis of the heart. A clinicopathologic study of 35 necropsy patients (group I) and review of 78 previously described necropsy patients (group II). Am J Med 1977;63:86-108.

143. Ratner SJ, Fenoglio JJ Jr, Ursell PC. Utility of endomyocardial biopsy in the diagnosis of cardiac sarcoidosis. Chest 1986;90:528-533.

144. Valantine H, McKenna WJ, Nihoyannopoulos P, Mitchell A, Foale RA, Davies MJ, Oakley CM. Sarcoidosis: a pattern of clinical and morphological presentation. Br Heart J 1987;57:256-263.

145. Sekiguchi M, Yazaki Y, Isobe M, Hiroe M. Cardiac sarcoidosis: diagnostic, prognostic, and therapeutic considerations. Cardiovasc Drugs Ther 1996;10:495-510.

146. Uemura A, Morimoto S, Hiramitsu S, Kato Y, Ito T, Hishida H. Histologic diagnostic rate of cardiac sarcoidosis: evaluation of endomyocardial biopsies. Am Heart J 1999;138:299-302.

147. Lemery R, McGoon MD, Edwards WD. Cardiac sarcoidosis: a potentially treatable form of myocarditis. Mayo Clin Proc 1985;60:549-554.

148. Valantine HA, Tazelaar HD, Macoviak J, Mullin AV, Hunt SA, Fowler MB, Billingham ME, Schroeder JS. Cardiac sarcoidosis: response to steroids and transplantation. J Heart Transplant 1987;6:244-250.

149. Oni AA, Hershberger RE, Norman DJ, Ray J, Hovaguimian H, Cobanoglu AM, Hosenpud JD. Recurrence of sarcoidosis in a cardiac allograft: control with augmented corticosteroids. J Heart Lung Transplant 1992;11:367-369.

150. Litovsky SH, Burke AP, Virmani R. Giant cell myocarditis: an entity distinct from sarcoidosis characterized by multiphasic myocyte destruction by cytotoxic T cells and histiocytic giant cells. Mod Pathol 1996;9:1126-1134.

151. Ferrans VJ, Rodriguez ER, McAllister HA Jr. Granulomatous inflammation of the heart. Heart Vessels Suppl 1985;1:262-270.

152. Rosenstein ED, Zucker MJ, Kramer N. Giant cell myocarditis: most fatal of autoimmune diseases. Semin Arthritis Rheum 2000;30:1-16.

153. Cooper LT Jr, Berry GJ, Shabetai R. Idiopathic giant-cell myocarditis—natural history and treatment. Multicenter Giant Cell Myocarditis Study Group Investigators. N Engl J Med 1997;336:1860-1866.

154. Davidoff R, Palacios I, Southern J, Fallon JT, Newell J, Dec GW. Giant cell versus lymphocytic myocarditis. A comparison of their clinical features and long-term outcomes. Circulation 1991;83:953-961.

155. Ren H, Poston RS Jr, Hruban RH, Baumgartner WA, Baughman KL, Hutchins GM. Long survival with giant cell myocarditis. Mod Pathol 1993;6:402-407.

156. Davies MJ, Pomerance A, Teare RD. Idiopathic giant cell myocarditis—a distinctive clinico-pathological entity. Br Heart J 1975;37:192-195.

157. Cooper LT Jr, Berry GJ, Rizeq M, Schroeder JS. Giant cell myocarditis. J Heart Lung Transplant 1995;14:394-401.

158. Tanaka M, Ichinohasama R, Kawahara Y, Esaki Y, Hirokawa K, Okishige K, Tanaka Y. Acute idio-pathic interstitial myocarditis: case report with special reference to morphological characteristics of giant cells. J Clin Pathol 1986;39:1209-1216.

159. Theaker JM, Gatter KC, Heryet A, Evans DJ, McGee JO. Giant cell myocarditis: evidence for the macrophage origin of the giant cells. J Clin Pathol 1985;38:160-164.

160. Avellini C, Alampi G, Cocchi V, Morritti MG, Leone O, Sabattini E, Pileri S, Piccaluga A. Acute idiopathic interstitial giant cell myocarditis. A histological and immunohistological study of a case. Pathologica 1991;83:229-235.

161. Ariza A, Lopez MD, Mate JL, Curos A, Villagrasa M, Navas-Palacios JJ. Giant cell myocarditis: monocytic immunophenotype of giant cells in a case associated with ulcerative colitis. Hum Pathol 1995;26:121-123.

Endomyocardial Biopsy in Myocarditis

Joseph G. Murphy, M.D., and Robert P. Frantz, M.D.

The accurate diagnosis of myocarditis rests on the finding of active inflammation involving cardiac myocytes and is made either at autopsy or ante mortem by endomyocardial biopsy findings.

WHAT IS THE PROBLEM WITH CURRENT DIAGNOSTIC TECHNIQUES FOR MYOCARDITIS?

Myocarditis is defined as an inflammatory condition of the heart muscle and is caused by multiple organisms and conditions. The diagnosis of myocarditis remains a challenge, with conflicting views among clinicians and investigators as to whether clinical or histologic diagnostic criteria should predominate.[1-4] When the clinical suspicion of myocarditis (sudden onset of heart failure or ventricular arrhythmias in association with or soon after a febrile illness) accords with the histologic diagnosis, there is little diagnostic problem. However, when the clinical presentation of myocarditis is not associated with biopsy evidence of myocyte damage and T-lymphocyte infiltration, this is a dilemma.

In the Myocarditis Treatment Trial,[5] most patients with clinically suspected myocarditis did not have biopsy evidence of myocarditis. In this trial, all patients underwent biopsy who had suspected myocarditis based on the new onset of unexplained heart failure during the 2 years preceding enrollment. The endomyocardial biopsy samples were reviewed according to the Dallas criteria by a panel of 7 pathologists and a consensus diagnosis was reached. The pathologists found histopathologic evidence of myocarditis on endomyocardial biopsy in just 214 of 2,233 patients (less than 10%). Other smaller series also reported a poor concordance between the clinical and histologic diagnoses of myocarditis, "possibly because the clinical diagnosis is wrong or the histologic criteria used by pathologists are inappropriate."[6]

The ongoing European Study of Epidemiology and Treatment of Cardiac Inflammatory Diseases (ESETCID) has expanded the light microscopic Dallas criteria for myocarditis by including immunohistochemical variables of myocardial inflammation.[7] Endomyocardial biopsy specimens are screened not only for infiltrating cells but also for the presence of persisting viral genome (enterovirus, cytomegalovirus, and adenovirus). This method shows inflammatory processes in the heart in 17.2% of the 3,055 patients screened. Only 182 of these patients showed a reduced ejection fraction below 45%, fulfilling the entrance criteria for the ESETCID trial. These data indicate that, in symptomatic patients, myocarditis should always be considered and relatively well-preserved left ventricular function does not exclude the diagnosis. In the ESETCID trial, viral genome was detected in 11.8% of patients (enterovirus 2.2%, cytomegalovirus 5.4%, adenovirus 4.2%).

ENDOMYOCARDIAL BIOPSY—THE TARNISHED STANDARD

Notwithstanding the above limitation, percutaneous endomyocardial biopsy remains the tarnished standard for the in vivo diagnosis of myocarditis.[8] In addition to light microscopy of endomyocardial biopsy samples, the diagnosis of specific viral myocarditis conditions has improved with the advent of immunohistochemistry and the molecular biology techniques of polymerase chain reaction, in situ hybridization, and Southern blot.[9,10] In addition, endomyocardial biopsy may be particularly valuable to exclude other noninflammatory causes of ventricular dysfunction such as amyloid heart disease and hemochromatosis (Fig. 15-1).[11-15] Patients who should be considered for endomyocardial biopsy include those with unexplained dilated cardiomyopathy, restrictive cardiomyopathy, and unexplained ventricular arrhythmias.[16-18] Conditions that may be diagnosed by endomyocardial biopsy are listed in Tables 15-1 and 15-2. The decision to perform an endomyocardial biopsy depends on the perceived probability that a biopsy could lead to a diagnosis that otherwise would not be made, and that this in turn will result in a treatment different from that recommended in the absence of biopsy results (Table 15-3). Brief descriptions of some scenarios in which endomyocardial biopsy may have major implications for management are outlined below.

GIANT CELL MYOCARDITIS

Endomyocardial biopsy is the only method permitting definitive antemortem diagnosis of giant cell myocarditis. Although this disorder is rare, prompt identification of such patients is critical. Mortality rates are high, usually owing to ventricular arrhythmia or progressive heart failure, and prompt referral to a transplant center is essential. Anecdotal reports suggest that such patients may respond to aggressive immunosuppression; randomized trials are under way and should be considered for these patients. Clues to the possibility of giant cell myocarditis include the presence of complex ventricular arrhythmias that may be associated with abrupt onset of cardiac failure. Because giant cell myocarditis may recur in the transplanted heart, vigilance is required even after transplantation.

HUMAN IMMUNODEFICIENCY VIRUS-INDUCED MYOCARDITIS

Human immunodeficiency virus (HIV) infection is a well-recognized cause of myocarditis, but the exact pathogenesis of the heart muscle disease in the acquired immunodeficiency syndrome is unclear. Possible causes of heart muscle damage include "a direct action of HIV on the myocardial tissue or to an autoimmune process induced by HIV, possibly in association with other cardiotropic viruses."[19]

Barbaro et al.[19] performed a prospective, long-term clinical and echocardiographic follow-up study of 952 asymptomatic HIV-positive patients to assess the incidence of dilated cardiomyopathy. All patients with an echocardiographic diagnosis of dilated cardio-

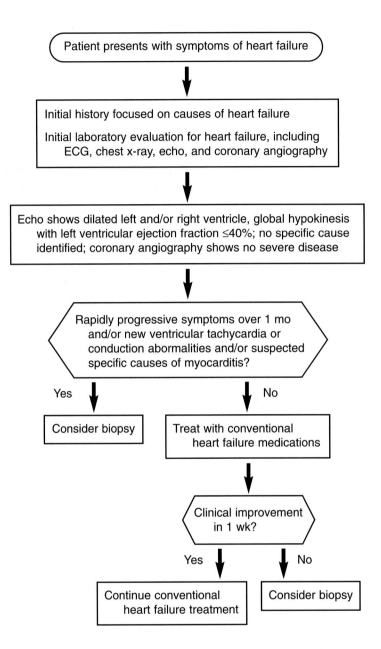

Fig. 15-1. Flow diagram for the work-up of patients with dilated cardiomyopathy. The timing of endomyocardial biopsy in patients who fail to improve on medical therapy is controversial. If the patient's left ventricular function and symptoms are stable after 1 week of treatment, additional time before endomyocardial biopsy could be considered, if appropriate in the treating physician's clinical judgment, to allow for delayed recovery to occur. *ECG*, electrocardiography; *echo*, echocardiography. (From Wu LA, Lapeyre AC III, Cooper LT. Current role of endomyocardial biopsy in the management of dilated cardiomyopathy and myocarditis. Mayo Clin Proc 2001;76:1030-1038. By permission of Mayo Foundation for Medical Education and Research.)

Table 15-1
Conditions That Can Be Diagnosed by Endomyocardial Biopsy

Arrhythmogenic right ventricular dysplasia
Amyloidosis
Sarcoidosis
Hemochromatosis
Myocarditis (eg, eosinophilic myocarditis, giant cell myocarditis)
Anthracycline cardiomyopathy
Storage diseases such as mucopolysaccharidoses
Carcinoid heart disease
Primary and metastatic neoplasms (eg, rhabdomyosarcoma, lymphoma)
Radiation-induced cardiac fibrosis
Cardiac allograft rejection

Table 15-2
Common Clinicopathologic Diagnoses in 1,230 Patients
With Initially Unexplained Cardiomyopathy

Diagnosis	Patients, no. (%)
Idiopathic dilated cardiomyopathy	616 (50)
Myocarditis	111 (9)
Ischemic cardiomyopathy	91 (7)
Infiltrative disease	59 (5)
Peripartum cardiomyopathy	51 (4)
Hypertension	49 (4)
Human immunodeficiency virus infection	45 (4)
Connective tissue disease	39 (3)
Substance abuse	37 (3)
Doxorubicin related	15 (1)
Other causes	111 (10)

From Wu LA, Lapeyre AC III, Cooper LT. Current role of endomyocardial
biopsy in the management of dilated cardiomyopathy and myocarditis.
Mayo Clin Proc 2001;76:1030-1038. By permission of Mayo Foundation
for Medical Education and Research.

myopathy underwent endomyocardial biopsy for histologic, immunohistologic, and virologic assessment. The mean follow-up period was 60 months, and an echocardiographic diagnosis of dilated cardiomyopathy was made in 76 patients (8%), yielding a mean annual incidence rate of 15.9 cases per 1,000 patients. The incidence of dilated cardiomyopathy was higher in patients with a CD4 count of less than 400 cells per μL (compared with a CD4 count of greater than or equal to 400 cells per μL) and in those who received therapy with zidovudine. A histologic diagnosis of myocarditis was made in 63 of the patients

Table 15-3
Signs and Symptoms in Patients With Congestive Heart Failure
Who Warrant an Endomyocardial Biopsy

Acute heart failure with symptoms refractory to current medical management
Rapidly decreasing left ventricular ejection fraction with no clear etiology despite conventional
  therapy for heart failure
Heart failure with acutely worsening rhythm disturbances, particularly ventricular tachycardia
New heart failure with conduction disturbances, particularly nodal block (not drug induced and
  negative Lyme serology)
Heart failure in the setting of peripheral eosinophilia, rash, and fever
Heart failure in the setting of clinical history and/or features of secondary causes where endo-
  myocardial biopsy may change or modify therapy:
  Collagen vascular diseases (systemic lupus erythematosus, scleroderma, Marfan syndrome,
    polyarteritis nodosum, dermatomyositis/polymyositis)
  Infiltrative and storage diseases (amyloid, sarcoid, hemochromatosis)
  Giant cell myocarditis
  Neoplasms

From Wu LA, Lapeyre AC III, Cooper LT. Current role of endomyocardial biopsy in the management of
  dilated cardiomyopathy and myocarditis. Mayo Clin Proc 2001;76:1030-1038. By permission of Mayo
  Foundation for Medical Education and Research.

(83%) with dilated cardiomyopathy. Inflammatory infiltrates were composed predominantly of CD3 and CD8 lymphocytes, with staining for major histocompatibility complex
class I antigens in 71% of the patients. In the myocytes of 58 patients, HIV nucleic acid
sequences were detected by in situ hybridization, and active myocarditis was documented
in 36 of the 58. Among these 36 patients, 6 were also infected with coxsackievirus group
B (17%), 2 with cytomegalovirus (6%), and 1 with Epstein-Barr virus (3%). Thus,
myocarditis was a common finding in HIV patients with echocardiographic evidence of
left ventricular dysfunction.

HEMOCHROMATOSIS

Hemochromatosis is an inherited disorder of iron metabolism. Typical manifestations
include diabetes, abnormal liver function, skin pigment changes, and dilated cardiomyopathy. Serum iron studies show marked increases of iron values. An endomyocardial
biopsy shows deposits of iron in the myocardium and allows the diagnosis of hemochromatosis to be made. This has significant implications for treatment and for screening of
family members.

AMYLOIDOSIS

Amyloidosis is a devastating disease that results from deposits of proteinaceous material in
various organs, including the heart. The precise nature of the material depends on the type

of amyloidosis (primary systemic, familial, or senile). Cardiac manifestations include exertional dyspnea, chest pain, atrial arrhythmias, conduction block, and congestive heart failure. Early in the course of cardiac involvement, left ventricular systolic function is relatively well preserved, whereas diastolic function is often abnormal, with a restrictive filling pattern. Increased wall thickness associated with low QRS voltage on the surface electrocardiogram must arouse suspicion regarding possible amyloidosis. Serum and urine immunoelectrophoresis should be performed, looking for a monoclonal gammopathy. However, this will be absent in familial and senile types of amyloidosis. Multiple possible biopsy sources such as fat aspirate or rectal biopsy may be considered, but if less invasive sites are not diagnostic, endomyocardial biopsy has a high sensitivity. Notification of the pathologist regarding the suspected diagnosis is important to be certain proper stains are performed. Patients with familial amyloidosis can be treated effectively with liver transplantation because the liver is the source of abnormal protein production. Combined heart-liver transplantation is often necessary, because cardiac involvement may be advanced at diagnosis. Selected patients with primary systemic amyloidosis may benefit from heart transplantation followed by stem cell (marrow) transplantation.

CARDIAC ALLOGRAFT REJECTION

Surveillance endomyocardial biopsies are essential in the management of cardiac transplant recipients. Such biopsies frequently allow the diagnosis and treatment of rejection before onset of symptoms, guide immunosuppressive strategies, and detect other conditions such as cytomegalovirus or toxoplasmosis infection. Accepted nomenclature for grading of cardiac allograft rejection is provided in Table 15-4.

HISTORY OF ENDOMYOCARDIAL BIOPSY

Cardiac biopsy was performed initially by means of thoracotomy beginning in the 1950s. A major advance was the development of the first percutaneous transvenous biopsy catheter. The original device consisted of 2 sharpened cups on a catheter shaft that closed when a control wire was pulled proximally. The disadvantages of this device were its size, which necessitated a surgical cutdown for venous entry, and its relative inflexibility, which made intracardiac manipulation difficult. The Stanford (Caves-Schultz) bioptome is a modification of the original design by Konno and is widely used for endomyocardial biopsy. This bioptome is relatively flexible and has a stainless steel shaft. The cutting jaws are activated by a control wire, but only 1 jaw moves while the other is fixed in position. The Stanford bioptome is designed for use via the right internal jugular vein. The curve of the shaft should be varied by the operator between biopsies to minimize repeated biopsies of the

Table 15-4
Endomyocardial Biopsy Rejection Grading

Grade	
0	No rejection
1	A = Focal (perivascular or interstitial infiltrate without necrosis)
	B = Diffuse but sparse infiltrate without necrosis
2	One focus only with aggressive infiltration and/or focal myocyte damage
3	A = Multifocal aggressive infiltrates and/or myocyte damage
	B = Diffuse inflammatory process with necrosis
4	Diffuse aggressive polymorphous ± infiltrate, ± edema, ± hemorrhage, ± vasculitis, with necrosis

same endomyocardial site. The Kawai bioptome is a flexible bioptome with a dial on the operator handle that controls tip movement.

An alternative strategy is to use a long sheath-guiding catheter inserted via the femoral vein in conjunction with an unguided cardiac bioptome. This strategy is used with the King bioptome and the long Stanford bioptome.

TECHNIQUE

Endomyocardial biopsies are performed most frequently via the right internal jugular or femoral vein. Biopsies usually are performed with local anesthesia, accompanied by conscious sedation if required. Children may require general anesthesia. Fluoroscopic guidance is used in the cardiac catheterization laboratory, but some operators prefer echocardiographic guidance, either alone or combined with fluoroscopy.

RIGHT INTERNAL JUGULAR VEIN APPROACH

The patient should be supine with the neck extended and the head turned fully to the left. Elevation of the feet on a foam wedge is useful if cardiac filling pressures are low. Careful identification of the triangle formed by the clavicle and the medial and lateral heads of the sternocleidomastoid muscle is essential. This may be facilitated by palpating and visualizing the neck while the patient slightly lifts the head from the table, resulting in activation of the appropriate muscles.

After sterile preparation and drape of the region, needle entry should be made in the upper third of the triangle, on a trajectory toward the ipsilateral nipple. A wheal is made under the skin (with a 21-gauge needle and 2% lidocaine), with gradually deeper injection along the anticipated approach to the internal jugular vein. Intermittent aspiration before advancement of the needle avoids intravascular injection of lidocaine and confirms entry to the vein. Presence of lidocaine in the syringe may result in the blood flash appearing bright, raising the question of inadvertent carotid cannulation. This can be resolved by replacement of the syringe with an empty syringe or one containing saline.

After confirmation of jugular vein location, a small nick in the skin should be made with a scalpel. The incision can be dilated slightly with blunt scissors to facilitate subsequent passage of a sheath. An 18-gauge needle with an attached syringe containing saline is then slowly advanced along the appropriate path toward the ipsilateral nipple. Pausing and aspirating while holding slight backward traction on the syringe helps the operator confirm venous cannulation. This needle is large enough to compress the vein, particularly if there is significant scar tissue from prior cannulations. This slight back and forth traction often helps achieve successful cannulation. If the vessel is difficult to locate, it may help to return to the 21-gauge needle to reconfirm location rather than guiding the 18-gauge needle in multiple directions. Particular caution is necessary when there is the temptation to direct the needle more medially, because inadvertent carotid artery puncture may occur. If this occurs, gentle pressure should be held over the puncture to reduce the risk of hematoma formation. Rarely, carotid dissection and occlusion or stroke related to emboli from thrombus or atheroma has been reported in association with inadvertent carotid puncture.

Use of ultrasound (SiteRite) should be strongly considered if there is any difficulty in locating the vein. Ultrasound can readily confirm the location of the vein and demonstrate relative location of the internal jugular vein and carotid artery. If there is doubt about which structure represents the vein, having the patient perform a Valsalva maneuver engorges the vein and makes it more obvious. Sometimes if the vein is collapsed or scarred, use of a Pediatric Introducer Set (Cook Inc., Bloomington, IN) helps, because the 18-gauge needle may compress the vein and make cannulation difficult. The Micropuncture set includes a 21-gauge needle, through which a 0.018-inch nitinol wire is advanced. A 4.0F catheter is placed over the wire. After removal of the inner dilator, a standard 0.038-inch J wire can then be placed, followed by a larger sheath. Fluoroscopy can confirm appropriate wire position, because occasionally the wire deflects toward the arm instead of advancing toward the right atrium. If multiple prior biopsies have been performed, passage of dilators of gradually increasing size from 6F up to the size of the required sheath facilitates placement.

A 9F sheath is required if a standard reusable Caves-Schultz-Scholten bioptome will be used. A 7F sheath is adequate for disposable bioptomes such as the Jawz or Bipal devices.

After placement, the sheath should be aspirated and flushed with saline. With fluoroscopic guidance, the bioptome is advanced with the tip curving medially until the tricuspid valve is crossed. Localization in the right ventricle can be confirmed by the occurrence of ventricular ectopic beats. This is not trivial; if the operator is not attentive, it is possible inadvertently to direct the bioptome down the inferior vena cava and medially into the liver and to obtain samples of liver. To direct the bioptome to the apical portion of the ventricular septum may require slight back and forth movement to keep the tip free, with slight rotation to redirect the tip. If any resistance is met, the bioptome should be withdrawn slightly and redirected. The bioptome should be advanced fully across the tricuspid valve, and, using fluoroscopy to visualize the heart borders, directed to the apical portion of the ventricular septum. Rotation of the fluoroscopy unit to a left anterior oblique position can help confirm appropriate direction of the bioptome, followed by return to the anteroposterior position to establish position relative to the tricuspid apparatus. Failure to advance the bioptome sufficiently distally in the right ventricle may result in damage to the tricuspid apparatus, leading to tricuspid insufficiency. This complication is unfortunately rather common in transplant recipients who have had dozens of biopsies. It is usually well tolerated, but sometimes it results in right-sided heart failure that is difficult to manage, particularly if there is an element of pulmonary hypertension.

After gentle advancement to the apical region of the ventricular septum, the bioptome should be withdrawn slightly, the jaws opened, and the bioptome advanced gently against the septum. For patients who have not had multiple prior biopsies, gentle pressure is adequate to obtain tissue (Fig. 15-2). This is particularly important in patients with dilated cardiomyopathy, who may have a thin-walled, soft myocardium. Patients with multiple prior biopsies may require slightly more pressure because of the presence of endomyocardial scar. Four or 5 specimens are generally obtained, placed promptly in appropriate preservative, and sent for pathologic review. The pieces should be inspected before submission. If multiple prior biopsies have been performed (eg, in cardiac transplant recipients), some of the pieces may appear pearly white, indicating that mostly scar and little myocardium is present. Such pieces are not helpful for pathologic examination, and better samples should be sought.

Excess force risks perforation of the right ventricle if the bioptome is not properly directed. Sharp pleuritic chest pain is a sign of likely perforation. If this occurs, blood pressure should be observed closely, and emergent echocardiography done to seek evidence of pericardial effusion. Equipment for placement of a pericardial catheter should be available.

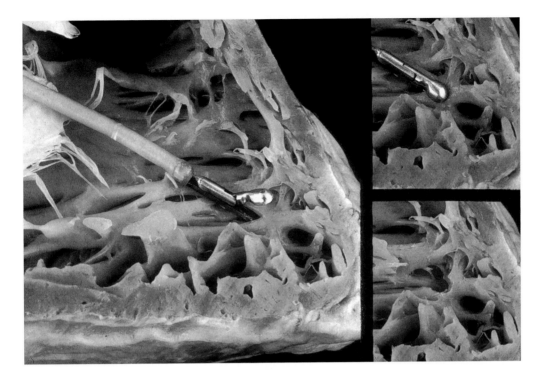

Fig. 15-2. Endomyocardial biopsy simulation in a cadaveric heart. (Courtesy of William D. Edwards, M.D.)

A hoarse voice due to injury of the recurrent laryngeal nerve has rarely been reported to occur after endomyocardial biopsy. This may be transient or occasionally may last for months.

Fistulae have been reported between the coronary artery and the right ventricle. These are visualized on surveillance coronary angiography and appear not to be associated with any clinical sequelae.

Choice of a bioptome reflects operator preference. The reusable Scholten bioptome is nicely steerable, holds its shape well, and has a blunt tip. However, it does require sterilization after each use and must be resharpened periodically. If it is used when it is dull, which may not be obvious by simple inspection, it may tear larger pieces of endocardium than desired. This is particularly true in cardiac transplant recipients who have had multiple biopsies and therefore have areas of scarring along the endocardium. Accordingly, if excess resistance is felt on efforts to withdraw the bioptome, it is best to release the jaws and reposition, rather than exerting heavier traction. The disposable bioptomes do not hold their shape as well as the Scholten bioptomes and are somewhat more awkward to position appropriately.

FEMORAL VEIN APPROACH

The femoral vein approach has some advantages and disadvantages relative to the jugular vein approach. Advantages include freedom from risks inherent in the jugular approach such as inadvertent carotid puncture. In addition, some patients prefer the femoral approach; it is less unpleasant than to have procedures through the neck. If multiple prior biopsies have been performed from the neck, scar tissue may begin to limit access and create more discomfort with sheath placement, in which case moving to the femoral approach may help. Disadvantages of the femoral approach include the need for a long sheath in which clots may develop, risk of deep venous thrombosis, and need for patients to remain supine for approximately 30 minutes after sheath removal. In addition, directing the bioptome across the tricuspid valve and to the appropriate region of the ventricle is difficult sometimes. The bioptomes used from the femoral approach may yield smaller samples than those from the neck, but usually they still provide adequate samples for accurate pathologic diagnosis.

After cannulation of the femoral vein by standard technique, a wire is advanced with fluoroscopic guidance. A 7 or 8F Mullins sheath of the type used for transseptal catheterization is advanced to the right ventricle. Sometimes putting some curvature on the end of the wire is necessary to help direct the system to the right ventricle. A Mullins sheath with a sidearm can facilitate aspiration and flushing of the sheath. Alternatively, a Mullins sheath without a sidearm and with a Tuohy-Borst hemostasis device of the type used for angioplasty can facilitate bioptome passes. The Mullins sheath should be positioned in the right ventricle pointing toward the apical portion of the ventricular septum. It may tend to sit too far down toward the inferior wall, in which case withdrawing it slightly may allow the bioptome to point more toward the septum. If there is doubt about the right ventricular location of the sheath, hooking it up to pressure helps to confirm right ventricular location.

With the Mullins tip free in the right ventricle, a long reusable Scholten bioptome or a disposable bioptome is passed to the right ventricular apical septum. Rotating the bioptome and moving it back and forth are necessary for proper positioning. Some forward pressure on the Mullins sheath and the bioptome is often necessary to seat the bioptome against the endocardium, because some of the forward pressure simply flexes the body of the bioptome. After the jaws are closed, *both* the bioptome and the Mullins sheath should be withdrawn gently until the bioptome comes free from the endocardium. Failure to hold back pressure on the Mullins sheath will pull the Mullins sheath over the bioptome and into the endocardium, risking right ventricular perforation if the bioptome does not come free easily. Once the bioptome is free, the Mullins sheath can be advanced slightly to maintain position in the right ventricle. It is important to aspirate and flush the sheath carefully after each pass of the bioptome to clear the

sheath of possible thrombus. Appropriate flushing of the sheath during exchanges min-
imizes the risk of entraining air. After retrieval of the specimens, the sheath should be
withdrawn into the inferior vena cava and then removed in the recovery room, where
local pressure ensures hemostasis.

A specially designed catheter produced by Cordis (Tampa Bay guiding catheter) sits
more easily in the right ventricle than a Mullins sheath. However, the bioptomes that fit
through this catheter are small, resulting in retrieval of small samples. They are often adequate for pathologic examination, and some operators prefer this system. Other
disposable bioptome and sheath systems are available.

ENDOMYOCARDIAL BIOPSY SPECIMEN PROCESSING

Multiple biopsy specimens (usually 5 to 8 samples) are taken from different biopsy sites in
the ventricular septum. There is a tendency for the bioptome to gravitate to the same biopsy
locations because the vascular entry site is fixed by the vascular sheath and the entry into
the right ventricle, by the tricuspid valve orifice. Biopsy specimens are placed in 10% formalin for light microscopy and 2.5% buffered glutaraldehyde if electron microscopy is
needed. Special preparation and immediate freezing may be required for immunologic
staining or molecular biologic studies of RNA or DNA.

THE DALLAS CRITERIA FOR THE HISTOLOGIC DIAGNOSIS
OF MYOCARDITIS

Before the acceptance of the Dallas criteria for the histologic diagnosis of myocarditis,
considerable interobserver variability existed in the interpretation of endomyocardial
biopsy samples. Shanes et al.[20] submitted biopsy specimens from 16 patients with dilated
cardiomyopathy to 7 experienced cardiac pathologists who independently reviewed the
same slides and assessed each for fibrosis, hypertrophy, nuclear changes on a 0 to 3 scale,
and mean lymphocyte count per high-power field. The prevalence of all observed variables varied widely; significant fibrosis ranged from 25% to 69%, hypertrophy from 19%
to 88%, nuclear changes from 31% to 94%, and abnormal lymphocyte count from 0% to
38%. One or more pathologists diagnosed definite or possible myocarditis in 11 of the 16
patients. Of these 11 patients, 3 pathologists agreed about 3 and 2 pathologists agreed
about 5. Myocarditis was diagnosed by 1 pathologist in 3 cases. The conclusion of this
study was that quantitative and standardized methods are needed to increase diagnostic
consistency in the histologic diagnosis of myocarditis.

COMPLICATIONS OF ENDOMYOCARDIAL BIOPSY

Endomyocardial biopsy is associated with an overall complication rate of 1% to 2% in most large series. However, these series include a high proportion of post cardiac transplant patients undergoing routine rejection surveillance, who may have a lower risk of complication than myocarditis patients. Myocarditis patients undergoing biopsy frequently have poor ventricular function and heart failure and are prone to ventricular arrhythmias. It is important to biopsy the interventricular septum and not the right ventricular apex, which may be only a few millimeters thick in some patients. Accurate anatomic localization of the biopsy site in the interventricular septum may be aided by biplane cardiac fluoroscopy or echocardiography.[21]

CARDIAC PERFORATION

The most important specific complication of endomyocardial biopsy is cardiac perforation, which can lead rapidly to cardiac tamponade and cardiac arrest. Cardiac perforation occurs in about 0.3% of patients. Patients with prior cardiac surgical procedures or post transplantation are relatively protected from cardiac perforation and tamponade by an adherent pericardium overlying the right ventricle.[22-24] Death due to endomyocardial biopsy occurs in approximately 1 of 1,000 procedures.

Cardiac perforation usually is heralded by the development of pleuritic chest pain. The presence of blood in the pericardial space frequently elicits a vasovagal-type reflex with bradycardia and hypotension. The biopsy specimen may be white and glistening, suggesting the presence of pericardium, and may float in formalin fixative owing to the presence of epicardial fat. Note that in patients who have had many previous myocardial biopsies such as cardiac transplant recipients, biopsy of a previous endomyocardial scar site may yield fibrotic-looking material that may simulate pericardium.

If myocardial perforation is suspected, systemic arterial pressure and right atrial pressure should be monitored for evidence of tamponade and an emergency echocardiogram should be performed. Fluoroscopy may show obliteration of the normal right-sided cardiac motion in tamponade, but findings on Doppler echocardiography are more specific and occur earlier in incipient tamponade. Emergency, percutaneous, echo-guided pericardial catheter drainage should be performed if evidence of incipient tamponade is present. Most perforations induced by endomyocardial biopsy are self-sealing and rarely require surgical exploration. The exceptions are in patients with severe pulmonary hypertension and coagulopathies, including patients receiving anticoagulant therapy. It is our practice to decline biopsy in patients with an international normalized ratio greater than 1.5 and in patients who have received heparin recently. Atropine, intravenous fluids, and inotropic agents are helpful temporizing measures before pericardiocentesis in patients with cardiac perforation.

THROMBOEMBOLISM

The risk of thromboembolism from either tissue or thrombus from the biopsy site is higher in left ventricular biopsy. Right-sided thromboembolism can be due to thrombus from the venous access sheath or air aspiration as a result of low central venous pressure, especially with the internal jugular approach.

In general, myocarditis that is not patchy will be diagnosed if 4 to 5 right ventricular biopsy samples are obtained. The possibility of some small added diagnostic yield by taking biopsy samples of the left ventricle in addition to the right is outweighed by the small attendant risk of systemic embolism. Transient nonsustained ventricular arrhythmias are common at the time of ventricular biopsy and indeed tend to confirm the ventricular location of the bioptome. Conduction disturbances may occur from mechanical trauma to the conduction system and are usually transient. Injury to the tricuspid valve may occur as a result of injury to the chordae tendineae.[25] Complications associated with internal jugular sheath placement include vasovagal reactions, pneumothorax, inadvertent carotid artery puncture, and hematoma formation.[22]

ENDOMYOCARDIAL BIOPSY IN CHILDREN

Pophal et al.[26] reviewed their experience with endomyocardial biopsy in children. This was a retrospective review of the morbidity and mortality of 1,000 consecutive endomyocardial biopsy procedures in 194 children (right ventricle 986, left ventricle 14) performed from July 1987 through March 1996. Indications for endomyocardial biopsy included heart transplant rejection surveillance (846) and evaluation of cardiomyopathy or arrhythmia for possible myocarditis (154). Thirty-seven procedures (4%) were performed on patients receiving intravenous inotropic support. There was 1 biopsy-related death, due to cardiac perforation, in a 2-week-old infant with dilated cardiomyopathy. There were 9 perforations of the right ventricle: 8 in patients with dilated cardiomyopathy and 1 in a transplant recipient. The transplant patient did not require immediate intervention; 2 patients required pericardiocentesis alone, and 6 underwent pericardiocentesis and surgical intervention. All 9 perforations were from the femoral venous approach ($P < 0.01$). Multivariate analysis demonstrated that the greatest risk of perforation occurred in children being evaluated for possible myocarditis ($P = 0.01$) and in those requiring positive inotropic support ($P < 0.01$). Other complications included arrhythmia ($n = 5$) and single cases of coronary-cardiac fistula, flail tricuspid leaflet, pneumothorax, hemothorax, endocardial stripping, and seizure. The authors concluded that the risk of endomyocardial biopsy is highest in sick children with suspected myocarditis receiving intravenous inotropic support. However, endomyocardial biopsy can be performed safely with low morbidity in pediatric heart transplant recipients.[27]

MAKING DECISIONS ABOUT ENDOMYOCARDIAL BIOPSY IN MYOCARDITIS

Most patients with dilated cardiomyopathy who have endomyocardial biopsy do not have any change in their clinical therapy as a result of the biopsy. About 80% to 90% of patients who have endomyocardial biopsy either because of new-onset heart failure or because of clinically suspected myocarditis have the nonspecific histologic finding of myocyte hypertrophy and fibrosis. About 10% to 20% of endomyocardial biopsies give definitive information for a specific diagnosis such as myocarditis, amyloidosis, sarcoidosis, or hemochromatosis. In less than half of the patients in whom a specific diagnosis is made, there is a change in clinical treatment based solely on the endomyocardial biopsy result.

The decision to proceed with an endomyocardial biopsy in a patient with suspected myocarditis should balance the expected gain from an accurate diagnosis with its attendant therapeutic implications against the small risk of a major procedural complication. Most patients with clinically suspected myocarditis do not have biopsy-proven myocarditis, and thus immunosuppressive therapy based solely on a clinical diagnosis of myocarditis is unwise. The Clinical Trial of Immunosuppressive Therapy for Myocarditis did not show a beneficial effect of immunosuppressive therapy (prednisone with either cyclosporine or azathioprine) on left ventricular function at 28 weeks in patients with biopsy-proven active myocarditis. The conclusion of this study does not apply to patients with other forms of histologically proven myocarditis that were not studied, including giant cell myocarditis, peripartum myocarditis, hypersensitivity myocarditis, and cardiac sarcoidosis.

ESETCID addresses some of the problems encountered in the Clinical Trial of Immunosuppressive Therapy for Myocarditis by distinguishing between different forms of myocarditis. Patients with cytomegalovirus-induced myocarditis will be treated by hyperimmunoglobulin or placebo. Patients with enterovirus-positive myocarditis will receive interferon-alfa or placebo. Patients with virus-negative myocarditis, which is considered autoimmune, will be treated with immunosuppression or placebo. The primary end point of this study will be an improvement in ejection fraction of more than 5%.

Hrobon et al.[28] used decision analysis to determine the efficacy (5-year risk reduction in mortality or transplantation) that a treatment for myocarditis would require to favor a biopsy-guided approach over conventional therapy. The prevalence of myocarditis among patients with dilated cardiomyopathy was estimated from the published literature (including or excluding borderline myocarditis) as 16% and 11%, respectively; sensitivity of endomyocardial biopsy diagnosis of myocarditis, 63% and 50%, respectively; probability of 5-year transplantation-free survival, 55%; specificity of endomyocardial biopsy diagnosis, 95.4%; mortality rate of endomyocardial biopsy, 0.4%; side effects resulting in withdrawal of immunosuppressive treatment, 4%; and 6-month mortality rate for immunosuppressive treatment, 0.1%.

The authors concluded that a therapy that decreased the rate of death or transplantation by 12.7% and 7.1% for patients, excluding or including borderline myocarditis, respectively, favored endomyocardial biopsy. Sensitivity analysis indicated that therapeutic efficacy was influenced by myocarditis prevalence and biopsy-related death but not by accuracy of biopsy or probability of immunosuppressive therapy side effects. Randomized trials powered to detect 7% and 25% reductions in death and transplantation would require 5,790 and 380 end points, respectively. Decreasing the rate of death or transplantation by 7.1% offsets therapy side effects, endomyocardial biopsy-related death, and inaccuracies in histologic diagnosis. Variables in this decision analysis that significantly affected outcome included the prevalence of myocarditis and the sensitivity of the diagnostic techniques.

The initial therapy for patients with suspected myocarditis is hospital admission for bed rest and electrocardiogram monitoring and vasodilators to decrease vascular resistance and lower left ventricular filling pressures. Patients with acute fulminant myocarditis and hemodynamic deterioration may benefit from short-term circulatory support with left ventricular-assist devices. The rationale for this approach is that short-term left ventricular support reduces wall stress and allows time for improvement in myocyte function.

Immunosuppressive therapy is not recommended in patients with acute infectious or postinfectious myocarditis, but a small subset of patients with noninfectious myocarditis due to giant cell myocarditis, scleroderma, lupus erythematosus, polymyositis, or sarcoidosis may benefit from immunosuppressive therapy.

A beneficial treatment of inflammatory heart disease is still difficult and not yet validated by a study with patient numbers sufficient to allow statistical analysis. The ESETCID addresses problems of etiology, pathogenesis, and specific treatment of myocarditis. It is the first multicenter, double-blind placebo-controlled randomized study, apart from the Myocarditis Treatment Trial, to distinguish between different forms of myocarditis. In the ESETCID, patients with acute or chronic myocarditis are treated specifically according to the etiology of the disease. This trial may yield a better understanding of the course of myocarditis, leading to more specific treatment, which may in turn decrease the number of patients with post-myocardial infarction heart muscle disease who require heart transplantation as a final therapeutic remedy.

CONCLUSION

Endomyocardial biopsy remains the tarnished standard for the diagnosis of myocarditis and should be considered in all patients with unexplained new-onset heart failure, particularly if complicated by ventricular tachycardia or high-grade heart block. The expectation of both clinician and patient should be that a specific diagnosis will be made in a minority of cases and that even smaller number of patients will have a change in clinical treatment. However, in this subset of patients endomyocardial biopsy may initiate lifesaving treatment.

REFERENCES

1. Fowles RE, Mason JW. Role of cardiac biopsy in the diagnosis and management of cardiac disease. Prog Cardiovasc Dis 1984;27:153-172.
2. Parrillo JE, Aretz HT, Palacios I, Fallon JT, Block PC. The results of transvenous endomyocardial biopsy can frequently be used to diagnose myocardial diseases in patients with idiopathic heart failure. Endomyocardial biopsies in 100 consecutive patients revealed a substantial incidence of myocarditis. Circulation 1984;69:93-101.
3. Davies MJ, Ward DE. How can myocarditis be diagnosed and should it be treated? Br Heart J 1992;68:346-347.
4. Caves PK, Stinson EB, Billingham M, Shumway NE. Percutaneous transvenous endomyocardial biopsy in human heart recipients. Experience with a new technique. Ann Thorac Surg 1973;16:325-336.
5. Mason JW, O'Connell JB, Herskowitz A, Rose NR, McManus BM, Billingham ME, Moon TE. A clinical trial of immunosuppressive therapy for myocarditis. The Myocarditis Treatment Trial Investigators. N Engl J Med 1995;333:269-275.
6. McKenna WJ, Davies MJ. Immunosuppression for myocarditis. N Engl J Med 1995;333:312-313.
7. Hufnagel G, Pankuweit S, Richter A, Schonian U, Maisch B. The European Study of Epidemiology and Treatment of Cardiac Inflammatory Diseases (ESETCID). First epidemiological results. Herz 2000;25:279-285.
8. Aretz HT, Billingham ME, Edwards WD, Factor SM, Fallon JT, Fenoglio JJ Jr, Olsen EG, Schoen FJ. Myocarditis. A histopathologic definition and classification. Am J Cardiovasc Pathol 1987;1:3-14.
9. Davydova J, Pankuweit S, Crombach M, Eckhardt H, Strache D, Faulhammer P, Maisch B. Detection of viral and bacterial protein in endomyocardial biopsies of patients with inflammatory heart muscle disease? Herz 2000;25:233-239.
10. Pankuweit S, Portig I, Eckhardt H, Crombach M, Hufnagel G, Maisch B. Prevalence of viral genome in endomyocardial biopsies from patients with inflammatory heart muscle disease. Herz 2000;25:221-226.
11. Sugrue DD, Holmes DR Jr, Gersh BJ, Edwards WD, McLaran CJ, Wood DL, Osborn MJ, Hammill SC. Cardiac histologic findings in patients with life-threatening ventricular arrhythmias of unknown origin. J Am Coll Cardiol 1984;4:952-957.
12. Billingham ME, Cary NR, Hammond ME, Kemnitz J, Marboe C, McCallister HA, Snovar DC, Winters GL, Zerbe A. A working formulation for the standardization of nomenclature in the diagnosis of heart and lung rejection: Heart Rejection Study Group. The International Society for Heart Transplantation. J Heart Transplant 1990;9:587-593.
13. Feldman AM, McNamara D. Myocarditis. N Engl J Med 2000;343:1388-1398.
14. Fenoglio JJ Jr, Ursell PC, Kellogg CF, Drusin RE, Weiss MB. Diagnosis and classification of myocarditis by endomyocardial biopsy. N Engl J Med 1983;308:12-18.
15. Lie JT. Myocarditis and endomyocardial biopsy in unexplained heart failure: a diagnosis in search of a disease. Ann Intern Med 1988;109:525-528.
16. Liangos O, Neure L, Kuhl U, Pauschinger M, Sieper J, Distler A, Schwimmbeck PL, Braun J. The possible role of myocardial biopsy in systemic sclerosis. Rheumatology (Oxford) 2000;39:674-679.

17. Jurkovich D, de Marchena E, Bilsker M, Fierro-Renoy C, Temple D, Garcia H. Primary cardiac lymphoma diagnosed by percutaneous intracardiac biopsy with combined fluoroscopic and transesophageal echocardiographic imaging. Cathet Cardiovasc Interv 2000;50:226-233.

18. Maisch B. Endomyocardial biopsy in myocarditis. [German.] Dtsch Med Wochenschr 2000;125 Suppl 1:S15.

19. Barbaro G, Di Lorenzo G, Grisorio B, Barbarini G. Incidence of dilated cardiomyopathy and detection of HIV in myocardial cells of HIV-positive patients. Gruppo Italiano per lo Studio Cardiologico dei Pazienti Affetti da AIDS. N Engl J Med 1998;339:1093-1099.

20. Shanes JG, Ghali J, Billingham ME, Ferrans VJ, Fenoglio JJ, Edwards WD, Tsai CC, Saffitz JE, Isner J, Furener S, Subramanian R. Interobserver variability in the pathologic interpretation of endomyocardial biopsy results. Circulation 1987;75:401-405.

21. Miller LW, Labovitz AJ, McBride LA, Pennington DG, Kanter K. Echocardiography-guided endomyocardial biopsy. A 5-year experience. Circulation 1988;78:III99-III102.

22. Deckers JW, Hare JM, Baughman KL. Complications of transvenous right ventricular endomyocardial biopsy in adult patients with cardiomyopathy: a seven-year survey of 546 consecutive diagnostic procedures in a tertiary referral center. J Am Coll Cardiol 1992;19:43-47.

23. Mason JW. Techniques for right and left ventricular endomyocardial biopsy. Am J Cardiol 1978;41:887-892.

24. Tsang TSM, Freeman WK, Barnes ME, Reeder GS, Packer DL, Seward JB. Rescue echocardiographically guided pericardiocentesis for cardiac perforation complicating catheter-based procedures. The Mayo Clinic experience. J Am Coll Cardiol 1998;32:1345-1350.

25. Braverman AC, Coplen SE, Mudge GH, Lee RT. Ruptured chordae tendineae of the tricuspid valve as a complication of endomyocardial biopsy in heart transplant patients. Am J Cardiol 1990;66:111-113.

26. Pophal SG, Sigfusson G, Booth KL, Bacanu SA, Webber SA, Ettedgui JA, Neches WH, Park SC. Complications of endomyocardial biopsy in children. J Am Coll Cardiol 1999;34:2105-2110.

27. Pass RH, Trivedi KR, Hsu DT. A new technique for endomyocardial biopsy in infants and small children. Cathet Cardiovasc Interv 2000;50:441-444.

28. Hrobon P, Kuntz KM, Hare JM. Should endomyocardial biopsy be performed for detection of myocarditis? A decision analytic approach. J Heart Lung Transplant 1998;17:479-486.

Treatment of Lymphocytic Myocarditis

Jay W. Mason, M.D.

MYOCARDITIS DUE TO ACTIVE INFECTION
    Viral Myocarditis
    Other Infections

MYOCARDITIS DUE TO POSTINFECTIOUS
AUTOIMMUNITY
    Immunosuppressive Therapy
    Other Therapies

NONINFECTIOUS AUTOIMMUNE MYOCARDITIS

MYOCARDITIS DUE TO TOXINS

SUMMARY

How to treat lymphocytic myocarditis has changed in the last 50 years from a simple, unanswered clinical question to a highly complex, but still unanswered, clinical and basic research inquiry. The early literature, which preceded the now huge basic science exploration of myocarditis, speculated on its immunologic causes and the potential utility of steroid therapy.[1,2] Clinical recognition of the many causes of myocarditis and fundamental basic research observations on disease mechanisms have led to a long list of potential therapies. Although only a few of them have been tested satisfactorily in clinical trials, therapies being considered are remarkably innovative and promising.

Therapy for lymphocytic myocarditis can be best understood if classified within broad categories of disease mechanisms (Table 16-1). Many of these therapies, especially those directed at autoimmunity, are as yet unproved, and, in fact, the disease mechanisms themselves are not fully understood. Much of the work on disease mechanisms has been done in animal models, which may not faithfully portray the disease as it occurs in humans or may represent a disease process that does not occur clinically. Thus, caution is required in translating experimental observations to the bedside.

MYOCARDITIS DUE TO ACTIVE INFECTION

VIRAL MYOCARDITIS

The term "viral myocarditis" has multiple meanings. It may refer to myocardial inflammation associated with active viral replication in the myocardium or to an autoimmune phase of myocarditis, which is thought to follow after active viral replication has ceased, or to both as a single, continuous disease entity. The term has become nearly synonymous with myocarditis because lymphocytic myocarditis, which is by far the most frequent form of myocarditis in most western and some eastern countries, is assumed, perhaps mistakenly, to be due to viral disease. To avoid confusion, it is prudent to reserve this term for active viral infection. "Postviral myocarditis" is an appropriate term for the autoimmune phase. When the origin is not clear, which is often the case in humans, "lymphocytic myocarditis" is the most appropriate term, because it describes the principal histologic finding without presuming a cause.

Viruses can infect the myocardium and induce heart failure and an interstitial inflammatory response during replication. This has been thoroughly delineated in animal models, and it has also been documented in humans by means of histologic examination and culture of myocardial biopsy specimens.

It is likely that most episodes of viral myocarditis spontaneously resolve without sequelae, as suggested by the high incidence of transient electrocardiographic changes that occur without associated heart failure during influenza epidemics. Thus, it appears that no

Table 16-1
Treatment of Lymphocytic Myocarditis

Etiology	Potential therapy
Infection	
Active virus	Direct antivirals, immune stimulation
Other	Direct antimicrobials
Postinfectious autoimmunity	Immune suppression, cytokine suppression
Autoimmunity	Immune suppression, cytokine suppression
Hypersensitivity	Withdrawal of agent, corticosteroids
Toxin	Withdrawal of agent, cytokine suppression, corticosteroids

therapy is needed in most cases of viral myocarditis, many or most of which go unrecognized. This recommendation must be tempered by the possibility that a proportion of cases of idiopathic dilated cardiomyopathy may result from remote or recent viral infection, as suggested by the late follow-up that Orinius[3] undertook in patients with upper respiratory coxsackievirus infections and by the finding of presumed viral RNA and DNA in the myocardium of patients with idiopathic dilated cardiomyopathy.[4-6] It is conceivable that if viral infection could be detected early in these cases, antiviral or other interventions might prevent subsequent development of idiopathic dilated cardiomyopathy.

Viral myocarditis would be expected to respond to direct antiviral chemotherapy. Enteroviruses (which include the coxsackieviruses) appear to account for the majority of cases in humans. Unfortunately, antivirals that specifically inhibit enteroviruses have not been tested adequately for clinical application. Specific inhibitors of influenza viruses (amantadine, rimantadine), herpesviruses (acyclovir, ganciclovir, foscarnet), and other non-human immunodeficiency viruses (ribavirin, lamivudine) now exist. In cases of myocarditis in which those viruses can be implicated, these drugs might be beneficial if administered during active viral infection. However, there is no proof of efficacy in humans as yet.

Nonspecific antiviral therapies have been tested or proposed for treatment of myocarditis. Immunoglobulin therapy, studied in children[7] and in adults,[8] appears promising, but it is not yet proved and may act against antibody-mediated autoimmunity rather than through viral suppression. Interferons also have the potential to ameliorate ongoing cardiotropic viral infections, but at present the only approved antiviral use is of interferon-α in condyloma acuminatum and hepatitis. A common myocyte membrane receptor for coxsackievirus and adenovirus has been proposed as a target for preventing development or spread of myocardial viral infection.[9]

Lymphocytic myocarditis is a well-recognized complication of acquired immuno-deficiency syndrome (AIDS). Its incidence varies from less than 10% to more than 50%.[10-13] Its etiology is debated. Human immunodeficiency virus myocardial infection, other coinfecting agents, or autoimmunity triggered by infection may be responsible. Because AIDS myocarditis is often associated with progressive dilated cardiomyopathy,[11] which is often lethal,[14] early detection and therapy may improve outcome. In addition to conventional therapy, possibly including angiotensin-converting enzyme inhibitors, aggressive antiretroviral therapy might be helpful. Immunosuppressive therapy has also been reported anecdotally to improve congestive failure in patients with AIDS-related myocarditis, but this approach is as yet unproved.

OTHER INFECTIONS

Although viral and postviral myocarditis appear to be the most frequent types in highly developed countries, other infectious agents are common elsewhere. The myocarditis of Chagas disease and diphtheritic myocarditis are thought to be the most frequent of the myocarditides worldwide. Chagas myocarditis usually develops long after the acute infection with *Trypanosoma cruzi* and is largely immune mediated. Antiprotozoal therapy with nifurtimox or benznidazole may help. Diphtheritic myocarditis is common in epidemics. In an outbreak in Kyrgyzstan,[15] 22% of patients with diphtheria developed myocarditis and the case-fatality rate was 3%. Diphtheria antitoxin combined with antibiotics (usually penicillin or erythromycin) is effective.

MYOCARDITIS DUE TO POSTINFECTIOUS AUTOIMMUNITY

The etiology of lymphocytic myocarditis in humans in developed countries is not clearly established. However, a good deal of circumstantial evidence points toward autoimmunity after viral infection as the major cause. Most cases of clinically suspected or biopsy-documented myocarditis in the United States fit into this category. Symptoms usually develop a few weeks after a viral infection. In the US Myocarditis Treatment Trial,[16] 89% of enrollees had had signs or symptoms of a possible viral prodrome.

IMMUNOSUPPRESSIVE THERAPY

In deciding if patients with lymphocytic myocarditis should be treated for a presumed autoimmune disorder, the first step is to rule out active viral infection. In most patients this distinction is not difficult because they present afebrile days or weeks after a virus-like illness or report no such prodrome. In a small proportion the viral symptoms are more recent and fever is present. There are no randomized studies of therapy in patients with presumed ongoing viral infection, but studies in mice demonstrate worsening of myocarditis when immunosuppression is instituted during the infectious phase.[17] Except as a last resort, immunosuppression should be withheld in patients who have ongoing viral infection.

Another reason to withhold or delay immunosuppression in the early phase of myocarditis is that at least some components of the early immune response are beneficial and should not be suppressed. In the Myocarditis Treatment Trial,[16] several indices of a heightened early immune response were associated with improved survival. One such relationship is illustrated in Figure 16-1, which shows reduced cumulative mortality in patients with higher concentrations of circulating cardiac IgG.

Efficacy of immunosuppression in the presumed autoimmune phase of lymphocytic myocarditis is not established. The Myocarditis Treatment Trial,[16] which is the only completed randomized trial of therapy in myocarditis defined by generally accepted histologic criteria, showed improvement in left ventricular ejection fraction in patients receiving immunosuppression, but the extent of improvement was no better than that observed in subjects who did not receive immunosuppressive drugs (Fig. 16-2). Furthermore, survival in the 2 treatment limbs was identical (Fig. 16-3).

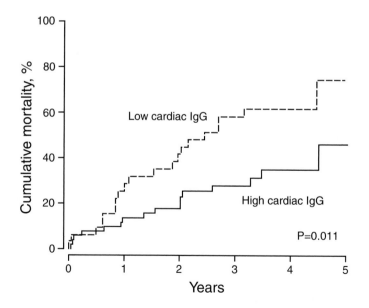

Fig. 16-1. In the US Myocarditis Treatment Trial, a high concentration of circulating cardiac-specific IgG was a univariate predictor of decreased mortality. It was not a significant predictor in a multivariate model. Nevertheless, this observation is consistent with beneficial effect of an early, appropriate immune response in myocarditis. (Modified from Mason JW. Immunopathogenesis and treatment of myocarditis: the United States Myocarditis Treatment Trial. J Card Fail 1996;2 Suppl 4:S173-S177. By permission of Elsevier Science.)

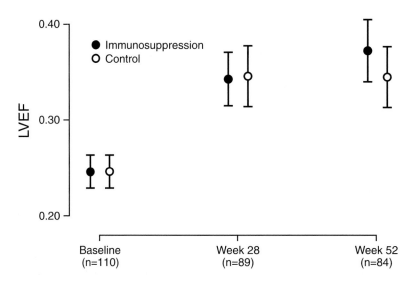

Fig. 16-2. In the US Myocarditis Treatment Trial, left ventricular ejection fraction (*LVEF*) increased significantly from baseline to week 28, and the increase was sustained to week 52. The extent of improvement was statistically equivalent in the immunosuppression and control groups. (From Mason et al.[16] By permission of the Massachusetts Medical Society.)

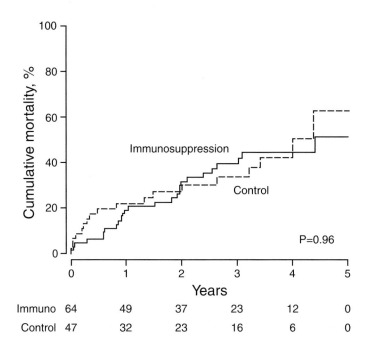

Fig. 16-3. There was no significant difference in mortality in the immunosuppression and control groups in the US Myocarditis Treatment Trial. The number of patients remaining in follow-up each year is displayed at the bottom of the graph. (From Mason et al.[16] By permission of the Massachusetts Medical Society.)

Garg and colleagues[18] performed a meta-analysis of 6 studies of immunosuppression in patients with myocarditis. They concluded that immunosuppression was not helpful. Reliability of this analysis is reduced by the fact that only 2 of the 6 studies were randomized controlled trials, and myocarditis was defined quite differently among the studies. In addition, all of the studies were relatively small, and each used a different form of immunosuppressive therapy.

The Myocarditis Treatment Trial remains the largest completed randomized trial of therapy for myocarditis. Nevertheless, the limits of its reliability should be understood. By design, the trial did not provide therapy tailored to specific causes of myocarditis, largely because specific therapies available today were not available at the time of the trial. The trial took place when there was an unusually prolonged cyclic reduction in the incidence of the most common cardiotropic virus infections. This accounts in part for the fact that it took 5 years to identify only 111 patients with biopsy-proven myocarditis in 31 enrollment centers. It may also account in part for the low incidence of biopsy specimens positive for myocarditis (only 10%) among the 2,233 patients suspected of having myocarditis. Thus, it is possible that the subjects enrolled in the trial had atypical causes of myocarditis. In addition, rigid adherence to the Dallas criteria[19] for histologic diagnosis of myocarditis may have excluded some treatment-responsive patients. Finally, the trial did not attract many cases of fulminant myocarditis. These patients may have a better prognosis when immunosuppressed (and, perhaps, without immunosuppression).[20]

Available information does not currently justify routine use of standard immunosuppressive therapy for lymphocytic myocarditis. However, a few exceptions seem appropriate. Immunosuppression should not be withheld as a potential life-saving measure in patients with cardiogenic shock who do not improve with conventional therapy. Patients without cardiogenic shock but who develop worsening heart failure are also candidates for a trial of immunosuppression. Patients who apparently responded to previous immunosuppressive therapy and develop recurrent myocarditis may be immunosuppressed again, and consideration should be given to use of different agents, larger doses, or a longer period of therapy.

Cardiopulmonary support has been used successfully in cases of cardiogenic shock due to acute and fulminant myocarditis. Kato et al.[21] reported on 9 patients with biopsy-confirmed myocarditis and cardiogenic shock treated with percutaneous cardiopulmonary support. All 9 patients improved hemodynamically and were weaned from the support device. Two patients died at days 13 and 113 of multiorgan failure and pneumonia. The remaining 7 were alive at a mean follow-up of 34 months. Kawahito and colleagues[22] reported on 6 patients who presented with cardiogenic shock 2 to 7 days after flu-like symptoms. The ejection fractions ranged from 15% to 30%. Five patients (83%) were weaned from support and dismissed. Ventricular-assist devices were used successfully as a bridge to transplantation in patients with lymphocytic myocarditis,[23] nonspecific myocarditis,[24] and giant cell myocarditis.[25]

Another category of patients with myocarditis in whom immunosuppression should be considered is the group presenting with life-threatening ventricular arrhythmias. Because myocarditis is often a self-limited process, in most cases it should be possible to avoid aggressive antiarrhythmic measures, such as ablation and cardioverter-defibrillator implantation, which are usually used for long-term suppression of arrhythmias. If a patient with myocarditis is facing the possibilities of those therapies, an attempt first to eliminate the arrhythmia by suppressing the inflammatory process is appropriate in some cases.

OTHER THERAPIES

The ongoing European Study of Epidemiology and Treatment of Cardiac Inflammatory Disease is a multicenter therapy trial based in Germany in which a recognition of the multiple etiologies of lymphocytic myocarditis is incorporated into the randomized treatment algorithm. Patients with evidence of active cytomegalovirus infection receive hyperimmune globulin, and if that is not effective, ganciclovir. Patients who have biopsy specimens containing enteroviral genomic material detected by polymerase chain reaction receive interferon-α. All others receive corticosteroids and azathioprine. None of these therapies are proven to be effective. The hope is that tailored therapy will be more likely to be successful.

Numerous new therapies have been proposed for treatment of lymphocytic myocarditis due to postinfectious autoimmunity (Table 16-2). Most of these new therapies are immunomodulatory. They attempt to suppress the evolution of the autoimmune process at an early stage (eg, FTY720), block immune mediators such as the cytokines (eg, anti-tumor necrosis factor-α antibodies), attack a specific molecular mechanism (T-cell antigen receptor-based DNA vaccines), or remove immune mediators from the circulation (eg, immunoadsorption). Other potential new therapies are derived from demonstrated success in prevention of adverse remodeling in congestive heart failure (eg, inhibition of angiotensin-converting enzyme). None of these new therapies were tested adequately in humans. Nevertheless, they represent the future in management of myocarditis and provide a reason for genuine optimism.

NONINFECTIOUS AUTOIMMUNE MYOCARDITIS

Autoimmune myocarditis also occurs independently of infectious insults. Immunoglobulin infiltration alone or in combination with cellular infiltration of the myocardium has been identified in several collagen vascular disorders, including rheumatoid arthritis, systemic lupus erythematosus, polyarteritis nodosa, dermatomyositis and polymyositis, scleroderma, and the CREST (calcinosis cutis, Raynaud phenomenon, esophageal dysfunction, sclero-

Table 16-2
New Therapies for Myocarditis Due to Postinfectious Autoimmunity

Therapy	Reference	Status
Intravenous immunglobulins	7,8	Uncontrolled trials in humans suggest efficacy
IgG adsorption	26	Effective in case-control studies in humans with idiopathic dilated cardiomyopathy
Anti-tumor-necrosis factor-α antibody	27	Effective as early therapy in mice
Nitric oxide inhibition	28	Pimobendan efficacy in mice may be mediated by inhibition of inducible nitric oxide synthase
T-cell antigen receptor-based DNA vaccines	29	Effective in murine autoimmune carditis
Tacrolimus	30-32	Effective in various murine models
FTY720	33	Reduces inflammatory infiltration in rats when administered early
Vesnarinone	34	Improves survival and reduces myocardial damage in mice by inhibiting natural killer cell activity
β-Adrenergic receptor blockers	35-37	Metoprolol is ineffective but carteolol is effective in improving CHF in murine models, a β_1-agonist is beneficial, no human studies
Calcium channel blockers	38	Amlodipine appears to be the most effective calcium antagonist in experimental models
α-Adrenergic receptor blockers	39	Helpful as early and protracted therapy
Angiotensin-converting enzyme inhibitors	40	Enzyme inhibitors and receptor blockers reduce myocardial injury in experimental myocarditis
Mu-Fang-Ji-Tang	41	Chinese herbal medicine improves CHF in murine myocarditis

CHF, congestive heart failure.

dactyly, and telangiectasia) syndrome.[42] There are no large series or controlled trials of therapy for myocarditis in these conditions. However, anecdotal experience showed that myocarditis is more likely to occur during heightened disease activity and to respond to the same therapies used to reduce that activity. Corticosteroids produce rapid and extensive improvement of ventricular function in some cases.

Numerous other disease-associated myocarditides are recognized, such as those associated with acute rheumatic fever and Kawasaki disease. Other disease-independent types of myocarditis, such as Dressler syndrome and postcardiotomy syndrome, are thought to have an autoimmune etiology. Any cardiac injury that releases myocellular proteins may be capable of inducing autoimmune carditis. Myosin is especially strongly implicated as a cause of autoimmune myocarditis.[43,44] In most of these conditions, corticosteroids and other immunosuppressive therapies acutely improve ventricular dysfunction, but long-term outcomes have not been studied adequately.

MYOCARDITIS DUE TO TOXINS

Numerous drugs and chemicals cause myocarditis. In some cases, these agents directly damage myocytes. Leak of intracellular contents into the interstitium induces inflammation and may also initiate a secondary autoimmune process. Other mechanisms undoubtedly exist. A hypersensitivity response to drugs and chemicals can be distinguished from direct toxicity by the presence of eosinophils. In either case, the most effective treatment is removal of the offending agent. Addition of corticosteroids may help when inflammation is unusually severe, ventricular dysfunction is markedly depressed, or recovery is delayed.

SUMMARY

Because lymphocytic myocarditis has multiple etiologies, therapy should be individualized according to the specific etiology. Unfortunately, efficacy of most therapies used or proposed for use in lymphocytic myocarditis has not been proven. Until this proof is available, specific and nonspecific antiviral measures should be considered for use in those relatively few patients who present with documented ongoing viral infection. Likewise, appropriate antimicrobial therapy is always indicated in lymphocytic myocarditis caused by bacterial and other organisms. The area of greatest controversy is the use of immunosuppressive and other immunomodulatory therapies for noninfectious and postinfectious myocarditis. Although this approach is unnecessary in many cases and ineffective in others, there are specific circumstances in which immunosuppression should be undertaken.

REFERENCES

1. Garrison RF, Swisher RC. Myocarditis of unknown etiology (Fiedler's ?) treated with ACTH: report of a case in a 7-year-old boy with improvement. J Pediatr 1953;42:591-599.

2. Ainger LE. Acute aseptic myocarditis: corticosteroid therapy. J Pediatr 1964;64:716-723.

3. Orinius E. The late cardiac prognosis after Coxsackie-B infection. Acta Med Scand 1968;183:235-237.

4. Bowles NE, Richardson PJ, Olsen EG, Archard LC. Detection of Coxsackie-B-virus-specific RNA sequences in myocardial biopsy samples from patients with myocarditis and dilated cardiomyopathy. Lancet 1986;1:1120-1123.

5. Giacca M, Severini GM, Mestroni L, Salvi A, Lardieri G, Falaschi A, Camerini F. Low frequency of detection by nested polymerase chain reaction of enterovirus ribonucleic acid in endomyocardial tissue of patients with idiopathic dilated cardiomyopathy. J Am Coll Cardiol 1994;24:1033-1040.

6. Weiss LM, Movahed LA, Billingham ME, Cleary ML. Detection of Coxsackievirus B3 RNA in myocardial tissues by the polymerase chain reaction. Am J Pathol 1991;138:497-503.

7. Drucker NA, Colan SD, Lewis AB, Beiser AS, Wessel DL, Takahashi M, Baker AL, Perez-Atayde AR, Newburger JW. Gamma-globulin treatment of acute myocarditis in the pediatric population. Circulation 1994;89:252-257.

8. McNamara DM, Rosenblum WD, Janosko KM, Trost MK, Villanueva FS, Demetris AJ, Murali S, Feldman AM. Intravenous immune globulin in the therapy of myocarditis and acute cardiomyopathy. Circulation 1997;95:2476-2478.

9. Liu PP, Opavsky MA. Viral myocarditis: receptors that bridge the cardiovascular with the immune system? Circ Res 2000;86:253-254.

10. Anderson DW, Virmani R, Reilly JM, O'Leary T, Cunnion RE, Robinowitz M, Macher AM, Punja U, Villaflor ST, Parrillo JE, Roberts WC. Prevalent myocarditis at necropsy in the acquired immuno-deficiency syndrome. J Am Coll Cardiol 1988;11:792-799.

11. Barbaro G, Di Lorenzo G, Grisorio B, Barbarini G. Incidence of dilated cardiomyopathy and detection of HIV in myocardial cells of HIV-positive patients. Gruppo Italiano per lo Studio Cardiologico dei Pazienti Affetti da AIDS. N Engl J Med 1998;339:1093-1099.

12. Barbaro G, Di Lorenzo G, Grisorio B, Barbarini G. Cardiac involvement in the acquired immuno-deficiency syndrome: a multicenter clinical-pathological study. Gruppo Italiano per lo Studio Cardiologico dei Pazienti Affetti da AIDS Investigators. AIDS Res Hum Retroviruses 1998;14:1071-1077.

13. Kaul S, Fishbein MC, Siegel RJ. Cardiac manifestations of acquired immune deficiency syndrome: a 1991 update. Am Heart J 1991;122:535-544.

14. De Castro S, d'Amati G, Gallo P, Cartoni D, Santopadre P, Vullo V, Cirelli A, Migliau G. Frequency of development of acute global left ventricular dysfunction in human immunodeficiency virus infection. J Am Coll Cardiol 1994;24:1018-1024.

15. Kadirova R, Kartoglu HU, Strebel PM. Clinical characteristics and management of 676 hospitalized diphtheria cases, Kyrgyz Republic, 1995. J Infect Dis 2000;181 Suppl 1:S110-S115.

16. Mason JW, O'Connell JB, Herskowitz A, Rose NR, McManus BM, Billingham ME, Moon TE. A clinical trial of immunosuppressive therapy for myocarditis. The Myocarditis Treatment Trial Investigators. N Engl J Med 1995;333:269-275.

17. Woodruff JF. Viral myocarditis. A review. Am J Pathol 1980;101:425-484.

18. Garg A, Shiau J, Guyatt G. The ineffectiveness of immunosuppressive therapy in lymphocytic myocarditis: an overview. Ann Intern Med 1998;129:317-322.

19. Aretz HT, Billingham ME, Edwards WD, Factor SM, Fallon JT, Fenoglio JJ Jr, Olsen EG, Schoen FJ. Myocarditis. A histopathologic definition and classification. Am J Cardiovasc Pathol 1987;1:3-14.

20. McCarthy RE III, Boehmer JP, Hruban RH, Hutchins GM, Kasper EK, Hare JM, Baughman KL. Long-term outcome of fulminant myocarditis as compared with acute (nonfulminant) myocarditis. N Engl J Med 2000;342:690-695.

21. Kato S, Morimoto S, Hiramitsu S, Nomura M, Ito T, Hishida H. Use of percutaneous cardiopulmonary support of patients with fulminant myocarditis and cardiogenic shock for improving prognosis. Am J Cardiol 1999;83:623-625, A10.

22. Kawahito K, Murata S, Yasu T, Adachi H, Ino T, Saito M, Misawa Y, Fuse K, Shimada K. Usefulness of extracorporeal membrane oxygenation for treatment of fulminant myocarditis and circulatory collapse. Am J Cardiol 1998;82:910-911.

23. Starling RC, Galbraith TA, Baker PB, Howanitz EP, Murray KD, Binkley PF, Watson KM, Unverferth DV, Myerowitz PD. Successful management of acute myocarditis with biventricular assist devices and cardiac transplantation. Am J Cardiol 1988;62:341-343.

24. Reiss N, el-Banayosy A, Posival H, Morshuis M, Minami K, Korfer R. Management of acute fulminant myocarditis using circulatory support systems. Artif Organs 1996;20:964-970.

25. Brilakis ES, Olson LJ, Berry GJ, Daly RC, Loisance D, Zucker M, Cooper LT Jr. Survival outcomes of patients with giant cell myocarditis bridged by ventricular assist devices. Asaio J 2000;46:569-572.

26. Muller J, Wallukat G, Dandel M, Bieda H, Brandes K, Spiegelsberger S, Nissen E, Kunze R, Hetzer R. Immunoglobulin adsorption in patients with idiopathic dilated cardiomyopathy. Circulation 2000;101:385-391.

27. Yamada T, Matsumori A, Sasayama S. Therapeutic effect of anti-tumor necrosis factor-alpha antibody on the murine model of viral myocarditis induced by encephalomyocarditis virus. Circulation 1994;89:846-851.

28. Iwasaki A, Matsumori A, Yamada T, Shioi T, Wang W, Ono K, Nishio R, Okada M, Sasayama S. Pimobendan inhibits the production of proinflammatory cytokines and gene expression of inducible nitric oxide synthase in a murine model of viral myocarditis. J Am Coll Cardiol 1999;33:1400-1407.

29. Matsumoto Y, Jee Y, Sugisaki M. Successful TCR-based immunotherapy for autoimmune myocarditis with DNA vaccines after rapid identification of pathogenic TCR. J Immunol 2000;164:2248-2254.

30. Kanda T, Nagaoka H, Kaneko K, Wilson JE, McManus BM, Imai S, Suzuki T, Murata K, Kobayashi I. Synergistic effects of tacrolimus and human interferon-alpha A/D in murine viral myocarditis. J Pharmacol Exp Ther 1995;274:487-493.

31. Hanawa H, Kodama M, Zhang S, Izumi T, Shibata A. An immunosuppressant compound, FK-506, prevents the progression of autoimmune myocarditis in rats. Clin Immunol Immunopathol 1992;62:321-326.

32. McManus BM, Han L, Caruso R, Stratta RJ, Wilson JE. Impact of FK 506 on myocarditis in the enteroviral murine model. Transplant Proc 1991;23:3365-3367.

33. Kitabayashi H, Isobe M, Watanabe N, Suzuki J, Yazaki Y, Sekiguchi M. FTY720 prevents development of experimental autoimmune myocarditis through reduction of circulating lymphocytes. J Cardiovasc Pharmacol 2000;35:410-416.

34. Matsui S, Matsumori A, Matoba Y, Uchida A, Sasayama S. Treatment of virus-induced myocardial injury with a novel immunomodulating agent, vesnarinone. Suppression of natural killer cell activity and tumor necrosis factor-alpha production. J Clin Invest 1994;94:1212-1217.

35. Rezkalla S, Kloner RA, Khatib G, Smith FE, Khatib R. Effect of metoprolol in acute coxsackievirus B3 murine myocarditis. J Am Coll Cardiol 1988;12:412-414.

36. Nishio R, Matsumori A, Shioi T, Wang W, Yamada T, Ono K, Sasayama S. Denopamine, a beta$_1$-adrenergic agonist, prolongs survival in a murine model of congestive heart failure induced by viral

myocarditis: suppression of tumor necrosis factor-alpha production in the heart.   J Am Coll Cardiol 1998;32:808-815.

37. Tominaga M, Matsumori A, Okada I, Yamada T, Kawai C. Beta-blocker treatment of dilated cardiomyopathy. Beneficial effect of carteolol in mice. Circulation 1991;83:2021-2028.

38. Wang WZ, Matsumori A, Yamada T, Shioi T, Okada I, Matsui S, Sato Y, Suzuki H, Shiota K, Sasayama S. Beneficial effects of amlodipine in a murine model of congestive heart failure induced by viral myocarditis. A possible mechanism through inhibition of nitric oxide production. Circulation 1997;95:245-251.

39. Yamada T, Matsumori A, Okada I, Tominaga M, Kawai C. The effect of alpha 1-blocker, bunazosin on a murine model of congestive heart failure induced by viral myocarditis. Jpn Circ J 1992;56:1138-1145.

40. Rezkalla S, Kloner RA, Khatib G, Khatib R. Beneficial effects of captopril in acute coxsackievirus B3 murine myocarditis. Circulation 1990;81:1039-1046.

41. Wang WZ, Matsumori A, Matoba Y, Matsui S, Sato Y, Hirozane T, Shioi T, Sasayama S. Protective effects of Mu-Fang-Ji-Tang against myocardial injury in a murine model of congestive heart failure induced by viral myocarditis. Life Sci 1998;62:1139-1146.

42. Ferrans VJ, Rodriguez ER. Cardiovascular lesions in collagen-vascular diseases. Heart Vessels Suppl 1985;1:256-261.

43. Neu N, Rose NR, Beisel KW, Herskowitz A, Gurri-Glass G, Craig SW. Cardiac myosin induces myocarditis in genetically predisposed mice. J Immunol 1987;139:3630-3636.

44. Rose NR. Viral damage or 'molecular mimicry'—placing the blame in myocarditis. Nat Med 2000;6:631-632.

Idiopathic Giant Cell Myocarditis

Leslie T. Cooper, Jr., M.D.

INTRODUCTION

Idiopathic giant cell myocarditis (IGCM) was first described by Saltykow[1] in a 37-year-old man who died suddenly after surgical drainage of an abscess. Since then, dozens of case reports and a few small series have documented that IGCM is a usually fatal disorder that generally affects young otherwise healthy individuals, although a minority of cases occur in association with autoimmune disorders or thymoma. From 1905 until 1987, all cases were described at autopsy, and survival was generally less than 3 months from symptom onset. In 1993, Ren et al.[2] described prolonged transplant-free survival in 3 patients with IGCM. Several patients whose disease was diagnosed by endomyocardial biopsy survived 1 or more years in association with immunosuppressive treatment.[3] This chapter reviews the pathophysiology, natural history, proposed diagnostic strategy, and treatment options for IGCM.

In the first half of the twentieth century, the term "giant cell myocarditis" was used to describe both granulomatous and diffuse inflammatory myocardial infiltrates that contained multinucleated giant cells.[4-6] Idiopathic granulomatous myocarditis with giant cells was described in several case reports as cardiac sarcoidosis or giant cell myocarditis.[7-9] Tesluk[10] first distinguished the well-organized, granulomatous lesions of cardiac sarcoidosis from a diffuse, nongranulomatous infiltrate, which he called giant cell myocarditis. Most authorities since have considered giant cell myocarditis as a distinct clinical and pathologic entity rather than a virulent form of isolated cardiac sarcoidosis.[11-13] This distinction does not result from a proven mechanistic difference between these disorders. Indeed, about half of the cases of cardiac sarcoidosis are isolated, with no evidence of extracardiac involvement.[14]

IGCM is a pathologic diagnosis (see Fig. 14-15 *A* and 14-15 *B*). A diffuse or multifocal inflammatory infiltrate consists of lymphocytes admixed with eosinophils and multinucleated giant cells. Myocyte damage must be evident in association with the inflammatory lesion.[15] Various degrees of fibrosis may be present.[12] Poorly formed granulomas may be seen in giant cell myocarditis, but well-organized follicular granulomas containing central giant cells exclude the diagnosis by definition. The lesions of active lymphocytic myocarditis may occasionally contain an isolated giant cell; nonetheless, giant cell myocarditis can usually be distinguished from lymphocytic myocarditis and granulomatous myocarditis, even on biopsy specimens (Table 17-1).

The differential diagnosis of IGCM includes drug reactions and systemic diseases (Table 17-2). Drug hypersensitivity reaction may manifest as IGCM, with evidence of hypersensitivity in other organs.[16,17] IGCM has been described after high-dose interleukin-2 treatment for lymphoma,[18] possibly as a result of cytokine imbalance. Giant cell myocarditis has been described in a case of measles myocarditis.[19]

Up to 20% of cases of giant cell myocarditis occur in individuals with other inflammatory or autoimmune disorders, especially inflammatory bowel disease (Table 17-3).[20-26] Interestingly, a small percentage of patients who present with giant cell myocarditis at

Table 17-1
**Pathologic Findings in Giant Cell Myocarditis, Cardiac Sarcoidosis,
and Lymphocytic Myocarditis**

Diagnosis	Definition	Gross pathology	Microscopic pathology	Comments
Giant cell myocarditis*	Widespread or serpiginous inflammation with myocyte necrosis in the absence of well-formed granulomas or specific etiology	Pale, flabby myocardium; dilation or hypertrophy may be present; treated cases may have extensive scar	Widespread or serpiginous inflammation with giant cells, lymphocytes, and often eosinophils; myocyte necrosis always present; poorly formed granulomas may be seen	See Tables 17-2 and 17-3 and text for differential diagnosis and associated disorders
Cardiac sarcoidosis[†]	Granulomatous myocarditis with no evidence of infectious or other specific cause	Sharply defined areas of granulomatous inflammation or scar; preferential involvement of papillary muscles, septum, and base of ventricles	Non-necrotizing granulomas, fibrosis with few eosinophils; myocyte necrosis is rare	Look for other organ involvement, anergy to common antigens, and ACE level to support diagnosis; exclude fungi, mycobacteria, and foreign body reaction with special studies
Lympho-cytic or idiopathic myocarditis[‡]	A predominantly lymphocytic infiltrate with associated myocyte damage in the absence of acute infarction	Focal or diffuse inflammatory lesions	First pathologic specimen may be active or borderline myocarditis, the latter having no myocyte damage; subsequent samples may be persistent, healing, or healed per "Dallas criteria"	Associated with coxsackie B, adenoviral, and hepatitis C viral infections; biopsy artifacts may resemble myocyte necrosis; rule out many specific causes

ACE, angiotensin-converting enzyme.
*Cooper et al. N Engl J Med 1997;336:1860-1866; Davies et al. Br Heart J 1975;37:192-195.
[†]Roberts et al. Am J Med 1977;63:86-108.
[‡]Bloom, editor. Diagnostic Criteria for Cardiovascular Pathology, 1997, p 365; Aretz et al. Am J Cardiovasc Pathol 1987;1:3-14.
From Cooper LT Jr. Giant cell myocarditis: diagnosis and treatment. Herz 2000;25:291-298.
 By permission of Urban & Vogel.

Table 17-2
Disorders That May Resemble Giant Cell Myocarditis

Disorder	Associated findings and diagnostic studies	
Sarcoidosis	Granulomatous myocarditis without specific cause; fibrosis may be prominent; myocyte necrosis is rare	Anergy to common antigens; angiotensin-converting enzyme level; look for other organ involvement
Wegener granulo-matosis	Granulomatous myocarditis; renal and upper and lower respiratory disease are generally present; vasculitis may affect the coronary arteries	c-ANCA, look for classic renal and respiratory findings
Foreign body reaction	Giant cells may be associated with myocardial reaction to pacemaker leads or ventricular-assist devices	
Hyper-sensitivity myocarditis	Diffuse, primarily interstitial infiltrate with numerous eosinophils; myocyte necrosis and giant cells are infrequent	Elevated liver function results, eosinophil count, and skin rash
Cardiac lymphoma	Hodgkin disease rarely reported with myocardial granulomas with giant cells*	Immunophenotyping, look for extracardiac involvement
Fungal myocarditis	Coccidioidomycosis, blastomycosis, actino-mycosis, and others from granulomas; seen in immunocompromised hosts, often with associated endocarditis or sepsis	Special stains such as Grocott methenamine silver and periodic acid-Schiff indicated
Measles	Rare complication of measles; may cause myocyte necrosis and giant cell myocarditis	Associated clinical findings
Syphilis	Gumma may rarely involve the myocardium; myocardial involvement is rarely isolated	Associated clinical findings; VDRL
Tuberculosis	Nodular, miliary, and diffuse infiltrative types; myocardial involvement is rarely isolated	Other organ involvement; PPD skin test
Rheumatic carditis	Interstitial granulomatous infiltrate without myocyte necrosis in active lesion	Jones criteria[†]

c-ANCA, antineutrophil cytoplasmic antibodies; PPD, purified protein derivative; VDRL, Venereal Disease Research Laboratory.
*Saphir O. Arch Pathol 1942;33:88.
[†]JAMA 1992;268:2069-2073.
From Cooper LT Jr. Giant cell myocarditis: diagnosis and treatment. Herz 2000;25:291-298. By permission of Urban & Vogel.

Table 17-3
Disorders Associated With Idiopathic Giant Cell Myocarditis

Inflammatory disorders
  Ulcerative colitis[24,26]
  Crohn disease[15]
  Orbital & skeletal myositis[27]
  Myasthenia gravis[22,28]
  Thyroiditis[13,29,30]
  Takayasu arteritis[31,32]
  Rheumatoid arthritis[33]
  Pernicious anemia[23]
  Alopecia totalis vitiligo[34]

Tumors
  Thymoma[28,35]
  Lung carcinoma[29]
  Lymphoma[36,37]
  Sarcoma[13]

Hypersensitivity reaction
  Silicone rubber[38]
  Antiseizure medication[17]

Miscellaneous
  Post-mitral valve surgery[39]
  Mitral stenosis-associated[40]

From Cooper LT Jr. Giant cell myocarditis: diagnosis and treatment. Herz 2000;25:291-298.
  By permission of Urban & Vogel.

autopsy or explantation have clinically unrecognized granulomatous inflammation in other organs, including the aorta, lungs, liver, and lymph nodes.[41] These cases suggest that IGCM can be the prime manifestation of a systemic granulomatous process. In our experience, several patients with fatal IGCM have had a granulomatous infiltrate in the lymph nodes or other organs. Therefore, the diagnosis of sarcoidosis or the presence of granulomatous infiltration in other organs does not exclude IGCM.[13,42]

Disorders that cause myocardial granulomas with associated giant cells may be mistaken for IGCM. Aschoff lesions of rheumatic myocarditis evolve into characteristic, focal interstitial granulomas with giant cells. Tuberculosis and cryptococcosis may also have giant cells within granulomatous lesions.[43-45] Special stains for organisms should be performed whenever there is a question of infection. Rarely, giant cells may be seen in syphilitic myocarditis.[45] Foreign body reaction, Wegener granulomatosis,[46,47] and systemic sarcoidosis must be considered in the differential diagnosis as well. These disorders usually have distinct clinical presentations and appropriate diagnostic studies usually prevent confusion with IGCM.

The tumor most commonly associated with giant cell myocarditis is thymoma, particularly the spindle cell type.[13] Myasthenia gravis and myositis are associated with thymoma and giant cell myocarditis individually and in combination.[20,22,27,31,48-52] The association of thymoma with giant cell myocarditis occurs almost exclusively in women.[28] IGCM once occurred 10 days after surgical resection of thymoma.[35] It has been postulated in the absence of direct evidence that alterations in immune function associated with thymoma predispose to giant cell myocarditis.[22] Associations with sarcoma arising from the thymus[13] and lymphoma[36] have also been described; however, lymphoproliferative disease of the heart may be difficult to distinguish from giant cell myocarditis if myocyte necrosis is present.

The incidence of giant cell myocarditis is low and varies with the population studied and method of diagnosis. In a Japanese autopsy registry, the incidence of giant cell myocarditis was 0.007% (25 of 377,841 cases from 1958 to 1977).[53] The incidence of giant cell myocarditis was a similarly low 3 of 12,815 necropsies from 1950 to 1963 at Oxford Infirmary.[11] The incidence is higher when all IGCM cases diagnosed by endomyocardial biopsy or other surgical specimens, explanted heart, and autopsy are included. Using all pathologic specimens, 5 large, heart failure referral centers in the United States encountered a case of giant cell myocarditis about every 21 months from 1993 to 1997 (Giant Cell Myocarditis Registry, unpublished data).

Until recently, no easily available source of authoritative information on IGCM has been maintained. In 2001, the Web site *www.gcminfo.org* was established to provide such a resource for affected individuals and their families. This site also provides links to other relevant sites concerned with inflammatory heart disease.

MECHANISMS OF GIANT CELL MYOCARDITIS

The cause of human giant cell myocarditis is not known but often presumed to be autoimmune. Useful data supporting an autoimmune mechanism come from the Lewis rat model of IGCM. Experimental IGCM can be produced in the Lewis rat by autoimmunization with myosin.[54] In this model, autoimmune giant cell myocarditis is mediated by CD4$^+$ T cells that produce interferon-γ and macrophages that produce tumor necrosis factor and nitric oxide.[55] The disease can be transferred by T lymphocytes.[56] The histologic changes and hemodynamic deterioration are associated with inducible nitric oxide synthetase expression and attenuated by aminoguanidine, an inhibitor of inducible nitric oxide synthetase.[57] The detrimental effect of nitric oxide in this model contrasts with the beneficial effects of nitric oxide in coxsackie viral myocarditis.[58] Also of interest, tumor necrosis factor-alpha stimulates multinucleation of macrophages into giant cells in vitro when it is secreted from macrophages, but not when it is added exogenously.[59]

Strain differences in rats with experimental giant cell myocarditis suggest that genetic factors play a major role in susceptibility to disease. Shioji and colleagues[60] reported the incidence, histopathology, and histocompatibility characteristics of 5 inbred strains of rats in which myocarditis was induced with porcine cardiac myosin. Immune-mediated myocarditis was induced in Lewis, Dahl (DIR/Eis) (RT-1), and Fisher rats but not in brown Norway rats or a second strain of Dahl rats (DIS/Eis) (RT-1). The disease was most severe in the Lewis rats and seemed to correlate with major histocompatibility complex class II region differences between the strains. Although 90% of cases in the Giant Cell Myocarditis Registry occurred in whites, firm conclusions regarding ethnic susceptibility cannot be drawn because these data may reflect the populations at the referral centers.[15]

Observations in human tissue suggest that IGCM is mediated by T lymphocytes as well.[12] In studies of paraffin-embedded tissue, infiltrating lymphocytes are almost always positive for T-cell antigens and giant cells are positive for macrophage antigens.[26,61,62] The T-cell subsets (helper and suppressor ratios) may vary during the evolution of the infiltrate. Electron microscopy has failed to find viral particles or other clues to the etiology of giant cell myocarditis.[62-64]

Data from the rat model of IGCM support aggressive immunosuppressive treatment early in the disease. Data from the rat model suggest that anti-T-lymphocyte antibodies and cyclosporine, but not prednisolone alone, prevent giant cell myocarditis.[65-67] From these observations, immunosuppression with muromonab-CD3 and cyclosporine would be a reasonable treatment for patients who have giant cell myocarditis.

DIAGNOSTIC STRATEGY

The diagnosis of giant cell myocarditis should be considered for all patients with subacute heart failure of unknown cause. Of the 63 Multicenter Giant Cell Myocarditis Registry patients,[15] 75% presented with congestive heart failure, 14% presented with ventricular arrhythmia, and lesser percentages presented with a syndrome mimicking acute myocardial infarction, heart block, or arterial embolization. The median time from symptom onset to presentation was 3 weeks. The median age was 42 years (range, 15 to 69 years), but patients younger than 15 years[68] and older than 70 years[11] have been reported. Men and women are affected equally, and cases have been described in many ethnic groups.

Common causes for heart failure and arrhythmia ought to be excluded per standard clinical practice. After a complete history, physical examination, electrocardiogram, and chest radiograph, an echocardiogram is usually done to exclude valvular and pericardial disease and cardiac masses. There are no specific echocardiographic findings to distinguish giant cell myocarditis from other forms of myocarditis, although the rapid decline in ejection fraction that may occur over several days in giant cell myocarditis patients is uncommon in lymphocytic myocarditis or cardiac sarcoidosis. Coronary angiography is superior to noninvasive stress imaging to exclude significant coronary stenosis or dissection. Magnetic resonance imaging or computed tomography may be done if clinically indicated to help exclude such disorders as arrhythmogenic right ventricular dysplasia or constrictive pericarditis.

Endomyocardial biopsy ought to be considered for patients with heart failure or ventricular arrhythmia of less than 3 months' duration who fail to improve despite optimal medical care. In most cases of lymphocytic myocarditis, the left ventricular ejection fraction improves with usual care,[69] whereas the ejection fraction in giant cell myocarditis rarely improves.[70] The development of ventricular tachycardia or heart block further increases the likelihood of giant cell myocarditis.[15,70,71] The presence of associated disorders such as thymoma, myasthenia gravis, myositis, or inflammatory bowel disease (Table 17-3) may provide valuable clues as well.

Because giant cell myocarditis usually affects the endocardium,[12] right ventricular endomyocardial biopsy may have a high sensitivity. In a substudy analysis of Giant Cell Myocarditis Registry subjects, Shields et al.[72] found that endomyocardial biopsy had 82% to 85% sensitivity for giant cell myocarditis compared to the standard of surgical pathology (autopsy, explanted heart, or apical wedge section). This compares favorably to the roughly 35% sensitivity of endomyocardial biopsy in lymphocytic myocarditis, a more common but generally less severe and widespread process.[73] However, the Shields et al. study included only subjects who had both endomyocardial biopsy and surgical specimens (ie, selected those with a particularly poor prognosis). The sensitivity of endomyocardial biopsy would likely be lower in an unselected population of heart failure subjects with giant cell myocarditis.

Sampling error is a concern in endomyocardial biopsy, and a minimum of 5 and sometimes more specimens ought to be obtained. Occasionally, the diagnostic lesion is seen only on additional cuts of the specimen blocks. Care must be taken to exclude hypersensitivity myocarditis, granulomatous myocarditis, foreign body reaction, and potential infectious causes by using standard diagnostic criteria and appropriate special stains.[74] Once the diagnosis of giant cell myocarditis is certain, then one can consider the use of immunosuppressive agents in addition to usual care.

Other diagnostic techniques that have been suggested for viral myocarditis or cardiac sarcoidosis have not been applied to giant cell myocarditis. For example, antibodies to cardiac myosin have been described for patients with acute and chronic myocarditis.[75]

Adenoviral and enteroviral DNA have been found in the hearts of patients with viral myocarditis.[76] Magnetic resonance imaging and newer echocardiographic techniques have been applied for myocarditis and cardiac sarcoidosis[77] in pilot studies. Nuclear imaging with gallium-67[78] to detect leukocytes or antimyosin antibodies to detect myocyte necrosis[73] has not been used systematically to diagnose giant cell myocarditis. Because of the rarity and severity of giant cell myocarditis, a highly specific noninvasive test would be of great value; however, such a development is unlikely without a much greater understanding of the cause of giant cell myocarditis.

TREATMENT OF GIANT CELL MYOCARDITIS

Giant cell myocarditis is rapidly progressive and frequently requires the concurrent management of congestive heart failure, tachyarrhythmias, heart block, and secondary renal and hepatic insufficiency. Supportive care may include standard pharmacologic therapy for congestive heart failure, a permanent or temporary pacemaker, an implantable cardiac defibrillator, and an intra-aortic balloon pump. The use of these drugs and devices should be dictated by standard clinical practice.

Ventricular-assist devices have been used to bridge the time until patients with giant cell myocarditis have heart transplantation. Ventricular-assist devices have been used successfully as a bridge to transplantation in patients with lymphocytic[79] or nonspecific myocarditis.[80] Brilakis et al.[81] reported a series of 9 patients from the Giant Cell Myocarditis Registry, who received ventricular-assist devices. Successful bridging to transplantation in 7 of 9 (78%) is similar to that reported for other recipients of assist devices. Post-transplantation survival of 57% (4 of 7) at 30 days and 29% (2 of 7) at 1 year was unexpectedly low. Poor post-transplantation survival may have been due to poor pre-transplantation condition of the patients. For a patient with giant cell myocarditis, the time to recovery has been bridged successfully with a biventricular Abiomed assist device (personal communication from patient).

Several case reports and the Giant Cell Myocarditis Registry suggest that treatment with certain combinations of immunosuppressants, but not steroids alone, prolongs transplant-free survival.[15,82-84] The median time to death or cardiac transplantation for all 63 Registry subjects was 5.5 months from onset of symptoms. Seventy percent of affected individuals died or required heart transplantation within 1 year, and the overall rate of death or cardiac transplantation was 89%.[15,85] Treatment with cyclosporine and steroid sometimes combined with azathioprine or muromonab-CD3 was associated with a median survival of 12.6 months compared with 3.0 months for those not treated with immunosuppressive agents ($P = 0.001$ by log-rank test).[15] No published data exist for the use of other immunosuppressive agents such as immunoglobulin, cyclophosphamide, tacrolimus, mycophenolate, or antithymocyte globulin for giant cell myocarditis.

These immunosuppressive treatment data must be interpreted cautiously. The data stem from a small registry, not a randomized controlled trial. They are subject to uncontrolled factors that could possibly lead to an observed treatment effect substantially larger than the actual treatment effect. As an example, it is possible that the giant cell myocarditis patients in this registry with longer transplant-free survival times were more likely to receive combined immunosuppression therapy than the patients with shorter times. If so, this would lead to a biased overestimate of the treatment effect.

The risks of aggressive immunosuppression in this setting are considerable. Cyclosporine can cause renal insufficiency, hypertension, liver function abnormalities, hirsutism, and gum enlargement. Muromonab-CD3 can cause profound hypotension, fever, chills, diarrhea, nausea, and vomiting. Long-term use of prednisone can cause osteoporosis and fractures, myopathy, cataracts, and glaucoma. Therefore, these drugs should be used to treat giant cell myocarditis by individuals experienced in their use at specialized centers.

Cardiac transplantation has been used with acceptable morbidity and mortality as a primary therapy for the management of giant cell myocarditis.[86-89] Enthusiasm for transplantation was tempered by several reports of post-transplantation recurrence of giant cell myocarditis (Fig. 17-1).[90-93] The 39 Giant Cell Myocarditis Registry patients who underwent heart transplantation had a 71% 5-year survival, despite a 25% post-transplantation histologic recurrence rate on surveillance endomyocardial biopsies. Therefore, overall post-transplantation survival for giant cell myocarditis patients is comparable to survival for patients who receive transplants for cardiomyopathy.[94]

THE GIANT CELL MYOCARDITIS TREATMENT TRIAL

To control for possible bias in the Registry survival data and to investigate the mechanisms of giant cell myocarditis, the multicenter Giant Cell Myocarditis Treatment Trial was organized. This study is a randomized, open-label trial of muromonab-CD3, cyclosporine, and steroids (prednisolone followed by prednisone) versus cyclosporine and steroids for giant cell myocarditis diagnosed by endomyocardial biopsy. The primary efficacy end point is to compare the rate of death, transplantation, and ventricular-assist device placement at 1 year (event-free survival) in the 2 groups. To investigate the mechanism of survival benefit, hemodynamic and immunohistologic assessments will be obtained before treatment and during the study. The secondary efficacy end points include 1) change in left ventricular ejection fraction measured by radionuclide angiography, 2) improvement in myocardial inflammatory infiltrate, and 3) functional status assessed by the Living With Heart Failure

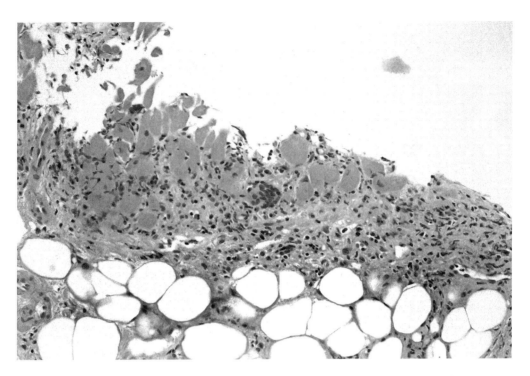

Fig. 17-1. Post-transplantation recurrence of giant cell myocarditis. (Courtesy of Edwina Duhing, MBBS, FRCPA.)

Questionnaire before and after 4 weeks of treatment. Adverse events will be monitored and assessed by an independent safety monitoring committee.

CONCLUSIONS

The prognosis of patients who have giant cell myocarditis is poor, but prolonged transplant-free survival may be possible with aggressive immunosuppression if treatment is started within several months of symptom onset. Because of possible bias in the retrospective Giant Cell Myocarditis Registry survival data and the substantial risks of treatment, the benefits of immunosuppression need to be confirmed in a prospective randomized trial. Consider the diagnosis of giant cell myocarditis for patients with less than 3 months of progressive congestive heart failure or ventricular arrhythmia. Patients with suspected IGCM might be referred to a center involved in the Giant Cell Myocarditis Treatment Trial. Despite a substantial rate of post-transplantation giant cell infiltration on surveillance biopsies, the post-transplantation survival of giant cell myocarditis patients is comparable to post-transplantation survival for cardiomyopathy patients.

REFERENCES

1. Saltykow S. Ueber diffuse Myokarditis. Virchows Arch Pathol Anat Berl 1905;182:1-39.

2. Ren H, Poston RS Jr, Hruban RH, Baumgartner WA, Baughman KL, Hutchins GM. Long survival with giant cell myocarditis. Mod Pathol 1993;6:402-407.

3. Menghini VV, Savcenko V, Olson LJ, Tazelaar HD, Dec GW, Kao A, Cooper LT Jr. Combined immunosuppression for the treatment of idiopathic giant cell myocarditis. Mayo Clin Proc 1999;74:1221-1226.

4. Jonas AF Jr. Granulomatous myocarditis. Bull Johns Hopkins Hosp 1939;64:45-65.

5. Saphir O. Myocarditis; general review, with analysis of 240 cases. Arch Pathol 1941;32:1000-1051; 1942;33:88-137.

6. Kean BH, Hoekenga MT. Giant cell myocarditis. Am J Pathol 1952;28:1095-1105.

7. Bernstein M, Konzelmann FW, Sidlick DM. Boeck's sarcoid; report of case with visceral involvement. Arch Intern Med 1929;44:721-734.

8. Scotti TM, McKeown CA. Sarcoidosis involving heart; report of case with sudden death. Arch Pathol 1948;46:289-300.

9. Johnson JB, Jason RS. Sarcoidosis of the heart; report of case and review of literature. Am Heart J 1944;27:246-258.

10. Tesluk H. Giant cell versus granulomatous myocarditis. Am J Clin Pathol 1956;26:1326-1333.

11. Whitehead R. Isolated myocarditis. Br Heart J 1965;27:220-230.

12. Litovsky SH, Burke AP, Virmani R. Giant cell myocarditis: an entity distinct from sarcoidosis characterized by multiphasic myocyte destruction by cytotoxic T cells and histiocytic giant cells. Mod Pathol 1996;9:1126-1134.

13. Davies MJ, Pomerance A, Teare RD. Idiopathic giant cell myocarditis—a distinctive clinico-pathological entity. Br Heart J 1975;37:192-195.

14. Fleming HA. Sarcoid heart disease. Br Heart J 1974;36:54-68.

15. Cooper LT Jr, Berry GJ, Shabetai R. Idiopathic giant-cell myocarditis—natural history and treatment. Multicenter Giant Cell Myocarditis Study Group Investigators. N Engl J Med 1997;336:1860-1866.

16. Daniels PR, Berry GJ, Tazelaar HD, Cooper LT. Giant cell myocarditis as a manifestation of drug hypersensitivity. Cardiovasc Pathol 2000;9:287-291.

17. Ishikawa H, Kaneko H, Watanabe H, Takagi A, Ming ZW. Giant cell myocarditis in association with drug-induced skin eruption. Acta Pathol Jpn 1987;37:639-644.

18. Truica CI, Hansen CH, Garvin DF, Meehan KR. Idiopathic giant cell myocarditis after autologous hematopoietic stem cell transplantation and interleukin-2 immunotherapy: a case report. Cancer 1998;83:1231-1236.

19. Frustaci A, Abdulla AK, Caldarulo M, Buffon A. Fatal measles myocarditis. Cardiologia 1990;35:347-349.

20. Klein BR, Hedges TR III, Dayal Y, Adelman LS. Orbital myositis and giant cell myocarditis. Neurology 1989;39:988-990.

21. de Jongste MJ, Oosterhuis HJ, Lie KI. Intractable ventricular tachycardia in a patient with giant cell myocarditis, thymoma and myasthenia gravis. Int J Cardiol 1986;13:374-378.

22. Burke JS, Medline NM, Katz A. Giant cell myocarditis and myositis. Associated with thymoma and myasthenia gravis. Arch Pathol 1969;88:359-366.

23. Kloin JE. Pernicious anemia and giant cell myocarditis. New association. Am J Med 1985;78:355-360.

24. McKeon J, Haagsma B, Bett JH, Boyle CM. Fatal giant cell myocarditis after colectomy for ulcerative colitis. Am Heart J 1986;111:1208-1209.

25. Weidhase A, Grone HJ, Unterberg C, Schuff-Werner P, Wiegand V. Severe granulomatous giant cell myocarditis in Wegener's granulomatosis. Klin Wochenschr 1990;68:880-885.

26. Ariza A, Lopez MD, Mate JL, Curos A, Villagrasa M, Navas-Palacios JJ. Giant cell myocarditis: monocytic immunophenotype of giant cells in a case associated with ulcerative colitis. Hum Pathol 1995;26:121-123.

27. Leib ML, Odel JG, Cooney MJ. Orbital polymyositis and giant cell myocarditis. Ophthalmology 1994;101:950-954.

28. Kilgallen CM, Jackson E, Bankoff M, Salomon RN, Surks HK. A case of giant cell myocarditis and malignant thymoma: a postmortem diagnosis by needle biopsy. Clin Cardiol 1998;21:48-51.

29. Benisch BM, Josephson M. Subacute (giant cell) thyroiditis and giant cell myocarditis in patient with carcinoma of lung. Chest 1973;64:764-765.

30. Burke JS, Medline NM, Katz A. Giant cell myocarditis and myositis: associated with thymoma and myasthenia gravis. Arch Pathol 1969;88:359-366.

31. Kennedy LJ Jr, Mitchinson MJ. Giant cell arteritis with myositis and myocarditis. Calif Med 1971;115:84-87.

32. Roberts WC, Wibin EA. Idiopathic panaortitis, supra-aortic arteritis, granulomatous myocarditis and pericarditis. A case of pulseless disease and possibly left ventricular aneurysm in the African. Am J Med 1966;41:453-461.

33. Roberts WC, Kehoe JA, Carpenter DF, Golden A. Cardiac valvular lesions in rheumatoid arthritis. Arch Intern Med 1968;122:141-146.

34. Theaker JM, Gatter KC, Brown DC, Heryet A, Davies MJ. An investigation into the nature of giant cells in cardiac and skeletal muscle. Hum Pathol 1988;19:974-979.

35. Glennon PE, Petersen ME, Sheppard MN. Fatal giant cell myocarditis after resection of thymoma. Heart 1996;75:531-532.

36. Hales SA, Theaker JM, Gatter KC. Giant cell myocarditis associated with lymphoma: an immuno-cytochemical study. J Clin Pathol 1987;40:1310-1313.

37. Helliwell TR, Edwards RH. Giant cell myocarditis associated with lymphoma (letter to the editor). J Clin Pathol 1988;41:598-599.

38. Kossovsky N, Cole P, Zackson DA. Giant cell myocarditis associated with silicone. An unusual case of biomaterials pathology discovered at autopsy using x-ray energy spectroscopic techniques. Am J Clin Pathol 1990;93:148-152.

39. Rabson AB, Schoen FJ, Warhol MJ, Mudge GH, Collins JJ Jr. Giant cell myocarditis after mitral valve replacement: case report and studies of the nature of giant cells. Hum Pathol 1984;15:585-587.

40. Gillie I, Fox H. Mitral stenosis together with a giant cell myocarditis limited to the left atrium. J Clin Pathol 1968;21:750-752.

41. Palmer HP, Michael IE. Giant-cell myocarditis with multiple organ involvement. Arch Intern Med 1965;116:444-447.

42. Dilling NV. Giant-cell myocarditis. J Pathol Bacteriol 1956;71:295-300.

43. Jones I, Nassau E, Smith P. Cryptococcosis of the heart. Br Heart J 1965;27:462-464.

44. Diefenbach WCL. Tuberculosis of the heart; review. Am Rev Tuberc 1950;62:390-402.

45. Saphir O. Nonrheumatic inflammatory diseases of the heart: C. Myocarditis. In: Gould SE, ed. Pathology of the heart. 2nd ed. Springfield, IL: Charles C Thomas, 1960:779-823.

46. Lie JT. Wegener's granulomatosis: histological documentation of common and uncommon manifestations in 216 patients. Vasa 1997;26:261-270.

47. McCrea PC, Childers RW. Two unusual cases of giant cell myocarditis associated with mitral stenosis and with Wegener's syndrome. Br Heart J 1964;26:490-498.

48. Schmid KO. Granulomatous giant cell polymyositis and myocarditis in benign thymoma. Verh Dtsch Ges Pathol 1965;49:248-253.

49. Namba T, Brunner NG, Grob D. Idiopathic giant cell polymyositis. Report of a case and review of the syndrome. Arch Neurol 1974;31:27-30.

50. Bourgeois-Droin C, Sauvanet A, Lemarchand F, De Roquancourt A, Cottenot F, Brocheriou C. Thymoma associated with myasthenia, erythroblastopenia, myositis and giant cell myocarditis. One case. Nouv Presse Med 1981;10:2097-2098; 2103-2104.

51. Tomimoto H, Akiguchi I, Kameyama M, Haibara H, Kitaichi M. Giant cell myositis and myocarditis associated with myasthenia gravis and thymoma—an autopsy case. Rinsho Shinkeigaku 1985;25:688-693.

52. Butany JW, McAuley P, Bergeron C, MacLaughlin P. Giant cell myocarditis and myositis associated with thymoma and leprosy. Can J Cardiol 1991;7:141-145.

53. Okada R, Wakafuji S. Myocarditis in autopsy. Heart Vessels Suppl 1985;1:23-29.

54. Kodama M, Matsumoto Y, Fujiwara M, Masani F, Izumi T, Shibata A. A novel experimental model of giant cell myocarditis induced in rats by immunization with cardiac myosin fraction. Clin Immunol Immunopathol 1990;57:250-262.

55. Okura Y, Yamamoto T, Goto S, Inomata T, Hirono S, Hanawa H, Feng L, Wilson CB, Kihara I, Izumi T, Shibata A, Aizawa Y, Seki S, Abo T. Characterization of cytokine and iNOS mRNA expression in situ during the course of experimental autoimmune myocarditis in rats. J Mol Cell Cardiol 1997;29:491-502.

56. Kodama M, Matsumoto Y, Fujiwara M. In vivo lymphocyte-mediated myocardial injuries demonstrated by adoptive transfer of experimental autoimmune myocarditis. Circulation 1992;85:1918-1926.

57. Hirono S, Islam MO, Nakazawa M, Yoshida Y, Kodama M, Shibata A, Izumi T, Imai S. Expression of inducible nitric oxide synthase in rat experimental autoimmune myocarditis with special reference to changes in cardiac hemodynamics. Circ Res 1997;80:11-20.

58. Badorff C, Fichtlscherer B, Rhoads RE, Zeiher AM, Muelsch A, Dimmeler S, Knowlton KU. Nitric oxide inhibits dystrophin proteolysis by coxsackieviral protease 2A through S-nitrosylation: a protective mechanism against enteroviral cardiomyopathy. Circulation 2000;102:2276-2281.

59. Sorimachi K, Akimoto K, Tsuru K, Ieiri T, Niwa A. The involvement of tumor necrosis factor in the multinucleation of macrophages. Cell Biol Int 1995;19:547-549.

60. Shioji K, Kishimoto C, Nakayama Y, Sasayama S. Strain difference in rats with experimental giant cell myocarditis. Jpn Circ J 2000;64:283-286.

61. Chow LH, Ye Y, Linder J, McManus BM. Phenotypic analysis of infiltrating cells in human myocarditis. An immunohistochemical study in paraffin-embedded tissue. Arch Pathol Lab Med 1989;113:1357-1362.

62. Cooper LT Jr, Berry GJ, Rizeq M, Schroeder JS. Giant cell myocarditis. J Heart Lung Transplant 1995;14:394-401.

63. Pyun KS, Kim YH, Katzenstein RE, Kikkawa Y. Giant cell myocarditis. Light and electron microscopic study. Arch Pathol 1970;90:181-188.

64. Tubbs RR, Sheibani K, Hawk WA. Giant cell myocarditis. Arch Pathol Lab Med 1980;104: 245-246.

65. Zhang S, Kodama M, Hanawa H, Izumi T, Shibata A, Masani F. Effects of cyclosporine, prednisolone and aspirin on rat autoimmune giant cell myocarditis. J Am Coll Cardiol 1993;21:1254-1260.

66. Hanawa H, Kodama M, Inomata T, Izumi T, Shibata A, Tuchida M, Matsumoto Y, Abo T. Anti-alpha beta T cell receptor antibody prevents the progression of experimental autoimmune myocarditis. Clin Exp Immunol 1994;96:470-475.

67. Kodama M, Hanawa H, Saeki M, Hosono H, Inomata T, Suzuki K, Shibata A. Rat dilated cardio-myopathy after autoimmune giant cell myocarditis. Circ Res 1994;75:278-284.

68. Goldberg GM. Myocarditis of giant-cell type in an infant. Am J Clin Pathol 1955;25:510-513.

69. Mason JW, O'Connell JB, Herskowitz A, Rose NR, McManus BM, Billingham ME, Moon TE. A clinical trial of immunosuppressive therapy for myocarditis. The Myocarditis Treatment Trial Investigators. N Engl J Med 1995;333:269-275.

70. Davidoff R, Palacios I, Southern J, Fallon JT, Newell J, Dec GW. Giant cell versus lymphocytic myocarditis. A comparison of their clinical features and long-term outcomes. Circulation 1991;83:953-961.

71. Okura Y, Dec GW, Hare JM, Berry GR, Tazelaar HD, Cooper LT. A Multicenter Registry comparison of cardiac sarcoidosis and idiopathic giant-cell myocarditis (abstract). Circulation 2000;102 Suppl 2:II-788.

72. Shields RC, Tazelaar HD, Berry GJ, Cooper LT. The role of right ventricular endomyocardial biopsy for idiopathic giant cell myocarditis. J Card Fail 2002;8:74-78.

73. Narula J, Khaw BA, Dec GW, Palacios IF, Newell JB, Southern JF, Fallon JT, Strauss HW, Haber E, Yasuda T. Diagnostic accuracy of antimyosin scintigraphy in suspected myocarditis. J Nucl Cardiol 1996;3:371-381.

74. Bloom S, Lie JT, Silver MD, eds. Diagnostic criteria for cardiovascular pathology: acquired diseases. Philadelphia: Lippincott-Raven Publishers, 1997:365.

75. Lauer B, Padberg K, Schultheiss HP, Strauer BE. Autoantibodies against human ventricular myosin in sera of patients with acute and chronic myocarditis. J Am Coll Cardiol 1994;23:146-153.

76. Martin AB, Webber S, Fricker FJ, Jaffe R, Demmler G, Kearney D, Zhang YH, Bodurtha J, Gelb B, Ni J, Bricker JT, Towbin JA. Acute myocarditis. Rapid diagnosis by PCR in children. Circulation 1994;90:330-339.

77. Shimada T, Shimada K, Sakane T, Ochiai K, Tsukihashi H, Fukui M, Inoue S, Katoh H, Murakami Y, Ishibashi Y, Maruyama R. Diagnosis of cardiac sarcoidosis and evaluation of the effects of steroid therapy by gadolinium-DTPA-enhanced magnetic resonance imaging. Am J Med 2001;110:520-527.

78. Hirose Y, Ishida Y, Hayashida K, Maeno M, Takamiya M, Ohmori F, Miyatake K, Uehara T, Nishimura T, Tachibana T. Myocardial involvement in patients with sarcoidosis. An analysis of 75 patients. Clin Nucl Med 1994;19:522-526.

79. Starling RC, Galbraith TA, Baker PB, Howanitz EP, Murray KD, Binkley PF, Watson KM, Unverferth DV, Myerowitz PD. Successful management of acute myocarditis with biventricular assist devices and cardiac transplantation. Am J Cardiol 1988;62:341-343.

80. Reiss N, El-Banayosy A, Posival H, Morshuis M, Minami K, Korfer R. Management of acute fulminant myocarditis using circulatory support systems. Artif Organs 1996;20:964-970.

81. Brilakis ES, Olson LJ, Daly RC, Cooper LT. Survival outcomes of patients with giant cell myocarditis bridged by ventricular assist devices (abstract). J Heart Lung Transplant 1999;18:43.

82. Costanzo-Nordin MR, Silver MA, O'Connell JB, Scanlon PJ, Robinson JA. Giant cell myocarditis: dramatic haemodynamic and histologic improvement with immunosuppressive therapy. Eur Heart J 1987;8 Suppl J:271-274.

83. Levy NT, Olson LJ, Weyand C, Brack A, Tazelaar HD, Edwards WD, Hammill SC. Histologic and cytokine response to immunosuppression in giant-cell myocarditis. Ann Intern Med 1998;128:648-650.

84. Desjardins V, Pelletier G, Leung TK, Waters D. Successful treatment of severe heart failure caused by idiopathic giant cell myocarditis. Can J Cardiol 1992;8:788-792.

85. Cooper LT Jr, Shabetai R. Immunosuppressive therapy for myocarditis (letter to the editor). N Engl J Med 1995;333:1713-1714.

86. Scott RL, Ratliff NB, Starling RC, Young JB. Recurrence of giant cell myocarditis in cardiac allograft. J Heart Lung Transplant 2001;20:375-380.

87. Nieminen MS, Salminen US, Taskinen E, Heikkila P, Partanen J. Treatment of serious heart failure by transplantation in giant cell myocarditis diagnosed by endomyocardial biopsy. J Heart Lung Transplant 1994;13:543-545.

88. Briganti E, Esmore DS, Federman J, Bergin P. Successful heart transplantation in a patient with histopathologically proven giant cell myocarditis (letter to the editor). J Heart Lung Transplant 1993;12:880-881.

89. Laruelle C, Vanhaecke J, Van de Werf F, Flameng W, Verbeken E, Meyns B, Vermeersch P, De Geest H. Cardiac transplantation in giant cell myocarditis. A case report. Acta Cardiol 1994;49:279-286.

90. Kong G, Madden B, Spyrou N, Pomerance A, Mitchell A, Yacoub M. Response of recurrent giant cell myocarditis in a transplanted heart to intensive immunosuppression. Eur Heart J 1991;12:554-557.

91. Gries W, Farkas D, Winters GL, Costanzo-Nordin MR. Giant cell myocarditis: first report of disease recurrence in the transplanted heart. J Heart Lung Transplant 1992;11:370-374.

92. Grant SC. Giant cell myocarditis in a transplanted heart (letter to the editor). Eur Heart J 1993;14:1437.

93. Grant SC. Recurrent giant cell myocarditis after transplantation (letter to the editor). J Heart Lung Transplant 1993;12:155-156.

94. Cooper LT, Olson LJ, Berry GJ, Tazelaar H. Post-transplantation survival of patients with idiopathic giant cell myocarditis (GCM) versus cardiomyopathy (CM) (abstract). J Am Coll Cardiol 1998;31 Suppl A:251A.

CHAPTER 18

Cardiac Sarcoidosis

Leslie T. Cooper, Jr., M.D.

INTRODUCTION

Sarcoidosis is an unusual cause of heart disease that occurs as isolated organ involvement and as part of systemic disease. The first case of cardiac sarcoidosis (CS) was reported in 1929 by Bernstein et al.[1] Publications in the subsequent 40 years consisted of isolated case reports and few notable case series.[2] These reports from the mid 20th century reveal the clinical features and syndromes associated with CS. Although the collection of published cases has defined the range of clinical presentations, they also reveal that the incidence and clinical features of the disease vary with the population studied and the diagnostic criteria used.[3-5] Some aspects of the genetics and immunology have been established, but the cause of sarcoidosis remains unknown.

The diagnosis of CS may be ascertained in multiple ways. Magnetic resonance imaging, gallium scintigraphy, endomyocardial biopsy, and serologic markers have been used in various select populations. Each technique has limitations. The incidence and prevalence of the disease vary within and between referral and community-based populations. For example, the range of reported rates of cardiac involvement for patients with systemic sarcoidosis extends from a low of 5% in North Americans with clinical symptoms to 78% in a Japanese autopsy series. Antemortem diagnosis is difficult owing to the low sensitivity of endomyocardial biopsy and lack of specificity of other noninvasive tests.

The present knowledge of CS is limited in many ways. Neither a sensitive and specific test to establish the diagnosis nor a means to predict disease progression exists. A key unanswered question is whether corticosteroids or other immunomodulatory agents can favorably alter the natural history of early CS. This chapter reviews the current state of our understanding of this unusual disease and suggests future directions for research into mechanisms, diagnosis, and treatment.

EPIDEMIOLOGY

The incidence of sarcoidosis in the United States has been estimated at 5.9 per 100,000 person-years for men and 6.3 per 100,000 person-years for women.[6] In the United States, the lifetime risk of sarcoidosis is estimated at 0.85% in whites and 2.4% in blacks.[7] Thus, the lifetime risk of CS with clinical symptoms developing is low.

Certain ethnic groups appear to have a high prevalence of sarcoidosis, and the presentation may vary with ethnicity. For example, Sweden, Denmark, Japan, and US blacks have particularly high prevalence rates, whereas Portugal, Saudi Arabia, Spain, and India have relatively low rates.[8,9] In a case series from Saudi Arabia, 16 of 21 cases of systemic sarcoidosis occurred in women, but there was no cardiac involvement.[10] In a large series from Baltimore, the rate of extrathoracic sarcoid was higher in African-American than in white patients (2.15 vs. 1.20 manifestations per patient, respectively).[11] From comparative autopsy data, the rate of cardiac involvement in sarcoid patients is higher in Japanese than in US patients.[12]

The frequency of cardiac involvement differs by sex too. Iwai and colleagues[12] compared autopsy records from Japan with those of 2 US medical centers. They found the rate of cardiac involvement was significantly higher in Japanese women older than age 50 years than in Japanese men. In black American women there was also a high incidence of cardiac involvement after age 40 years. In a series of 43 cases from Johns Hopkins Hospital consisting of 33 black Americans and 10 whites, there was also a female predominance (18 males, 25 females).[13] In contrast, the male-to-female ratio of cardiac involvement in whites autopsied with a diagnosis of sarcoidosis was 1:1.[12] Similarly, in a clinical study of 270 cases (249 whites) of CS from the United Kingdom, there were equal numbers of men and women.[14]

CS usually presents in relatively young adults, but rare cases have been reported in children[15] and in the elderly. In Fleming's[14] series from England, patient age ranged from 18 to 88 years, with a peak between ages 25 and 55 years. The majority of patients at Johns Hopkins Hospital presented between ages 30 and 49 years.[13] In Sekiguchi's[16] series, the majority of female patients presented between ages 40 and 59 years, whereas most males presented between ages 20 and 39 years.

In systemic sarcoidosis, the lungs are the most commonly affected organ, but important extrapulmonary manifestations involve the skin (including erythema nodosum), lymph nodes, eye (uveitis), central and peripheral nervous system, and heart.[17] Autopsy data from the 1970s suggested that clinical myocardial involvement occurs infrequently, in about 5% of patients with sarcoidosis.[3] However, the rate of electrocardiographic abnormalities in Japanese patients with systemic sarcoidosis was higher than in control cases at 22.1%, suggesting that a substantial proportion had asymptomatic cardiac involvement.[4] Furthermore, the observed rate of cardiac involvement is also much higher in autopsy series, confirming that many cases of cardiac involvement are clinically silent.[18]

The clinical picture of the disease probably depends on ethnicity, sex, duration of the illness, and the extent of organ involvement. Frequently, extracardiac involvement is subclinical in patients who present with cardiac symptoms.[19] In the author's experience, only about one-third of patients with clinical myocardial involvement have clinical evidence of extracardiac disease.

ETIOLOGY

Because the etiology of sarcoidosis is unknown, the diagnosis remains one of exclusion. As such, there is no one test to confirm the diagnosis. Indeed, sarcoidosis' clinical heterogeneity probably reflects multiple disease etiologies. CS may represent a final common clinical and histopathologic presentation for several pathologic sequences. Acknowledging the limitations of our understanding, it is worthwhile summarizing the major studies in epidemiology and immunogenetics in systemic sarcoidosis. Few data exist for isolated cardiac disease, and these are noted when available.

Boeck used the term "sarkoid" in 1899 to describe cutaneous lesions because he thought the lesions resembled sarcoma (reviewed in reference 17). Associations with malignant neoplasms have been described since, suggesting that sarcoidosis might be a form of or a marker for malignancy. Epithelioid granulomas were observed in the regional lymph nodes of a small percentage of patients with carcinomas or in association with non-Hodgkin lymphoma;[20,21] however, a large well-controlled study of 555 sarcoidosis cases in Denmark failed to demonstrate an excess rate of malignancy in sarcoid patients.[22] Currently, the trend of investigation is away from malignancy associations and toward identification of environmental triggers in genetically susceptible individuals.

Infectious and environmental agents have been considered in the search for a cause. Early investigators thought that sarcoidosis could be a variant of tuberculosis.[23] Other putative infectious agents include *Borrelia burgdorferi*, *Propionibacterium acnes*, *Mycoplasma*, and several viruses (Table 18-1). Environmental agents that could induce a granulomatous response include aluminum, zirconium, and talc. An epidemiologic report suggested that

Table 18-1
Examples of Agents Suggested to Be Involved in the Etiology of Sarcoidosis*

Type of agent
    Infectious agents
        Viruses (herpes, Epstein-Barr, retrovirus, coxsackie B
            virus, cytomegalovirus)
        Borrelia burgdorferi
        Propionibacterium acnes
        Mycobacterium tuberculosis and other mycobacteria
        Mycoplasma
    Inorganic agents
        Aluminum
        Zirconium
        Talc
    Organic agents
        Pine tree pollen
        Clay

*This table does not include beryllium, which causes berylliosis and not sarcoidosis.
From Hunninghake et al.[17] By permission of PCA Publishing.

exposure to wood stoves and fireplaces, both rurally linked risk factors, was associated with the development of sarcoidosis.[24] The argument for a transmissible agent is supported by the development of sarcoidosis in a transplant recipient who received tissue from a donor with sarcoidosis.[25]

The argument for an environmental cause or person-to-person transmission is further strengthened by the observation that sarcoidosis cases cluster temporally. Clustering has been observed in the Isle of Man,[26,27] and among firefighters[28] and health care workers.[29] Furthermore, some cases occur in families,[30-32] and there is evidence to suggest a seasonal clustering in the winter and early spring.[33] Taken together these data suggest that an environmental or infectious trigger(s) may play a role in some cases of sarcoidosis.

Arguments for a genetic predisposition come from familial clustering, race as a risk factor, and studies of the major histocompatibility complex genes. The most common genotype frequencies in sarcoidosis are class I human leukocyte antigen (HLA)-A1 and B8 and class II HLA-DR.[34-36] The polymorphism for tumor necrosis factor (TNF)-beta (TNFB*1) is associated with good prognosis in pulmonary sarcoidosis.[37] Genetic studies demonstrated an association of certain alleles for angiotensin-converting enzyme (ACE) genotype, interferon (IFN) regulatory factor 4, and interleukin (IL)-1 alpha in certain groups with systemic sarcoidosis.[38,39] The data for cardiac involvement are limited to a report by Takashige et al.[40] that demonstrated a TNF-alpha (A2) gene polymorphism was more common in Japanese patients with CS than in normal controls (RR 11.51, $P = 0.001$). These associations of allelic polymorphisms with phenotype and prognosis may explain some individual differences in susceptibility to disease.

The cellular pathophysiology of sarcoidosis is an area of active research. Studies of pulmonary sarcoidosis suggest that CD4$^+$ T lymphocytes accumulate at sites of inflammation. These cells release cytokines, including IFN-gamma and IL-2,[41] suggesting a T$_H$1-type T-cell response. Alveolar macrophages are also active, secreting cytokines and growth factors. A T$_H$1-type response seems to favor the formation of granulomas in the lung.[42] The pathway that leads to granuloma resolution and fibrosis is not well understood. Knowledge of these cellular mechanisms of disease may guide rational, targeted therapeutic trials; however, at the present time, neither the antigenic stimulus nor the mechanism of persistent inflammation and fibrosis is known.

To better define the causes of sarcoidosis, the National Heart, Lung, and Blood Institute sponsored a case-control study of sarcoidosis (ACCESS).[43] This multicenter, observational study includes a comprehensive investigation of genetic, environmental, infectious, and primary immune factors in sarcoidosis. The study has the power to permit testing of multiple hypotheses; 720 cases will be compared with an equal number of matched controls. Enrollment in this study is ongoing.

DIAGNOSIS

Sarcoidosis may be seen first in the heart and has various common clinical presentations. Because it is a rare cause of common clinical syndromes, the diagnosis is frequently overlooked. The 4 clinical syndromes associated with CS are congestive heart failure from systolic or diastolic left ventricular dysfunction, syncope or presyncope from tachyarrhythmias or bradyarrhythmias, pericarditis with or without constrictive physiology, and secondary right ventricular failure from pulmonary disease. Asymptomatic electrocardiographic changes such as right bundle branch block or ventricular ectopy are probably the most common manifestation, but these are nonspecific and usually should not initiate a search for CS.

In patients who initially present with cardiac symptoms and no history of sarcoidosis, a careful family history may reveal affected members. The physical examination may reveal manifestations of extracardiac sarcoidosis including uveitis, erythema nodosum, or lymphadenopathy. Chest radiograph may reveal bilateral hilar adenopathy (stage I) or more advanced stages of pulmonary sarcoidosis. The electrocardiogram is frequently abnormal, with degrees of heart block or tachyarrhythmias (Table 18-2).

The observed complications in a series of 300 cases of cardiac sarcoid are summarized in Table 18-3. Ventricular arrhythmia occurred in 45%, supraventricular arrhythmia in 28%, complete heart block in 26%, and sudden death in 16%. The overall rate of death was 46% (138 of 300). In the series of 43 cases from Johns Hopkins Hospital, cardiomyopathy was seen in 49%, syncope in 33%, tachyarrhythmia in 28%, and pericardial disease in 7% of cases.[13] Mortality was similar in a series of 36 cases from Japan, in which 47% (17 patients) died. The cause of death was congestive heart failure in 11 (65%), sudden death in 3 (18%), fatal arrhythmia in 2 (12%), and cerebral embolism in 1 (6%). A limitation of these data is that time-dependent analysis of the risk of morbidity and death is not available.

Confirmation of CS is extremely challenging because the sensitivity of endomyocardial biopsy is about 25%. The diagnosis is established by noncaseating granulomas on a tissue sample (see Figure 14-5 *B*; see color plate 25, p. 340). In a study by Uemura and colleagues,[44] only 5 of 26 patients (19%) with clinical sarcoidosis and suspected cardiac involvement had diagnostic endomyocardial biopsies. The frequency of a positive biopsy result was higher in those with dilated cardiomyopathy (DCM) than in those with conduction disturbances and normal left ventricular ejection fraction. In select populations, the diagnostic rate may be somewhat higher.[45] The low sensitivity of endomyocardial biopsy is likely because the focal nature of the infiltrates results in sampling error.[3]

Once a granulomatous infiltrate is confirmed in a patient with suspected CS, other causes of granulomatous lesions must be excluded by appropriate serologic studies and special stains. The major causes of myocardial granuloma are listed in Table 18-4. Fungal

Table 18-2
Electrocardiographic Findings and Their Frequency in Cardiac Sarcoidosis

Finding	A (*n* = 30)	B (*n* = 15)	C (*n* = 59)	Total (*n* = 104)
SA block	1 (3)	1 (7)	1 (2)	3 (3)
AV block				
I	4 (13)	2 (13)	10 (17)	16 (15)
II	1 (3)	0 (0)	6 (10)	7 (7)
III	17 (57)	6 (40)	27 (46)	50 (48)
RBBB	8 (27)	9 (60)	30 (51)	47 (45)
IRBBB	2 (7)	2 (13)	1 (2)	5 (5)
LBBB	1 (3)	9 (0)	3 (5)	4 (4)
LAD	5 (17)	7 (47)	13 (22)	25 (24)
Abnormal Q	4 (13)	2 (13)	4 (7)	10 (10)
PSVT	0 (0)	0 (0)	1 (2)	1 (1)
PVC	5 (17)	6 (40)	16 (27)	27 (26)
VT	12 (40)	4 (27)	10 (17)	26 (25)
ST–T change	1 (3)	4 (27)	7 (12)	12 (12)
LVH	0 (0)	2 (13)	1 (2)	3 (3)
Low voltage	2 (7)	0 (0)	0 (0)	2 (2)

AV, atrioventricular; IRBBB, incomplete right bundle branch block; LAD, left axis deviation; LBBB, left bundle branch block; LVH, left ventricular hypertrophy; PSVT, paroxysmal supraventricular tachycardia; PVC, premature ventricular contraction; RBBB, right bundle branch block; SA, sinoatrial; VT, ventricular tachycardia.

*$P < 0.05$.

Documented case reports and the author's own cases were analyzed in 3 groups: A, autopsy-proven fatal myocardial sarcoidosis; B, biopsy-proven cases with myocardial sarcoidosis; C, clinically diagnosed sarcoidosis cases with apparent cardiac involvement, although the presence of sarcoid granulomas was not confirmed. Percentages in parentheses.

(From Yazaki Y et al. Report for the Intractable Disease Division, Public Health Bureau, Ministry of Health and Welfare of Japan, 1993.)

From Sekiguchi et al.[56] By permission of Kluwer Academic Press.

myocarditis usually occurs in the immunocompromised host in association with endocarditis. Mycobacteria may be identified on acid-fast stain; tuberculosis is suggested by a positive tuberculin test result. Antineutrophil cytoplasmic autoantibodies usually are found in Wegener granulomatosis. Idiopathic giant cell myocarditis usually has prominent myocyte necrosis and eosinophils in a widespread inflammatory infiltrate, but granulomas are not prominent.

Noninvasive tests and serologic markers may support the diagnosis of CS, but the ideal screening and confirmatory tests do not exist. Serum ACE concentrations were first recognized as a biochemical marker of sarcoidosis in 1975.[46] Epithelial cells in the sarcoid

Table 18-3
Complications in 300 Patients With Cardiac Sarcoid

Complication	Patients, %
Ventricular arrhythmia	45
Supraventricular arrhythmia	28
Complete heart block	26
Heart failure	24
Right bundle branch block	23
Partial heart block	23
Mitral systolic murmur	22
Sudden death	16
Left bundle branch block	15
Simulating myocardial infarction	5
Pericarditis	3
Transplantation of heart	1

From Fleming HA. Cardiac sarcoidosis. Lung Biology in Health and Disease 1994;73:323-334. By permission of Marcel Dekker.

Table 18-4
Differential Diagnosis of Cardiac Sarcoidosis

Wegener granulomatosis
Foreign body reaction
Rheumatic carditis (Aschoff nodules)
Atypical drug reaction
Infectious agents
    Mycobacteria, fungal myocarditis, and visceral larval migrans (*T gondi*)
Idiopathic giant cell myocarditis

granulomas produce ACE, the value of which is then increased in serum. The clinical utility of serum ACE as a diagnostic tool in CS is limited because ACE can be increased in other granulomatous disorders and diabetes. Furthermore, although ACE values may decrease with steroid treatment, this decrease does not always correlate with clinical improvement in pulmonary sarcoidosis.[47] Hypercalcemia can also support the diagnosis.

Magnetic resonance imaging has been used to diagnose cardiac abnormalities in patients with systemic sarcoidosis. In 16 patients with biopsy-proven sarcoidosis, gadolinium-enhanced, cardiac magnetic resonance imaging showed enhanced signal intensity in the left ventricle of 8 patients (50%).[48] These abnormalities improved in all 8 patients after 1 month of prednisone therapy. Cardiac abnormalities on magnetic resonance imaging are also common in nonspecific myocarditis,[49] which would limit the specificity of this technique in a more general population. It is not known whether improvement on magnetic resonance imaging correlates with improved clinical outcome.

Positron emission tomography was used to document myocardial disease in patients with suspected CS.[50] The rate of positive results was 100% compared with 80% by ^{99m}Tc-sestamibi single photon emission computed tomography and 50% by ^{67}Ga scintigraphy. Only 10 of the 16 patients in this study had cardiac involvement suspected on clinical or histologic grounds. The usefulness of this technique needs to be confirmed in larger studies with defined standard criteria for cardiac involvement.

The presentation of biopsy-proven CS is somewhat different than the presentation of lymphocytic myocarditis (LM) and DCM. The clinical and electrocardiographic presentation of 29 patients with sarcoidosis and granulomas on endomyocardial biopsy were compared to LM and DCM diagnosed by biopsy. Subjects with CS had higher rates of ventricular tachycardia, heart block, and syncope (Tables 18-5 and 18-6). Although this study was limited because of possible selection bias, the findings are consistent with results of most published series. Of note, only 33% of the subjects in this series reported extracardiac involvement.

Because of the difficulty in confirming myocardial sarcoidosis, we recommend the following approach to diagnostic evaluation. Patients from high prevalence groups who develop DCM complicated by ventricular tachycardia or heart block are at risk for CS. If enlarged lymph nodes or cutaneous lesions are present, biopsy should be done, because the risk of skin or lymph node biopsy is usually lower than the risk of endomyocardial biopsy. The presence of CS may be presumed if granulomas are present and other causes such as tuberculosis and histoplasmosis are excluded. Gadolinium-enhanced magnetic resonance imaging may be considered in this setting. If more easily accessible lesions are not available, endomyocardial biopsy should be performed and a minimum of 5 samples obtained.

Table 18-5
Patient Characteristics

Characteristic	CS (n = 29)	DCM (n = 58)	LM (n = 27)
Age at onset, y*	47.7 ± 11.9	48.2 ± 12.5	46.8 ± 17.8
Male, %	55.2	72.4	59.3
White, %	24.1	94.8	100
Black, %	41.4	3.4	0
EF, %*	28.8 ± 14.4	26.2 ± 12.1	35.2 ± 18.1

CS, cardiac sarcoidosis; DCM, dilated cardiomyopathy; EF, ejection fraction; LM, lymphocytic myocarditis.
*Mean ± SD.
Modified from Cooper et al.[60] By permission of Monduzzi Editore Spa.

Table 18-6
Symptoms at Hospital Presentation

Symptom	Patients, %		
	CS	DCM	LM
Left-sided heart failure	41.4	84.5	63.0
Right-sided heart failure	6.9	0	0
Both-sided heart failure	13.8	1.7	3.7
Palpitation	24.1	5.2	11.1
Syncope	31.0	0	11.1

CS, cardiac sarcoidosis; DCM, dilated cardiomyopathy; LM, lymphocytic myocarditis.
Modified from Cooper et al.[60] By permission of Monduzzi Editore Spa.

TREATMENT

Supportive treatment of cardiac disease due to CS is similar to treatment of similar syndromes resulting from other causes. For DCM with class II to III congestive heart failure, ACE inhibitors and nonselective β-adrenergic receptor blockers are the mainstay of therapy. Diuretics should be used as needed to maintain optimal preload. We do not routinely use digoxin because of the risk of heart block and proarrhythmia, although limited data exist for or against its use in this population.

Symptomatic heart block is common and is usually treated with a permanent pacemaker, although isolated case reports suggest that prednisone therapy may occasionally improve conduction disturbance. If a patient with compensated DCM develops heart block, β-adrenergic receptor blocker therapy risks progression to complete heart block. In that setting, the decision to withdraw the β-adrenergic receptor blocker or to place a pacemaker and maximize β blockade depends on the individual circumstances.

Ventricular arrhythmias may be difficult to manage with antiarrhythmic therapy, and many patients with symptomatic, sustained ventricular tachycardia receive an automatic implantable cardiac defibrillator.[51,52] Early case reports suggested efficacy of quinidine,[15] but currently amiodarone or therapy guided by electrophysiologic study is common for cardiomyopathy.

Case reports and small case series suggest heart transplantation is effective for refractory arrhythmias or end-stage cardiomyopathy due to CS.[53] A limitation to transplantation is functional impairment of other organs from sarcoidosis. Sarcoidosis can occur after transplantation in the lung,[54] but this is not considered a contraindication to cardiac transplantation.

An area of debate is the role of corticosteroids in the management of CS. There are no prospective data to answer many key questions, including the timing, intensity, and duration of treatment; how different populations respond to treatment; and the risks of recurrence after tapering or discontinuing steroid therapy. Small, retrospective case series suggest that corticosteroids may prolong survival in sarcoidosis patients who received a pacemaker.[55] However, treatment efficacy early in the disease is difficult to assess because there is sometimes a substantial rate of spontaneous remissions. Furthermore, late in the disease, extensive fibrosis develops that will not reverse with corticosteroids.

Expert opinion forms the basis of treatment recommendations. Sekiguchi et al.[56] recommended 30 mg/day or 60 mg every other day for initial treatment of CS. The dose may be tapered to 5 to 10 mg/day and continued for life. Prednisone usually was started at a somewhat higher dose of 60 mg/day by the group at Johns Hopkins, with a taper of 5 mg every 2 weeks. A maintenance dose of 10 to 15 mg was usually continued "for months or years."[13] We generally treat according to the Hopkins recommendations, if there are no contraindications.

People who are intolerant of steroids may be considered for methotrexate. Chloroquine and tetracycline benefit patients with cutaneous sarcoidosis,[57] but their role in cardiac disease is unknown. Methotrexate has considerable hepatic toxicity and teratogenic effects. This is relevant because many of the CS patients are women of childbearing age.

PROGNOSIS

Few direct comparisons are available of survival in CS and in other disorders. One series[58] from Japan suggested that survival in CS is worse than in DCM; however, patients in that series had frequent extracardiac lesions (53%) and few granulomas on biopsy. These patients may have presented at a late stage when fibrosis had replaced active granuloma. In contrast, a study by Felker et al.[59] suggested that there was no significant difference in survival between CS and DCM. This study was particularly compelling because all patients were diagnosed by endomyocardial biopsy.

In our experience,[60] survival in biopsy-proven CS was similar to survival in DCM and LM (Fig. 18-1). The probability of death estimated from date of biopsy was 72.5% for CS at 1,207 days and 72.5% for LM at 1,199 days and 73.4% at 1,067 days. The P values by log-rank test for survival comparisons were 0.667, CS versus LM; 0.428, CS versus DCM; and 0.503, CS versus combined LM and DCM.

Our study was limited because the population of CS patients was gathered from a multicenter registry, whereas the DCM and LM populations were from a single referral center. Comparison of groups gathered from different referral sources raises the possibility of referral and selection bias. Prognosis may also depend on ethnicity, but no comparative data exist and our series was too small to answer this question. Nonetheless, a strength of our study was that all CS patients had diagnostic granulomas, indicating that the disease was active and suggesting we intervened at an early stage.

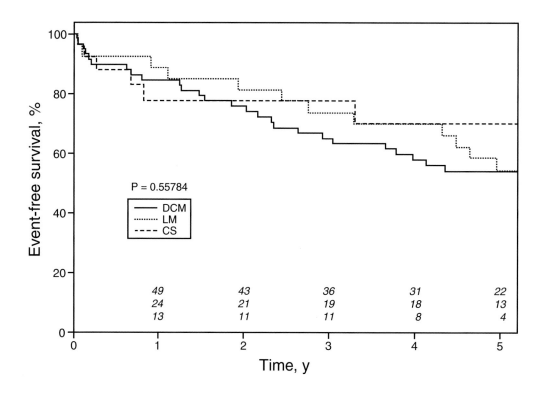

Fig. 18-1. Survival in cardiac sarcoidosis (*CS*), dilated cardiomyopathy (*DCM*), and lymphocytic myocarditis (*LM*) groups by Kaplan-Meier method. *P* value calculated by log-rank test. (From Cooper et al.[60] By permission of Monduzzi Editore Spa.)

FUTURE DIRECTIONS

Progress in our understanding of CS is limited primarily by the rarity of the disease. No single center can accumulate sufficient experience to perform prospective clinical trials. Therefore, expert opinion based on personal experience and the scant published literature forms the basis for present therapeutic guidelines. Fortunately, the multicenter ACCESS study sponsored by the National Institutes of Health should provide essential mechanistic insights and accelerate progress in cardiac and systemic disease.

The triggers of disease activity ought to be better defined. Prevention of disease may someday include avoidance of exposure to key environmental stimuli or vaccine-based prevention in genetically predisposed individuals. Progress in these areas will begin once the influence of ethnicity, sex, and genetic factors on the natural history is better defined by longitudinal surveillance of the ACCESS cohort.

The benefit of immunosuppression in addition to comprehensive supportive care needs to be confirmed in a multicenter, prospective clinical trial. Clearly, for such a trial to be feasible, the method of diagnosis for cardiac disease must be established unequivocally. There are promising but yet unproved noninvasive tests, including magnetic resonance imaging and positron emission tomography, that may emerge as part of composite clinical and test-based diagnostic criteria. To estimate statistical power for a trial, time-dependent analyses of "hard" event rates (death, need for pacemaker or automatic implantable cardiac defibrillator) need to be defined in men and women of several ethnic groups. With the results of the ACCESS project, the feasibility of prospective clinical studies will be known.

REFERENCES

1. Bernstein M, Konzelmann FW, Sidlick DM. Boeck's sarcoid: report of a case with visceral involvement. Ann Intern Med 1929;44:721-734.
2. Longcope WT, Freiman DG. A study of sarcoidosis based on combined investigation of 160 cases including 30 autopsies from Johns Hopkins Hospital and Massachusetts General Hospital. Medicine (Baltimore) 1952;31:1-132.
3. Roberts W, McAllister H, Ferrans V. Sarcoidosis of the heart. A clinicopathologic study of 35 necropsy patients (group I) and review of 78 previously described necropsy patients (group II). Am J Med 1977;63:86-108.
4. Numao Y, Sekiguchi M, Fruie T, Matsui Y, Izumi T, Mikami R. A study of cardiac involvement in 963 cases of sarcoidosis by EKG and endomyocardial biopsy. In: Williams WJ, Davies BH, eds. Sarcoidosis and other granulomatous diseases: eighth international conference on sarcoidosis and other granulomatous diseases. Cardiff, Wales: Alpha Omega Publishers, 1980:607-614.
5. Matsui Y, Iwai K, Tachibana T, Fruie T, Shigematsu N, Izumi T, Homma AH, Mikami R, Hongo O, Hiraga Y, Yamamoto M. Clinicopathological study of fatal myocardial sarcoidosis. Ann NY Acad Sci 1976;278:455-469.
6. Henke CE, Henke G, Elveback LR, Beard CM, Ballard DJ, Kurland LT. The epidemiology of sarcoidosis in Rochester, Minnesota: a population-based study of incidence and survival. Am J Epidemiol 1986;123:840-845.
7. Rybicki BA, Major M, Popovich J Jr, Maliarik MJ, Iannuzzi MC. Racial differences in sarcoidosis incidence: a 5-year study in a health maintenance organization. Am J Epidemiol 1997;145:234-241.
8. Mana J, Badrinas F, Morera J, Fite E, Manresa F, Fernandez-Nogues F. Sarcoidosis in Spain. Sarcoidosis 1992;9:118-122.
9. James DG. Sarcoidosis and other granulomatous disorders. Lung Biology in Health and Disease 1994, vol 73.
10. Samman Y, Ibrahim M, Wali S. Sarcoidosis in the Western Region of Saudi Arabia. Sarcoidosis Vas Diffuse Lung Dis 1999;16:215-218.
11. Johns CJ, Schonfeld SA, Scott PP, Zachary JB, MacGregor MI. Longitudinal study of chronic sarcoidosis with low-dose maintenance corticosteroid therapy. Outcome and complications. Ann NY Acad Sci 1986;465:702-712.
12. Iwai K, Sekiguchi M, Hosoda Y, DeRemee RA, Tazelaar HD, Sharma OP, Maheshwari A, Noguchi TI. Racial difference in cardiac sarcoidosis incidence observed at autopsy. Sarcoidosis 1994;11:26-31.

13. Johns CJ, Paz H, Kasper EK, Baughman K. Myocardial sarcoidosis: course and management. Sarcoidosis 1992;9 Suppl 1:231-236.

14. Fleming HA. Cardiac sarcoidosis. Clin Dermatol 1986;4:143-149.

15. Serwer GA, Edwards SB, Benson DW Jr, Anderson PA, Spach M. Ventricular tachyarrhythmia due to cardiac sarcoidosis in a child. Pediatrics 1978;62:322-325.

16. Sekiguchi M, Kaneko M, Hiroe M, Hirosawa K. Recent trends in cardiac sarcoidosis research in Japan. Heart Vessels Suppl 1985;1:45-49.

17. Hunninghake GW, Costabel U, Ando M, Baughman R, Cordier JF, du Bois R, Eklund A, Kitaichi M, Lynch J, Rizzato G, Rose C, Selroos O, Semenzato G, Sharma OP. ATS/ERS/WASOG statement on sarcoidosis. American Thoracic Society/European Respiratory Society/World Association of Sarcoidosis and Other Granulomatous Disorders. Sarcoidosis Vasc Diffuse Lung Dis 1999;16:149-173.

18. Silverman KJ, Hutchins GM, Bulkley BH. Cardiac sarcoid: a clinicopathologic study of 84 unselected patients with systemic sarcoidosis. Circulation 1978;58:1204-1211.

19. Fleming HA. Myocardial sarcoidosis. Lancet 1973;1:106.

20. Brincker H. Sarcoid reactions in malignant tumours. Cancer Treat Rev 1986;13:147-156.

21. Rømer FK. Sarcoidosis and cancer. Lung Biology in Health and Disease 1994;73:401-415.

22. Rømer FK, Hommelgaard P, Schou G. Sarcoidosis and cancer revisited: a long-term follow-up study of 555 Danish sarcoidosis patients. Eur Respir J 1998;12:906-912.

23. Hosoda Y, Okada M. History of sarcoidosis. Semin Respir Med 1992;13:359-367.

24. Kajdasz DK, Lackland DT, Mohr LC, Judson MA. A current assessment of rurally linked exposures as potential risk factors for sarcoidosis. Ann Epidemiol 2001;11:111-117.

25. Heyll A, Meckenstock G, Aul C, Sohngen D, Borchard F, Hadding U, Modder U, Leschke M, Schneider W. Possible transmission of sarcoidosis via allogeneic bone marrow transplantation. Bone Marrow Transplant 1994;14:161-164.

26. Parkes SA, Baker SB, Bourdillon RE, Murray CR, Rakshit M. Epidemiology of sarcoidosis in the Isle of Man—1: a case controlled study. Thorax 1987;42:420-426.

27. Hills SE, Parkes SA, Baker SB. Epidemiology of sarcoidosis in the Isle of Man—2: evidence for space-time clustering. Thorax 1987;42:427-430.

28. Kern DG, Neill MA, Wrenn DS, Varone JC. Investigation of a unique time-space cluster of sarcoidosis in firefighters. Am Rev Respir Dis 1993;148:974-980.

29. Edmondstone WM. Sarcoidosis in nurses: is there an association? Thorax 1988;43:342-343.

30. Buck AA, McKusick VA. Epidemiologic investigations of sarcoidosis: III. Serum proteins, syphilis, association with tuberculosis: familial aggregation. Am J Hyg 1961;74:174-188.

31. Sharma OP, Neville E, Walker AN, James DG. Familial sarcoidosis: a possible genetic influence. Ann NY Acad Sci 1976;278:386-400.

32. Harrington DW, Major M, Rybicki B, Popovich J, Maliarik M, Iannuzzi MC. Familial sarcoidosis: analysis of 91 families. Sarcoidosis 1994;11 Suppl 1:240-243.

33. Bardinas F, Morera J, Fite E, Plasencia A. Seasonal clustering of sarcoidosis. Lancet 1989;2:455-456.

34. Pasturenzi L, Martinetti M, Cuccia M, Cipriani A, Semenzato G, Luisetti M. HLA class I, II, and III polymorphism in Italian patients with sarcoidosis. The Pavia-Padova Sarcoidosis Study Group. Chest 1993;104:1170-1175.

35. Gardner J, Kennedy HG, Hamblin A, Jones E. HLA associations in sarcoidosis: a study of two ethnic groups. Thorax 1984;39:19-22.

36. Lenhart K, Kolek V, Bartova A. HLA antigens associated with sarcoidosis. Dis Markers 1990;8:23-29.

37. Yamaguchi E, Itoh A, Hizawa N, Kawakami Y. The gene polymorphism of tumor necrosis factor-beta, but not that of tumor necrosis factor-alpha, is associated with the prognosis of sarcoidosis. Chest 2001;119:753-761.

38. Maliarik MJ, Rybicki BA, Malvitz E, Sheffer RG, Major M, Popovich J Jr, Iannuzzi MC. Angiotensin-converting enzyme gene polymorphism and risk of sarcoidosis. Am J Respir Crit Care Med 1998;158:1566-1570.

39. Rybicki BA, Maliarik MJ, Malvitz E, Sheffer RG, Major M, Popovitch J Jr, Iannuzzi MC. Influence of T cell receptor and cytokine genes on sarcoidosis susceptibility in African Americans. Hum Immunol 1999;60:867-874.

40. Takashige N, Naruse TK, Matsumori A, Hara M, Nagai S, Morimoto S, Hiramitsu S, Sasayama S, Inoko H. Genetic polymorphisms at the tumour necrosis factor loci (TNFA and TNFB) in cardiac sarcoidosis. Tissue Antigens 1999;54:191-193.

41. Moller DR. Cells and cytokines involved in the pathogenesis of sarcoidosis. Sarcoidosis Vasc Diffuse Lung Dis 1999;16:24-31.

42. Agostini C, Adami F, Semenzato G. New pathogenetic insights into the sarcoid granuloma. Curr Opin Rheumatol 2000;12:71-76.

43. ACCESS Research Group. Design of a case control etiologic study of sarcoidosis (ACCESS). J Clin Epidemiol 1999;52:1173-1186.

44. Uemura A, Morimoto S, Hiramitsu S, Kato Y, Ito T, Hishida H. Histologic diagnostic rate of cardiac sarcoidosis: evaluation of endomyocardial biopsies. Am Heart J 1999;138:299-302.

45. Ratner SJ, Fenoglio JJ Jr, Ursell PC. Utility of endomyocardial biopsy in the diagnosis of cardiac sarcoidosis. Chest 1986;90:528-533.

46. Lieberman J. Elevation of serum angiotensin-converting-enzyme (ACE) level in sarcoidosis. Am J Med 1975;59:365-372.

47. Turner-Warwick M, McAllister W, Lawrence R, Britten A, Haslam PL. Corticosteroid treatment in pulmonary sarcoidosis: do serial lavage lymphocyte counts, serum angiotensin converting enzyme measurements, and gallium-67 scans help management? Thorax 1986;41:903-913.

48. Shimada T, Shimada K, Sakane T, Ochiai K, Tsukihashi H, Fukui M, Inoue S, Katoh H, Murakami Y, Ishibashi Y, Maruyama R. Diagnosis of cardiac sarcoidosis and evaluation of the effects of steroid therapy by gadolinium-DTPA-enhanced magnetic resonance imaging. Am J Med 2001;110:520-527.

49. Gagliardi MG, Polletta B, Di Renzi P. MRI for the diagnosis and follow-up of myocarditis. Circulation 1999;99:458-459.

50. Okumura W, Iwasaki T, Ueda T, Seki R, Miyajima A, Hatori T, Sato H, Toyama T, Suzuki T, Matsubara K, Otake H, Aoyagi K, Inoue T, Endo K, Nagai R. Usefulness of ^{18}F-FDG PET for diagnosis of cardiac sarcoidosis. [Japanese.] Kaku Igaku 1999;36:341-348.

51. Bajaj AK, Kopelman HA, Echt DS. Cardiac sarcoidosis with sudden death: treatment with the automatic implantable cardioverter defibrillator. Am Heart J 1988;116:557-560.

52. Winters SL, Cohen M, Greenberg S, Stein B, Curwin J, Pe E, Gomes JA. Sustained ventricular tachycardia associated with sarcoidosis: assessment of the underlying cardiac anatomy and the prospective utility of programmed ventricular stimulation, drug therapy and an implantable antitachycardia device. J Am Coll Cardiol 1991;18:937-943.

53. Valantine HA, Tazelaar HD, Macoviak J, Mullin AV, Hunt SA, Fowler MB, Billingham ME, Schroeder JS. Cardiac sarcoidosis: response to steroids and transplantation. J Heart Transplant 1987;6:244-250.

54. Martinez FJ, Orens JB, Deeb M, Brunsting LA, Flint A, Lynch JP III. Recurrence of sarcoidosis following bilateral allogeneic lung transplantation. Chest 1994;106:1597-1599.

55. Takada K, Ina Y, Yamamoto M, Satoh T, Morishita M. Prognosis after pacemaker implantation in cardiac sarcoidosis in Japan. Clinical evaluation of corticosteroid therapy. Sarcoidosis 1994;11:113-117.

56. Sekiguchi M, Yazaki Y, Isobe M, Hiroe M. Cardiac sarcoidosis: diagnostic, prognostic, and therapeutic considerations. Cardiovasc Drugs Ther 1996;10:495-510.

57. Bachelez H, Senet P, Cadranel J, Kaoukhov A, Dubertret L. The use of tetracyclines for the treatment of sarcoidosis. Arch Dermatol 2001;137:69-73.

58. Yazaki Y, Isobe M, Hiramitsu S, Morimoto S, Hiroe M, Omichi C, Nakano T, Saeki M, Izumi T, Sekiguchi M. Comparison of clinical features and prognosis of cardiac sarcoidosis and idiopathic dilated cardiomyopathy. Am J Cardiol 1998;82:537-540.

59. Felker GM, Thompson RE, Hare JM, Hruban RH, Clemetson DE, Howard DL, Baughman KL, Kasper EK. Underlying causes and long-term survival in patients with initially unexplained cardiomyopathy. N Engl J Med 2000;342:1077-1084.

60. Cooper LT, Okura Y, Hare JM, Grogan M. Survival in biopsy-proven cardiac sarcoidosis is similar to survival in lymphocytic myocarditis and dilated cardiomyopathy. In: Kimchi A, ed. Heart disease: new trends in research, diagnosis and treatment. Englewood, NJ: Medimond Medical Publications, 2001:491-496.

The Eosinophil
in Cardiac Disease

Lambert A. Wu, M.D., Leslie T. Cooper, Jr., M.D.,
Gail M. Kephart, B.S., and Gerald J. Gleich, M.D.

Eosinophils were first described by Wharton-Jones[1] as coarse granule cells in 1846. It was not until Ehrlich's[2] 1879-1880 paper that these cells became known as "eosinophils." The association between eosinophils and clinical diseases has been known for many years, but only recently, through more detailed analyses, has their role in the pathogenesis of disease been elucidated.

The first section of this chapter discusses the development and pathophysiology of the eosinophil, and the remainder focuses primarily on eosinophil-associated myocardial diseases.

EOSINOPHILIC DEVELOPMENT AND CELLULAR COMPOSITION

In the bone marrow, eosinophils develop from CD34[+] precursor cells containing cell-surface interleukin (IL)-5 receptors. The actual stimulus for the expression of these receptors is unknown. IL-5 stimulates these precursors to produce several granule proteins. Chief among these is major basic protein (MBP).[3] The direct precursor of MBP produced in translation of MBP mRNA transcripts is proMBP.[4,5] As the eosinophil matures and differentiates, proMBP aggregates into large, uncondensed granules where it undergoes post-translation processing into MBP.[6] MBP then condenses into dense granules that appear to form the core of the mature eosinophil. In addition to stimulating the synthesis of MBP, IL-5 stimulates the eosinophil precursor cell to synthesize other granule proteins.[3,7]

Migration from the bone marrow through the sinusoidal endothelium requires IL-5.[8] During this migration process, eosinophils increase their expression of β_2 integrin, thereby increasing IL-5–mediated eosinophil release. Another protein, eotaxin, is required for the mobilization of eosinophils from bone marrow and appears to have synergistic effects when combined with IL-5.[9] Eotaxin may also induce the migration of eosinophil progenitor cells to peripheral tissues.[10]

Once in the circulation, eosinophils can migrate selectively into diseased tissues. To do so, they must first go through a complex process that includes contacting, tethering, and rolling along the endothelial cells of the vessel wall. In vitro studies have shown that during this process, tethering and adhesion require interaction between P-selectin and vascular cell adhesion molecule (VCAM)-1 on the endothelial cell and very late activation antigen-4 on the eosinophil.[11-13] IL-4 stimulates expression of P-selectin and VCAM-1 on endothelial cells.[14] Blocking of P-selectin, VCAM-1, and very late activation antigen-4 with antibodies abolished tethering of eosinophils to endothelial cells; antibodies to α_4 and β_2 integrins on eosinophils blocked firm binding of eosinophils. However, in vivo experiments with mice showed that IL-4 increases VCAM-1 expression but does not alter P-selectin expression. Additionally, mice treated with IL-4 and deficient in P-selectin still show leukocyte recruitment and this is blocked by antibodies to α_4 integrin.[15] Thus, in

IL-4–mediated tethering and adhesion, VCAM-1 and very late activation antigen-4 appear to play more important roles than P-selectin.

Once firmly bound, the eosinophil changes morphology to migrate between endothelial cells and extrude into the extravascular space. At the cellular level, C5a anaphylatoxin activates eosinophil adhesion and assists in the transmigration of eosinophils, whereas C3a is specific for eosinophil chemotaxis.[16,17] In addition, specific eosinophil eotaxins— eotaxins 1, 2, and 3—are important eosinophil chemoattractants.[18-27] After migration between endothelial cells, the eosinophil must cross the basement membrane. This requires that the eosinophil express matrix metalloproteinases (MMP), particularly MMP-9.[28-30] The tissue inhibitor of MMP prevents this migration.[30] Once in the extravascular space, the eosinophil is guided to its destination by chemoattractants, chiefly eotaxin. Eotaxin was initially discovered in a guinea pig model of asthma.[31] Murine and human eotaxins have been found.[18,32] The expression of eotaxin mRNA in endothelial cells is stimulated by tumor necrosis factor-α and IL-1.[20]

Once at its intended site, the eosinophil is activated by cytokines and immunoglobulin receptors[33,34] and this activation depends critically on β_2 integrins, especially MAC-1 (αMβ2).[35] For example, β_2 integrins, cytokines, and immunoglobulins mediate an increase of the eosinophil life span and eosinophil degranulation.[33,36-38] Additionally, these stimulants promote eosinophil superoxide anion production. Platelet-activating factor may also serve as an endogenous eosinophil stimulant.[39] In studies utilizing platelet-activating factor antagonists, IgG- and IL-5-induced eosinophil superoxide production and degranulation were inhibited.[39]

Once at the site of inflammation, eosinophils can promote proinflammatory and cytotoxic effects. The granules stored within the eosinophil contain the MBP dense core surrounded by the eosinophil matrix, which is composed of the other granule proteins— namely, eosinophil peroxidase, eosinophil cationic protein, and eosinophil-derived neurotoxin.[40] These granule proteins have various effects, including ribonuclease activity,[41,42] formation of toxic pores in target cells,[43] and degranulation of other cells, including basophils and mast cells. Eosinophils are also capable of chemoattractant production, such as platelet-activating factor and eotaxin, and cytokine production.[35,44] Eosinophilic proteins such as eosinophil peroxidase are also capable of producing cytotoxic substances, including hydrogen peroxide and hypohalous acids.[40]

EOSINOPHIL-ASSOCIATED MYOCARDIAL DISEASES

Various terms are used to categorize eosinophilic endomyocardial diseases, resulting in a large number of descriptors—for example, hypereosinophilic myocarditis, Löffler endocarditis, endomyocardial fibrosis, tropical obliterative endomyocardial fibrosis, and eosinophilic endomyocardial disease.

In this section, the eosinophilic myocarditides are grouped according to general categories, such as those associated with systemic disease (hypereosinophilic syndrome, Churg-Strauss syndrome, and malignancies); those associated with drugs (hypersensitivity eosinophilic myocarditis); those associated with parasitic infections; and the specific entity of acute necrotizing eosinophilic myocarditis.

EOSINOPHILIC MYOCARDITIS: ASSOCIATION WITH SYSTEMIC DISEASES
Eosinophilic Myocarditis in the Hypereosinophilic Syndrome (HES)
HES is a general term encompassing a disease state characterized by a marked increase in peripheral eosinophils, infiltration of multiple organ systems with mature eosinophils, and resultant multiorgan dysfunction.[45,46] Organ systems involved may include the skin, liver, intestinal tract, nervous system, and lung. However, it is involvement of the heart that is most critical for morbidity and mortality.[46]

Case reports describing eosinophilic myocarditis in the setting of HES have been published. The first description was from Löffler[47] in 1936, in which he presented 2 patients with eosinophilia and heart failure due to fibrous thickening of the endocardium. In 1948, Davies[48] reported a case series consisting of 36 Ugandan patients with heart failure and endocardial thickening. This latter entity became known as Davies tropical endomyocardial fibrosis and is not consistently associated with eosinophilia.

Different clinical and pathologic manifestations of HES myocarditis include endocardial fibrosis, valvular regurgitation due to endocardial fibrosis of the valvular apparatuses, right- and left-sided congestive heart failure, and systemic thromboembolization due to thrombus formation on the endocardial surface.[45]

Myocarditis Associated With Churg-Strauss Syndrome
In 1951, Churg and Strauss first described allergic angiitis and granulomatosis, now commonly referred to as the Churg-Strauss syndrome.[49] This syndrome is characterized by necrotizing vasculitis, extravascular granulomata, and tissue infiltration with eosinophils. The annual incidence has been estimated at 2.4 cases per 1,000,000 people,[50] and case reports and case series have been published.[51-55] Criteria were published by the American College of Rheumatology to increase the sensitivity and specificity of distinguishing Churg-Strauss from other vasculitides.[56] The 6 criteria include peripheral eosinophilia of 10% or more in the leukocyte differential, biopsy-proven extravascular eosinophils, asthma, paranasal sinus abnormality, mononeuropathy or polyneuropathy, and nonfixed pulmonary infiltrates.

As in other diseases with eosinophilic infiltration of multiple organs, cardiac involvement can be the major cause of morbidity and mortality. Numerous clinical signs and symptoms of cardiac involvement may be seen.[53,57-63] These include presentation with heart failure, pulmonary embolism, myocardial infarction, and signs and symptoms associated with constrictive pericarditis.[53,58]

Eosinophilic Myocarditis Associated With Cancer

Reports in the literature demonstrated the association of tissue and blood eosinophilia with cancer of the lung,[64-70] the gastrointestinal tract,[71-74] the genitourinary tract,[75-91] and the skin.[85,92] Eosinophilic myocarditis in this setting has been described.[68,93,94]

Endomyocardial Fibrosis: Eosinophilic Versus Tropical

Endomyocardial fibrosis is a pathologic diagnosis, describing the replacement of endocardium with thick collagen tissue overlying a looser framework of connective tissue in the involved endomyocardium.[95] Although pathologically descriptive, the term "endomyocardial fibrosis" belies the dynamic pathophysiology, especially that of the eosinophil, which contributes to this "end result" and to the debate in distinguishing the 2 entities frequently associated with this pathologic finding: Löffler endomyocardial fibrosis and Davies endomyocardial fibrosis (tropical endomyocardial fibrosis).

As alluded to above, Löffler[47] initially described endomyocardial fibrosis in the setting of myocardial eosinophil infiltration within the context of the hypereosinophilic syndrome. The patients in whom this type of endomyocardial fibrosis develops (Löffler endomyocardial fibrosis) are generally male; from geographic regions with temperate climates; and clinically demonstrate fever, rash, weight loss, congestive heart failure, restrictive physiology, and systemic embolization.[46,96,97] Eosinophilia and myocardial infiltration with eosinophils are the rule. However, by the time of necropsy or endomyocardial biopsy, the eosinophilic infiltrations may have already stopped, leaving only the remaining endomyocardial fibrosis.

The pathophysiology of endomyocardial disease in HES is associated strikingly with cardiac deposition of eosinophil granule protein initially onto the endocardium and later on the mural thrombi and on myocardial cells.[98] Analyses of cardiac tissue from 18 autopsies and biopsies of patients with HES-associated endomyocardial disease revealed dramatic MBP and eosinophil cationic protein deposition, especially during the acute phase of the disease. Surprisingly, MBP deposition in subendocardial fibrous tissue may persist and provide a signal indicative of eosinophil involvement. Because MBP causes platelet activation,[99] inhibits the capacity of endothelial cell surface thrombomodulin to generate the natural anticoagulant (activated protein C),[99] and activates cardiac mast cells,[100] its deposition may stimulate clot formation directly, with subsequent embolization and encroachment on the ventricular cavity.

Tropical endomyocardial fibrosis (Davies endomyocardial fibrosis) is distributed geographically along the tropical and subtropical regions of Africa, India, and South America.[101,102] The sex distribution is approximately equal, and children and young adults are affected most.[103,104] Eosinophilia and eosinophilic infiltration of myocardium are not distinct features of this disease.[97,101,105]

HYPERSENSITIVITY MYOCARDITIS

With the increasing use of medications, iatrogenic causes of hypersensitivity myocarditis from drugs need to be understood and considered. The incidence of hypersensitivity myocarditis is unknown. One series[106] reported 16 cases of hypersensitivity myocarditis in 3,373 consecutive autopsy cases.

The first series of patients describing the association of myocarditis with drug therapy was published in 1942 by French and Weller.[107] They reported on 126 patients who developed eosinophilic infiltration and interstitial myocarditis after sulfonamide administration. Subsequently, numerous published case reports have had similar findings in patients treated with various medications.[106,108-120] These are listed in Table 19-1. The mechanism of hypersensitivity myocarditis is thought to be a delayed hypersensitivity reaction.[106,121] Hypersensitivity myocarditis associated with eosinophilia is generally independent of drug dosage, and drugs can also have a direct, dose-related toxic effect on myocardium, causing a myocarditis unassociated with eosinophils.[122]

Clinically, patients may present with symptoms characteristic of a drug hypersensitivity reaction, including nonspecific skin rash, malaise, fever, and eosinophilia.[120] More specific signs and symptoms referable to the heart include conduction abnormalities and tachyarrhythmias, sudden death, and increased concentrations of cardiac enzymatic markers such as creatine kinase and the creatine kinase-MB isozyme.[106,120,122, 123] Acute fulminant myocarditis with hemodynamic instability has also been described.[106,116] The onset of hypersensitivity myocarditis after initiation of the offending medication is highly variable, with onsets hours to months after a medication is started.[106,116]

Further evaluation with noninvasive testing, including echocardiography, may show a dilated cardiomyopathy with regional or global wall motion abnormalities. Endomyocardial biopsy may be performed for histologic evidence.[124-126] However, if endomyocardial biopsy is used, the procedural risks versus benefits must be understood.

Treatment mainly consists of withdrawal of the suspected offending medication, which should not only be therapeutic but also diagnostic.[106,122] Perhaps most importantly, a high level of clinical awareness is required to diagnose this entity.

ACUTE NECROTIZING EOSINOPHILIC MYOCARDITIS

A few patients have been reported who presented with an aggressive form of hypereosinophilic-associated myocarditis: acute necrotizing eosinophilic myocarditis. All 3 patients with acute necrotizing eosinophilic myocarditis without extracardiac abnormality had viral prodromes, allergic diatheses, and rapidly deteriorating courses ending in death.[127] These

Table 19-1
Drugs Associated With Hypersensitivity Myocarditis

Antibiotics	Anti-inflammatory
Amphotericin B	Indomethacin
Ampicillin	Oxyphenbutazone
Chloramphenicol	Phenylbutazone
Penicillin	
Tetracycline	Diuretics
Streptomycin	Acetazolamide
	Chlorthalidone
Sulfonamides	Hydrochlorothiazide
Sulfadiazine	Spironolactone
Sulfisoxazole	
	Others
Anticonvulsants	Amitriptyline
Phenytoin	Methyldopa
Carbamazepine	Sulfonylureas
	Tetanus toxoid
Antituberculous	Clozapine
Isoniazid	
Para-aminosalicylic acid	

From Kounis NG, Zavras GM, Soufras GD, Kitrou MP. Hypersensitivity myocarditis. Ann Allergy 1989;62:71-74. By permission of the American College of Allergy, Asthma, and Immunology.

cases differed from prior reports of eosinophilia-associated heart disease in which a more chronic myocarditis occurred in the setting of systemic disease and extracardiac involvement. As its name implies, this form of eosinophilic heart disease is characterized by an acute onset and rapid progression of hemodynamic compromise and systolic ventricular failure. Mortality is high, with patients typically dying within days to weeks.

On histopathologic study, extensive inflammatory infiltration with eosinophils is seen in the setting of extensive myocyte necrosis (Fig. 19-1; see color plate 37). Analyses of 2 children who died of this disease showed massive eosinophil infiltration and degranulation with deposition of MBP onto necrotic myocardial cells.[128] Electron microscopic study showed extensive areas of myocardial necrosis in the presence of degenerating eosinophils, the latter characterized by loss of the cytoplasmic membrane with release of eosinophil granules to the extracellular milieu. Immunosuppressive therapy, especially intravenous glucocorticoids in massive doses, may be beneficial in these patients,[130] although they usually present acutely ill and often die.

EOSINOPHILIC MYOCARDITIS ASSOCIATED WITH PARASITIC INFECTIONS

Parasites that cause myocarditis associated with eosinophilic infiltration are listed in Table 19-2. Eosinophilia may occur in patients infected with helminthic parasites as an immune

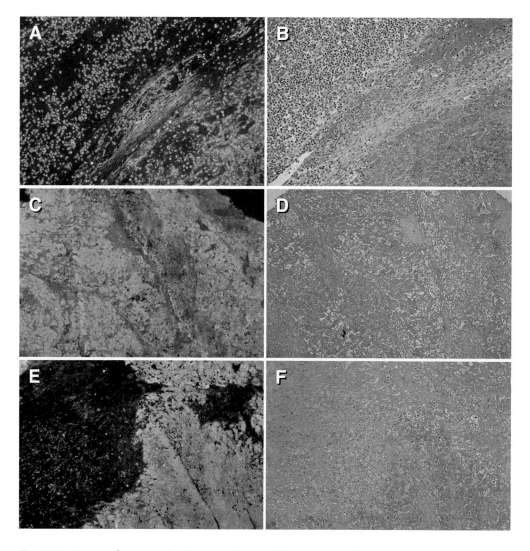

Fig. 19-1. Immunofluorescent localization of eosinophil granule major basic protein in heart tissue. See color plate 37.

response during which cytotoxic granule proteins may kill these organisms and damage cardiac tissues as bystanders.[131-133] Additionally, protozoal disease may be associated with eosinophilic myocarditis. Chief among these is Chagas myocarditis caused by the protozoan *Trypanosoma cruzi*. The prevalence of trypanosomiasis is highest in Central and South America; an estimated 20 million people are infected with this parasite.[134-136] The disease is transmitted to humans through the reduviid insect acting as the vector.[137-139] Once the reduviid bug bites the human host, trypanosomes present in the reduviid bug feces gain entry by breaks in the skin or mucosa, particularly the conjunctiva.

Table 19-2
Parasitic Infections Associated With Eosinophilic Myocarditis

Protozoal
  Trypanosoma cruzi (Chagas disease)
  Toxoplasma gondii (toxoplasmosis)

Metazoal
  Trichinella spiralis (trichinosis)
  Toxocara canis (visceral larva migrans)
  Echinococcus granulosus (hydatid cyst)
  Schistosomiasis

Clinically, infected patients undergo acute, latent, and chronic phases. During the acute phase, patients present with myalgia, fever, diaphoresis, hepatosplenomegaly, and myocarditis with congestive heart failure.[136,138] These symptoms may last for months and generally resolve. During the latent phase, symptoms usually are not present, although there can be a subclinical progression of cardiomyopathy. As cardiomyopathy progresses, patients may develop overt heart failure, thromboembolic phenomena from apical aneurysms, conduction abnormalities such as right bundle branch block and left anterior fascicular block, arrhythmias (atrial and ventricular), and sudden cardiac death.[140-144]

Gross cardiac pathologic features may include dilated and hypertrophied cardiac chambers and left ventricular or apical aneurysm formation with thrombus.[134,135,144] On histologic examination, extensive fibrosis is seen in the setting of a chronic mononuclear cellular infiltrate.[136,139] The mononuclear cell infiltrate is composed chiefly of lymphocytes, macrophages, and plasma cells.[145-149]

Eosinophils have been associated with these lesions, and activated eosinophils with their extruded granule constituents have been reported in the disrupted myofibrillar lesions.[145-152] Finding actual parasites in these lesions is unusual and has brought into question whether the cardiac disruption is due to autoimmune phenomena.[153-155]

TREATMENT

Treatment for the eosinophilic myocarditides depends on the underlying cause. In patients with eosinophilic myocarditis in the setting of systemic disease (such as hypereosinophilic syndrome and Churg-Strauss syndrome), high-dose corticosteroid therapy is beneficial. Mural thrombus may be an additional feature that requires anticoagulation therapy. In patients with endomyocardial fibrosis, surgical treatment may be required, involving myocardial stripping, valve replacement, and thrombectomy.[156-159] For patients with hypersensitivity myocarditis, the offending medication must be withdrawn and treatment with high-dose corticosteroids is recommended. For patients with eosinophilic myocarditis associated with parasitic infections, treatment with antiparasitic medications may be of benefit. Use of immunosuppressive therapies specifically for eosinophilic myocarditis is still experimental.

SUMMARY

In this chapter, we have discussed the elegant mechanisms by which the eosinophil develops from its conception in the bone marrow, through its maturation, and finally to its attachment, extrusion, and homing into areas of inflammation in the myocardium. We have also discussed the role of the eosinophil in myocardial diseases, including eosinophilic myocarditis associated with systemic diseases such as HES, Churg-Strauss, and cancer; hypersensitivity myocarditis; acute necrotizing eosinophilic myocarditis; and eosinophilic myocarditis associated with parasitic infections. Although treatment currently consists of corticosteroids or therapies specifically directed toward underlying primary diseases (or both), the future may hold possibilities for alternative immunosuppressive regimens for the eosinophilic myocarditides.

REFERENCES

1. Wharton-Jones T. The blood-corpuscle considered in its different phases of development in the animal series. Memoir I. Vertebrata. Philos Trans R Soc Lond 1846;136:63-87.
2. Ehrlich P. Methodologische Beiträge zur Physiologie und Pathologie der verschiedenen Formen der Leukocyten. Z Klin Med Berl 1879-1880;1:553-560.
3. Plager DA, Loegering DA, Weiler DA, Checkel JL, Wagner JM, Clarke NJ, Naylor S, Page SM, Thomas LL, Akerblom I, Cocks B, Stuart S, Gleich GJ. A novel and highly divergent homolog of human eosinophil granule major basic protein. J Biol Chem 1999;274:14464-14473.
4. Barker RL, Gleich GJ, Pease LR. Acidic precursor revealed in human eosinophil granule major basic protein cDNA. J Exp Med 1988;168:1493-1498.
5. Popken-Harris P, McGrogan M, Loegering DA, Checkel JL, Kubo H, Thomas LL, Moy JN, Sottrup-Jensen L, Snable JL, Kikuchi MT, Gleich GJ. Expression, purification, and characterization of the recombinant proform of eosinophil granule major basic protein. J Immunol 1995;155:1472-1480.
6. Popken-Harris P, Checkel J, Loegering D, Madden B, Springett M, Kephart G, Gleich GJ. Regulation and processing of a precursor form of eosinophil granule major basic protein (ProMBP) in differentiating eosinophils. Blood 1998;92:623-631.
7. Gleich GJ. Mechanisms of eosinophil-associated inflammation. J Allergy Clin Immunol 2000;105:651-663.
8. Palframan RT, Collins PD, Severs NJ, Rothery S, Williams TJ, Rankin SM. Mechanisms of acute

eosinophil mobilization from the bone marrow stimulated by interleukin 5: the role of specific adhesion molecules and phosphatidylinositol 3-kinase. J Exp Med 1998;188:1621-1632.

9. Palframan RT, Collins PD, Williams TJ, Rankin SM. Eotaxin induces a rapid release of eosinophils and their progenitors from the bone marrow. Blood 1998;91:2240-2248.

10. Kim YK, Uno M, Hamilos DL, Beck L, Bochner B, Schleimer R, Denburg JA. Immunolocalization of CD34 in nasal polyposis. Effect of topical corticosteroids. Am J Respir Cell Mol Biol 1999;20:388-397.

11. Robinson SD, Frenette PS, Rayburn H, Cummiskey M, Ullman-Cullere M, Wagner DD, Hynes RO. Multiple, targeted deficiencies in selectins reveal a predominant role for P-selectin in leukocyte recruitment. Proc Natl Acad Sci U S A 1999;96:11452-11457.

12. Dobrina A, Menegazzi R, Carlos TM, Nardon E, Cramer R, Zacchi T, Harlan JM, Patriarca P. Mechanisms of eosinophil adherence to cultured vascular endothelial cells. Eosinophils bind to the cytokine-induced ligand vascular cell adhesion molecule-1 via the very late activation antigen-4 integrin receptor. J Clin Invest 1991;88:20-26.

13. Bochner BS, Luscinskas FW, Gimbrone MA Jr, Newman W, Sterbinsky SA, Derse-Anthony CP, Klunk D, Schleimer RP. Adhesion of human basophils, eosinophils, and neutrophils to interleukin 1-activated human vascular endothelial cells: contributions of endothelial cell adhesion molecules. J Exp Med 1991;173:1553-1557.

14. Patel KD. Eosinophil tethering to interleukin-4-activated endothelial cells requires both P-selectin and vascular cell adhesion molecule-1. Blood 1998;92:3904-3911.

15. Hickey MJ, Granger DN, Kubes P. Molecular mechanisms underlying IL-4-induced leukocyte recruitment in vivo: a critical role for the alpha 4 integrin. J Immunol 1999;163:3441-3448.

16. DiScipio RG, Daffern PJ, Jagels MA, Broide DH, Sriramarao P. A comparison of C3a and C5a-mediated stable adhesion of rolling eosinophils in postcapillary venules and transendothelial migration in vitro and in vivo. J Immunol 1999;162:1127-1136.

17. Daffern PJ, Pfeifer PH, Ember JA, Hugli TE. C3a is a chemotaxin for human eosinophils but not for neutrophils. I. C3a stimulation of neutrophils is secondary to eosinophil activation. J Exp Med 1995;181:2119-2127.

18. Garcia-Zepeda EA, Rothenberg ME, Ownbey RT, Celestin J, Leder P, Luster AD. Human eotaxin is a specific chemoattractant for eosinophil cells and provides a new mechanism to explain tissue eosinophilia. Nat Med 1996;2:449-456.

19. Kato M, Kephart GM, Talley NJ, Wagner JM, Sarr MG, Bonno M, McGovern TW, Gleich GJ. Eosinophil infiltration and degranulation in normal human tissue. Anat Rec 1998;252:418-425.

20. Lilly CM, Nakamura H, Kesselman H, Nagler-Anderson C, Asano K, Garcia-Zepeda EA, Rothenberg ME, Drazen JM, Luster AD. Expression of eotaxin by human lung epithelial cells: induction by cytokines and inhibition by glucocorticoids. J Clin Invest 1997;99:1767-1773.

21. Lamkhioued B, Renzi PM, Abi-Younes S, Garcia-Zepada EA, Allakhverdi Z, Ghaffar O, Rothenberg MD, Luster AD, Hamid Q. Increased expression of eotaxin in bronchoalveolar lavage and airways of asthmatics contributes to the chemotaxis of eosinophils to the site of inflammation. J Immunol 1997;159:4593-4601.

22. Ghaffar O, Hamid Q, Renzi PM, Allakhverdi Z, Molet S, Hogg JC, Shore SA, Luster AD, Lamkhioued B. Constitutive and cytokine-stimulated expression of eotaxin by human airway smooth muscle cells. Am J Respir Crit Care Med 1999;159:1933-1942.

23. Teran LM, Mochizuki M, Bartels J, Valencia EL, Nakajima T, Hirai K, Schroder JM. Th1- and Th2-type cytokines regulate the expression and production of eotaxin and RANTES by human lung fibroblasts. Am J Respir Cell Mol Biol 1999;20:777-786.

24. Mochizuki M, Bartels J, Mallet AI, Christophers E, Schroder JM. IL-4 induces eotaxin: a possible mechanism of selective eosinophil recruitment in helminth infection and atopy. J Immunol 1998;160:60-68.

25. Li L, Xia Y, Nguyen A, Lai YH, Feng L, Mosmann TR, Lo D. Effects of Th2 cytokines on chemokine expression in the lung: IL-13 potently induces eotaxin expression by airway epithelial cells. J Immunol 1999;162:2477-2487.

26. White JR, Imburgia C, Dul E, Appelbaum E, O'Donnell K, O'Shannessy DJ, Brawner M, Fornwald J, Adamou J, Elshourbagy NA, Kaiser K, Foley JJ, Schmidt DB, Johanson K, Macphee C, Moores K, McNulty D, Scott GF, Schleimer RP, Sarau HM. Cloning and functional characterization of a novel human CC chemokine that binds to the CCR3 receptor and activates human eosinophils. J Leukoc Biol 1997;62:667-675.

27. Shinkai A, Yoshisue H, Koike M, Shoji E, Nakagawa S, Saito A, Takeda T, Imabeppu S, Kato Y, Hanai N, Anazawa H, Kuga T, Nishi T. A novel human CC chemokine, eotaxin-3, which is expressed in IL-4-stimulated vascular endothelial cells, exhibits potent activity toward eosinophils. J Immunol 1999;163:1602-1610.

28. Ohno I, Ohtani H, Nitta Y, Suzuki J, Hoshi H, Honma M, Isoyama S, Tanno Y, Tamura G, Yamauchi K, Nagura H, Shirato K. Eosinophils as a source of matrix metalloproteinase-9 in asthmatic airway inflammation. Am J Respir Cell Mol Biol 1997;16:212-219.

29. Okada S, Kita H, George TJ, Gleich GJ, Leiferman KM. Migration of eosinophils through basement membrane components in vitro: role of matrix metalloproteinase-9. Am J Respir Cell Mol Biol 1997;17:519-528.

30. Kumagai K, Ohno I, Okada S, Ohkawara Y, Suzuki K, Shinya T, Nagase H, Iwata K, Shirato K. Inhibition of matrix metalloproteinases prevents allergen-induced airway inflammation in a murine model of asthma. J Immunol 1999;162:4212-4219.

31. Jose PJ, Griffiths-Johnson DA, Collins PD, Walsh DT, Moqbel R, Totty NF, Truong O, Hsuan JJ, Williams TJ. Eotaxin: a potent eosinophil chemoattractant cytokine detected in a guinea pig model of allergic airways inflammation. J Exp Med 1994;179:881-887.

32. Rothenberg ME, Luster AD, Leder P. Murine eotaxin: an eosinophil chemoattractant inducible in endothelial cells and in interleukin 4-induced tumor suppression. Proc Natl Acad Sci U S A 1995;92:8960-8964.

33. Motegi Y, Kita H. Interaction with secretory component stimulates effector functions of human eosinophils but not of neutrophils. J Immunol 1998;161:4340-4346.

34. Kita H, Adolphson CR, Gleich GJ. Biology of eosinophils. In: Middleton E Jr, Reed CE, Ellis EF, Adkinson NF Jr, Yunginger JW, Busse WW, eds. Allergy: principles & practice. 5th ed. Vol 1. St. Louis: Mosby, 1998:242-260.

35. Kita H. The eosinophil: a cytokine-producing cell? J Allergy Clin Immunol 1996;97:889-892.

36. Kim JT, Schimming AW, Kita H. Ligation of Fc gamma RII (CD32) pivotally regulates survival of human eosinophils. J Immunol 1999;162:4253-4259.

37. Kaneko M, Horie S, Kato M, Gleich GJ, Kita H. A crucial role for beta 2 integrin in the activation of eosinophils stimulated by IgG. J Immunol 1995;155:2631-2641.

38. Nagata M, Sedgwick JB, Kita H, Busse WW. Granulocyte macrophage colony-stimulating factor augments ICAM-1 and VCAM-1 activation of eosinophil function. Am J Respir Cell Mol Biol 1998;19:158-166.

39. Bartemes KR, McKinney S, Gleich GJ, Kita H. Endogenous platelet-activating factor is critically involved in effector functions of eosinophils stimulated with IL-5 or IgG. J Immunol 1999;162:2982-2989.

40. Rothenberg ME. Eosinophilia. N Engl J Med 1998;338:1592-1600.

41. Slifman NR, Loegering DA, McKean DJ, Gleich GJ. Ribonuclease activity associated with human eosinophil-derived neurotoxin and eosinophil cationic protein. J Immunol 1986;137:2913-2917.

42. Gleich GJ, Loegering DA, Bell MP, Checkel JL, Ackerman SJ, McKean DJ. Biochemical and functional similarities between human eosinophil-derived neurotoxin and eosinophil cationic protein:

homology with ribonuclease. Proc Natl Acad Sci U S A 1986;83:3146-3150.

43. Young JD, Peterson CG, Venge P, Cohn ZA. Mechanism of membrane damage mediated by human eosinophil cationic protein. Nature 1986;321:613-616.

44. Moqbel R, Levi-Schaffer F, Kay AB. Cytokine generation by eosinophils. J Allergy Clin Immunol 1994;94:1183-1188.

45. Parrillo JE, Borer JS, Henry WL, Wolff SM, Fauci AS. The cardiovascular manifestations of the hypereosinophilic syndrome. Prospective study of 26 patients, with review of the literature. Am J Med 1979;67:572-582.

46. Parrillo JE. Heart disease and the eosinophil. N Engl J Med 1990;323:1560-1561.

47. Löffler W. Endocarditis parietalis fibroplastica mit Bluteosinophilie: Ein eigenartiges Krankheitsbild. Schweiz Med Wochenschr 1936;66:817-820.

48. Davies JNP. Endocardial fibrosis in Africans. East Afr Med J 1948;25:10-14.

49. Churg J, Strauss L. Allergic granulomatosis, allergic angiitis, and periarteritis nodosa. Am J Pathol 1951;27:277-301.

50. Watts RA, Carruthers DM, Scott DG. Epidemiology of systemic vasculitis: changing incidence or definition? Semin Arthritis Rheum 1995;25:28-34.

51. Chumbley LC, Harrison EG Jr, DeRemee RA. Allergic granulomatosis and angiitis (Churg-Strauss syndrome). Report and analysis of 30 cases. Mayo Clin Proc 1977;52:477-484.

52. Sehgal M, Swanson JW, DeRemee RA, Colby TV. Neurologic manifestations of Churg-Strauss syndrome. Mayo Clin Proc 1995;70:337-341.

53. Lanham JM, Graham MF, Schaberg DE. Hiring the handicapped—an 18-year success story. Occup Health Saf 1978;47:40-42, 50.

54. Guillevin L, Cohen P, Gayraud M, Lhote F, Jarrousse B, Casassus P. Churg-Strauss syndrome. Clinical study and long-term follow-up of 96 patients. Medicine (Baltimore) 1999;78:26-37.

55. Ramakrishna G, Connolly HM, Tazelaar HD, Mullany CJ, Midthun DE. Churg-Strauss syndrome complicated by eosinophilic endomyocarditis. Mayo Clin Proc 2000;75:631-635.

56. Masi AT, Hunder GG, Lie JT, Michel BA, Bloch DA, Arend WP, Calabrese LH, Edworthy SM, Fauci AS, Leavitt RY, Lightfoot RW Jr, McShane DJ, Mills JA, Stevens MB, Wallace SL, Zvaifler NJ. The American College of Rheumatology 1990 criteria for the classification of Churg-Strauss syndrome (allergic granulomatosis and angiitis). Arthritis Rheum 1990;33:1094-1100.

57. Wishnick MM, Valensi Q, Doyle EF, Balian A, Genieser NB, Chrousos G. Churg-Strauss syndrome. Development of cardiomyopathy during corticosteroid treatment. Am J Dis Child 1982;136:339-344.

58. Davison AG, Thompson PJ, Davies J, Corrin B, Turner-Warwick M. Prominent pericardial and myocardial lesions in the Churg-Strauss syndrome (allergic granulomatosis and angiitis). Thorax 1983;38:793-795.

59. Sasaki A, Hasegawa M, Nakazato Y, Ishida Y, Saitoh S. Allergic granulomatosis and angiitis (Churg-Strauss syndrome). Report of an autopsy case in a nonasthmatic patient. Acta Pathol Jpn 1988;38:761-768.

60. Lanham JG, Cooke S, Davies J, Hughes GR. Endomyocardial complications of the Churg-Strauss syndrome. Postgrad Med J 1985;61:341-344.

61. Hellemans S, Dens J, Knockaert D. Coronary involvement in the Churg-Strauss syndrome. Heart 1997;77:576-578.

62. Terasaki F, Hayashi T, Hirota Y, Okabe M, Suwa M, Deguchi H, Kitaura Y, Kawamura K. Evolution to dilated cardiomyopathy from acute eosinophilic pancarditis in Churg-Strauss syndrome. Heart Vessels 1997;12:43-48.

63. Kozak M, Gill EA, Green LS. The Churg-Strauss syndrome. A case report with angiographically documented coronary involvement and a review of the literature. Chest 1995;107:578-580.

64. Majumdar NK, Zahn DW. Pulmonary malignancy and eosinophilia: a discussion and a case report. Am Rev Tuberc 1957;75:644-647.

65. Serafini F. Circulatory and tissue eosinophilia in pulmonary tumor patients. [Italian.] Gaz Int Med Chir 1962;67:2673-2681.

66. Viola MV, Chung E, Mukhopadhyay MG. Eosinophilia and metastatic carcinoma. Med Ann Dist Columbia 1972;41:1-3.

67. Wasserman SI, Goetzl EJ, Ellman L, Austen KF. Tumor-associated eosinophilotactic factor. N Engl J Med 1974;290:420-424.

68. Barrett AJ, Barrett A. Bronchial carcinoma with eosinophilia and cardiomegaly. Br J Dis Chest 1975;69:287-292.

69. Muller E, Kolb E. Local responses in primary and secondary human lung cancers. I. Patterns of cellular (eosinophils and macrophages) and extracellular (acid mucopolysaccharide) reactions. Br J Cancer 1979;40:403-409.

70. Kappis M. Hochgradige Eosinophilie des Blutes bei einem malignen Tumor der rechten Lunge. München Med Wochenschr 1907;54:881-883.

71. Yoon IL. The eosinophil and gastrointestinal carcinoma. Am J Surg 1959;97:195-200.

72. Böhmig R. Das Krebsstroma und seine morphologischen Reaktionsformen. Beitr Path Anat Allg Path 1929;83:333-382.

73. Döderlein A. Spezielle Untersuchungen über eosinophile Leukozyten beim Krebs. Arch Geschwulstforsch 1955;8:111-125.

74. Isaacson NH, Rapoport P. Eosinophilia in malignant tumors: its significance. Ann Intern Med 1946;25:893-902.

75. Divack DM, Janovski NA. Eosinophilia encountered in female genital organs. Am J Obstet Gynecol 1962;84:761-763.

76. Bettazzi G. Sull'eosinofilia locale nei tumori maligni. Arch Ital Anat Istol Pat 1932;3:249-266.

77. Przewoski E. Ueber die locale Eosinophilie beim Krebs nebst Bemerkungen uber die Bedeutung der eosinophilen. Zentralbl Allg Pathol 1896;5:177-191.

78. Weill P. Uber die Beildung von granulierten Leukozyten im Karzinomgewebe. Virchows Arch Pathol Anat 1919;226:212-227.

79. Schoch EO. Eosinophilie in Probeexzisionen, ein prognostisch günstiges Zeichen für die Strahlenbehandlung der Portiokarzinome. München Med Wochenschr 1925;72:380.

80. Fluhmann CF. Carcinoma of the cervix uteri: a clinical and pathological study. Am J Obstet Gynecol 1927;13:174-184.

81. Kalberer HJ. Beiträge zum Studium histologischer Kriterien der Strahlensensibilität von Portiokarzinomen. Schweiz Med Wochenschr 1927;8:645.

82. Lahm W. Die Prognose des bestrahlten Uteruscarcinoms im Lichte der mikroskopischen Untersuchung. Strahlentherapie 1927;25:22-75.

83. Lahm W. Uber die lokale Eosinophilie bei Karzinom. Zentralbl Gynäkol 1927;51:669-672.

84. Goforth JL, Snoke PO. A consideration of body resistance to neoplasia: with a report of a case of carcinoma of the cervix of long duration and with distant metastases. Am J Med Sci 1928;175:504-510.

85. Böhmig R. Das Krebsstroma und seine morphologischen Reaktionsformen. Beitr Path Anat Allg Path 1929;83:333-382.

86. Scarpitti C. Studio dello stroma nell'evoluzione del cancro dell'utero e suo valore prognostico. Ann Ostet Ginec 1932;54:661-704.

87. Sala AM, Stein RJ. A case of carcinoma of the cervix with a blood picture simulating chronic aleukemic eosinophilic leukemia. Am J Cancer 1937;29:125-127.

88. Gill AJ. Local eosinophilia in malignant neoplasms. J Lab Clin Med 1944;29:820-824.

89. Linnell F, Mansson B. The prognostic value of eosinophilic leucocytes in the stroma of carcinoma of the cervix uteri. Acta Radiol 1954;41:453-456.

90. Bjersing L, Borglin N. Eosinophilia in the myometrium of the human uterus. Acta Path Microbiol Scand 1962;54:353-364.

91. Lasersohn JT, Thomas LB, Smith RR, Ketcham AS, Dillon JS. Carcinoma of the uterine cervix: a study of surgical, pathological and autopsy findings. Cancer 1964;17:338-351.

92. Ormos P. Eosinophil cells in carcinoma. [German.] Orvosi Hetil 1932;76:53-55.

93. Brink AJ, Weber HW. Fibroplastic parietal endocarditis with eosinophilia: Löffler's endocarditis. Am J Med 1963;34:52-70.

94. Sheperd AJ, Walsh CH, Archer RK, Wetherley-Mein G. Eosinophilia, splenomegaly and cardiac disease. Br J Haematol 1971;20:233-239.

95. Chopra P, Narula J, Talwar KK, Kumar V, Bhatia ML. Histomorphologic characteristics of endomyocardial fibrosis: an endomyocardial biopsy study. Hum Pathol 1990;21:613-616.

96. Weller PF, Bubley GJ. The idiopathic hypereosinophilic syndrome. Blood 1994;83:2759-2779.

97. Spyrou N, Foale R. Restrictive cardiomyopathies. Curr Opin Cardiol 1994;9:344-348.

98. Tai PC, Ackerman SJ, Spry CJ, Dunnette S, Olsen EG, Gleich GJ. Deposits of eosinophil granule proteins in cardiac tissues of patients with eosinophilic endomyocardial disease. Lancet 1987;1:643-647.

99. Rohrbach MS, Wheatley CL, Slifman NR, Gleich GJ. Activation of platelets by eosinophil granule proteins. J Exp Med 1990;172:1271-1274.

100. Patella V, de Crescenzo G, Marino I, Genovese A, Adt M, Gleich GJ, Marone G. Eosinophil granule proteins are selective activators of human heart mast cells. Int Arch Allergy Immunol 1997;113:200-202.

101. Valiathan MS. Endomyocardial fibrosis. Natl Med J India 1993;6:212-216.

102. Vijayaraghavan G, Balakrishnan M, Sadanandan S, Cherian G. Pattern of cardiac calcification in tropical endomyocardial fibrosis. Heart Vessels Suppl 1990;5:4-7.

103. Child JS, Perloff JK. The restrictive cardiomyopathies. Cardiol Clin 1988;6:289-316.

104. Gupta PN, Valiathan MS, Balakrishnan KG, Kartha CC, Ghosh MK. Clinical course of endomyocardial fibrosis. Br Heart J 1989;62:450-454.

105. Shaper AG. What's new in endomyocardial fibrosis? Lancet 1993;342:255-256.

106. Taliercio CP, Olney BA, Lie JT. Myocarditis related to drug hypersensitivity. Mayo Clin Proc 1985;60:463-468.

107. French AJ, Weller CV. Interstitial myocarditis following clinical and experimental use of sulfonamide drugs. Am J Pathol 1942;18:109-121.

108. Billingham M. Morphologic changes in drug-induced heart disease. In: Bristow MR, ed. Drug-induced heart disease. Amsterdam: Elsevier/North-Holland Biomedical Press, 1980:127-149.

109. Waugh D. Myocarditis, arteritis, and focal hepatic, splenic, and renal granulomas apparently due to penicillin sensitivity. Am J Pathol 1952;28:437-447.

110. Hodge PR, Lawrence JR. Two cases of myocarditis associated with phenylbutazone therapy. Med J Aust 1957;1:640-641.

111. Field JB, Federman DD. Sudden death in a diabetic subject during treatment with BZ-55 (Carbutamide). Diabetes 1957;6:67-70.

112. Chatterjee SS, Thakre MW. Fiedler's myocarditis: report of a fatal case following intramuscular injection of streptomycin. Tubercle 1958;39:240-241.

113. Lilienfeld A, Hochstein E, Weiss W. Acute myocarditis with bundle branch block due to sulfonamide sensitivity. Circulation 1950;1:1060-1064.

114. Kline IK, Kline TS, Saphir O. Myocarditis in senescence. Am Heart J 1963;65:446-457.

115. Kerwin AJ. Fatal myocarditis due to sensitivity to phenindione. Canad Med Assoc J 1964;90:1418-1419.

116. Langsjoen PH, Stinson JC. Acute fatal allergic myocarditis: report of a case. Dis Chest 1965;48:440-441.

117. Banerjee D. Myocarditis in penicillin sensitivity. Indian Heart J 1968;20:73-75.

118. Plafker J. Penicillin-related nephritis and myocarditis: a case report. South Med J 1971;64:852-854.

119. Herman JE, Fleischmann P. Unusual evidence of myocardial involvement during a hypersensitivity reaction to oral penicillin. Isr J Med Sci 1978;14:848-851.

120. Fenoglio JJ Jr, McAllister HA Jr, Mullick FG. Drug related myocarditis. I. Hypersensitivity myocarditis. Hum Pathol 1981;12:900-907.

121. Kounis NG. A review: drug-induced bronchospasm. Ann Allergy 1976;37:285-291.

122. Anonymous. Myocarditis related to drug hypersensitivity (editorial). Lancet 1985;2:1165-1166.

123. Lie JT, Hunt D. Eosinophilic endomyocarditis complicating acute myocardial infarction. Involvement of the cardiac conduction system. Arch Intern Med 1974;134:754-757.

124. Fenoglio JJ Jr, Ursell PC, Kellogg CF, Drusin RE, Weiss MB. Diagnosis and classification of myocarditis by endomyocardial biopsy. N Engl J Med 1983;308:12-18.

125. Nippoldt TB, Edwards WD, Holmes DR Jr, Reeder GS, Hartzler GO, Smith HC. Right ventricular endomyocardial biopsy: clinicopathologic correlates in 100 consecutive patients. Mayo Clin Proc 1982;57:407-418.

126. Kim CH, Vlietstra RE, Edwards WD, Reeder GS, Gleich GJ. Steroid-responsive eosinophilic myocarditis: diagnosis by endomyocardial biopsy. Am J Cardiol 1984;53:1472-1473.

127. Herzog CA, Snover DC, Staley NA. Acute necrotising eosinophilic myocarditis. Br Heart J 1984;52:343-348.

128. deMello DE, Liapis H, Jureidini S, Nouri S, Kephart GM, Gleich GJ. Cardiac localization of eosinophil-granule major basic protein in acute necrotizing myocarditis. N Engl J Med 1990;323:1542-1545.

129. Wright RS, Simari RD, Orszulak TA, Edwards WD, Gleich GJ, Reeder GS. Eosinophilic endomyocardial disease presenting as cyanosis, platypnea, and orthodeoxia. Ann Intern Med 1992;117:482-483.

130. Aggarwal A, Bergin P, Jessup P, Kaye D. Hypersensitivity myocarditis presenting as cardiogenic shock (letter to the editor). J Heart Lung Transplant 2001;20:1241-1244.

131. Capron M. Eosinophils and parasites. Ann Parasitol Hum Comp 1991;66 Suppl 1:41-45.

132. Davidson RA. Immunology of parasitic infections. Med Clin North Am 1985;69:751-758.

133. Butterworth AE. Cell-mediated damage to helminths. Adv Parasitol 1984;23:143-235.

134. Hagar JM, Rahimtoola SH. Chagas' heart disease in the United States. N Engl J Med 1991;325:763-768.

135. Rossi MA. Comparison of Chagas' heart disease to arrhythmogenic right ventricular cardiomyopathy. Am Heart J 1995;129:626-629.

136. Hagar JM, Rahimtoola SH. Chagas' heart disease. Curr Probl Cardiol 1995;20:825-924.

137. Sadigursky M, von Kreuter BF, Ling PY, Santos-Buch CA. Association of elevated anti-sarcolemma, anti-idiotype antibody levels with the clinical and pathologic expression of chronic Chagas myocarditis. Circulation 1989;80:1269-1276.

138. Morris SA, Tanowitz HB, Wittner M, Bilezikian JP. Pathophysiological insights into the cardiomyopathy of Chagas' disease. Circulation 1990;82:1900-1909.

139. Mota EA, Guimaraes AC, Santana OO, Sherlock I, Hoff R, Weller TH. A nine year prospective study of Chagas' disease in a defined rural population in northeast Brazil. Am J Trop Med Hyg 1990;42:429-440.

140. Espinosa RA, Pericchi LR, Carrasco HA, Escalante A, Martinez O, Gonzalez R. Prognostic indicators of chronic chagasic cardiopathy. Int J Cardiol 1991;30:195-202.

141. Rossi MA. Microvascular changes as a cause of chronic cardiomyopathy in Chagas' disease. Am Heart J 1990;120:233-236.

142. Casado J, Davila DF, Donis JH, Torres A, Payares A, Colmenares R, Gottberg CF. Electrocardiographic abnormalities and left ventricular systolic function in Chagas' heart disease. Int J Cardiol 1990;27:55-62.

143. Carrasco HA, Guerrero L, Parada H, Molina C, Vegas E, Chuecos R. Ventricular arrhythmias and left ventricular myocardial function in chronic chagasic patients. Int J Cardiol 1990;28:35-41.

144. Bestetti RB, Freitas OC, Muccillo G, Oliveira JS. Clinical and morphological characteristics associated with sudden cardiac death in patients with Chagas' disease. Eur Heart J 1993;14:1610-1614.

145. Mazza S, Jörg ME, Canal Feijoo EJ. Primer caso crónico mortal de forma cardíaca de enfermedad de Chagas demostrado en Santiago del Estero. Invest Enferm de Chagas 1938;38:3-75.

146. Romana C. Anatomia patologica, patogenia e immunologia. In: Romaña C, ed. Enfermedad de Chagas. Buenos Aires: López Libreros, 1963:97-146.

147. Koberle F. Chagas' disease and Chagas' syndromes: the pathology of American trypanosomiasis. Adv Parasitol 1968;6:63-116.

148. Andrade Z, Andrade S. Patologia. In: Brener Z, Andrade Z, eds. Trypanosoma cruzi e doenca de Chagas. Rio de Janeiro: Guanabara Koogan, 1979:199-248.

149. Molina HA, Kierszenbaum F. A study of human myocardial tissue in Chagas' disease: distribution and frequency of inflammatory cell types. Int J Parasitol 1987;17:1297-1305.

150. Lundeberg KR. A fatal case of Chagas disease occurring in a man 77 years of age. Am J Trop Med 1938;18:185-196.

151. Laranja FS, Dias E, Nobrega G, Miranda A. Chagas' disease. A clinical, epidemiologic, and pathologic study. Circulation 1956;14:1035-1060.

152. Lorenzana R. Chronic Chagas' myocarditis. Report of a case. Am J Clin Pathol 1967;48:39-43.

153. Mengel JO, Rossi MA. Chronic chagasic myocarditis pathogenesis: dependence on autoimmune and microvascular factors. Am Heart J 1992;124:1052-1057.

154. Sanchez JA, Milei J, Yu ZX, Storino R, Wenthold R Jr, Ferrans VJ. Immunohistochemical localization of laminin in the hearts of patients with chronic chagasic cardiomyopathy: relationship to thickening of basement membranes. Am Heart J 1993;126:1392-1401.

155. Reis DD, Jones EM, Tostes S, Lopes ER, Chapadeiro E, Gazzinelli G, Colley DG, McCurley TL. Expression of major histocompatibility complex antigens and adhesion molecules in hearts of patients with chronic Chagas' disease. Am J Trop Med Hyg 1993;49:192-200.

156. de Oliveira SA, Pereira Barreto AC, Mady C, Dallan LA, da Luz PL, Jatene AD, Pileggi F. Surgical treatment of endomyocardial fibrosis: a new approach. J Am Coll Cardiol 1990;16:1246-1251.

157. Davies J, Sapsford R, Brooksby I, Olsen EG, Spry CJ, Oakley CM, Goodwin JF. Successful surgical treatment of two patients with eosinophilic endomyocardial disease. Br Heart J 1981;46:438-445.

158. Dubost C, Maurice P, Gerbaux A, Bertrand E, Rulliere R, Vial F, Barrillon A, Prigent C, Carpentier A, Soyer R. The surgical treatment of constrictive fibrous endocarditis. Ann Surg 1976;184:303-307.

159. Metras D, Coulibaly AO, Ouattara K. The surgical treatment of endomyocardial fibrosis: results in 55 patients. Circulation 1985;72:II274-II279.

Chagas Heart Disease

James M. Hagar, M.D., and Shahbudin H. Rahimtoola, M.B.

INTRODUCTION

American trypanosomiasis and its etiologic agent *Trypanosoma cruzi* were first described by Carlos Chagas in 1909.[1,2] Chagas single-handedly characterized this new disease in all of its aspects by first discovering the causative agent and its vector and then seeking out and describing human cases of infection.[3]

Chagas was assigned as a malaria officer in the state of Minas Gerais in Brazil in 1908 (Fig. 20-1), where he observed bloodsucking reduviids infesting the dwellings of the local people. In the gut of the reduviids he discovered a new species of trypanosome, which he named after his colleague and mentor Oswaldo Cruz. Using only the crude methods available to him, he fully elucidated its life cycle and its pathogenicity in wild and domestic animals. Postulating that a human disease might be caused by this trypanosome, he cultured the trypanosome from a specimen from a 9-month-old child with an acute febrile illness and facial swelling and later from adults with cardiac disorders, which he then transmitted back into experimental animals. He described in detail the epidemiologic, microbiologic, and pathologic features of the disease,[4,5] including cardiac involvement. He later reported the clinical features of late cardiac and gastrointestinal tract involvement and correctly estimated their high prevalence, years before the development of electrocardiography and serologic testing for the disease.[6]

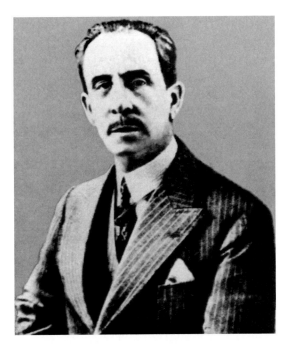

Fig. 20-1. Photograph of Carlos Chagas. (Photo from Chagas Filho, 1959.) (From Lewinsohn R.[3] By permission of the Royal Society of Tropical Medicine and Hygiene.)

Cardiac involvement is the most frequent manifestation of Chagas disease and is a form of chronic myocarditis. This chapter presents an overview of Chagas heart disease, reviewing its epidemiology, pathology and pathogenesis, clinical features, and treatment. In particular, we focus on advances in the understanding of the disease, our own experience with Chagas disease outside an endemic area, and advances in prevention and treatment.

EPIDEMIOLOGY

T cruzi, the etiologic agent of Chagas disease, is a hemoflagellate protozoan transmitted by the bite of a bloodsucking insect of the family Reduviidae, subfamily Triatominae (Fig. 20-2). Free-living reduviids transmit *T cruzi* infection in an enzootic cycle to a wide variety of wild animal hosts, such as rodents, opossums, and raccoons, and to domestic animals,[7] which serve as reservoirs of infection. Although most of the known species of reduviids harbor *T cruzi* in their gut, not all are capable of adapting to human habitation, and only a dozen species are epidemiologically important vectors of *T cruzi* infection in humans. Differences

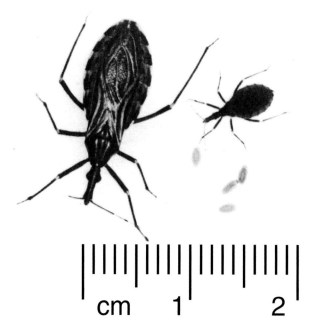

Fig. 20-2. Rodnius prolixus, one of the major vectors of *Trypanosoma cruzi* in Central America. Eggs, immature nymph, and adult forms are shown. (From Kirchhoff LV, Neva FA. *Trypanosoma* species [Chagas' disease]. In: Mandell GL, Douglas RG Jr, Bennett JE, eds. Principles and practice of infectious diseases. 2nd ed. New York: Wiley, 1985:1531-1537. By permission of the publisher.)

among species influence their ability to transmit *T cruzi* to humans and the types of measures likely to be most effective in their control.[8]

The types of housing found in impoverished rural areas of Central and South America facilitate transmission of *T cruzi* from reduviids to humans. Earthen floors, thatched roofs, and cracks in walls provide shelter for reduviids to live and breed in abundance.[9] More modern types of dwellings (eg, brick or stucco with concrete floors and metal roofs) are less likely to support breeding of reduviids. *T cruzi* is transmitted most often to humans when a reduviid takes its blood meal from a human victim, often during sleep. Bites are often on the face or other exposed skin. The reduviid defecates as it feeds, depositing *T cruzi*-laden feces near the bite. The victim then scratches the bite, inoculating *T cruzi* into the bite. Transmission through blood transfusion is the second most frequent method of transmission and is discussed below. Maternal-fetal transmission occurs in up to 10% of cases of chronic maternal infection and frequently results in spontaneous abortion or premature birth.[10,11]

T CRUZI LIFE CYCLE AND BIOLOGY

T cruzi completes its life cycle in a complex series of transformations within its insect vector and mammalian host. Reduviids acquire *T cruzi* by feeding on the blood of infected animals, in the form of free-living trypomastigotes, which have a membrane and flagellum. These develop in the insect's hindgut into metacyclic trypomastigotes, a form in which they are capable of infecting an animal host. Once the trypomastigotes invade the host via the feces of the reduviid, they enter macrophages in cutaneous tissues and multiply as intracellular amastigote (leishmanial) forms, which lack a membrane or flagellum. With the death of the macrophage, released amastigotes infect additional macrophages while others become trypomastigotes and circulate in peripheral blood. Ultimately, these invade remote tissues for which they exhibit varying degrees of tropism, particularly skeletal and cardiac muscle, and continue to multiply as amastigotes (Fig. 20-3).

PARASITE GENETICS AND HOST FACTORS

There is a great deal of variability in the morphology, antigenicity, and infectivity of different strains of *T cruzi* from patient to patient and between regions. Distinct strains of *T cruzi* can be identified according to their zymodemes, the electrophoretic classification of enzyme subtypes,[12] which may correlate with clinical differences in disease manifestations and resistance to antiparasitic drugs. Surface glycoproteins may also play a role in determining *T cruzi* invasiveness or virulence. Genetic polymorphisms can be identified within the *T cruzi* genome by using polymerase chain reaction (PCR)-based methods. PCR can be used to classify strains according to their zymodeme[13] and thus their virulence.[14] One small study found that different clinical forms of the disease are the result of genetic variability

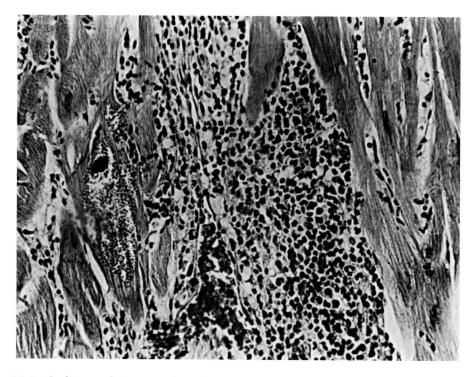

Fig. 20-3. Cardiac muscle in acute Chagas disease. An infected myocyte has become distended with *Trypanosoma cruzi* amastigotes, formed a pseudocyst, and ruptured. There is intense inflammatory reaction at this site. (Courtesy of Dr. Maria de Lourdes Higuchi.) (From Hagar and Rahimtoola.[38] By permission of Mosby-Year Book.)

in *T cruzi* strains.[15] Currently, genetic typing of *T cruzi* is useful mainly to study evolutionary development and geographic distribution of strains,[16] but one day it could be used to determine prognosis, end-organ disease, or drug sensitivity. The *T cruzi* Genome Project[17] is a multinational collaborative effort to sequence and provide a database for the genome of a *T cruzi* strain, *T cruzi* polymorphisms, and expressed sequence tags. This project undoubtedly will contribute greatly to knowledge in many areas, such as identifying new targets for pharmacotherapy.[18]

Host immunologic factors and environmental conditions are also important in determining the pattern and severity of disease that develops in an infected individual. Although human data are scant, in experimental animals, factors such as elevated environmental temperature[19] and protein malnutrition[20] alter the host immune response and tissue injury. Repeated reinfection and variation in the initial inoculum affect the severity of the infection and modify host immunity.[21] Intercurrent infection, especially viral infection, markedly enhances host susceptibility and the disease process. Overall, it is the balance among parasite tropism and invasiveness and host defenses that determines the pattern, severity, and course of the resulting cardiac disease.[22]

EPIDEMIOLOGY OF HUMAN CHAGAS DISEASE

Natural reservoirs of *T cruzi* can be found throughout most of the western hemisphere, as far north as Maryland and northern California, and as far south as the southern portions of Chile and Argentina. It has not been found outside of the Americas or in the Caribbean. Human infection with *T cruzi* is frequent throughout nearly all of South America, Central America,[23] and southern Mexico.[24] Human infection becomes less frequent at more northern latitudes; it is much less common in northern Mexico and is extremely rare in the southwestern United States. Although reduviid species are widely distributed in North America and frequently carry *T cruzi*,[25] infection acquired in the United States (other than laboratory- and transfusion-acquired infection) is extremely rare, with only 5 such cases reported.[26-29] This is mostly the result of better housing, but it may also result from differences in reduviid behavior and infectivity of *T cruzi* strains in temperate climates.

Estimates from the World Health Organization, based on seroepidemiologic studies, conservatively place the number of infected persons at 18 to 20 million,[30] with 90 million living in zones where transmission of *T cruzi* is endemic. An estimated 550,000 new cases and 50,000 deaths related to Chagas disease occur annually. In endemic countries, the overall prevalence of human infection averages about 10%, and in highly endemic rural areas rates ranging from 20% to 75% have been found. The prevalence of infection varies widely even among cities and provinces within one country, due to variations in climate, housing conditions, public health measures, and urbanization.

The number of cases of clinical Chagas disease and the number of case fatalities are not well known, because there is no case reporting in most areas. Individuals are exposed to *T cruzi* early and repeatedly throughout life, and the prevalence of infection in cross-sectional studies increases rapidly beginning in infancy and childhood. For example, in a highly endemic region of rural Venezuela, 16% of children aged 5 to 9 years had positive serologic results, increasing to 56% by ages 20 to 24 years, and 74% by age 65 years.[31] The prevalence of infection actually declines in the middle and older age groups, probably due to premature cardiovascular death in those infected.[32] The prevalence of right bundle branch block, an indicator of cardiac involvement, increased rapidly in the third decade of life among seropositive individuals, reaching 85% by age 50 years. Overall, 17% of the population had signs or symptoms of overt heart disease, nearly all attributable to Chagas disease. Chagas heart disease is the most common cause of dilated cardiomyopathy in endemic countries. In highly endemic areas it is the leading cause of cardiovascular death[33] and the leading cause of all deaths among persons ages 25 to 44 years.[34]

T cruzi infection and Chagas heart disease are sometimes encountered outside of endemic countries. In the United States, *T cruzi* infection has been found in as many as 4.9% of immigrants from highly endemic areas,[35] although the prevalence was lower in other surveys and depends on the demographic mix of subjects. A study at our institution found 1.1% of 988 blood donors positive for *T cruzi* by complement fixation, with 0.2% of those from endemic areas positive by radioimmunoprecipitation assay.[36] Reports of Chagas heart disease in the United States include our series of 42 cases,[37,38] and 8 additional cases.[39-45] Estimates of the number of infected persons residing in the United States have ranged from 400,000 to 500,000.[35,46]

The country of origin of persons with Chagas disease found in a nonendemic country is determined by the relative proportion of immigrants from each country, their socio-economic status, and the prevalence of infection in those countries. Thus, our patients were most frequently from Central America, followed by Mexico, and the smallest number were from South America[35] (Table 20-1). Cases of Chagas disease and asymptomatic *T cruzi* infection have been reported from numerous other nonendemic countries around the world as a result of worldwide immigration.[47]

TRANSFUSION-ACQUIRED CHAGAS DISEASE

Transfusion-acquired Chagas disease has long been a serious problem in endemic areas; transfusion is the second most frequent route of human infection. Transfusion-related transmission occurs outside of rural areas or even internationally because of population migration. The prevalence of *T cruzi* infection among blood donors in endemic countries

Table 20-1
Country of Origin of North American Patients With Chagas Heart Disease and Proportions of United States Immigrants From Endemic Areas

Origin	Immigrant population from endemic countries, no. (%)	
	LAC + USC series	2000 census*
Mexico	12 (29)	7,841 (67)
Central America	26 (62)	1,948 (17)
El Salvador	17 (40)	765 (7)
Guatemala	4 (10)	327 (3)
Nicaragua	3 (7)	245 (2)
Honduras	2 (5)	250 (2)
South America	4 (10)	1,876 (16)
Argentina	2 (5)	89 (1)
Colombia	1 (2)	435 (4)
Bolivia	1 (2)	44 (0.4)

*U.S. Census Bureau. The Foreign-Born Population (Table 3-4). Country or Area of Birth of the Foreign-Born Population From Latin America and Northern America: 2000. Published February 2000. <http://www.census.gov/population/socdemo/foreign/pp1-145/tab03-4.xls>. Numbers of persons in thousands. LAC + USC is Los Angeles County + University of Southern California Medical Center.

has been studied widely and indicates the prevalence of *T cruzi* infection in the population. Reported rates vary from less than 1% to more than 60%, depending on the region and whether the population studied is primarily an urban or a rural one.[48]

A recipient of infected blood develops persistent seropositivity, indicating transmission of chronic infection, in 14% to 49% of cases.[49,50] A few persons infected in this way develop fulminant acute Chagas disease, usually infants and the immunocompromised.[51] Most have no sign of disease or develop a mild nonspecific febrile illness that is easily over-looked.[52] They are not discovered until cardiac or gastrointestinal tract disease develops decades later.

In areas where there is a significant prevalence of infection, there is general agreement that screening of all donated units is necessary to eliminate transfusion-related transmission of *T cruzi*. Such screening is now required by law in nearly all endemic countries, and it is being implemented well in most.[53] Transfusion-acquired Chagas disease also occurs in the United States and other nonendemic countries, usually after transfusion of infected blood to immunocompromised individuals.[54,55] The optimum strategy for screening of donated units in these areas continues to be debated. In some areas, screening of all donated units may be necessary. In our institution, a screening geographic questionnaire is used, which identifies approximately 40% of donors as being at higher risk of *T cruzi* infection; only blood from these donors undergoes serologic screening.[56] Among such individuals, 0.5%, representing 0.2% of the entire population, were positive for *T cruzi* (confirmed by radioimmunoprecipitation assay).[57] This appears to be a reasonable strategy, although there are rare cases without a geographic history, which represent disease acquired within the United States.[58] In other areas of the United States the prevalence of *T cruzi* in the blood supply is negligible.[59] Thus, the best strategy to prevent transfusion-related disease may be different in each institution.

PREVENTION AND ERADICATION OF CHAGAS DISEASE

Public health preventive measures are the most important means of controlling the devastating impact of Chagas disease. The goal of these programs is to prevent new cases in children and young adults through interruption of insect-borne transmission and elimination of transfusion-related transmission. Spraying of housing twice yearly with residual pesticides coupled with entomologic surveillance can successfully eradicate domiciliary transmission and is the cornerstone of current control efforts in most countries. Permanent improvement in the quality of housing available in rural areas is a more long-term solution. When pursued intensively, as in the case of the cooperative multinational Southern Cone Initiative and similar projects,[60] disease transmission to humans has been markedly reduced or interrupted altogether.[61] Complete elimination of human *T cruzi* transmission in many of these countries is predicted within the next 5 years.[62]

PATHOLOGY AND PATHOPHYSIOLOGY OF CHAGAS HEART DISEASE

PATHOLOGIC FINDINGS

The acute and chronic phases of Chagas heart disease differ markedly in their pathologic appearance and pathogenesis. Cases of acute human Chagas disease with myocarditis bear many similarities to the commonly studied murine model of acute Chagas myocarditis. Such cases are characterized by intense inflammatory pancarditis and have abundant mononuclear and polymorphonuclear cells (Fig. 20-3). Amastigote forms and parasitic pseudocysts are easily found in cardiac muscle cells, skeletal muscle, central nervous system, and autonomic ganglia. Myocytolysis and edema are evident and may be direct effects of the parasite or mediated by eosinophils and neutrophils.[63]

Chronic Chagas heart disease presents a picture of chronic myocarditis, which is located focally but affects multiple areas. Scattered mononuclear inflammatory infiltrates are always found although they may be infrequent. There is focal and diffuse loss of myocytes (Fig. 20-4), ultimately leading to replacement with fibrosis (Fig. 20-5). These confluent areas of dense fibrosis replace muscle tissue and lead to the segmental wall motion abnormalities characteristic of the disease.[64,65] Irregular myocyte hypertrophy is found in other areas. This process of inflammation and fibrosis is widespread throughout ventricles and atria but has a particular predilection for the cardiac conduction system and the apex of the left ventricle. Degradation of extracellular collagen struts and dilatation of coronary microvessels are prominent. Such pathologic features are unique to Chagas myocarditis and are quite different from the findings in idiopathic dilated cardiomyopathy.[66]

The resulting loss of myocytes in confluent areas and extracellular collagen degradation routinely lead to segmental thinning and akinesis. This often results in the classic narrow-necked left ventricular aneurysm at the apex, which may be large or small and often contains mural thrombus. Aneurysms can be found at other sites, such as adjacent to the mitral annulus. Localized areas of thinning and akinesis are frequently present throughout the left or right ventricle. When myocardial involvement is diffuse, a picture of dilated cardiomyopathy develops.

Another unique characteristic is the early and preferential involvement of the cardiac conduction system at all stages of the disease.[67,68] The anterior fascicle of the left bundle and of the right bundle typically are involved, showing chronic fibrosis and progressive obliteration, as in the right bundle branch shown in Figure 20-6. This leads to the characteristic electrocardiogram (ECG) abnormalities of right bundle branch block or left anterior fascicular block (or both), found in up to 80% of patients with cardiac disease. These abnormalities frequently progress to complete atrioventricular block, sometimes with little other overt evidence of myocardial damage. The sinus node may be involved.[69]

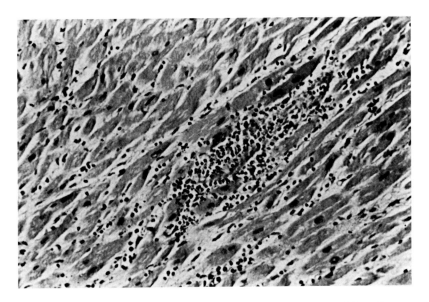

Fig. 20-4. Ventricular myocardium in chronic Chagas disease. There are scattered foci of mononuclear cell infiltrate and focal cytolysis without fibrosis. (From Suarez JA, Puigbo JJ, Nava Rhode JR, Valero JA, Yepez CG. Study of 210 cases of cardiomyopathies in Venezuela. In: Acquatella H, Pulido PA, eds. Miocardiopatias. Barcelona: Salvat Editores, 1982:5.)

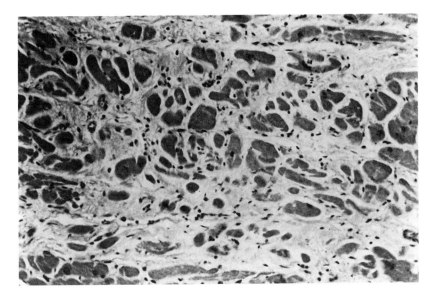

Fig. 20-5. The late stage of chronic Chagas heart disease. There is interstitial fibrosis and replacement of myocardium. Inflammatory cells are infrequent. (From Suarez JA, Puigbo JJ, Nava Rhode JR, Valero JA, Yepez CG. Study of 210 cases of cardiomyopathies in Venezuela. In: Acquatella H, Pulido PA, eds. Miocardiopatias. Barcelona: Salvat Editores, 1982:5.)

AUTONOMIC DYSFUNCTION

Loss of cardiac innervation is a frequent and unique pathologic feature of Chagas heart disease. This abnormality develops early in the course of the disease, preceding other evidence of cardiac involvement, and is a unique feature of Chagas heart disease that distinguishes it from other cardiomyopathic disorders.[70] Pathologically, abnormalities may be found in acute and chronic Chagas disease,[71] including periganglionitis, perineuritis, damage to neuron sheaths, direct parasitism of neurons, and a reduced number of vagal ganglion cells.[72] Clinically, autonomic dysfunction manifests as abnormal cardiovascular and baroreceptor

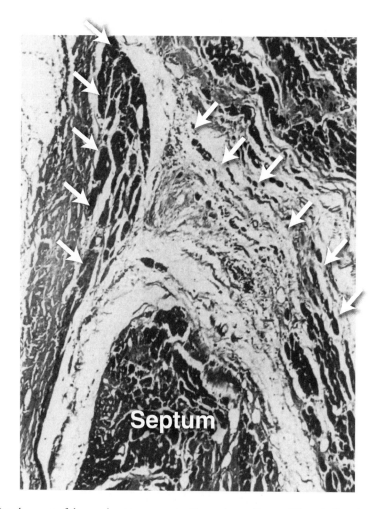

Fig. 20-6. Involvement of the conducting system in Chagas heart disease. There is fibrosis and destruction of the initial portion of the right bundle branch (*on right*) that extends into the septum. The left bundle (*on left*) is relatively spared. This process explains the typical findings of right bundle branch block. (Courtesy of Dr. Maria de Lourdes Higuchi.) (From Hagar and Rahimtoola.[38] By permission of Mosby-Year Book.)

reflexes. When this process occurs in the gastrointestinal tract, megaesophagus or mega-colon results,[73] characterized by severe dysfunction and dilatation of the respective organs but without the extensive tissue destruction seen in the myocardium. Whether cardiac autonomic dysfunction is clinically important or how it might contribute to the development of the cardiomyopathy is still uncertain.

PERSISTENCE OF INFECTION IN THE CHRONIC PHASE

Amastigote forms are extremely rare in conventionally stained histologic sections of cardiac tissues from patients in the chronic phase of the disease. When they are present, they appear to bear little relation to the pathologic features encountered. However, immunohisto-chemical staining, confocal microscopy, and DNA labeling consistently show *T cruzi* antigens and DNA in cardiac tissues in chronic Chagas heart disease, and those areas are clearly associated with foci of inflammatory infiltrate.[74,75] Endomyocardial biopsies confirm the continuing presence of *T cruzi* amastigotes and antigens in 85% to 92% of patients in the chronic phase.[76,77] In animal models, clearance of *T cruzi* DNA is associated with disappearance of inflammatory changes.[78] *T cruzi* DNA is found in the peripheral blood in 80% to 85% of chronically infected individuals, when sensitive PCR-based methods are used for its detection.[79] Thus, parasites and parasitic antigens are present much more frequently than was recognized in the past, strongly supporting the concept that persistent parasitism is the major stimulus driving ongoing tissue injury and progression of the disease.

IMMUNE RESPONSES

Cell-mediated and humoral immunity play major roles in all phases of cardiac *T cruzi* infection. In the acute phase of the disease, foci of intense polymorphonuclear and eosinophilic inflammation predominate, with a major role for CD8+ cytotoxic T lymphocytes[80] and macrophages.[81] In chronic disease, the intensity of inflammatory exudate is less and is predominantly mononuclear, although eosinophils may be associated with foci of cytolysis. Antibodies directed toward trypomastigotes are a major mechanism of host resistance.[82] In acute and chronic disease, CD4+ Th1 lymphocytes are the main effector cell, providing helper cell functions and producing interferon-γ, a stimulus for induction of nitric oxide synthase.[83] Cytotoxic CD8+ T lymphocytes in the myocardial interstitium, once sensitized to trypanosomal antigens, may produce myocyte injury and perpetuate the immune response by elaborating cytokines that stimulate macrophage migration into the tissues.

Mechanisms used by the parasites to produce tissue injury directly have been studied. Entry of *T cruzi* into host cells requires specific recognition sites, its trans-sialidase activity,[84] which is a major virulence factor, and the complement system.[85] *T cruzi* also induces apoptosis in host cells.[86]

The host immune response to *T cruzi* undoubtedly contributes to tissue injury, but *T cruzi* epitopes might also trigger host autoimmune responses by virtue of molecular mimicry. Antibodies have been described that react with antigens common to *T cruzi* and striated muscle,[87] peripheral nerve,[88] and cholinergic[89] and beta-adrenergic[90] receptors, which alter their function, although such studies have often lacked reproducibility.[91] T lymphocytes from infected humans and mice exert a negative inotropic effect[92] or produce myocarditis[93] in normal animals. Shared epitopes between *T cruzi* trypomastigotes and cardiomyocytes have been described.[94,95] Antibodies to a lymphocyte-activating antigen that depress lymphocyte proliferation[96] may explain the decreased cellular immune response to *T cruzi* antigens found in patients with advanced Chagas disease.[97] *T cruzi* kinetoplast DNA can be incorporated stably into human macrophage cell lines, altering their membrane antigens and allowing specific recognition by antibodies from *T cruzi*-infected patients.[98] These are fascinating hypotheses, but it has not been proven that such mechanisms are responsible for any of the pathologic changes found in cardiac tissues in human Chagas disease.[99]

EXTRACELLULAR MATRIX

The progressive loss of myocytes in chronic Chagas heart disease is associated with a concomitant increase in cardiac fibrosis, replacing necrotic myocytes and surrounding viable myocytes and blood vessels. There is progressive deposition of fibronectin, laminin, and type III and IV collagen in areas of inflammatory cell infiltration, which expand and distort the extracellular matrix[100] and could interfere with myocardial function. *T cruzi*-infected mesenchymal and endothelial cells secrete soluble factors that directly stimulate fibroblast proliferation and collagen formation[101] and an abnormal extracellular matrix.[102]

The normal extracellular matrix may be a site of injury in Chagas disease. Proteases from parasites and activated macrophages degrade native collagen and other matrix proteins.[103] There is progressive focal destruction of the collagen matrix throughout the course of the disease (Fig. 20-7), which is particularly prominent in the left ventricular apex.[104] Such extracellular matrix damage would lead to fiber slippage, apical thinning, segmental wall motion abnormalities, and adverse ventricular remodeling.

MICROVASCULAR ABNORMALITIES

Abnormalities of the coronary microvasculature have been hypothesized to contribute to the pathogenesis of Chagas heart disease. Basement membrane thickening was described in the myocardial microvessels of some patients with advanced cardiac disease.[105] Vascular proliferation and focal reversible vasoconstriction are found in the mouse model of acute *T cruzi* infection.[106] Clinically, endothelial function of large and small coronary vessels is abnormal in patients with Chagas heart disease.[107] Such structural and functional

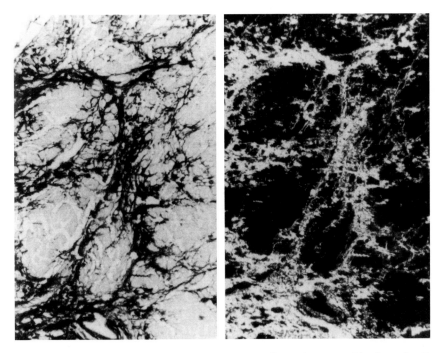

Fig. 20-7. Pattern of interstitial fibrosis encasing myocyte bundles and coronary blood vessels. Picrosirius red stain (*Left*) and polarized light (*Right*). (From Rossi MA. The pattern of myocardial fibrosis in chronic Chagas' heart disease. Int J Cardiol 1991;30:335-340. By permission of Elsevier Science Publishers.)

changes could be the result of infection of endothelial cells with *T cruzi*,[108] the action of *T cruzi* neuraminidase, or the autocrine or paracrine (or both) action of cytokines[109] and endothelin-1[110] elaborated by infected cells. Such microvascular alterations could lead to hyperresponsiveness to vasoconstrictor stimuli, microvascular ischemia, and focal myocytolysis.[111]

CLINICAL FEATURES OF CHAGAS HEART DISEASE

Cardiac involvement is typically present at all stages of Chagas disease. *Acute Chagas disease* is uncommon and is characterized by a febrile illness sometimes associated with facial or unilateral palpebral edema (Romaña sign) or localized indurated swelling at the site of inoculation (chagoma). Acute myocarditis is usually present at this stage but is rarely detected. Clinically evident acute myocarditis develops in approximately 1% of cases, and it is fatal in about 10%.[112] The remainder, who have no signs or symptoms of disease, enter the *indeterminate phase* of chronic infection.[113]

Such persons remain infected for life, with persistence of the parasite in tissues and measurable parasitemia in most. Active myocarditis and fibrosis are frequently present in this phase[114,115] and correlate with increasing severity of subsequent clinical disease.[116] Myocardial damage is thus a steadily progressive, cumulative, but variable process in the indeterminate phase of Chagas disease. This progression of myocardial damage leads to overt end-organ damage, most often cardiac, after a latent period of at least 15 to 20 years.

The percentage of infected individuals ultimately developing heart disease depends on how carefully the disease is sought. Approximately 30% to 40% of infected individuals develop detectable cardiac abnormalities during their lifetime,[117,118] such as an abnormal ECG or echocardiogram, whereas overt symptomatic cardiac involvement develops in 10% to 20%.[119] Of the remainder, usually classified as indeterminate, many actually have subclinical cardiac involvement when studied carefully.[120] Therefore, clinically evident Chagas heart disease represents only the tip of the iceberg of the cardiomyopathy.

It is sometimes useful to classify patients with Chagas disease according to the extent and severity of end-organ involvement (and thus prognosis). One such system[121] takes into account the early manifestations of disease, such as minor segmental wall motion abnormalities, autonomic dysfunction, and diastolic dysfunction (Table 20-2). However, a

Table 20-2
Clinical Classification of Chagas Heart Disease

Stage	Symptoms	ECG	Heart size	LVEF	LV wall motion	Autonomic function
I						
A	None	Normal	Normal	Normal	Normal	Normal
B	None	Normal	Normal	Normal	Mild abnormalities or diastolic dysfunction	May be abnormal
II	Minimal	Conduction abnormalities or PVCs	Normal	Normal	Segmental akinesis or aneurysm	May be abnormal
III	CHF, arrhythmias	Conduction abnormalities, pathologic Q waves, complex arrhythmias	Enlarged	Reduced	Global dysfunction with segmental WMA	Usually abnormal

CHF, congestive heart failure; ECG, electrocardiogram; LV, left ventricle; LVEF, left ventricular ejection fraction; PVCs, premature ventricular complexes; WMA, wall motion abnormalities.
Modified from Puigbó et al.[121] By permission of the publisher.

clinically based classification does not take into account the extent and severity of cardiac inflammation and parasitism, which may influence treatment and outcomes. With advances in laboratory testing, such information may provide additional clinical utility.

When *T cruzi* infection of the heart is demonstrated by pathologic examination of cardiac tissues, the diagnosis is certain. All other cases must meet a strict case definition that requires a combination of epidemiologic, serologic, and clinical criteria.[122] This is particularly important in populations where Chagas disease is uncommon relative to other forms of heart disease. The case definition we have used[37,38] requires 4 criteria be met: 1) a history of residence in an area endemic for Chagas disease, 2) an unequivocally positive serologic test for *T cruzi* by 2 methods, 3) a clinical syndrome compatible with Chagas heart disease, and 4) no evidence of another cardiac disorder to which the findings can be attributed.

LABORATORY DIAGNOSIS OF CHAGAS DISEASE

T cruzi infection can be diagnosed by finding the parasite, its antigens, or its DNA in blood or tissues or by a positive serologic test. Historically, the reference method of detection has been xenodiagnosis, in which laboratory-raised reduviids feed on blood of individuals with suspected *T cruzi* infection and are then examined after 4 to 6 weeks for the presence of trypomastigotes. Although specific, xenodiagnosis is cumbersome and has poor sensitivity in the chronic phase of the disease.[123] Instead, PCR-based methods to detect *T cruzi* nuclear or kinetoplast minicircle DNA sequences in blood or tissue have replaced xenodiagnosis for the direct diagnosis of *T cruzi* infection in most research centers. The sensitivity of PCR is greater than that of xenodiagnosis, with the most sensitive assays able to detect < 1 parasite/mL;[124] its sensitivity is 80% or higher in chronic infection but is still lower than that of serologic tests. PCR testing promises to be most useful for diagnosis of the disease when there is an equivocal or even negative serologic result[125] and for monitoring the effectiveness of antiparasitic drug therapy.

Serologic testing for Chagas disease is the mainstay of clinical diagnosis. Numerous methods are available to detect IgG antibodies to *T cruzi* trypomastigote antigens, which begin to appear within 3 to 6 weeks of infection and remain for life. Although useful in diagnosis, their titer and the change in titer over time do not correlate with disease activity. Testing is usually performed by 2 different methods to enhance the accuracy. The complement fixation, or Guerreiro-Machado, test was the first test developed and is still in use. It has a sensitivity of more than 90% and a specificity of more than 99% in cases of late disease.[126] In acute disease, however, the sensitivity is as low as 60%. The indirect immunofluorescence test is a simple slide test that is performed easily and is more sensitive than the complement fixation test,[127] although low titer false-positive results sometimes occur in patients infected with leishmaniasis or with nonpathogenic trypanosome strains. Enzyme-linked immunosorbent assay is simple and can be automated, and widely used commercially available kits have a 98% to 100% sensitivity and a 93% to 100% specificity.[128] However, the newer enzyme immunoassay has a nearly 100% sensitivity and specificity.[129] More specialized antibody tests have been used for specific research purposes.[130,131] The radioimmunoprecipitation[132] and enzyme immunoassays with their high specificity are most useful as a confirmatory test in populations with a low incidence of positivity, such as blood donors in nonendemic areas.

CLINICAL MANIFESTATIONS OF CHAGAS HEART DISEASE

Because the panmyocarditis of Chagas heart disease progressively involves the various cardiac tissues, patients may present with a wide variety of clinical manifestations. The most important of these are ventricular arrhythmias, congestive heart failure, thromboembolism, and complete atrioventricular block.

In early cardiac disease, when the cumulative extent of myocardial damage is small (stage IA and IB), ventricular abnormalities are minimal or absent and the ECG is normal. These patients are typically asymptomatic and have a good prognosis. When myocardial damage is more advanced (stage II), areas of abnormal wall motion may be evident and conduction abnormalities usually are present due to lesions within the His-Purkinje system. In such patients, global ventricular function is preserved, but sudden cardiac death or complete atrioventricular block may develop. Nonspecific symptoms such as chronic fatigue, weakness, palpitations, and chest pain[133] may be present. Such chest pain is vague and atypical of myocardial ischemia, but it sometimes prompts diagnostic evaluation. When the extent of myocardial damage is severe (stage III), the disease manifests as myocardial dysfunction that may be segmental, typically a ventricular aneurysm, or global, resembling a dilated cardiomyopathy. The clinical manifestations at this stage are those of severe congestive heart failure, ventricular arrhythmias, systemic thromboembolism, and complete heart block. However, the severity of symptoms frequently does not correlate with the degree of structural abnormality present; asymptomatic patients with profoundly abnormal ventricles are encountered frequently, whereas some with milder disease may have prominent constitutional symptoms.

The initial clinical manifestations of the 34 women and 8 men in our series are shown in Table 20-3. Most had received treatment for other presumed cardiac diagnoses, usually coronary artery disease or idiopathic dilated cardiomyopathy, before Chagas disease was considered.

ECG ABNORMALITIES

Involvement of the conduction system is ubiquitous and progressive when there is cardiac involvement. It was the study of Chagas heart disease that led to our modern understanding of the pathologic features of right bundle branch block and the discovery of the fascicular blocks.[134] The characteristic ECG abnormalities of right bundle branch block or

Table 20-3
Clinical Presentation of North American Patients With Chagas Heart Disease*

Clinical presentation	Patients, no. (%)
Atrioventricular block	9 (21)
Congestive heart failure	8 (19)
Chest pain	6 (14)
Conduction abnormality on ECG	8 (19)
Aborted sudden death	3 (7)
Sustained ventricular tachycardia	3 (7)
Embolic event	3 (7)
Other	2 (5)

ECG, electrocardiogram.

*Age at diagnosis (mean ± SEM) = 52 ± 2 years; duration of prior symptoms = 20 ± 6 months (range, 0 to 108); and no symptoms before initial presentation = 10 (24%).

Modified from Hagar and Rahimtoola.[37] By permission of the Massachusetts Medical Society.

left anterior fascicular block (or both) are found in up to 80% of patients with overt cardiac disease in our patients and in 2 other large series (Table 20-4). Conduction abnormalities were present in all of those in our series who had ventricular aneurysm or severe ventricular dysfunction. The prevalence of right bundle branch block in some endemic areas is so high that it has been used as a marker for Chagas heart disease in some studies. The presence of right bundle branch block (complete, incomplete, or induced by the antiarrhythmic agent ajmaline[135]) or left anterior fascicular block virtually always indicates the presence of significant myocarditis,[136] although the extent of myocardial damage may vary. Left bundle branch block is infrequent. This apparent preference for the right bundle branch and anterior fascicle is explained by the anatomic vulnerability of these highly localized conducting tissues (Fig. 20-6).

Ventricular premature beats occur in virtually all patients with Chagas heart disease, and generally they become more frequent and complex with more advanced disease.[137] Sinus bradycardia is not infrequent, indicating sinus node involvement or autonomic neuropathy, but does not indicate an adverse prognosis. Atrial fibrillation, on the other hand, usually is associated with severe left ventricular dysfunction. Patients who have isolated right bundle branch block as their only ECG abnormality may have a more benign prognosis, whereas those with left anterior fascicular block tend to have more extensive wall motion abnormalities and ventricular arrhythmias.[138]

Pathologic Q waves, primary T-wave changes, and ST-segment elevation were frequent in our patients and always indicate the presence of extensive wall motion abnormalities or ventricular aneurysm.[139,140] Such ECG abnormalities, which resemble myocardial infarction or ischemia (or both), are prominent in advanced cases of Chagas heart disease and may confuse the clinician unfamiliar with Chagas disease.

Table 20-4
Electrocardiographic Findings in 3 Series of Patients With Chagas Heart Disease

	Patients		
	Hagar and Rahimtoola[38]	Laranja et al.[118]	Puigbo et al.[31]
	No.	%	%	%
Conduction abnormality*				
Bundle branch block				
RBBB	20	47	51	45
Without LAD	8	18		19
With LAD	12	29		26
LBBB	4	10	5	7
Left anterior hemiblock only	11	26	–	26
No conduction abnormality	7	17	–	18
Arrhythmias				
Complete heart block	3	7	8	–
Atrial fibrillation with slow response	4	10	7	–
Second degree AV block	2	5	4	6
Ventricular ectopic beats	26	62	47	35
Sinus bradycardia	7	17	–	–
Other abnormalities				
Q wave MI pattern	18	43	14	10
Anteroseptal	6			
Anterolateral	2			
Lateral	5			
Inferolateral	4			
Inferior	1			
With ST elevation (simulating acute MI)	6	14		–
Primary T-wave inversion	19	45	23	66
ST depression	2	5		

AV, atrioventricular; LAD, left axis deviation; LBBB, left bundle branch block; MI, myocardial infarction; RBBB, right bundle branch block.
*Complete and incomplete bundle branch blocks classified together.
From Hagar and Rahimtoola.[38] By permission of Mosby-Year Book.

MYOCARDIAL ABNORMALITIES

Chagas heart disease is unique among the cardiomyopathies in causing marked segmental wall motion abnormalities and aneurysms of the left ventricle. These abnormalities result in a high incidence of malignant ventricular arrhythmias and systemic thromboembolism in patients with Chagas disease. The classic lesion of Chagas disease is a localized aneurysm of the left ventricular apex, with relatively normal surrounding wall motion (Fig. 20-8 through 20-10). This results in a narrow neck when visualized by echocardiography or ventriculography;[141] when present, this can usually distinguish an aneurysm of Chagas heart disease from one due to coronary artery disease.[142] The aneurysms and segmental abnormalities are thought to result from localized destruction of extracellular matrix collagen along with myocyte loss, which leads to focal weakening of the ventricular wall. The apical location is particularly vulnerable because of the nature of the collagen structure at this location, normal apical thinning, and a relatively increased wall stress, which would promote the gradual development of aneurysmal dilatation of the weakened segment. Regional dyssynergia caused by segmental conduction abnormalities could also contribute to aneurysm formation.

Echocardiography has proved useful to identify the presence and extent of end-organ damage. Areas of segmental hypokinesis or akinesis are commonly found early in the chronic phase,[143] even in those with normal ECGs who would otherwise be given a diagnosis of indeterminate phase disease. Right ventricular abnormalities may be present,[144] and diastolic dysfunction frequently is found. In time, the disease results in progressively larger areas of akinesis or aneurysm, declining systolic dysfunction, mitral insufficiency, and overt congestive heart failure.

Table 20-5
Left Ventricular Function and Coronary Arteriographic Findings
in North American Patients With Chagas Heart Disease

Finding	Patients, no. (%)
Left ventricular function	
Global systolic function abnormal*	20 (48)
Wall motion abnormalities	30 (71)
Left ventricular aneurysm (coronary arteriogram in 14, normal in all)	15 (36)
Segmental wall motion abnormality without aneurysm Apical akinesis 6, apical hypokinesis 1	7 (16)
Diffuse hypokinesis	8 (19)
Multiple abnormalities	7 (17)
Both left ventricular wall motion and global function normal	12 (29)
Coronary arteriography (n = 25)	
Normal	23
Minimal atherosclerotic disease	2†

*Ejection fraction < 50% by contrast ventriculography (n = 21) or radionuclide angiography (n = 6); echocardiographic fractional shortening < 28% (n = 15).
†Less than 60% obstruction small diagonal in 1; < 50% obstruction distal right coronary artery.
From Hagar and Rahimtoola.[38] By permission of Mosby-Year Book.

In our series, 71% of patients had left ventricular abnormalities—most often an aneurysm (Table 20-5). Wall motion abnormalities were often multiple. Nearly half of patients with ventricular aneurysms had normal overall left ventricular function. Aneurysms usually involved the apex and sometimes the posterolateral wall. Aneurysms varied in size and morphology from fingertip-sized outpouchings to massive structures (Fig. 20-8 through 20-10).

The segmental nature of the myocardial abnormalities extended to myocardial perfusion scintigraphy. All 10 patients studied with exercise and redistribution thallium perfusion scans had abnormal studies.[145] Fixed defects were found in 2 patients, a reversible defect in 1, and both fixed and reversible defects in 4. These defects corresponded to areas of abnormal left ventricular wall motion or aneurysm, although none had coronary artery disease in any artery supplying these regions. Such a study is shown in Figure 20-11. There was also reverse redistribution in 1 or more segments in 3 cases, which is a frequent finding when there is cardiac involvement,[146] but which does not correspond to areas of abnormal wall motion. Fixed defects might be expected where there is focal myocyte loss and fibrosis; the finding of reversible defects could be interpreted as supporting a microvascular ischemia hypothesis. Practically, it means that myocardial perfusion imaging cannot be used to exclude coronary artery disease in patients with Chagas heart disease.

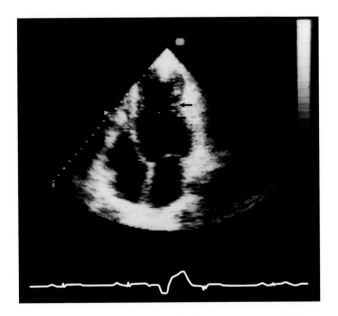

Fig. 20-8. Two-dimensional echocardiogram, apical 4-chamber view. There is a large but relatively narrow-necked apical aneurysm with mural thrombus (*arrow*). (From Hagar and Rahimtoola.[38] By permission of Mosby-Year Book.)

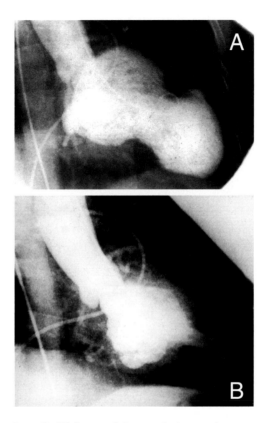

Fig. 20-9. Diastolic (*A*) and systolic (*B*) frames of cineventriculogram demonstrate a classic narrow-necked apical aneurysm. Basal akinesis is also present. From an asymptomatic patient with right bundle branch block. (From Hagar and Rahimtoola.[38] By permission of Mosby-Year Book.)

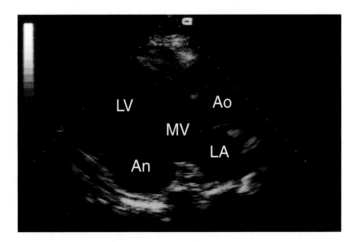

Fig. 20-10. Two-dimensional echocardiogram in parasternal long-axis view shows a large basal posterior aneurysm (*An*) and a small pericardial effusion discovered incidentally in a patient presenting with tuberculous pericarditis. *Ao*, aorta; *LA*, left atrium; *LV*, left ventricle; *MV*, mitral valve. (From Hagar and Rahimtoola.[38] By permission of Mosby-Year Book.)

Stress   Redistribution

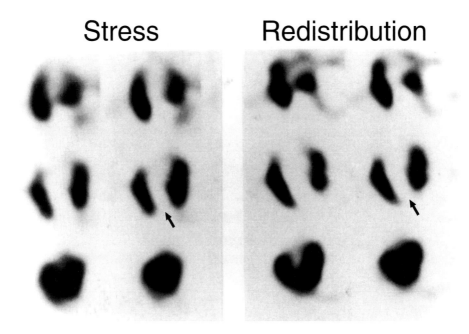

Fig. 20-11. Exercise and redistribution thallium perfusion images in Chagas disease from a patient with a large apical aneurysm who presented with cerebral embolus. There is a large fixed apical defect (*arrows*) without redistribution. (From Hagar and Rahimtoola.[38] By permission of Mosby-Year Book.)

VENTRICULAR ARRHYTHMIAS

The pathology of Chagas heart disease is highly conducive to the development of ventricular arrhythmias. Malignant ventricular arrhythmias and sudden cardiac death are the most frequent causes of death in Chagas disease, occurring more often than in dilated cardio-myopathy.[147] Life-threatening arrhythmias may be the first manifestation of the disease, as in several of our patients. Ventricular ectopy is remarkably frequent in all stages of the disease, even when there is no other evidence of cardiac involvement.[148] Ectopy is dense and temporally unvarying, with patients often having tens of thousands of ectopic beats per day.[149] In our series, 14% of patients presented with aborted sudden death, and sustained ventricular tachycardia or sudden death occurred subsequently in 39% of patients with left ventricular aneurysm or dysfunction.

The severity and complexity of ventricular ectopy are related to the extent of myocardial disease. Nonsustained ventricular tachycardia has been found by ambulatory monitoring in 10% of patients with mild wall motion abnormalities, in 56% of those with severe wall motion abnormalities or aneurysms without heart failure, and in 87% of those with advanced congestive heart failure.[137] The 25 patients in our series who had ambulatory ECG monitoring all had frequent ventricular premature beats. Nonsustained ventricular tachycardia was found in 9, of whom 5 had inducible sustained ventricular tachycardia on subsequent programmed ventricular stimulation. However, 6 other patients with inducible ventricular tachycardia and 4 with subsequent spontaneous ventricular tachycardia or sudden death had no ventricular tachycardia on a single 24-hour ECG.

Electrophysiologic testing in asymptomatic patients with cardiac involvement has shown that sinus node dysfunction is present in 18%, pacing-induced atrioventricular block in 41%, and multiple sites of conducting system dysfunction often coexist.[150] Sustained ventricular tachycardia is inducible with programmed ventricular stimulation in most patients who present with sustained ventricular arrhythmias and in half of those who have symptomatic nonsustained ventricular tachycardia.[151] The sites of origin of ventricular tachycardia are typically left ventricular or septal, are frequently at the edge of an area of abnormal wall motion, and may be multiple. When the sites of earliest activation of ventricular tachycardia within aneurysms have been examined histologically, these sites contain subendocardial islets of viable but often damaged myocytes interdigitated with areas of dense fibrous connective tissue.[152] Treatment of arrhythmias and the role of invasively guided antiarrhythmic therapy are discussed in a later section.

CONGESTIVE HEART FAILURE

Congestive heart failure is a late manifestation of Chagas heart disease that indicates an extensive amount of irreversible myocardial damage and structural abnormality. Congestive heart failure usually develops after age 40 years and tends to occur later in the course of the disease than symptomatic atrioventricular block or ventricular aneurysm. When congestive heart failure does develop in a patient younger than age 30 years, it indicates a particularly fulminant form of the disease, with aggressive myocarditis and a poor prognosis.[153]

Diastolic dysfunction is frequently found by echocardiography in patients with Chagas disease and develops early in the course of the disease. It manifests as impaired isovolumic relaxation and diminished ventricular filling and is usually not associated with segmental wall motion abnormalities or systolic dysfunction.[154] Nearly one-half of patients who would otherwise be classified as indeterminate phase have this abnormality, as do nearly all with symptomatic cardiac disease. The clinical and prognostic significance of diastolic dysfunction in Chagas disease is uncertain, but it should be taken as evidence of cardiac involvement in seropositive patients if other causes of diastolic dysfunction are excluded.

THROMBOEMBOLISM

Thromboembolism, arterial and venous, appears to be quite frequent in advanced Chagas disease, and its occurrence is probably underdiagnosed.[155,156] At autopsy, 73% of patients have left or right ventricular mural thrombi, with evidence of pulmonary or systemic embolization in 60%.[157] The apical aneurysm typical of Chagas disease is particularly prone to the formation of thrombi[158] and is associated with a high incidence of thromboembolic events.

Three of the patients in our series presented with systemic thromboembolic events as the initial manifestation of their disease (Table 20-3). During follow-up, 1 patient had an acute myocardial infarction and another had unstable angina with marked transient T-wave changes; both patients had left ventricular mural thrombi and normal coronary arteries, suggesting coronary artery embolism.[159]

ATRIOVENTRICULAR BLOCK

In cross-sectional studies it has been appreciated that the conduction block in Chagas heart disease progresses steadily over time: from incomplete to complete right bundle branch block, left anterior fascicular block, and finally to complete atrioventricular block. In these studies, complete atrioventricular block is found in approximately 1% of all sero-positive individuals, 5% to 8% of those who meet criteria for heart disease (Table 20-4), and 20% to 30% of patients with advanced cardiac disease. Many of these patients have nearly normal ventricular function and a good prognosis with permanent pacing. On the other hand, complete heart block commonly develops in patients with advanced heart failure and may be manifest when antiarrhythmic drug treatment is required. Syncope or near-syncope is the usual symptom on presentation. Some cases of unexplained cardiac death in rural areas may also be due to atrioventricular block. In our series, 9 patients (21%) had symptomatic second degree or third degree block at diagnosis. Ultimately, 15 patients (36%) required permanent pacemaker insertion, usually VVI or VVIR, for these indications. Left ventricular aneurysm or dysfunction was not more frequent in patients who received pacemakers, and congestive heart failure, arrhythmic events, and death did not develop more frequently during follow-up.

CARDIOVASCULAR AUTONOMIC DYSFUNCTION

Cardiovascular autonomic dysfunction is found frequently in patients with Chagas disease, consistent with the autonomic nervous system abnormalities described earlier. Although such abnormalities are sometimes found in dilated cardiomyopathy of any cause, they are more frequent and more severe and develop earlier in Chagas disease. Reported abnormalities include blunted hemodynamic response to exercise,[160] postural hypotension,[161] and diminished heart rate variability,[162] predominantly due to parasympathetic denervation. Abnormal responses to baroreflex testing,[163] handgrip,[164] atropine,[165] and the Valsalva maneuver[166] are frequently found at all stages of the disease. Plasma norepinephrine concentrations correlated with increasing degrees of autonomic dysfunction.[167] Such abnormalities are sometimes found in the absence of other signs of heart disease, but they are more frequent when some degree of cardiac or gastrointestinal tract disease is present.[168] The clinical significance of such autonomic abnormalities is uncertain, but some have suggested a relationship to the development of sudden cardiac death.[169]

PROGNOSIS AND NATURAL HISTORY

Infection with *T cruzi* significantly shortens the life expectancy of affected persons. Mortality rates vary greatly between geographic regions, suggesting that environmental factors, comorbid infections, or trypanosome strain may influence the severity or progression of disease.[170] In a rural Venezuelan population with a prevalence of infection of 47% studied for 4 years, heart disease developed in initially seropositive patients at a rate of 1.1%/year.[171] Mortality due to Chagas heart disease in this period was 7% in those younger than age 50 years and 3% in the entire group, accounting for 69% of all deaths. Death typically results a minimum of 15 years after infection, with most persons dying of Chagas heart disease between age 25 and 45 years. Chagas disease is by far the leading cause of death in this young age group in endemic areas, making it a major public health problem.

The cause of death in Chagas heart disease is sudden cardiac death in approximately 50% of patients, congestive heart failure in 40%, and cerebral embolism in 10%. Among the patients in our series, 9 of the 11 deaths were sudden. Sudden death is more frequent than death from congestive heart failure in younger patients, in stage II patients (segmental wall motion abnormalities without heart failure),[172] and in those with complex and sustained ectopy on ambulatory ECG.[173] Sudden death in Chagas heart disease, usually due to ventricular tachycardia or fibrillation, is frequent in endemic countries; autopsy studies of fatal traffic accidents and sudden death often reveal that Chagas heart disease is the sole finding.[172] Half of those dying suddenly are asymptomatic before death, and death is the first sign of Chagas disease. Nearly all such individuals have significant, often extensive, ventricular abnormalities and conduction system disease.[174,175]

The presence of congestive heart failure is the strongest predictor of subsequent mortality in all studies. Mortality in such patients is high, probably higher than in patients with congestive heart failure from other etiologies.[176] Ten-year survival in a typical study was 9% after development of congestive heart failure (stage III) compared with 65% in those with ECG abnormalities without heart failure (stage II), and it was normal in seropositive patients with a normal ECG (stage I).[177] Among those who have congestive heart failure, maximum oxygen consumption, functional class, and ejection fraction predict survival.[178]

In our series (average follow-up, 56 ± 9 months), 5-year survival was 64%[38] (Fig. 20-12). Five-year survival was 30% in those with left ventricular dysfunction versus 88% in those with normal function. No deaths occurred in patients without either ventricular aneurysm or systolic dysfunction versus 42% survival in patients having either one. Factors associated with decreased survival are shown in Table 20-6. Congestive heart failure at initial presentation and its occurrence during follow-up were the 2 historical features most strongly associated with a fatal outcome. In a multivariate model, initial congestive heart failure and the presence of either left ventricular aneurysm or systolic dysfunction (P = 0.03) were the only independent predictors of subsequent death.

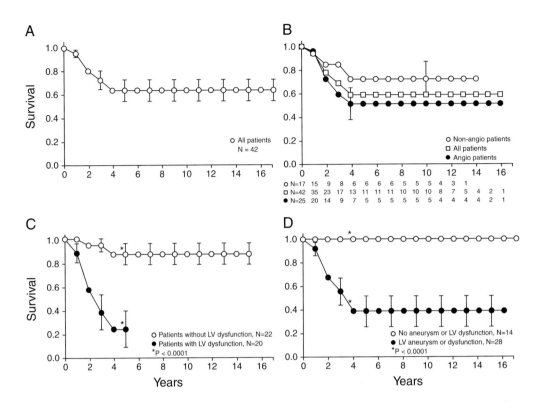

Fig. 20-12. Actuarial survival of Chagas heart disease patients seen in the United States. *A*, Survival of the entire group. *B*, Survival of patients having or not having coronary angiography (see text). *C*, Survival of patients with and without left ventricular (*LV*) dysfunction. *D*, Survival of patients with either LV aneurysm or dysfunction or without either. (*A* and *C* from Hagar and Rahimtoola.[38] By permission of Mosby-Year Book. *B* and *D* from Hagar and Rahimtoola.[37] By permission of the Massachusetts Medical Society.)

DIAGNOSIS OF CHAGAS HEART DISEASE OUTSIDE OF ENDEMIC AREAS

To correctly diagnose and treat Chagas heart disease, clinicians outside of endemic areas must become familiar with its protean manifestations and aware of its true prevalence. North American physicians may believe that Chagas heart disease does not exist there or that it is found only in persons from South America. With increased awareness on the part of North American clinicians, it is likely that Chagas heart disease will be recognized more often and earlier.

One reason for problems in diagnosis is that Chagas disease may mimic other forms of heart disease, particularly coronary artery disease, and commonly used noninvasive tests cannot reliably distinguish them. Chest pain is a frequent complaint of patients with Chagas disease. Although it is usually atypical of angina, it may prompt diagnostic evaluation. ECG changes suggestive of myocardial infarction or ischemia are quite typical of this disease. Further complicating matters, radionuclide perfusion scans are consistently abnormal in Chagas heart disease, with abnormalities consistent with myocardial infarction or

Table 20-6
Univariate Predictors of Survival in North American Patients With Chagas Heart Disease

Feature	Patients with feature, %	RR	P*
Congestive heart failure on initial presentation	24	4.8	0.002[†]
Aneurysm or LV dysfunction present	67	2.4	0.002[†]
LV dysfunction present	48	5.8	0.001
ST-segment elevation present on ECG	14	2.8	0.002
Pathologic Q waves present on ECG	43	4.5	0.01
Congestive heart failure during follow-up	26	3.4	0.04
Left atrial enlargement	31	3.4	0.02
Moderate or severe mitral regurgitation present[‡]	19	2.5	0.007

	Mean of patients dying	Mean of patients surviving	P
LV end-diastolic volume index[‡]	200 ± 25 mL[§]	102 ± 8 mL	0.006
Left atrial dimension[‡]	47 ± 3 mm[§]	40 ± 2 mm	0.05

ECG, electrocardiogram; LV, left ventricular; RR, relative risk.
*From linear regression of survival time with log-rank test ($n = 42$).
[†]Variables independently predicting survival in multivariate model.
[‡]Mitral regurgitation greater than 1+ (1-4+ scale) by 2-D color Doppler echocardiography or cineventricu-lography ($n = 42$). Left atrial dimension by M-mode echocardiogram ($n = 31$). Mean ± SEM.
[§]Mean differences significant $P < 0.05$ by Student t test.
From Hagar and Rahimtoola.[38] By permission of Mosby-Year Book.

ischemia (or both). In fact, 55% of our patients had been treated previously by physicians for other presumed diagnoses, usually coronary artery disease, for periods up to 9 years. Although the clinical syndromes, ECG, and ventricular abnormalities in our North American patients do not differ from those in endemic countries, the clinical findings of Chagas heart disease usually are attributed to coronary artery disease or dilated cardiomyopathy in a country where these diseases are much more prevalent. Coronary angiography may be necessary to exclude atherosclerotic heart disease in nonendemic countries, especially in older patients and in those with segmental wall motion abnormalities.

Finally, the criteria for the diagnosis of Chagas disease in populations with a low prevalence of infection are problematic. Some patients with cardiac disorders have low-level positive or equivocal serologic tests for *T cruzi*, and others who have never resided in an endemic area have false-positive results. Such patients should not be considered to have definite Chagas heart disease. Additional serologic or parasitologic testing is useful in such cases. This emphasizes the importance of the case definition described above, which requires epidemiologic, serologic, and clinical criteria to be met. Although not appropriate in all populations, the use of such a definition is essential in populations where the number of false-positive serologic results exceeds the number of cases of Chagas disease or where other forms of cardiomyopathy are far more frequent than Chagas heart disease.

TREATMENT

Management of patients with Chagas heart disease is mostly oriented toward treating and preventing its complications: congestive heart failure, atrioventricular block, thromboembolism, and malignant ventricular arrhythmias. The role of antiparasitic drugs in all phases of *T cruzi* infection has begun to expand as our understanding of the disease has increased, but many important questions about their use will remain unanswered until randomized trials can be done.

TREATMENT OF CONGESTIVE HEART FAILURE

Congestive heart failure in Chagas heart disease responds to digitalis, diuretics, and vasodilators as in heart failure due to other cardiomyopathic disorders. There is little evidence to suggest that outcome is improved with pharmacologic therapy, and the ominous prognosis associated with development of congestive heart failure has already been discussed. Angiotensin-converting enzyme inhibitors are useful to improve symptoms in patients with advanced Chagas cardiomyopathy and to reduce neurohormonal activation,[179,180] but there is no evidence that their use improves survival. Long-term anticoagulation therapy is almost certainly appropriate in patients with severe left ventricular dysfunction or left ventricular aneurysm, in view of the high incidence of thromboembolism and the morbidity that results from it. However, routine anticoagulation therapy is not often used in endemic areas because of socioeconomic factors, and controlled trials of its benefits are therefore not available. Second-generation β-blockers (bisoprolol, metoprolol CR/XL, or carvedilol) may be tried in those with chronic heart failure.

MANAGEMENT OF HEART BLOCK WITH PACING

Experience with permanent ventricular pacing in Chagas disease is extensive in South American tertiary care centers. In general, the symptomatic status and probably the longevity of patients with Chagas disease are improved by permanent ventricular pacing.[181] Single-chamber ventricular pacing is generally used, and dual-chamber or rate-responsive pacing offers little additional benefit for most patients.[182] Mortality in patients with permanent pacemakers depends mainly on the severity of the underlying myocardial disease and averages 5% per year.

MANAGEMENT OF VENTRICULAR ARRHYTHMIAS

Ventricular tachyarrhythmias are clearly the most serious and difficult to treat of the complications of Chagas disease, dubbed a "tachycardiomyopathy" by some authors.[183] At present, there is no consensus on the indications, efficacy, or choice of the available antiarrhythmic agents and treatments. What is generally agreed is that ventricular arrhythmias often are highly malignant, drug therapy is frequently disappointing, and none of the available agents is very effective at preventing arrhythmic events in patients with advanced Chagas heart disease.

Invasively guided antiarrhythmic drug therapy seems to offer a good method for risk stratification and drug selection in patients with symptomatic or high-grade ventricular arrhythmias (or both). Sustained ventricular tachycardia is inducible in more than 80% of patients with clinical sustained ventricular tachycardia and in 50% of those with non-sustained ventricular tachycardia or presenting with syncope; a prolonged HV interval is also found in a third.[184] Arrhythmias that are inducible frequently can be rendered noninducible by drug therapy,[185] which has been found to prolong survival.[186] However, only 29% of all patients studied were in this category. In the remainder, sustained ventricular tachycardia was noninducible or an effective drug could not be identified. Nonpharmacologic therapy or empiric therapy with amiodarone typically is used in such patients.

In our series, 9 of 15 patients studied with programmed ventricular stimulation (indications of nonsustained ventricular tachycardia in 6, syncope or near-syncope in 4, aborted sudden death in 3, and sustained ventricular tachycardia in 2) had inducible sustained ventricular tachycardia or ventricular fibrillation. They were treated with invasively guided antiarrhythmic therapy or, failing this, an implantable cardioverter defibrillator or left ventricular aneurysmectomy. There has been only 1 sudden death in this group. Two patients had inducible monomorphic ventricular tachycardia that terminated spontaneously; 1 of these had sudden death. Four patients had no inducible arrhythmia and were treated with empiric antiarrhythmic therapy; 3 of the 4 subsequently died suddenly. Three of 5 patients treated empirically with amiodarone subsequently died suddenly. This experience, in patients with advanced disease, emphasizes the highly malignant nature of the arrhythmias, the limitations of pharmacotherapy, the value of an invasively guided approach in some cases, and the need to treat high-risk individuals even if tachycardia is noninducible on electrophysiologic testing.

Essentially all known antiarrhythmic drugs have been used in patients with Chagas heart disease.[187] Unfortunately, these trials usually have been uncontrolled, noninvasively guided or empiric, and short-term. No drug has been shown to prolong survival in a randomized trial. In comparative studies using ambulatory electrocardiography, Haedo et al.[188] and Rosenbaum et al.[189] showed that amiodarone is the most effective of the antiarrhythmic agents and is well tolerated. Patients with malignant arrhythmias treated with amiodarone and followed for 26 months with ambulatory ECG had few arrhythmic events.[190] In another study,[191] there was a low risk of recurrence or death when the ejection fraction was above 30%, but there was a 100% recurrence rate and an 80% mortality in functional class III-IV patients with an ejection fraction less than 30%. An implantable defibrillator would be more appropriate in such patients. Proarrhythmia appears to be common in patients with Chagas disease[192] and occurred in 4 of our patients. Proarrhythmia has been reported with all agents, including amiodarone.[193] This is emphasized by a report of 10 patients with Chagas heart disease who died during ambulatory ECG monitoring. In 6 of 10 patients, the terminal event was torsades de pointes due to type IA antiarrhythmic drugs.[194] These data support the concept that drug therapy cannot prevent arrhythmic death in patients with Chagas heart disease and highlight the need for a greater use of nonpharmacologic therapies.

The implantable cardioverter-defibrillator has been used successfully in small numbers of patients with Chagas heart disease.[195] Implantable defibrillator placement may be the optimum therapy for survivors of sudden cardiac death syndrome whose arrhythmia cannot be induced during programmed ventricular stimulation or cannot be suppressed with pharmacologic therapy. Nonsustained ventricular tachycardia is frequent in such patients, and additional antiarrhythmic drug therapy frequently is required to reduce inappropriate discharges. Chagas disease patients with implantable defibrillators respond similarly to coronary disease patients,[196] although they tend to experience more shocks.[197] The effect of defibrillator implantation on survival has not been determined. Successful transcoronary[198] and radio frequency catheter ablation[199,200] have been reported in a few cases. These therapies might be considered in patients with refractory arrhythmias who have normal left ventricular function and who are not candidates for aneurysmectomy or an implantable defibrillator.

Aneurysmectomy is an effective treatment for refractory ventricular arrhythmias if there is a localized aneurysm and left ventricular function is preserved.[201,202] Two patients in our series with discrete apical aneurysms and normal overall ventricular function were treated with aneurysmectomy for life-threatening ventricular arrhythmias. These patients subsequently remained free of events for 14 and 18 years until presenting with global ventricular dysfunction, congestive heart failure, and recurrent arrhythmias. This indicates the effectiveness of aneurysmectomy in this subset of patients and the relentlessly progressive nature of myocardial damage in Chagas disease.

ANTIPARASITIC THERAPY FOR *T CRUZI* INFECTION

The 2 best studied antitrypanosomal agents for treatment of *T cruzi* infection in humans are nifurtimox and benznidazole. The adult dose of benznidazole is 5 mg/kg per day for 30 to 60 days. Nifurtimox, which is no longer manufactured, is given in an adult dose of 10 mg/kg per day for 60 to 120 days, although gastrointestinal tract toxicity may limit the duration of therapy. Both drugs may cause leukopenia and polyneuritis. Redox cycling of these agents generates reactive oxygen species toxic to *T cruzi* because it lacks antioxidant enzymes.[203] In the United States, benznidazole is available from the Centers for Disease Control.

The indications for antiparasitic therapy have changed considerably and continue to evolve. Antiparasitic therapy is indicated for 1) all patients with acute phase disease, 2) children and young adults with indeterminate phase disease, 3) adults in the indeterminate phase or with early manifestations of heart disease, 4) infection resulting from laboratory accidents or operations, and 5) reactivation of infection in transplant recipients and other immunosuppressed individuals. Use in those with established heart disease is uncertain.

Treatment with benznidazole or nifurtimox in the acute phase produces long-term negative xenodiagnosis in 90% of patients and negative serologic results in about 80%.[204] However, the rate of parasitologic cure can be as low as 20% in some highly resistant strains.[205] In early indeterminate phase infection, 58% to 62% of schoolchildren treated with benznidazole had negative serologic results after 3 to 4 years.[206,207] Persons who achieve negative serologic results and xenodiagnosis (or PCR) after treatment of acute disease can be considered cured of their *T cruzi* infection, and late end-organ disease does not appear to develop in such patients.

Things are more complicated in the chronic phase. Treatment in the chronic phase results in negative xenodiagnosis in 90% to 98% of cases[208] but rarely results in a negative serologic finding.[209] This represents persistent antibodies cross-reacting with antigenic determinants in intestinal flora or continuing parasitemia below the level of detection of xenodiagnosis. It is important to make this distinction; otherwise parasitologic cure cannot be ascertained. To overcome this limitation, investigators have used highly purified or recombinant *T cruzi* antigens, immunoabsorption of serum samples,[210] the complement-mediated lysis test,[211] or an enzyme-linked immunosorbent assay directed against a panel of anti-Galalpha epitopes[212] to determine parasitologic cure. Detection of *T cruzi* DNA by PCR may be the ideal approach to determine parasitologic cure.[125]

PCR demonstrated the elimination of parasitemia in 67% of patients in the chronic phase and treated with benznidazole, and it was more sensitive than repeated xenodiagnosis.[213] Thus, a third of individuals with persistently negative xenodiagnosis after treatment, who previously would have been considered cured, actually have persistent parasitemia. One study found that in none of the patients treated with benznidazole was the parasite eliminated.[214] In another study, 9 of 10 patients treated with benznidazole for acute disease had persistence of myocarditis on biopsy after 11 months, in spite of negative results of xenodiagnosis, and cardiac disease later developed in several.[215] Thus, the application of PCR and other methods has redefined parasitologic cure and demonstrated the frequent ineffectiveness of drug therapy.

In the chronic phase, evidence suggests that antiparasitic treatment might prevent late end-organ damage in humans, as it does in animals.[216,217] In chronically infected patients treated with benznidazole and followed for 8 years, cardiac disease developed much less frequently than in untreated patients.[218] The role of drug therapy to halt the progression of disease in patients with overt cardiac disease, however, is not well studied. Antiparasitic drugs might be expected to benefit patients with mild or moderate cardiac disease who have a life expectancy of at least several years, given the progressive nature of the cardiac damage, but this is speculative.

New and better antiparasitic drugs are needed. Many other agents have been used empirically to treat Chagas disease but have proven ineffective or excessively toxic. Keto-conazole, although minimally effective alone,[219] may enhance the effectiveness of benznidazole.[220] Allopurinol, which inhibits *T cruzi* purine metabolism, is modestly effective in vivo and in vitro against *T cruzi* and is well tolerated;[221] it may be useful in cases resistant to conventional agents. Thioridazine and other phenothiazines are highly effective antitrypanosomal agents.[222] Their neuropsychiatric side effects preclude their clinical use, but they may serve as a starting point for new drug design. Newer molecular modeling techniques[223] have led to development of a highly effective inhibitor of a *T cruzi* cysteine protease that is undergoing clinical trials.[224]

Attempts to develop an effective human vaccine to *T cruzi* have been unsuccessful. Such a vaccine would be useful in endemic areas where transmission of *T cruzi* still occurs. One vaccine has been partially protective in dogs, but its effectiveness is short-lived and incomplete.[225]

T CRUZI AND IMMUNOSUPPRESSION

Given the importance of host immune mechanisms, especially CD4+ lymphocytes, in pro-tection against *T cruzi*, it is not surprising that immunosuppressive therapy may lead to reactivation or progression of clinical disease, as seen in experimental models.[226] In humans such reactivation may be fulminant or may have unusual manifestations such as brain abscess or panniculitis. Clinically evident reactivation is uncommon in patients undergoing immunosuppressive therapy for hematologic malignancies and collagen vascular diseases; thus, routine administration of prophylactic antiparasitic therapy is not recommended. However, corticosteroid treatment is known to increase levels of parasitemia,[227] and monitoring of parasitemia during treatment may be advisable in some patients.

After renal and bone marrow transplantation in patients with chronic *T cruzi* infection, reactivation occurs in 20% to 25%.[228] Reactivation is diagnosed more reliably by measure-ment of parasitemia than by serologic testing, which is frequently negative.[229] In such patients, it is recommended that serologic status and parasitemia be monitored routinely and any parasitemia or change in serologic status be treated promptly before clinical disease develops.[230] Recipients of organs from *T cruzi*-infected donors have a relatively low rate of infection; they should also be monitored and treated as needed.

CARDIAC TRANSPLANTATION

In transplant centers that have significant populations of patients with Chagas disease, Chagas disease is not considered a contraindication to cardiac transplantation, although special concerns must be addressed. Immunosuppression frequently results in acute reactivation of disease, even if antiparasitic therapy is administered prophylactically.[231] Such infection may be particularly fulminant and is often associated with characteristic skin lesions[232] or central nervous system disease.[233] Trypanosomes frequently are present in endomyocardial biopsy specimens in such cases, but standard serologic tests may not parallel the activity of the disease. This acute reactivation generally responds well to treatment with a short course of nifurtimox or benznidazole. In view of the acute toxicity of the available antiparasitic agents, most centers administer such therapy to cardiac transplant patients only when endomyocardial biopsies or clinical findings suggest reactivation of disease.

Several small series found excellent long-term survival in Chagas heart disease patients undergoing cardiac transplantation.[234,235] However, there is a higher incidence of lymphoid and solid tumors in patients who have Chagas disease than in other transplant patients.[236] Careful regulation or reduction of the level of immunosuppression may reduce the incidence of this complication.

CONCLUSION

Chagas disease is a major public health problem in Central and South America that is only recently being controlled through intensive public health measures and improved housing. Cardiac involvement is its most frequent and serious manifestation. As a result of immigration, Chagas heart disease is now encountered outside of endemic countries, especially in the United States.

The manifestations of Chagas heart disease are diverse and are the result of progressive damage to the myocardium, extracellular matrix, cardiac autonomic innervation, and possibly the coronary microvessels. Chagas heart disease often mimics ischemic heart disease and commonly used noninvasive tests cannot reliably distinguish them in populations where the latter is far more common. Prognosis depends largely on the extent of myocardial damage and is poor when left ventricular dysfunction or aneurysm or both are present. Ventricular arrhythmias in these patients are exceptionally malignant. Aggressive public health measures and advances in the understanding of the pathobiology of the disease hold the promise that this fascinating and deadly disease can be eliminated.

REFERENCES

1. Chagas C. Neue Trypanosomiasis. Arch Schiffs Tropen-Hygiene 1909;13:120-122.

2. Chagas C. Ueber eine neue Trypanosomiasis des Menschen. Arch Schiffs Tropen-Hygiene 1909;13:351-353.

3. Lewinsohn R. Carlos Chagas (1879-1934): the discovery of *Trypanosoma cruzi* and of American trypanosomiasis (foot-notes to the history of Chagas's disease). Trans R Soc Trop Med Hyg 1979;73:513-523.

4. Chagas C. Nova Tripanozomiaze humana. Estudios sobre a morfolojia e o ciclo evolutivo do *Schizotrypanum cruzi* n. gen., n. sp., ajente etiolojio de nova entidade morbida do homen. Mem do Inst Oswaldo Cruz 1909;1:159-218.

5. Chagas C. Nova entidade morbida do homen. Rezumo geral de estudos etiologicos e clinicos. Mem do Inst Oswaldo Cruz 1911;3:219-275.

6. Chagas C, Villela E. Forma cardiaca da Trypanosomiase Americana. Mem do Inst Oswaldo Cruz 1922;14:5-61.

7. de Gorodner OL, Mendivil GT, Risso A, Risso JJ, Petraglia G, De Francesco C, Bustamante A. [Natural Chagas' disease in dogs. Serologic, anatomopathologic and electrocardiographic studies of the chronic indeterminate phase of the infection.] Medicina 1985;45:535-538.

8. Zeledón R. Epidemiology, modes of transmission and reservoir hosts of Chagas' disease. Ciba Found Symp 1974;20:51-77.

9. Anonymous. Immunology of Chagas' disease. Bull World Health Organ 1974;50:459-472.

10. Zaidenberg M. [Congenital Chagas' disease in the province of Salta, Argentina, from 1980 to 1997.] Rev Soc Bras Med Trop 1999;32:689-695.

11. Blanco SB, Segura EL, Gurtler RE. [Control of congenital transmission of *Trypanosoma cruzi* in Argentina.] Medicina (B Aires) 1999;59 Suppl 2:138-142.

12. Barnabe C, Brisse S, Tibayrenc M. Population structure and genetic typing of *Trypanosoma cruzi*, the agent of Chagas disease: a multilocus enzyme electrophoresis approach. Parasitology 2000;120:513-526.

13. Blanco A, Montamat EE. Genetic variation among *Trypanosoma cruzi* populations. J Exp Zool 1998;282:62-70.

14. Espinoza B, Vera-Cruz JM, Gonzalez H, Ortega E, Hernandez R. Genotype and virulence correlation within Mexican stocks of *Trypanosoma cruzi* isolated from patients. Acta Trop 1998;70:63-72.

15. Vago AR, Andrade LO, Leite AA, d'Avila Reis D, Macedo AM, Adad SJ, Tostes S Jr, Moreira MC, Filho GB, Pena SD. Genetic characterization of *Trypanosoma cruzi* directly from tissues of patients with chronic Chagas disease: differential distribution of genetic types into diverse organs. Am J Pathol 2000;156:1805-1809.

16. Oliveira RP, Melo AI, Macedo AM, Chiari E, Pena SD. The population structure of *Trypanosoma cruzi*: expanded analysis of 54 strains using eight polymorphic CA-repeat microsatellites. Mem Inst Oswaldo Cruz 1999;94 Suppl 1:65-70.

17. Oswaldo Cruz Institute. Department of Biochemistry and Molecular Biology. United Web Project to Biotechnology in Latin-America and the Caribbean. Retrieved December 17, 2001, from the World Wide Web: http://www.dbbm.fiocruz.br.

18. Levin MJ. [Contribution of the *Trypanosoma cruzi* Genome Project to the understanding of the pathogenesis of Chagas disease.] Medicina (B Aires) 1999;59 Suppl 2:18-24.

19. Dimock KA, Davis CD, Kuhn RE. Effect of elevated environmental temperature on the antibody response of mice to *Trypanosoma cruzi* during the acute phase of infection. Infect Immun 1991;59:4377-4382.

20. Machado CR, Moraes-Santos T, Machado AB. Cardiac noradrenalin in relation to protein malnutrition in chronic experimental Chagas' disease in the rat. Am J Trop Med Hyg 1984;33:835-838.

21. Marinho CR, D'Imperio Lima MR, Grisotto MG, Alvarez JM. Influence of acute-phase parasite load on pathology, parasitism, and activation of the immune system at the late chronic phase of Chagas' disease. Infect Immun 1999;67:308-318.

22. Higuchi MD. Chronic chagasic cardiopathy: the product of a turbulent host-parasite relationship. Rev Inst Med Trop Sao Paulo 1997;39:53-60.

23. Cedillos RA. Current knowledge of the epidemiology of Chagas' disease in Central America and Panama. In: Brenner RR, Stoka AM, eds. Chagas' disease vectors. Volume I: Taxonomic, ecological, and epidemiological aspects. Boca Raton, FL: CRC Press, 1988:41-56.

24. Goldsmith RS, Zarate RJ, Zarate LG, Kagan I, Jacobson LB. Clinical and epidemiologic studies of Chagas' disease in rural communities in Oaxaca State, Mexico, and a seven-year follow-up: I. Cerro del Aire. Bull Pan Am Health Organ 1985;19:120-138.

25. Kagan IG, Norman L, Allain D. Studies of *Trypanosoma cruzi* isolated in the United States: a review. Rev Biol Trop 1966;14:55-73.

26. Woody NC, Woody HB. American trypanosomiasis (Chagas' disease). First indigenous case in the United States. JAMA 1955;159:676-677.

27. Greer DA. Found. Two cases of Chagas' disease. Tex Health Bull 1956;9:11-13.

28. Schiffler RJ, Mansur GP, Navin TR, Limpakarnjanarat K. Indigenous Chagas' disease (American trypanosomiasis) in California. JAMA 1984;251:2983-2984.

29. Herwaldt BL, Grijalva MJ, Newsome AL, McGhee CR, Powell MR, Nemec DG, Steurer FJ, Eberhard ML. Use of polymerase chain reaction to diagnose the fifth reported US case of autochthonous transmission of *Trypanosoma cruzi*, in Tennessee, 1998. J Infect Dis 2000;181:395-399.

30. World Health Organization. Special programme for research and training in tropical diseases. Tropical disease research: progress 1995-96: thirteenth programme report UNDP/World Bank/WHO Special Programme for Research & Training in Tropical Diseases (TDR). Geneva: World Health Organization, 1997.

31. Puigbo JJ, Rhode JR, Barrios HG, Suarez JA, Yepez CG. Clinical and epidemiological study of chronic heart involvement in Chagas' disease. Bull World Health Organ 1966;34:655-669.

32. Maguire JH, Mott KE, Lehman JS, Hoff R, Muniz TM, Guimaraes AC, Sherlock I, Morrow RH. Relationship of electrocardiographic abnormalities and seropositivity to *Trypanosoma cruzi* within a rural community in northeast Brazil. Am Heart J 1983;105:287-294.

33. Maguire JH, Hoff R, Sherlock I, Guimaraes AC, Sleigh AC, Ramos NB, Mott KE, Weller TH. Cardiac morbidity and mortality due to Chagas' disease: prospective electrocardiographic study of a Brazilian community. Circulation 1987;75:1140-1145.

34. Amorim DS. Chagas' disease. Prog Cardiol 1979;8:235-279.

35. Kirchhoff LV, Gam AA, Gilliam FC. American trypanosomiasis (Chagas' disease) in Central American immigrants. Am J Med 1987;82:915-920.

36. Kerndt PR, Waskin HA, Kirchhoff LV, Steurer F, Waterman SH, Nelson JM, Gellert GA, Shulman IA. Prevalence of antibody to *Trypanosoma cruzi* among blood donors in Los Angeles, California. Transfusion 1991;31:814-818.

37. Hagar JM, Rahimtoola SH. Chagas' heart disease in the United States. N Engl J Med 1991;325:763-768.

38. Hagar JM, Rahimtoola SH. Chagas' heart disease. Curr Probl Cardiol 1995;20:825-924.

39. Massumi RA, Gooch A. Chagas' myocarditis. Arch Intern Med 1965;116:531-536.

40. Kirchhoff LV, Neva FA. Chagas' disease in Latin American immigrants. JAMA 1985;254:3058-3060.

41. Pearlman JD. Chagas' disease in northern California. No longer an endemic diagnosis. Am J Med 1983;75:1057-1060.

42. Feit A, El-Sherif N, Korostoff S. Chagas' disease masquerading as coronary artery disease. Arch Intern Med 1983;143:144-145.

43. Lorenzana R. Chronic Chagas' myocarditis. Report of a case. Am J Clin Pathol 1967;48:39-43.

44. Shafii A. Chagas' disease with cardiopathy and hemiplegia. N Y State J Med 1977;77:418-419.

45. Case Records of the Massachusetts General Hospital Case 32-1993. A native of El Salvador with tachycardia and syncope. N Engl J Med 1993;329:488-496.

46. Milei J, Mautner B, Storino R, Sanchez JA, Ferrans VJ. Does Chagas' disease exist as an undiagnosed form of cardiomyopathy in the United States? Am Heart J 1992;123:1732-1735.

47. Frank M, Hegenscheid B, Janitschke K, Weinke T. Prevalence and epidemiological significance of Trypanosoma cruzi infection among Latin American immigrants in Berlin, Germany. Infection 1997;25:355-358.

48. Schmunis GA. Trypanosoma cruzi, the etiologic agent of Chagas' disease: status in the blood supply in endemic and nonendemic countries. Transfusion 1991;31:547-557.

49. Cerisola JA, Rabinovich A, Alvarez M, Di Corleto CA, Pruneda J. [Chagas' disease and blood transfusion.] Bol Oficina Sanit Panam 1972;73:203-221.

50. Zuna H, La Fuente C, Valdez E, Recacoechea M, Franco JL, Romero A, Bermudez H. [Prospective study of the transmission of Trypanosoma cruzi by blood in Bolivia.] Ann Soc Belg Med Trop 1985;65 Suppl 1:107-113.

51. Shikanai-Yasuda MA, Lopes MH, Tolezano JE, Umezawa E, Amato Neto V, Barreto AC, Higaki Y, Moreira AA, Funayama G, Barone AA, et al. [Acute Chagas' disease: transmission routes, clinical aspects and response to specific therapy in diagnosed cases in an urban center. Rev Inst Med Trop Sao Paulo 1990;32:16-27.

52. Schmuñis GA. Chagas' disease and blood transfusion. In: Rondanelli EG, ed. Blood transfusion and infectious disease. Padua: Piccin, 1989:197-218.

53. Schmuñis GA. [Risk of Chagas disease through transfusions in the Americas.] Medicina (B Aires) 1999;59 Suppl 2:125-134.

54. Grant IH, Gold JW, Wittner M, Tanowitz HB, Nathan C, Mayer K, Reich L, Wollner N, Steinherz L, Ghavimi F, O'Reilly RJ, Armstrong D. Transfusion-associated acute Chagas disease acquired in the United States. Ann Intern Med 1989;111:849-851.

55. Nickerson P, Orr P, Schroeder ML, Sekla L, Johnston JB. Transfusion-associated Trypanosoma cruzi infection in a non-endemic area. Ann Intern Med 1989;111:851-853.

56. Appleman MD, Shulman IA, Saxena S, Kirchhoff LV. Use of a questionnaire to identify potential blood donors at risk for infection with Trypanosoma cruzi. Transfusion 1993;33:61-64.

57. Shulman IA, Appleman MD, Saxena S, Hiti AL, Kirchhoff LV. Specific antibodies to Trypanosoma cruzi among blood donors in Los Angeles, California. Transfusion 1997;37:727-731.

58. Leiby DA, Fucci MH, Stumpf RJ. Trypanosoma cruzi in a low- to moderate-risk blood donor population: seroprevalence and possible congenital transmission. Transfusion 1999;39:310-315.

59. Barrett VJ, Leiby DA, Odom JL, Otani MM, Rowe JD, Roote JT, Cox KF, Brown KR, Hoiles JA, Saez-Alquezar A, Turrens JF. Negligible prevalence of antibodies against Trypanosoma cruzi among blood donors in the southeastern United States. Am J Clin Pathol 1997;108:499-503.

60. Schofield CJ, Dias JC. The Southern Cone Initiative against Chagas disease. Adv Parasitol 1999;42:1-27.

61. Lorca M, Schenone H, Contreras MC, Garcia A, Rojas A, Valdes J. [Evaluation of vectors of Chagas' disease eradication programs in Chile by serological study of children under 10 years old.] Bol Chil Parasitol 1996;51:80-85.

62. Moncayo A. Progress towards the elimination of transmission of Chagas disease in Latin America. World Health Stat Q 1997;50:195-198.

63. Parada H, Carrasco HA, Anez N, Fuenmayor C, Inglessis I. Cardiac involvement is a constant

finding in acute Chagas' disease: a clinical, parasitological and histopathological study. Int J Cardiol 1997;60:49-54.

64. Oliveira JS, Mello De Oliveira JA, Frederique U Jr, Lima Filho EC. Apical aneurysm of Chagas's heart disease. Br Heart J 1981;46:432-437.

65. Anselmi A, Pifano F, Suarez JA, Gurdiel O. Myocardiopathy in Chagas' disease. I. Comparative study of pathologic findings in chronic human and experimental Chagas' myocarditis. Am Heart J 1966;72:469-481.

66. Higuchi ML, Fukasawa S, De Brito T, Parzianello LC, Bellotti G, Ramires JA. Different micro-circulatory and interstitial matrix patterns in idiopathic dilated cardiomyopathy and Chagas' disease: a three dimensional confocal microscopy study. Heart 1999;82:279-285.

67. Mello de Oliveira JA, Meira Oliveira JS, Koberle F. Pathologic anatomy of the His-Tawara system and electrocardiographic abnormalities in chronic Chagas' heart disease. Arq Bras Cardiol 1972;25:17-25.

68. Andrade ZA, Andrade SG, Oliveira GB, Alonso DR. Histopathology of the conducting tissue of the heart in Chagas' myocarditis. Am Heart J 1978;95:316-324.

69. Andrade ZA, Camara EJ, Sadigursky M, Andrade SG. [Sinus node involvement in Chagas' disease.] Arq Bras Cardiol 1988;50:153-158.

70. Machado CR, Camargos ER, Guerra LB, Moreira MC. Cardiac autonomic denervation in congestive heart failure: comparison of Chagas' heart disease with other dilated cardiomyopathy. Hum Pathol 2000; 31:3-10.

71. Almeida HdeO, Teixeira VP, Gobbi H, Araujo WF. [Qualitative changes in the intracardiac auto-nomic nervous system in chronic Chagas' disease patients.] Arq Bras Cardiol 1983;41:171-174.

72. Mott KE, Hagstrom JWC. The pathologic lesions of the cardiac autonomic nervous system in chronic Chagas' myocarditis. Circulation 1965;31:273-286.

73. Kirchhoff LV. American trypanosomiasis (Chagas' disease). Gastroenterol Clin North Am 1996;25:517-533.

74. Higuchi ML, De Brito T, Reis MM, Barbosa A, Bellotti G, Pereira-Barreto AC, Pileggi F. Correlation between *Trypanosoma cruzi* parasitism and myocardial inflammatory infiltrate in human chronic chagasic myocarditis: light microscopy and immunohistochemical findings. Cardiovasc Pathol 1993;2:101-106.

75. Mortara RA, de Silva S, Patricio FR, Higuchi ML, Lopes ER, Gabbai AA, Carnevale P, Rocha A, Ferreira MS, Souza MM, de Franco MF, Turcato G Jr, Ferraz Neto BH. Imaging *Trypanosoma cruzi* within tissues from chagasic patients using confocal microscopy with monoclonal antibodies. Parasitol Res 1999;85:800-808.

76. Bellotti G, Bocchi EA, de Moraes AV, Higuchi ML, Barbero-Marcial M, Sosa E, Esteves-Filho A, Kalil R, Weiss R, Jatene A, Pileggi F. In vivo detection of *Trypanosoma cruzi* antigens in hearts of patients with chronic Chagas' heart disease. Am Heart J 1996;131:301-307.

77. Anez N, Carrasco H, Parada H, Crisante G, Rojas A, Fuenmayor C, Gonzalez N, Percoco G, Borges R, Guevara P, Ramirez JL. Myocardial parasite persistence in chronic chagasic patients. Am J Trop Med Hyg 1999;60:726-732.

78. Zhang L, Tarleton RL. Parasite persistence correlates with disease severity and localization in chronic Chagas' disease. J Infect Dis 1999;180:480-486.

79. Chiari E. Chagas disease diagnosis using polymerase chain reaction, hemoculture and serologic methods. Mem Inst Oswaldo Cruz 1999;94 Suppl 1:299-300.

80. Sato MN, Yamashiro-Kanashiro EH, Tanji MM, Kaneno R, Higuchi ML, Duarte AJ. CD8+ cells and natural cytotoxic activity among spleen, blood, and heart lymphocytes during the acute phase of *Trypanosoma cruzi* infection in rats. Infect Immun 1992;60:1024-1030.

81. Brener Z, Gazzinelli RT. Immunological control of *Trypanosoma cruzi* infection and pathogenesis of Chagas' disease. Int Arch Allergy Immunol 1997;114:103-110.

82. Reed SG. Immunology of *Trypanosoma cruzi* infections. Chem Immunol 1998;70:124-143.

83. Hoft DF, Schnapp AR, Eickhoff CS, Roodman ST. Involvement of CD4(+) Th1 cells in systemic immunity protective against primary and secondary challenges with *Trypanosoma cruzi*. Infect Immun 2000;68:197-204.

84. Pereira ME, Zhang K, Gong Y, Herrera EM, Ming M. Invasive phenotype of *Trypanosoma cruzi* restricted to a population expressing trans-sialidase. Infect Immun 1996;64:3884-3892.

85. Rimoldi MT, Tenner AJ, Bobak DA, Joiner KA. Complement component Clq enhances invasion of human mononuclear phagocytes and fibroblasts by *Trypanosoma cruzi* trypomastigotes. J Clin Invest 1989;84:1982-1989.

86. Barcinski MA, Dos Reis GA. Apoptosis in parasites and parasite-induced apoptosis in the host immune system: a new approach to parasitic diseases. Braz J Med Biol Res 1999;32:395-401.

87. Acosta AM, Santos-Buch CA. Autoimmune myocarditis induced by *Trypanosoma cruzi*. Circulation 1985;71:1255-1261.

88. Khoury EL, Ritacco V, Cossio PM, Laguens RP, Szarfman A, Diez C, Arana RM. Circulating antibodies to peripheral nerve in American trypanosomiasis (Chagas' disease). Clin Exp Immunol 1979;36:8-15.

89. Goin JC, Borda ES, Auger S, Storino R, Sterin-Borda L. Cardiac M(2) muscarinic cholinoceptor activation by human chagasic autoantibodies: association with bradycardia. Heart 1999;82:273-278.

90. Sterin-Borda L, Gorelik G, Postan M, Gonzalez Cappa S, Borda E. Alterations in cardiac beta-adrenergic receptors in chagasic mice and their association with circulating beta-adrenoceptor-related autoantibodies. Cardiovasc Res 1999;41:116-125.

91. Baig MK, Salomone O, Caforio AL, Goldman JH, Amuchastegui M, Caiero T, McKenna WJ. Human chagasic disease is not associated with an antiheart humoral response. Am J Cardiol 1997;79:1135-1137.

92. Gorelik G, Borda E, Postan M, Gonzalez Cappa S, Sterin-Borda L. T lymphocytes from *T. cruzi*-infected mice alter heart contractility: participation of arachidonic acid metabolites. J Mol Cell Cardiol 1992;24:9-20.

93. Laguens RP, Cabeza Meckert PM, Chambo JG. [Immunologic studies on a murine model of Chagas disease.] Medicina 1989;49:197-202.

94. Felix JC, von Kreuter BF, Santos-Buch CA. Mimicry of heart cell surface epitopes in primary anti-*Trypanosoma cruzi* Lyt2+ T lymphocytes. Clin Immunol Immunopathol 1993;68:141-146.

95. Levin MJ, Mesri E, Benarous R, Levitus G, Schijman A, Levy-Yeyati P, Chiale PA, Ruiz AM, Kahn A, Rosenbaum MB, Torres HN, Segura EL. Identification of major *Trypanosoma cruzi* antigenic determinants in chronic Chagas' heart disease. Am J Trop Med Hyg 1989;41:530-538.

96. Hernandez-Munain C, De Diego JL, Alcina A, Fresno M. A *Trypanosoma cruzi* membrane protein shares an epitope with a lymphocyte activation antigen and induces crossreactive antibodies. J Exp Med 1992;175:1473-1482.

97. Cetron MS, Basilio FP, Moraes AP, Sousa AQ, Paes JN, Kahn SJ, Wener MH, Van Voorhis WC. Humoral and cellular immune response of adults from northeastern Brazil with chronic *Trypanosoma cruzi* infection: depressed cellular immune response to *T. cruzi* antigen among Chagas' disease patients with symptomatic versus indeterminate infection. Am J Trop Med Hyg 1993;49:370-382.

98. Simoes-Barbosa A, Barros AM, Nitz N, Arganaraz ER, Teixeira AR. Integration of *Trypanosoma cruzi* kDNA minicircle sequence in the host genome may be associated with autoimmune serum factors in Chagas disease patients. Mem Inst Oswaldo Cruz 1999;94 Suppl 1:249-252.

99. Kierszenbaum F. Chagas' disease and the autoimmunity hypothesis. Clin Microbiol Rev 1999;12:210-223.

100. Andrade SG, Grimaud JA, Stocker-Guerret S. Sequential changes of the connective matrix components of the myocardium (fibronectin and laminin) and evolution of cardiac fibrosis in mice infected with *Trypanosoma cruzi*. Am J Trop Med Hyg 1989;40:252-260.

101. Wyler DJ, Libby P, Prakash S, Prioli RP, Pereira ME. Elaboration by mammalian mesenchymal cells infected with *Trypanosoma cruzi* of a fibroblast-stimulating factor that may contribute to chagasic cardiomyopathy. Infect Immun 1987;55:3188-3191.

102. Morris SA, Wittner M, Weiss L, Hatcher VB, Tanowitz HB, Bilezikian JP, Gordon PB. Extracellular matrix derived from *Trypanosoma cruzi* infected endothelial cells directs phenotypic expression. J Cell Physiol 1990;145:340-346.

103. Santana JM, Grellier P, Schrevel J, Teixeira AR. A *Trypanosoma cruzi*-secreted 80 kDa proteinase with specificity for human collagen types I and IV. Biochem J 1997;325:129-137.

104. Factor SM, Tanowitz H, Wittner M, Ventura MC. Interstitial connective tissue matrix alterations in acute murine Chagas' disease. Clin Immunol Immunopathol 1993;68:147-152.

105. Sanchez JA, Milei J, Yu ZX, Storino R, Wenthold R Jr, Ferrans VJ. Immunohistochemical localization of laminin in the hearts of patients with chronic chagasic cardiomyopathy: relationship to thickening of basement membranes. Am Heart J 1993;126:1392-1401.

106. Tanowitz HB, Morris SA, Factor SM, Weiss LM, Wittner M. Parasitic diseases of the heart I: acute and chronic Chagas' disease. Cardiovasc Pathol 1992;1:7-15.

107. Torres FW, Acquatella H, Condado JA, Dinsmore R, Palacios IF. Coronary vascular reactivity is abnormal in patients with Chagas' heart disease. Am Heart J 1995;129:995-1001.

108. Morris SA, Bilezikian JP, Hatcher V, Weiss LM, Tanowitz HB, Wittner M. *Trypanosoma cruzi*: infection of cultured human endothelial cells alters inositol phosphate synthesis. Exp Parasitol 1989;69:330-339.

109. Tanowitz HB, Gumprecht JP, Spurr D, Calderon TM, Ventura MC, Raventos-Suarez C, Kellie S, Factor SM, Hatcher VB, Wittner M, Berman JW. Cytokine gene expression of endothelial cells infected with *Trypanosoma cruzi*. J Infect Dis 1992;166:598-603.

110. Tanowitz HB, Wittner M, Morris SA, Zhao W, Weiss LM, Hatcher VB, Braunstein VL, Huang H, Douglas SA, Valcic M, Spektor M, Christ GJ. The putative mechanistic basis for the modulatory role of endothelin-1 in the altered vascular tone induced by *Trypanosoma cruzi*. Endothelium 1999;6:217-230.

111. Ramos SG, Rossi MA. Microcirculation and Chagas' disease: hypothesis and recent results. Rev Inst Med Trop Sao Paulo 1999;41:123-129.

112. Pan American Health Organization. Health Conditions in the Americas. (Scientific Publication 524.) Vol. 1. Washington, DC: Pan American Health Organization, 1990:160-164.

113. Ribeiro AL, Rocha MO. [Indeterminate form of Chagas disease: considerations about diagnosis and prognosis.] Rev Soc Bras Med Trop 1998;31:301-314.

114. Carrasco Guerra HA, Palacios-Pru E, Dagert de Scorza C, Molina C, Inglessis G, Mendoza RV. Clinical, histochemical, and ultrastructural correlation in septal endomyocardial biopsies from chronic chagasic patients: detection of early myocardial damage. Am Heart J 1987;113:716-724.

115. Mady C, Barretto AC, Stolf N, Lopes EA, Dauar D, Wajngarten M, Martinelli Filho M, Macruz R, Pileggi F. [Endomyocardial biopsy in the indeterminate form of Chagas' disease.] Arq Bras Cardiol 1981;36:387-390.

116. Higuchi ML, De Morais CF, Pereira Barreto AC, Lopes EA, Stolf N, Bellotti G, Pileggi F. The role of active myocarditis in the development of heart failure in chronic Chagas' disease: a study based on endomyocardial biopsies. Clin Cardiol 1987;10:665-670.

117. Coura JR. Evolutive patterns in Chagas' disease and the life span of *Trypanosoma cruzi* in human infections. In: New approaches in American trypanosomiasis research. (Scientific Publication 318.) Washington, DC: Pan American Health Organization, 1976:378-382.

118. Laranja FS, Dias E, Nobrega G, Miranda A. Chagas' disease: a clinical, epidemiologic, and patho-logic study. Circulation 1956;14:1035-1060.

119. Pan American Health Organization. Status of Chagas' disease in the region of the Americas. Epidemiologic Bulletin, Pan American Health Organization 1984;5:5-9.

120. Barretto AC, Azul LG, Mady C, Ianni BM, De Brito Vianna C, Belloti G, Pileggi F. [Indeterminate form of Chagas' disease. A polymorphic disease.] Arq Bras Cardiol 1990;55:347-353.

121. Puigbó JJ, Giordano H, Suárez C, Acquatella H, Combellas I. Clinical aspects in Chagas' disease. In: Madoery RJ, Madoery C, Cámera MI, eds. Actualizaciones en la Enfermedad de Chagas. Buenos Aires: Organismo Oficial del Congreso Nacional de Medicina, 1993:27-38.

122. Mahmoud AA, Warren KS. Algorithms in the diagnosis and management of exotic diseases. IV. American trypanosomiasis. J Infect Dis 1975;132:121-124.

123. Schenone H, Alfaro E, Reyes H, Taucher E. [Value of xenodiagnosis in chronic Chagasic infection.] Bol Chil Parasitol 1968;23:149-154.

124. Ribeiro-dos-Santos G, Nishiya AS, Sabino EC, Chamone DF, Saez-Alquezar A. An improved, PCR-based strategy for the detection of *Trypanosoma cruzi* in human blood samples. Ann Trop Med Parasitol 1999;93:689-694.

125. Gomes ML, Galvao LM, Macedo AM, Pena SD, Chiari E. Chagas' disease diagnosis: comparative analysis of parasitologic, molecular, and serologic methods. Am J Trop Med Hyg 1999;60:205-210.

126. Camargo E, Hoshino-Shimizu S, Macedo V, Peres BA, Castro C. [Serologic diagnosis of human *Trypanosoma cruzi* infection. Comparative study of complement fixation, immunofluorescence, hemagglutination and flocculation tests in 3,624 serum samples.] Rev Inst Med Trop Sao Paulo 1977;19:254-260.

127. Camargo ME. American trypanosomiasis (Chagas' disease). In: Balows A, Hausler WJ Jr, Ohashi M, Turano A, eds. Laboratory diagnosis of infectious diseases: principles and practice. Vol. 1. New York: Springer-Verlag, 1988:744-753.

128. Oelemann WM, Teixeira MD, Verissimo Da Costa GC, Borges-Pereira J, De Castro JA, Coura JR, Peralta JM. Evaluation of three commerical enzyme-linked immunosorbent assays for diagnosis of Chagas' disease. J Clin Microbiol 1998;36:2423-2427.

129. Winkler MA, Brashear RJ, Hall HJ, Schur JD, Pan AA. Detection of antibodies to *Trypanosoma cruzi* among blood donors in the southwestern and western United States. II. Evaluation of a supplemental enzyme immunoassay and radioimmunoprecipitation assay for confirmation of seroreactivity. Transfusion 1995;35:219-225.

130. Matsumoto TK, Hoshino-Shimizu S, Nakamura PM, Andrade HF Jr, Umezawa ES. High resolution of *Trypanosoma cruzi* amastigote antigen in serodiagnosis of different clinical forms of Chagas' disease. J Clin Microbiol 1993;31:1486-1492.

131. Reis DD, Gazzinelli RT, Gazzinelli G, Colley DG. Antibodies to *Trypanosoma cruzi* express idio-typic patterns that can differentiate between patients with asymptomatic or severe Chagas' disease. J Immunol 1993;150:1611-1618.

132. Leiby DA, Wendel S, Takaoka DT, Fachini RM, Oliveira LC, Tibbals MA. Serologic testing for *Trypanosoma cruzi*: comparison of radioimmunoprecipitation assay with commercially available indirect immunofluorescence assay, indirect hemagglutination assay, and enzyme-linked immunosorbent assay kits. J Clin Microbiol 2000;38:639-642.

133. dos Santos VM, da Cunha SF, dos Santos JA, dos Santos TA, dos Santos LA, da Cunha DF. [Frequency of precordialgia in chagasic and non-chagasic women.] Rev Soc Bras Med Trop 1998;31:59-64.

134. Rosenbaum MB, Alvarez AJ. The electrocardiogram in chronic chagasic myocarditis. Am Heart J 1955;50:492-527.

135. Chiale PA, Przybylski J, Laino RA, Halpern MS, Sanchez RA, Gabrieli A, Elizari MV, Rosenbaum MB. Electrocardiographic changes evoked by ajmaline in chronic Chagas' disease with manifest myocarditis. Am J Cardiol 1982;49:14-20.

136. Bestetti RB, Pinto LZ, Soares EG, Muccillo G, Oliveira JS. Changes in electrocardiographic patterns at different stages of Chagas' heart disease in rats. Clin Sci (Colch) 1991;80:33-37.

137. Carrasco HA, Guerrero L, Parada H, Molina C, Vegas E, Chuecos R. Ventricular arrhythmias and left ventricular myocardial function in chronic chagasic patients. Int J Cardiol 1990;28:35-41.

138. Migliore RA, Guerrero FT, Adaniya ME, Miguez G, Iannariello JH, Tamagusuku H, Posse RA. [Differences between patients with right bundle branch block and left anterior hemiblock in Chagas myocardiopathy.] Medicina 1992;52:17-22.

139. Bittencourt LA, Carvalhal SS, Miguel A Jr. [Electrocardiographic signs of apical lesions in Chagas' heart disease.] Arq Bras Cardiol 1975;28:437-442.

140. Barretto AC, Bellotti G, Deperon SD, Arteaga-Fernandez E, Mady C, Ianni BM, Pileggi F. [The value of the electrocardiogram in evaluating myocardial function in patients with Chagas' disease.] Arq Bras Cardiol 1989;52:69-73.

141. Albanesi Filho FM, Gomes Filho JB. [Apical left ventricular involvement in chronic Chagas' cardiopathy: clinical and ventriculographic aspects.] Arq Bras Cardiol 1989;52:115-120.

142. Acquatella H, Schiller NB. Echocardiographic recognition of Chagas' disease and endomyocardial fibrosis. J Am Soc Echocardiogr 1988;1:60-68.

143. Acquatella H, Schiller NB, Puigbo JJ, Giordano H, Suarez JA, Casal H, Arreaza N, Valecillos R, Hirschhaut E. M-mode and two-dimensional echocardiography in chronic Chagas' heart disease. A clinical and pathologic study. Circulation 1980;62:787-799.

144. Marin-Neto JA, Marzullo P, Sousa AC, Marcassa C, Maciel BC, Iazigi N, L'Abbate A. Radionuclide angiographic evidence for early predominant right ventricular involvement in patients with Chagas' disease. Can J Cardiol 1988;4:231-236.

145. Hagar JM, Tubau JF, Rahimtoola SH. Chagas' heart disease in the USA: thallium abnormalities mimic coronary artery disease (abstract). Circulation 1991;84 Suppl 2:II-631.

146. Marin-Neto JA, Marzullo P, Marcassa C, Gallo Junior L, Maciel BC, Bellina CR, L'Abbate A. Myocardial perfusion abnormalities in chronic Chagas' disease as detected by thallium-201 scintigraphy. Am J Cardiol 1992;69:780-784.

147. Parada H, Carrasco H, Guerrero L, Molina C, Checos R, Martinez O. [Clinical and paraclinical differences between chronic Chagas' cardiomyopathy and primary dilated cardiomyopathies.] Arq Bras Cardiol 1989;53:99-104.

148. Pereira Barretto AC, Bellotti G, Sosa E, Grupi C, Mady C, Ianni BM, Fernandez EA, Pileggi F. [Arrhythmias and the indeterminate form of Chagas' disease.] Arq Bras Cardiol 1986;47:197-199.

149. Chiale PA, Halpern MS, Nau GJ, Przybylski J, Tambussi AM, Lazzari JO, Elizari MV, Rosenbaum MB. Malignant ventricular arrhythmias in chronic chagasic myocarditis. Pacing Clin Electrophysiol 1982;5:162-172.

150. Pimenta J, Miranda M, Pereira CB. Electrophysiologic findings in long-term asymptomatic chagasic individuals. Am Heart J 1983;106:374-380.

151. de Paola AA, Horowitz LN, Miyamoto MH, Pinheiro R, Ferreira DF, Terzian AB, Cirenza C, Guiguer N Jr, Portugal OP. Angiographic and electrophysiologic substrates of ventricular tachycardia in chronic Chagasic myocarditis. Am J Cardiol 1990;65:360-363.

152. Milei J, Pesce R, Valero E, Muratore C, Beigelman R, Ferrans VJ. Electrophysiologic-structural correlations in chagasic aneurysms causing malignant arrhythmias. Int J Cardiol 1991;32:65-73.

153. Correa de Araujo R, Bestetti RB, Godoy RA, Oliveira JS. Chronic Chagas' heart disease in children and adolescents: a clinicopathologic study. Int J Cardiol 1985;9:439-455.

154. Combellas I, Puigbo JJ, Acquatella H, Tortoledo F, Gomez JR. Echocardiographic features of impaired left ventricular diastolic function in Chagas's heart disease. Br Heart J 1985;53:298-309.

155. Bestetti R. Stroke in a hospital-derived cohort of patients with chronic Chagas' disease. Acta Cardiol 2000;55:33-38.

156. Samuel J, Oliveira M, Correa De Araujo RR, Navarro MA, Muccillo G. Cardiac thrombosis and thromboembolism in chronic Chagas' heart disease. Am J Cardiol 1983;52:147-151.

157. Arteaga-Fernandez E, Barretto AC, Ianni BM, Mady C, Lopes EA, Vianna Cd, Bellotti G, Pileggi F. [Cardiac thrombosis and embolism in patients having died of chronic Chagas cardiopathy.] Arq Bras Cardiol 1989;52:189-192.

158. Fernandes SO, de Oliveira MS, Teixeira Vd, Almeida Hd. [Endocardial thrombosis and type of left vortical lesion in chronic Chagasic patients.] Arq Bras Cardiol 1987;48:17-19.

159. De Morais CF, Higuchi ML, Lage S. Chagas' heart disease and myocardial infarct. Incidence and report of four necropsy cases. Ann Trop Med Parasitol 1989;83:207-214.

160. Gallo Junior L, Morelo Filho J, Maciel BC, Marin Neto JA, Martins LE, Lima Filho EC. Functional evaluation of sympathetic and parasympathetic system in Chagas' disease using dynamic exercise. Cardiovasc Res 1987;21:922-927.

161. Neto JA, Gallo L Jr, Manco JC, Rassi A, Amorim DS. Postural reflexes in chronic Chagas's heart disease. Heart rate and arterial pressure responses. Cardiology 1975;60:343-357.

162. Junqueira Junior LF. Ambulatory assessment of cardiac autonomic function in Chagas' heart disease patients based on indexes of R-R interval variation in the Valsalva maneuver. Braz J Med Biol Res 1990;23:1091-1102.

163. Junqueira Junior LF, Gallo Junior L, Manco JC, Marin-Neto JA, Amorim DS. Subtle cardiac autonomic impairment in Chagas' disease detected by baroreflex sensitivity testing. Braz J Med Biol Res 1985;18:171-178.

164. Marin-Neto JA, Maciel BC, Gallo Junior L, Junqueira Junior LF, Amorim DS. Effect of parasympathetic impairment on the haemodynamic response to handgrip in Chagas's heart disease. Br Heart J 1986;55:204-210.

165. Davila DF, Donis JH, Navas M, Fuenmayor AJ, Torres A, Gottberg C. Response of heart rate to atropine and left ventricular function in Chagas' heart disease. Int J Cardiol 1988;21:143-156.

166. Fuenmayor AJ, Rodriguez L, Torres A, Donis J, Navas M, Fuenmayor AM, Davila D. Valsalva maneuver: a test of the functional state of cardiac innervation in Chagasic myocarditis. Int J Cardiol 1988;18:351-356.

167. Iosa D, DeQuattro V, Lee DD, Elkayam U, Palmero H. Plasma norepinephrine in Chagas' cardioneuromyopathy: a marker of progressive dysautonomia. Am Heart J 1989;117:882-887.

168. Marin-Neto JA, Bromberg-Marin G, Pazin-Filho A, Somoes MV, Maciel BC. Cardiac autonomic impairment and early myocardial damage involving the right ventricle are independent phenomena in Chagas' disease. Int J Cardiol 1998;65:261-269.

169. Junqueira Junior LF. [Possible role of autonomic heart dysfunction in sudden death associated with Chagas disease.] Arq Bras Cardiol 1991;56:429-434.

170. Pinto Dias JC. Epidemiology of Chagas' disease in Brazil. In: Brenner RR, Stoka AM, eds. Chagas' disease vectors. Volume I: Taxonomic, ecological, and epidemiological aspects. Boca Raton, FL: CRC Press, 1988:57-84.

171. Puigbo JJ, Nava Rhode JR, Carcia Barrios H, Gil Yepez C. A 4-year follow-up study of a rural community with endemic Chagas' disease. Bull World Health Organ 1968;39:341-348.

172. Lopes ER, Chapadeiro E, Almeida HO, Rocha A. Contribuicao ao estudo da anatomia patologica dos coracoes de chagasicos falecidos subitamente. Rev Soc Bras Med Trop 1975;9:269-282.

173. Espinosa RA, Pericchi LR, Carrasco HA, Escalante A, Martinez O, Gonzalez R. Prognostic indicators of chronic chagasic cardiopathy. Int J Cardiol 1991;30:195-202.

174. Andrade Z, Lopes ER, Prata SP. [Changes in the heart conduction system in Chagasic patients suffering sudden death.] Arq Bras Cardiol 1987;48:5-9.

175. Prata A, Lopes ER, Chapadeiro E. [Characteristics of unexpected sudden death in Chagas disease.] Rev Soc Bras Med Trop 1986;19:9-12.

176. Bestetti RB, Muccillo G. Clinical course of Chagas' heart disease: a comparison with dilated cardiomyopathy. Int J Cardiol 1997;60:187-193.

177. Espinosa R, Carrasco HA, Belandria F, Fuenmayor AM, Molina C, Gonzalez R, Martinez O. Life expectancy analysis in patients with Chagas' disease: prognosis after one decade (1973-1983). Int J Cardiol 1985;8:45-56.

178. Mady C, Cardoso RH, Barretto AC, da Luz PL, Bellotti G, Pileggi F. Survival and predictors of survival in patients with congestive heart failure due to Chagas' cardiomyopathy. Circulation 1994;90:3098-3102.

179. Roberti RR, Martinez EE, Andrade JL, Araujo VL, Brito FS, Portugal OP, Horowitz SF. Chagas cardiomyopathy and captopril. Eur Heart J 1992;13:966-970.

180. Khoury AM, Davila DF, Bellabarba G, Donis JH, Torres A, Lemorvan C, Hernandez L, Bishop W. Acute effects of digitalis and enalapril on the neurohormonal profile of chagasic patients with severe congestive heart failure. Int J Cardiol 1996;57:21-29.

181. Greco OT, Ardito RV, Garzon SA, Bilaqui A, Bellini AJ, Ribeiro Rde A, Jacob JL, Nicolau JC, Ayoub JC, De Lima ER, et al. [Follow-up of 991 patients with multiprogrammable artificial cardiac pacemaker.] Arq Bras Cardiol 1987;49:327-331.

182. Martinelli Filho M, D'Orio SD, Nadalin E, Siqueira SF, Costa R, Scanavacca M, Sosa EA, Bellotti G, Pileggi F. [Pacemaker with mechanical sensors. Accumulated experience in long-term follow-up.] Arq Bras Cardiol 1990;55:189-194.

183. Brugada P. [Chagas' disease and tachycardiomyopathy.] Arq Bras Cardiol 1991;56:5-7.

184. Barbosa EC, Albanesi Filho FM, Ginefra P, da Rocha PJ, Boghossian SH, Musse NS, Gomes Filho JB. [Evaluation of syncope in patients with chronic Chagas heart disease.] Arq Bras Cardiol 1991;57:301-305.

185. Mendoza I, Camardo J, Moleiro F, Castellanos A, Medina V, Gomez J, Acquatella H, Casal H, Tortoledo F, Puigbo J. Sustained ventricular tachycardia in chronic chagasic myocarditis: electrophysiologic and pharmacologic characteristics. Am J Cardiol 1986;57:423-427.

186. Giniger AG, Retyk EO, Laino RA, Sananes EG, Lapuente AR. Ventricular tachycardia in Chagas' disease. Am J Cardiol 1992;70:459-462.

187. Elizari MV, Chiale PA. Cardiac arrhythmias in Chagas' heart disease. J Cardiovasc Electrophysiol 1993;4:596-608.

188. Haedo AH, Chiale PA, Bandieri JD, Lazzari JO, Elizari MV, Rosenbaum MB. Comparative anti-arrhythmic efficacy of verapamil, 17-monochloracetylajmaline, mexiletine and amiodarone in patients with severe chagasic myocarditis: relation with the underlying arrhythmogenic mechanisms. J Am Coll Cardiol 1986;7:1114-1120.

189. Rosenbaum M, Posse R, Sgammini H, Nunez Burgos J, Chiale PA, Pastori JD, Gonzalez Zuelgaray J, Brunetto JF, Califano JE. [Comparative multicenter clinical study of flecainide and amiodarone in the treatment of ventricular arrhythmias associated with chronic Chagas cardiopathy.] Arch Inst Cardiol Mex 1987;57:325-330.

190. Chiale PA, Halpern MS, Nau GJ, Tambussi AM, Przybylski J, Lazzari JO, Elizari MV, Rosenbaum MB. Efficacy of amiodarone during long-term treatment of malignant ventricular arrhythmias in patients with chronic chagasic myocarditis. Am Heart J 1984;107:656-665.

191. Scanavacca MI, Sosa EA, Lee JH, Bellotti G, Pileggi F. [Empiric therapy with amiodarone in patients with chronic Chagas cardiomyopathy and sustained ventricular tachycardia.] Arq Bras Cardiol 1990;54:367-371.

192. Mendoza I, Marquez J, Moleiro F. Como tratan los expertos la arritmias ventriculares en la enfermedad de Chagas. Avances Cardiologicos 1990;10:14.

193. Curti HV, Sanches PC, Bittencourt LA, Manigot DA, Jorge PA, Carvalhal S. [Ventricular tachycardia caused by the use of amiodarone. Report of a case.] Arq Bras Cardiol 1981;36:49-51.

194. Mendoza I, Moleiro F, Marques J. [Sudden death in Chagas' disease.] Arq Bras Cardiol 1992;59:3-4.

195. Valero de Pesce EM, Favaloro M, Pesce RA, Favaloro RG. Automatic implantable cardioverter-defibrillator: 4 year experience. Rev Arg Cardiol 1991;59:4.

196. Muratore C, Rabinovich R, Iglesias R, Gonzalez M, Daru V, Liprandi AS. Implantable cardioverter defibrillators in patients with Chagas' disease: are they different from patients with coronary disease? Pacing Clin Electrophysiol 1997;20:194-197.

197. Rabinovich R, Muratore C, Iglesias R, Gonzalez M, Daru V, Valentino M, Liprandi AS, Luceri R. Time to first shock in implantable cardioverter defibrillator (ICD) patients with Chagas cardiomyopathy. Pacing Clin Electrophysiol 1999;22:202-205.

198. de Paola AA, Gomes JA, Miyamoto MH, Fo EE. Transcoronary chemical ablation of ventricular tachycardia in chronic chagasic myocarditis. J Am Coll Cardiol 1992;20:480-482.

199. Sosa E, Scanavacca M, D'Avila A, Bellotti G, Pileggi F. Radiofrequency catheter ablation of ventricular tachycardia guided by nonsurgical epicardial mapping in chronic Chagasic heart disease. Pacing Clin Electrophysiol 1999;22:128-130.

200. Rosas F, Velasco V, Arboleda F, Santos H, Orjuela H, Sandoval N, Caicedo V, Correa J, Fontaine G. Catheter ablation of ventricular tachycardia in Chagasic cardiomyopathy. Clin Cardiol 1997;20:169-174.

201. Lamourier EN, Herrmann JL, Martinez EE, Buffolo E, De Andrade JC, Korkes H, Schubsky V, Ferreira C, Barcellini A, Portugal OP. [Aneurysmectomy as the treatment for refractory tachycardias in patients with ventricular arrhythmias of chagasic etiology.] Arq Bras Cardiol 1975;28:549-555.

202. Blandon R, De Leon LE, Gonzalez B. [Surgical treatment of cardiac arrhythmia refractory to medication in a patient with chronic chagasic cardiopathy.] Rev Med Panama 1986;11:164-170.

203. Stoppani AO. [The chemotherapy of Chagas disease.] Medicina (B Aires) 1999;59 Suppl 2:147-165.

204. Cerisola JA. Chemotherapy of Chagas' infection in man. In: Brener Z, ed. Symposium on Chagas' disease. (Scientific Publication 347.) Washington, DC: Pan American Health Organization, 1977:35-47.

205. Andrade SG, Rassi A, Magalhaes JB, Ferriolli Filho F, Luquetti AO. Specific chemotherapy of Chagas disease: a comparison between the response in patients and experimental animals inoculated with the same strains. Trans R Soc Trop Med Hyg 1992;86:624-626.

206. de Andrade AL, Zicker F, de Oliveira RM, Almeida Silva S, Luquetti A, Travassos LR, Almeida IC, de Andrade SS, de Andrade JG, Martelli CM. Randomised trial of efficacy of benznidazole in treatment of early *Trypanosoma cruzi* infection. Lancet 1996;348:1407-1413.

207. Sosa Estani S, Segura EL, Ruiz AM, Velazquez E, Porcel BM, Yampotis C. Efficacy of chemotherapy with benznidazole in children in the indeterminate phase of Chagas' disease. Am J Trop Med Hyg 1998;59:526-529.

208. Coura JR, de Abreu LL, Willcox HP, Petana W. [Comparative controlled study on the use of benznidazole, nifurtimox and placebo, in the chronic form of Chagas' disease, in a field area with interrupted transmission. I. Preliminary evaluation.] Rev Soc Bras Med Trop 1997;30:139-144.

209. Ferreira H de O. Treatment of the undetermined form of Chagas disease with nifurtimox and benznidazole. Rev Soc Bras Med Trop 1990;23:209-211.

210. Gazzinelli RT, Galvao LM, Krautz G, Lima PC, Cancado JR, Scharfstein J, Krettli AU. Use of *Trypanosoma cruzi* purified glycoprotein (GP57/51) or trypomastigote-shed antigens to assess cure

for human Chagas' disease. Am J Trop Med Hyg 1993;49:625-635.

211. Galvao LM, Nunes RM, Cancado JR, Brener Z, Krettli AU. Lytic antibody titre as a means of assessing cure after treatment of Chagas disease: a 10 years follow-up study. Trans R Soc Trop Med Hyg 1993;87:220-223.

212. Antas PR, Medrano-Mercado N, Torrico F, Ugarte-Fernandez R, Gomez F, Correa Oliveira R, Chaves AC, Romanha AJ, Araujo-Jorge TC. Early, intermediate, and late acute stages in Chagas' disease: a study combining anti-galactose IgG, specific serodiagnosis, and polymerase chain reaction analysis. Am J Trop Med Hyg 1999;61:308-314.

213. Britto C, Cardoso A, Silveira C, Macedo V, Fernandes O. Polymerase chain reaction (PCR) as a laboratory tool for the evaluation of the parasitological cure in Chagas disease after specific treatment. Medicina (B Aires) 1999;59 Suppl 2:176-178.

214. Braga MS, Lauria-Pires L, Arganaraz ER, Nascimento RJ, Teixeira AR. Persistent infections in chronic Chagas' disease patients treated with anti-*Trypanosoma cruzi* nitroderivatives. Rev Inst Med Trop Sao Paulo 2000;42:157-161.

215. Inglessis I, Carrasco HA, Anez N, Fuenmayor C, Parada H, Pacheco JA, Carrasco HR. [Clinical, parasitological and histopathologic follow-up studies of acute Chagas patients treated with benznidazole.] Arch Inst Cardiol Mex 1998;68:405-410.

216. Andrade SG, Stocker-Guerret S, Pimentel AS, Grimaud JA. Reversibility of cardiac fibrosis in mice chronically infected with *Trypanosoma cruzi*, under specific chemotherapy. Mem Inst Oswaldo Cruz 1991;86:187-200.

217. Andrade SG, Magalhaes JB, Pontes AL. [Therapy of the chronic phase of the experimental infection by *Trypanosoma cruzi* with benznidazole and nifurtimox.] Rev Soc Bras Med Trop 1989;22:113-118.

218. Viotti R, Vigliano C, Armenti H, Segura E. Treatment of chronic Chagas' disease with benznidazole: clinical and serologic evolution of patients with long-term follow-up. Am Heart J 1994;127:151-162.

219. Brener Z, Cancado JR, Galvao LM, da Luz ZM, Filardi Ld, Pereira ME, Santos LM, Cancado CB. An experimental and clinical assay with ketoconazole in the treatment of Chagas disease. Mem Inst Oswaldo Cruz 1993;88:149-153.

220. Araujo MS, Martins-Filho OA, Pereira ME, Brener Z. A combination of benznidazole and ketoconazole enhances efficacy of chemotherapy of experimental Chagas' disease. J Antimicrob Chemother 2000;45:819-824.

221. Marr JJ. Purine analogs as chemotherapeutic agents in leishmaniasis and American trypanosomiasis. J Lab Clin Med 1991;118:111-119.

222. Rivarola HW, Fernandez AR, Enders JE, Fretes R, Gea S, Suligoy M, Palma JA, Paglini-Oliva P. Thioridazine treatment modifies the evolution of *Trypanosoma cruzi* infection in mice. Ann Trop Med Parasitol 1999;93:695-702.

223. Urbina JA. Chemotherapy of Chagas' disease: the how and the why. J Mol Med 1999;77:332-338.

224. Harth G, Andrews N, Mills AA, Engel JC, Smith R, McKerrow JH. Peptide-fluoromethyl ketones arrest intracellular replication and intercellular transmission of *Trypanosoma cruzi*. Mol Biochem Parasitol 1993;58:17-24.

225. Basombrio MA, Segura MA, Mora MC, Gomez L. Field trial of vaccination against American trypanosomiasis (Chagas' disease) in dogs. Am J Trop Med Hyg 1993;49:143-151.

226. Sinagra A, Riarte A, Lauricella M, Segura EL. Reactivation of experimental chronic *T cruzi* infection after immunosuppressive treatment by cyclosporine A and betametasone. Transplantation 1993;55:1431-1434.

227. Rassi A, Neto VA, de Siqueira AF, Leite MS. [Nifurtimox as a prophylactic drug to prevent reactivation in chronic chagasic patients treated with corticoid for associated diseases.] Rev Soc Bras Med Trop 1998;31:249-255.

228. Cantarovich F, Vazquez M, Garcia WD, Abbud Filho M, Herrera C, Villegas Hernandez A. Special infections in organ transplantation in South America. Transplant Proc 1992;24:1902-1908.

229. Riarte A, Luna C, Sabatiello R, Sinagra A, Schiavelli R, De Rissio A, Maiolo E, Garcia MM, Jacob N, Pattin M, Lauricella M, Segura EL, Vazquez M. Chagas' disease in patients with kidney transplants: 7 years of experience 1989-1996. Clin Infect Dis 1999;29:561-567.

230. Dictar M, Sinagra A, Veron MT, Luna C, Dengra C, De Rissio A, Bayo R, Ceraso D, Segura E, Koziner B, Riarte A. Recipients and donors of bone marrow transplants suffering from Chagas' disease: management and preemptive therapy of parasitemia. Bone Marrow Transplant 1998;21:391-393.

231. Boullon F, Sinagra A, Riarte A, Lauricella M, Barra J, Besanson M, Lejour C, Lopez Blanco O, Favaloro R, Segura EL. Experimental cardiac transplantation and chronic Chagas' disease in dogs. Transplant Proc 1988;20 Suppl 1:432-437.

232. Libow LF, Beltrani VP, Silvers DN, Grossman ME. Post-cardiac transplant reactivation of Chagas' disease diagnosed by skin biopsy. Cutis 1991;48:37-40.

233. Leiguarda R, Roncoroni A, Taratuto AL, Jost L, Berthier M, Nogues M, Freilij H. Acute CNS infection by *Trypanosoma cruzi* (Chagas' disease) in immunosuppressed patients. Neurology 1990;40:850-851.

234. Bocchi EA, Bellotti G, Mocelin AO, Uip D, Bacal F, Higuchi ML, Amato-Neto V, Fiorelli A, Stolf NA, Jatene AD, Pileggi F. Heart transplantation for chronic Chagas' heart disease. Ann Thorac Surg 1996;61:1727-1733.

235. de Carvalho VB, Sousa EF, Vila JH, da Silva JP, Caiado MR, Araujo SR, Macruz R, Zerbini EJ. Heart transplantation in Chagas' disease. 10 years after the initial experience. Circulation 1996;94:1815-1817.

236. Bocchi EA, Higuchi ML, Vieira ML, Stolf N, Bellotti G, Fiorelli A, Uip D, Jatene A, Pileggi F. Higher incidence of malignant neoplasms after heart transplantation for treatment of chronic Chagas' heart disease. J Heart Lung Transplant 1998;17:399-405.

Cardiac Involvement in Acute Rheumatic Fever

**Jagat Narula, M.D., Ph.D., Ragavendra Baliga, M.D.,
Navneet Narula, M.D., Prem Chopra, M.D., and
Y. Chandrashekhar, M.D.**

Acute rheumatic fever (RF) is a noninfectious, systemic, immunologic delayed complication of group A β-hemolytic streptococcal pharyngitis.[1,2] RF has ravaged humankind since the industrial revolution.[3] The disease was widely prevalent in the early and midpart of the 20th century in the industrialized nations.[4,5] Although the disease has been contained effectively,[6,7] it continues to surface intermittently even in these countries.[8,9] It remains the most important cardiovascular scourge in the developing world. No temporal changes in group A streptococcal infections and carrier rates have been observed, and the rise and fall and resurgence of RF in the developed countries remain inexplicable. These epidemiologic trends constitute a major challenge to physicians who care for RF patients and to researchers who try to unravel the pathogenetic basis of the disease.[10] Because RF evolves into rheumatic heart disease (RHD), it becomes imperative to manage and prevent acute occurrences of the disease effectively. This disease entity has been extensively discussed in cardiovascular texts, and we limit our discussion to the advances and emerging trends in the diagnosis, pathogenesis, and management of RF.

PATHOGENESIS OF RHEUMATIC CARDITIS

The association between RF and streptococcal pharyngitis has been known since the beginning of the 20th century. However, the exact mechanism by which this infection leads to acute RF and carditis remains an enigma, particularly because only certain strains of the bacteria have been implicated and only certain individuals are susceptible. An *interaction* between group A streptococcal pharyngitis and genetic susceptibility of the affected individual probably results in an autoimmune process by which multisystem connective tissue involvement occurs.

GENETIC SUSCEPTIBILITY OF THE HOST

Numerous observations suggest that the development of acute RF is modulated by the genetic constitution of the host. Only certain individuals with group A streptococcal infection develop RF and recurrences of RF. The affected individuals exhibit an exaggerated immunologic response to group A streptococcal antigens. Further, only certain class II histocompatibility antigens are more commonly associated with rheumatic individuals than normal controls. The host variables that influence responses are not clearly understood, and no group is known to be free of the risk of RF when exposed to susceptible strains of group A streptococci.

Late in the 19th century, Newsholme[11] was the first to suggest that RF has a hereditary pattern. Later surveys by the British Medical Council also revealed that certain families had a higher incidence of RF.[12] Pickles[13] reported RF or mitral stenosis in 23 of 53 descendants of a patient who had RF. These observations led Schwentker[14] to explore genetic factors. He reported that RF occurred 4 to 8 times more frequently in relatives of patients with the disease. A widely quoted study in twins suggested that genetic factors play an important role in the pathogenesis of RF,[15] with a concordance rate of 2.5% in dizygotic twins and 19% in monozygotic twins; arthritis and Sydenham chorea were more concordant in monozygotic than in dizygotic twins.[16] Thus, genetic factors seem to play a role not only in susceptibility to RF but also in determining the clinical sequela. In early studies certain ethnic populations, such as the Irish population in New York, had a higher incidence of RF. More recently, Native Americans, African Americans, Hispanics, Samoans in Hawaii, and the Maori population in New Zealand have been found to have a higher incidence of RF and a more serious illness compared with whites.[17-22] These observations in the Maori population have been made in all socioeconomic classes and that in the African American population in the same economic class, suggesting that hereditary factors play an important role in the pathogenesis of RF.

The pathogenesis of RF has been ascribed to *hyperimmune responsiveness* to streptococcal antigens. The hyperimmune response disappears within 2 years in poststreptococcal glomerulonephritis and in patients with RF without mitral valve involvement, whereas it persists in patients with residual mitral valve disease. This has been supported by the observation that the immune response to streptococcal cell wall carbohydrate in genetically related animals produces antibodies that are idiotypically related and that the idiotypic determinants segregate in a mendelian manner. In humans, Sasazuki et al.[23] found that high and low antibody responders to streptococcal cardohydrate segregated to different families in recessive and dominant fashion, respectively. The gene controlling the low responders to streptococcal cell wall carbohydrate antigen was linked closely to a human leukocyte antigen (HLA) gene.

With the awareness that HLA antigens and genetic predisposition to disease are linked, several investigators examined the association between HLA antigens and RF. Genes that encode the HLA molecules are present on the short arm of chromosome 6. HLA antigens associated with RF include DR1, DR2, DR3, DR4, DR7, DR16, DQw2, and DRw53[7,24-26] but vary among populations (Table 21-1). RF is also associated with some B-cell antigens. For example, the D8/17 is identical in almost all patients with RF compared with 15% of controls. The D8/17 antibody recognizes a non-HLA antigen.[34,35] These data suggest that the DR locus is closely linked to the candidate gene. However, no single trait has been identified that can distinguish individuals susceptible to RF from among the general population. The identification of clear genetic markers of susceptibility to RF is important because it allows targeting of susceptible individuals for primary prevention.

Table 21-1
Genetic Susceptibility in Rheumatic Fever

Ethnicity or race	HLA C1 antigens	Patients, no.	Controls, % positive	Patients, % positive	Study
White	DR4	24	32	63	Ayoub et al., 1986[7]
White	DR4	33	32	52	Anastasiou-Nana et al., 1986[27]
African American	DR2	48	23	54	Ayoub et al., 1986[7]
Black African	DR1	120	3	13	Maharaj et al., 1987[28]
Indian (South Asian)	DR3	134	26	50	Jhinghan et al., 1986[26]
Indian (South Asian)	DQw2	54	32	63	Taneja et al., 1989[29]
Brazilian	DR7	40	26	58	Guilherme et al., 1991[30]
	DRw53		39	73	
Brazilian	DR16	24	34	83	Weidebach et al., 1994[31]
Arab	DR4	40	12	65	Rajapakse et al., 1987[32]
Turkish	DR3	107	23	49	Ozkan et al., 1993[33]
	DR7		33	57	

PATHOGENETIC CHARACTERISTICS OF GROUP A STREPTOCOCCI

Group A streptococcal infection can result in human illnesses ranging from sore throat to invasive infections such as necrotizing fasciitis and toxic shock syndrome to postinfectious sequelae such as glomerulonephritis and RF. The development of RF requires colonization of the pharynx by group A streptococcal infection, whereas cutaneous infection by streptococcus has not been shown to cause RF. The evidence that RF is a sequela of streptococcal pharyngitis includes the following. The epidemiology of RF mirrors that of streptococcal pharyngitis, depending on the time interval between the pharyngitis and the onset of RF; antibodies to streptolysin O (ASO) and hyaluronidase are almost always present; and recurrent attack of RF is always preceded by a streptococcal infection.

Group A streptococci produce virulence factors that can elicit both cellular and humoral responses in the mammalian host. The surface M protein is one of the major virulence factors for these organisms because it protects the bacteria from phagocytosis by the mammalian cells and elicits immune responses that play a role in the pathogenesis of RF and RHD. More than 100 M-protein serotypes of group A streptococci cause RF; however, these strains vary in their potential to induce RF. Studies have shown that there is no association between pharyngitis caused by some serotypes of group A streptococci such as M2, 4, and 28 and RF.[36] M-types 1, 3, 5, 6, 14, 18, 19, 24, 27, and 29 are associated with RF.[37] Furthermore, the RF strains tend to be rich in M protein, tend to induce an intense M-type-specific immune response, and share epitopes with human tissue. Others have disputed the role of M types in the pathogenesis of acute RF. In some areas of high endemicity of RF and group A streptococcal infection, the M type has not been detected or has come from an M strain traditionally associated with cutaneous disease. Although many of the RF-associated strains originate from just a few M types, it is believed that rheumatogenicity is strain related rather than M-type-associated. However, it has been suggested that any group A streptococci can acquire the ability to cause RF by horizontal gene transfer from other bacteria.

The mechanism by which group A streptococci produce RF remains an enigma, and efforts to determine the mechanism have been hampered by the absence of an animal model of the disease. It is widely believed that group A streptococcal infection induces RF in a susceptible individual by a complex interaction among the strain of the bacterial agent and the genetic constitution of the human host and the autoimmune response of the host.

AUTOIMMUNE SEQUELAE TO STREPTOCOCCAL INFECTION

The autoimmune theory has credence because there is a relatively long latent period between the onset of streptococcal pharyngeal infection and RF and numerous antigenic similarities exist between various components of the human tissue and constituents of group A streptococcus. Further, patients with RF have higher titers of antibodies to streptococcal antigens than those with uncomplicated streptococcal infection, and patients with RF exhibit an exaggerated cellular reactivity to streptococcal antigens.

Components of the streptococcal cell wall (including group A carbohydrate and M protein) and of the cell membrane share antigenic determinants with various constituents of the human heart (Table 21-2). The M protein is an α-helical coiled coil molecule that extends from the surface with its hypervariable NH_2-terminus and contains type-specific epitopes evoking antibodies that correlate with protection against the homologous serotype.

Table 21-2
Potential Antigenic Targets in Acute Rheumatic Fever

Antigen	Potential antigenic targets
Hyaluronate capsule of the streptococcus	Valve glycoproteins
Streptococcal membrane antigens	Myocardial and smooth muscle sarcolemma
Streptococcal M protein	Cardiac myosin, tropomyosin, keratin, vimentin

The M protein has randomly repeated sequences of hepatic periodicity.[38] These repeat regions within the M protein are grouped into 4 domains of A, B, C, or D. The size, sequence, and number vary between different serotypes of group A streptococcus. The *emm* gene is located in a regulon controlled by the upstream positive regulator *mga*. Depending on the serotype, the regulon may contain 1, 2, or 3 *emm* and *emm*-like genes. In serotypes containing only 1 *emm* gene, deletion or interruption of the *emm* gene results in an avirulent organism that can no longer resist phagocytosis. In serotypes expressing several *emm*-like genes, each may partially contribute to phagocytosis resistance, but among the many defined surface proteins of group A streptococci, only antibodies against the M protein are opsonic. The streptococcal M proteins also elicit antibodies that can cross-react with other α-helical molecules, including human myosin, tropomyosin, keratin, and vimentin. A fascinating study reported T-cell clones from valvular lesions of RHD patients that recognize both M-protein synthetic peptides and a heart tissue protein fraction.[39]

Immune responses, both humoral[40,41] and cellular, are more vigorous in patients with RF than in the normal population. Two of the streptococcal antigens, the pepsin-generated fraction of M protein PepM5 and a streptococcal pyrogenic exotoxin, are believed to behave as superantigens. These antigens do not bind to antigen-binding clefts in T or B cells and can amplify an immune response by clonal expansion of T and B cells and release of cytokines and adhesion molecules, which could help localize immune responses to certain tissues. Finally, superantigenic stimulation may help T cells respond to antigens like M proteins, which they might not do in the absence of such stimulation.

PATHOLOGIC CHARACTERISTICS OF RHEUMATIC CARDITIS

The histologic hallmark of the disease is the Aschoff body, which is pathognomonic of rheumatic carditis. The typical Aschoff body is a granulomatous lesion (Fig. 21-1; see color plate 38) that usually measures less than 1 mm and is found in the endocardium and the perivascular regions of the myocardial interstitium.[42] The Aschoff body consists of a central area of fibrinoid necrosis surrounded or infiltrated by histiocytes called Anitschkow cells or Aschoff cells, lymphocytes, plasma cells, polymorphonuclear cells, and, rarely, mast cells. The Aschoff cell has a basophilic cytoplasm, sharply outlined vesicular nucleus, and condensed chromatin. On longitudinal section, the chromatin appears like a caterpillar. In transverse section, the chromatin appears as a dark spot surrounded by a clear area producing a nucleus shaped like an owl eye. The Anitschkow cell is not specific for RF and may be found in the normal as well as other inflammatory and noninflammatory conditions of myocardium. When an Aschoff cell reveals 2 or more nuclei, then it is designated as an Aschoff giant cell.

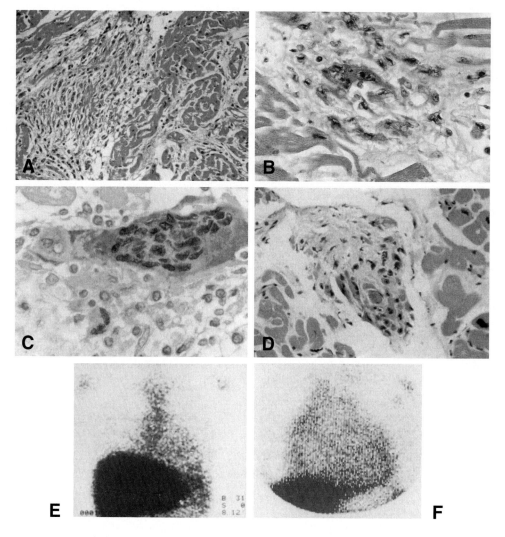

Fig. 21-1. Myocardial involvement in rheumatic fever (RF). Aschoff nodules are the pathologic hallmark of RF. An Aschoff nodule is present in ventricular and atrial endomyocardium and comprises perivascular fibrinoid necrosis-associated mononuclear and histiocytic cellular infiltration. Histiocytic infiltration is intermixed with giant cells or Aschoff cells, which have abundant cytoplasm and characteristic one or multiple nuclei. *A,* Perivascular interstitial Aschoff nodule at low magnification (x10), as observed in the left ventricular myocardium of a boy who died of acute RF at age 11 years. *B,* Higher magnification (x40) of the same lesion demonstrates Aschoff giant cells; the centrally located Aschoff cells are multinucleated. *C,* The giant cells are of monocyte-macrophage origin as revealed by immunostaining with α-chemotrypsin (x40). Objective evidence of rheumatic myocarditis in life has been obtained by endomyocardial biopsy and gamma imaging techniques. *D,* Presence of Aschoff nodule in biopsy specimen is pathognomonic or diagnostic of rheumatic carditis (x40). *E,* Gallium-67 nuclear imaging allows the detection of myocardial inflammation noninvasively. *F,* Nuclear imaging with antimyosin antibody, which identifies myocyte necrosis, is less sensitive and suggests that rheumatic myocarditis is a more infiltrative than degenerative disorder. (*A, B, D,* Hematoxylin and eosin.) See color plate 38. (*C* and *F* from Massell and Narula.[2] By permission of the publisher. *E* was a gift from Jose Calegaro, M.D., Brasilia, Brazil.)

The Aschoff body develops in different phases: exudative and proliferative or granulo-matous.[43-45] The exudative phase occurs up to 2 to 3 weeks after the onset of RF. In this phase there is fibrinoid change in the collagen with or without associated acute inflamma-tion. In the granulomatous phase there is a full-blown Aschoff nodule. The granulomatous phase lasts 1 to 6 months after the onset of the disease. The Aschoff bodies may be seen in the left atrial appendicular endocardium years after the initial illness. However, their per-sistence is rarely encountered in the myocardial interstitium in chronic RHD, and their pathologic presence may actually represent a missed clinical event.

PERICARDITIS

The pericarditis in RF is of the fibrinous variety (Fig. 21-2; see color plate 39). Grossly, the pericardial surface varies from slightly red to white and demonstrates thick, fibrinous, stringy to shaggy exudates that result in the characteristic bread-and-butter appearance. Microscopically, there is fibrinous exudate with acute and chronic inflammation. Aschoff nodules can be seen in the pericardium. The exudate is almost always modest and does not result in a large effusion or a pericardial tamponade. The pericarditis resolves with time, and neither adhesions nor evolution into pericardial constriction occurs.

MYOCARDITIS

Grossly, the heart may look normal or at times there is enlargement of the heart involving the atria and the ventricles. Histologically, there is interstitial edema with nonspecific inflammation. Cardiac myocytes are affected only occasionally. The Aschoff bodies are located within the interstitium in the perivascular region about a small artery. The Aschoff bodies are preferentially found in the ventricular septum, posterior wall of the left ventricle, posterior papillary muscle of left ventricle, pulmonary conus, and left atrium.

ENDOCARDITIS

Endocarditis is the most frequent and clinically significant complication of rheumatic cardi-tis and is responsible for chronic rheumatic valvulitis. In acute rheumatic carditis the valves have friable, small, fibrinous, verrucous vegetations seen on the atrial aspect of the atrio-ventricular valves and ventricular surface of the semilunar valves along the lines of closure[46] (Fig. 21-3; see color plate 40). They are also found on the chordae tendineae. The vegeta-tions are 1 to 2 mm and firmly attached to the valves and have an associated inflammation consisting of lymphocytes, histiocytes, and occasional plasma cells, polymorphonuclear leukocytes, eosinophils, and mast cells. The valve appears edematous and becomes vascu-larized with muscular arterioles and capillaries. Aschoff bodies are seldom observed.

Acute rheumatic mitral endocarditis results in mitral regurgitation that contributes to ventricular dilatation and congestive heart failure (CHF). When there are no vegetations, there is a mixed inflammatory infiltrate involving the valve. The inflammation extends to the chordae. During evolution to chronic disease, there is granulation tissue formation with thickening and eventual fibrosis of the cusps with commissural fusion. The chordae tendineae also thicken and fuse. The mitral valve is most commonly involved, followed by the aortic valve. Involvement of the tricuspid and pulmonic valves is rare. In addition to valvular endocardium and covering of the chordae, the posterior wall of the left atrium demonstrates an area of endocardial thickening called the MacCallum patch. This is

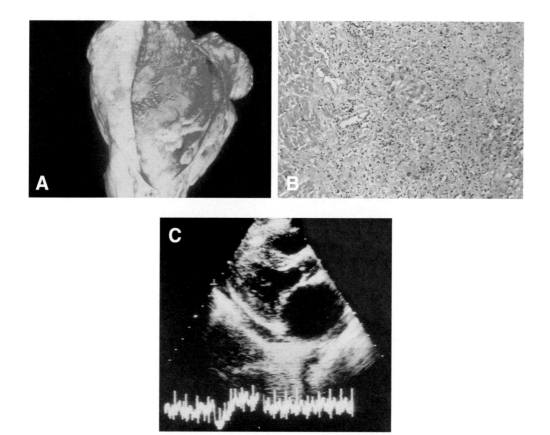

Fig. 21-2. Pericardial involvement in rheumatic fever. Pericarditis is typically fibrinous, and removal of the parietal pericardial layer imparts an appearance as if bread slices have been pulled apart in a buttered sandwich (*A*). Apart from fibrinous exudates, lymphomononuclear cells are seen on microscopic examination with the rare presence of Aschoff nodules, as seen in the center of the photomicrograph (*B*). Clinical presence of pericardial rub indicates the pericardial involvement in rheumatic fever. (Hematoxylin and eosin; x40.) Echocardiographically, pericardial effusion may be associated (*C*). Occasionally, a rub masks the underlying regurgitant murmurs and the echocardiogram becomes a useful diagnostic aid. See color plate 39. (*A* and *C* from Massell and Narula.[2] By permission of the publisher.)

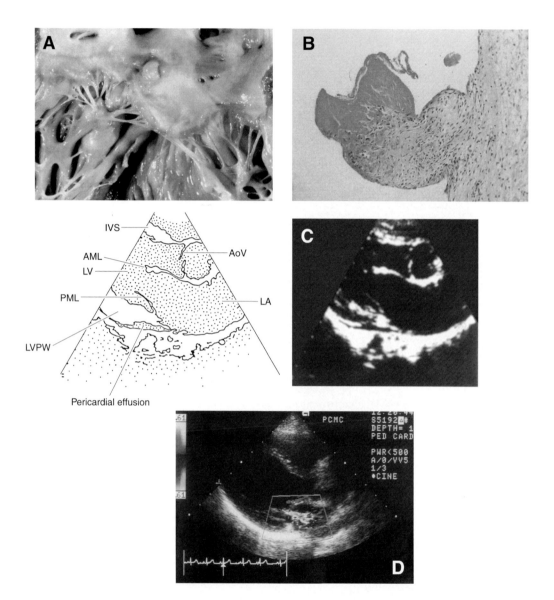

Fig. 21-3. Endocardial involvement in rheumatic fever. Acute valvulitis is the only pathologic abnormality that leads to permanent damage. Endocardial involvement results in development of tiny vegetations on the valve surfaces, which are noninfective and nonfragile. The vegetations comprise fibrinous material on the surface and reveal pallisading mononuclear cellular infiltration at the base of the vegetation. *A,* Gross macroscopic appearance of rheumatic vegetations on the atrial side of the mitral valve. *B,* Microscopic section through one of the vegetations; Aschoff cells are occasionally observed in the infiltrate. Noninvasive diagnosis of endocardial involvement is made currently by echocardiographic examination. (Hematoxylin and eosin; x10.) *C,* Presence of small nodular vegetations on the valve surfaces is proposed as ultrasonic counterpart of pathologic nodules. *D,* Consequent valvular regurgitation can be appreciated best by Doppler studies (eg, mitral regurgitation shown here). Regurgitation has also been described as evidence of subclinical carditis in rheumatic fever patients with no evidence of clinical carditis. See color plate 40. (*C* from Vasan et al.[59] By permission of the American Heart Association. *D* from Massell and Narula.[2] By permission of the publisher.)

formed as a result of the jet lesion of mitral regurgitation rather than representing a direct inflammatory process.[47]

VASCULITIS IN RHEUMATIC CARDITIS

The muscular arteries within the myocardium are involved in RF. There are periadventitial Aschoff bodies. The media of the arteries can show fibrinoid necrosis with palisading histiocytes and other inflammatory cells in approximately one-third of cases. The presence of Aschoff bodies in the media has not been described, but they can be seen periadventitially. The small arterioles and veins can show histiocytic infiltration.

The aortic involvement in RF is controversial.[45] In well-documented cases, perivascular lymphocytic infiltration of the adventitial vessels is seen. Scattered Aschoff cells are present, but Aschoff bodies do not occur. The arterioles are thickened and extend into the media. The media shows fibrinoid necrosis and histiocytic inflammation. The intima may also show fibrinoid necrosis with histiocytes and neutrophils.

IMMUNOPHENOTYPIC CHARACTERISTICS OF CARDITIC LESIONS

The presence of the different proportions of the cell types in the Aschoff nodules has been evaluated immunophenotypically. The Aschoff cells and giant cells are macrophages of histiocyte lineage.[48] Besides macrophages, other infiltrating cells are predominantly T lymphocytes; fewer B cells are present. The other cell types present in Aschoff nodules include a variable number of fibroblasts that depend on the stage of healing.[49] Marboe et al.[50] studied the rheumatic lesions in an endomyocardial biopsy (EMB) before and after anti-inflammatory treatment with prednisone and aspirin. They showed a higher prevalence of infiltrating T cells in pretreatment biopsies; helper T cells were 2-fold more prevalent than the cytotoxic T cells. Other cell types included macrophages, B cells, and mast cells. After treatment, the overall cellularity was decreased. Although the T cells were still the most common cell type, the ratio of helper T cells decreased significantly. Macrophages were present in the biopsy specimens after treatment, but B cells and mast cells became rare.

Most rheumatic valves have a predominance of T cells and there is a relative paucity of B cells. Most T cells in the valves are helper cells, and only a small proportion are cytotoxic T cells. Immunologic cross-reactivity has been demonstrated between streptococcal proteins and different cellular components of cardiac valvular tissue. Valvular interstitial cells show strong positive staining with antibody to antistreptococcal monoclonal antibody and also with antivimentin monoclonal antibody. It has been suggested that the intermediate filament may be a prominent valvular intracellular target of the antistreptococcal antibodies because preincubation of antistreptococcal antibodies with purified vimentin eliminated all valvular staining.[49] Immunologic cross-reactivity has been shown between streptococcal cell membranes and human heart valve fibroblasts.[51]

CLINICAL CHARACTERISTICS OF RHEUMATIC CARDITIS

Although RF is a multisystem disorder, only cardiac involvement results in permanent damage. Cardiac involvement has been reported to occur in from nearly one-third to almost all cases in retrospective hospital-based studies; these studies have not differentiated recurrences from first attacks of RF.[52] On the other hand, the prevalence has ranged between one-third and one-half of RF patients in prospective series.[53-55] Clinical carditis was diagnosed in three-fourths of RF patients in the resurgence of disease in the United States,[9] possibly due to more virulent streptococcal strains. Echocardiography is inherently more sensitive in detecting subclinical valvular regurgitation and it inflates the prevalence of carditis in RF. Accordingly, in the Utah series echo-detected carditis occurred in 90% of RF patients.[9]

Patients who have rheumatic carditis can present clinically as having subclinical cardiac involvement or acute overt or even fulminant CHF with mitral (MR) or aortic regurgitation (AR) of variable severity. The presentation as having chronic carditis and CHF is more common in younger patients, whereas joint involvement is more common in older patients.[2] Introduction of penicillin has rendered carditis milder. Rheumatic carditis is an early manifestation of RF and usually develops within the first 2 weeks of the onset of RF.[56,57] Although rheumatic carditis typically[58] involves all 3 layers of heart, including pericardium, myocardium, and endocardium, and pericardial and myocardial involvement can contribute to clinical presentation, rheumatic carditis cannot be diagnosed unequivocally without valvular involvement.

CLINICAL PRESENTATION OF PATIENTS WITH ENDOCARDITIS OR VALVULITIS

The clinical diagnosis of rheumatic endocarditis is derived predominantly from the presence of mitral or aortic valve (or both) regurgitation murmurs. Mitral valve involvement occurs in almost all patients with rheumatic carditis and coexists with aortic valve disease in up to 25%. Isolated aortic valve disease is uncommon and may occur in up to 5% of patients. Although pathologic tricuspid valve involvement may be seen in 30% to 50% of patients, clinical tricuspid valve involvement is rare in the first attack of RF,[58] and pulmonary valve involvement is almost never recognized clinically. The mitral valve involvement is recognized by a blowing, pansystolic MR murmur, which is usually grade II-IV and radiates to the axilla. MR murmur is occasionally associated with an apical, low pitched, short mid-diastolic murmur rumble without a presystolic accentuation—referred to as Carey Coombs murmur. MR is often mild-to-moderate in severity and resolves without residua if recurrent attacks are prevented. Severity of MR portends development of chronic valvular heart disease. AR in rheumatic carditis is usually mild. Valvular stenosis never occurs in acute rheumatic carditis and its presence offers evidence for chronic RHD.

MR in RF occurs as a result of a combination of active inflammatory valvulitis, valve prolapse, annular dysfunction or dilatation, and ventricular enlargement. Patients with mild-to-moderate MR show left ventricular dilatation with mild or no annular dilatation.[59] On the other hand, patients with more severe MR demonstrate marked annular dilatation, chordal elongation, and anterior mitral leaflet prolapse.[60,61] Rarely, the chordal rupture may result in flail leaflets and severe acute MR.[62] Because mild-to-moderate MR frequently disappears on follow-up in a majority of RF patients,[53,57,63,64] it is likely that functional rather than structural alterations in the mitral valve and annulus result in the pathogenesis of MR. AR may accrue from valvulitis and inflammatory involvement of the aortic annulus and only occasionally from aortic valve prolapse.

CLINICAL CHARACTERISTICS OF MYOCARDIAL INVOLVEMENT

Myocarditis is often indicated by cardiomegaly or CHF or both. New-onset cardiomegaly or a recent change in cardiac size (especially if it improves once the carditis resolves) suggests myocarditis, more so in the absence of a significant pericardial effusion. Although CHF in RF patients traditionally has been ascribed to severe myocardial inflammation, observations indicated that myocyte damage is not the primary cause of CHF.[9,65] There is so little myocardial damage in patients dying of RF that it is difficult to explain cause of death. Similarly, EMB in patients with rheumatic carditis does not show significant evidence of myocyte damage.[66] In addition, echocardiographic left ventricular ejection fraction and indices of myocardial contractility remain normal in patients with rheumatic carditis even in the presence of CHF.[59,65] Further, CHF occurs only in the presence of hemodynamically significant valvular lesions, and rapid clinical improvement is observed after mitral valve replacement during active carditis.[65] Therefore, it is usually the case that CHF in RF is caused by severe MR.

CLINICAL RECOGNITION OF PERICARDITIS

Clinical pericardial involvement occurs in up to 15% of patients during the acute stage of RF. The diagnosis is determined by the presence of a pericardial friction rub. Pericarditis in RF always occurs in the presence of valvular involvement. Occasionally, pericardial rub can mask the appreciation of underlying valvular murmurs and echocardiographic study may help diagnosis. If valvular involvement is not apparent after resolution of friction rub, one can safely conclude that the pericarditis was not of rheumatic origin.[2] Rheumatic pericarditis is often associated with a serosanguineous or hemorrhagic effusion, which usually resolves without residua. Only isolated reports have described the occurrence of pericardial tamponade[67] or pericardial constriction.[68]

DIAGNOSIS OF RHEUMATIC CARDITIS

THE JONES CRITERIA

The Jones criteria provide clinical guidelines for the diagnosis of RF and carditis. In the original criteria proposed by Jones,[69] the manifestations of RF were divided into major and minor categories. Major manifestations were most likely to lead to a specific diagnosis and included carditis, joint symptoms, subcutaneous nodules, and chorea. Because of the tendency for recurrences, evidence of previous RF or RHD was also considered a major manifestation. Minor manifestations, although suggestive of RF, were not considered sufficient for the diagnosis of RF; minor manifestations included clinical signs (such as fever and erythema marginatum) and laboratory markers of acute inflammation (such as leukocytosis, increased erythrocyte sedimentation rate, or C-reactive protein). Presence of *2 major* or *1 major and 2 minor* manifestations was considered diagnostic for rheumatic activity. Because a previous history of definite RF or RHD was considered a major criterion, only minor manifestations were sufficient for the diagnosis of an RF recurrence.

The Jones criteria were modified on several occasions.[70-73] In the first modification,[70] joint symptoms were classified into objective evidence of arthritis and subjective complaint of arthralgia; arthritis replaced joint symptoms as a major manifestation and arthralgia was included in the list of minor manifestations. The history of previous RF or RHD was downgraded to the minor category and, therefore, documentation of at least 1 major manifestation became necessary for the diagnosis of an RF recurrence. Erythema marginatum was upgraded to a major criterion. In addition, the preceding evidence of group A β-hemolytic streptococcal pharyngitis was introduced as a minor manifestation.[70] Importance of the preceding streptococcal infection was further emphasized in the subsequent revision of the Jones criteria, wherein demonstration of streptococcal origin became mandatory for the diagnosis of RF. It was presumed that the exclusion of clinical syndromes of nonstreptococcal origin enhanced the specificity of the Jones criteria for the diagnosis of RF.[71] Although the inclusion of this criterion increased the specificity of diagnosis, at least one-fourth of the RF cases diagnosed by earlier versions of the Jones criteria could not be diagnosed by the criteria requiring the demonstration of streptococcal etiology.[74] Such patients usually presented in the relatively late phase of the disease or with delayed manifestations of RF (such as chorea) when evidence of preceding streptococcal infection had already subsided. Therefore, the late manifestations of RF were subsequently exempted from the requirement of demonstration of prior streptococcal infection.[72]

In the Jones criteria, diagnosis of a primary episode of rheumatic carditis depends on the presence of a significant apical systolic murmur (suggestive of mitral valve regurgitation) or basal diastolic murmur (suggestive of aortic incompetence) or both, the clinical presence of pericarditis, or unexplained CHF. Rheumatic cardiac involvement is tacitly believed to be invariably present in an RF recurrence if the initial episode involved the heart.[66,71] The recurrence of carditis, however, requires evidence of pericarditis or an obvious change in previous cardiac findings indicative of myocardial and valvular involvement.[59] Changes in the cardiac findings at follow-up include the appearance of new murmur, a change in previous murmur, or an obvious radiographic increase in cardiac size.

The clinical diagnosis of rheumatic carditis requires evidence of carditis as 1 major manifestation and another major or 2 minor manifestations in the presence of laboratory markers of preceding streptococcal infection. Occasionally, 1 of these requirements may not be obvious, precluding the fulfillment of the Jones criteria,[66,73,75,76] especially when carditis is the sole manifestation of RF and during a recurrence of RF. For instance, when carditis assumes an insidious course and the patient seeks medical attention late in the course of disease, the signs of carditis are unmistakable but the supportive clinical findings and antistreptococcal antibody titers have resolved already. During an acute episode of recurrent rheumatic activity, the carditis could be apparent as florid CHF, but owing to lack of knowledge of the patient's previous cardiac status, a change in cardiac findings may not be established. Unlike a primary RF episode, mere presence of unexplained CHF is not sufficient for the diagnosis of active rheumatic carditis by the revised Jones criteria. The diagnosis of acute carditis as the cause of CHF rather than decompensated chronic progressive valvular disease is critical because *use of steroids may be lifesaving in active carditis* but of no benefit in valvular disease. Steroids may be associated with markedly increased risk of infectious complications. The diagnosis of recurrent carditis in a patient with previous RHD, in the absence of overt CHF, becomes even more difficult when the previous cardiac findings are not available for comparison. However, carditis is likely to be present because recurrent episodes of RF have been reported to almost always replicate a preceding episode. These difficulties led to a radical change in the 1992 Update[73] of the Jones criteria when the previous history of RF or RHD was excluded from the list of minor manifestations, allowing the applicability of the Jones criteria to only primary episodes of RF. This change represented a return to the intent of the original proposal by Jones,[69] which did not require strict application of the criteria for the diagnosis of a recurrence of RF.

NECESSITY FOR THE REVISION OF THE JONES CRITERIA

As discussed above, the Jones criteria have been revised repeatedly by the American Heart Association to improve the specificity of the criteria. Most of the changes were made without prospective studies and based on the perceived effects of the previous revision. Actually, a computer software maintenance paradigm was applied to the original publication of Jones criteria and the 4 revisions were categorized as corrective (error correction) and perfective (enhancement in response to user needs). The only adaptive (response to new knowledge) change in the criteria was made in 1954 when a laboratory aid was included for establishing the streptococcal origin of the disease. This change signaled a landmark improvement in the Jones criteria. It is apparent that solution to improving diagnostic accuracy is not repackaging of the clinical criteria but the inclusion of the laboratory aids of incremental diagnostic utility. Although numerous diagnostic techniques have been used for the detection of pericardial, myocardial, and valvular involvement in cardiac diseases, their role and clinical applicability in RF have not been evaluated. Inclusion of these commonly used diagnostic techniques for the diagnosis of RF should be particularly useful because clinical and auscultatory skills are waning in the countries where the frequency of RF has decreased. It is expected that even an empirical inclusion of these techniques in the Jones criteria will further stimulate the likelihood of research.

Furthermore, the brunt of the RF is borne by the Third World countries. It is known that recurrences of the disease are common in these geographic areas owing to lack of health care facilities, detection, and prevention of disease. The data from tertiary care centers in developing countries demonstrate that the majority of active RF patients present with a recurrence of disease. The last version of the Jones criteria does not provide clear guidelines for the diagnosis of recurrence of RF. It is feared that lack of guidelines results in either overdiagnosis of RF or many cases of RF missed. In fact, clinicians in the developing countries have continued to use the penultimate modification of the Jones criteria,[72] which is likely to be more applicable in their clinical context. Because the American Heart Association–American College of Cardiology guidelines establish worldwide standards for the diagnosis and management of various cardiovascular disorders, it becomes mandatory that diagnosis of RF recurrences be included in the guidelines.

ROLE OF CONTEMPORARY DIAGNOSTIC TECHNIQUES IN RHEUMATIC CARDITIS

Echocardiography in Rheumatic Carditis

Several studies have attempted to evaluate the role of echocardiography in the detection of carditis. In the Utah outbreak of RF, carditis was diagnosed clinically in 72% of RF patients. Doppler echocardiographic evidence of MR was also observed in an additional 19% of patients who had RF with isolated arthritis or pure chorea but no clinically detectable carditis (CDC).[9] In a subsequent larger study from the same center,[77] nonclinical echocardiographic cardiac (NCEC) involvement was detected in 47% of RF patients presenting with isolated polyarthritis. Similar results were reported in a study from a Middle Eastern country. Valvular involvement was observed with color flow Doppler examination in all patients with RF and polyarthritis but no CDC.[78,79] In contrast, a study from New Zealand found Doppler evidence of valvular involvement in 100% of RF patients compared with 79% by clinical auscultation;[80] all NCEC patients developed audible murmurs within the 2 weeks of follow-up. Doppler echocardiography, therefore, may allow earlier diagnosis but eventually may not necessarily be superior. This contention was supported by a larger prospective study from India that did not find incremental diagnostic benefit of Doppler echocardiographic examination in the patients with no CDC.[59]

It is presumed that patients in developing countries seek medical attention in a relatively late phase of their disease when clinical valvular involvement has become easily observed. Furthermore, most of the RF episodes in developing countries are recurrences in the patients with established RHD. The ability of Doppler echocardiography to detect subclinical recurrence of carditis in the presence of preexisting RHD remains obscure unless there is a development of obvious change in Doppler findings from a previous echocardiogram. It is unreasonable to expect a previous echocardiogram and availability of records for comparison in developing countries.

Use of echocardiography for the detection of valvulitis has significant advantages but also presents logistic problems. The most important advantages are identification of patients with rheumatic carditis and prevention of the patients with carditis from misclassification with a more benign prognosis that requires an abbreviated secondary prophylactic regimen. Although the clinical diagnosis of MR and AR forms the basis of diagnosis of rheumatic carditis, valvular regurgitation may not always be detected by routine clinical auscultation. Even in the golden era of clinical examination, some patients in the Irvington House reports with no CDC in the first attack of RF had RHD on follow-up.[56,81] Clinical auscultatory skills of physicians in training are discouragingly suboptimal,[82-85] at least in countries where RF is declining. Accordingly, the role of Doppler echocardiography is inversely proportional to the degree of clinical skills of the examiner. Doppler echocardiographic examination not only identifies valvular regurgitation not detectable with clinical examination[9,77-80,86] but also allows visualization of valve structure and detection of non-rheumatic cases of valvular dysfunction, such as mitral valve prolapse.

However, the logistic problems of allowing the use of echocardiography for the detection of rheumatic carditis include the likelihood of detecting carditis in almost every RF patient (because of the sensitivity of Doppler echocardiography for the diagnosis of clinically inaudible trivial MR) or overdiagnosis of physiologic valvular regurgitation as organic dysfunction. Also, availability of echocardiographic facilities is a remote possibility in the developing countries where a majority of the RF-RHD patients live. Doppler echocardiographic evidence of trivial-to-mild MR can be observed in up to half[87] and tricuspid regurgitation in up to three-fourths of the normal population; even AR has been reported in normal people.[88] The prevalence of regurgitation is likely to be higher by color flow Doppler examination and in febrile patients (with hyperdynamic circulation) suspected to have RF. Various authors have tried to distinguish benign valvular regurgitation from organic rheumatic valvular dysfunction,[89,90] and have proposed the importance of demonstration of a holosystolic jet of mitral regurgitation, which extends beyond the plane of valve leaflets in 2 echo planes.[80,86] It is expected that during the course of the disease the organic valvular involvement[59] would persist, progress in severity, or involve other unaffected valves. Although such a trend may improve the specificity of abnormal echocardiographic findings, it will delay the diagnostic process perhaps to a point that the murmurs become clinically audible.

Nodular structures on inflamed valves have been observed on transthoracic echocardiographic examination[59] and proposed as the ultrasonic counterparts of pathologic endocardial verrucae. These nodules are gone on follow-up in the majority of patients and have been suggested as evidence of rheumatic carditis. However, the diagnostic utility of valvular nodules needs to be validated prospectively, especially because they are observed in only a maximum of one-third of patients with clinical rheumatic carditis. In summary, in the absence of a standard for the diagnosis of rheumatic carditis, the diagnostic accuracy of Doppler echocardiographic findings can only be evaluated by actual development of residual heart disease on follow-up.

The diagnosis of carditis by Doppler echocardiography is made in 90% to 100% of RF patients, which is significantly higher than the incidence of CDC. However, the utility of a test that diagnoses carditis in almost every patient with RF is questionable. Universal prevalence of carditis suggests that the disease almost always affects the heart valves with variable severity, diagnosis of which was not possible previously. Even if echocardiographic diagnosis of subclinical carditis is appropriately made, it is unlikely to modify the management of RF because the use of corticosteroids is not indicated in patients with mild carditis. NCEC is not likely to facilitate assessment of prognosis either, because the benign prognosis in patients without carditis was established in clinical studies[56,64,81,91-98] and RF patients with NCEC[59] are expected to demonstrate good prognosis similar to the clinically non-carditic group.

Endomyocardial Biopsy in Rheumatic Carditis

Because myocarditis is an essential component of cardiac involvement in RF,[2] a large prospective study of 54 RF patients[66] investigated the role of biopsy in the diagnosis of rheumatic carditis. The histologic characteristics of carditis in EMB specimens were established in patients with first episode of RF and were compared with EMB specimens from patients with quiescent chronic RHD. Perivascular histiocytic aggregates resembling Aschoff nodules were identified less frequently. Minor interstitial or myocyte alterations were more often observed than the histiocytic aggregates. The cardiac myocytes were focally degenerated, occasionally myofibrillolytic, and rarely necrotic, but the degenerative foci often lacked cellular infiltrates. Deposition of fibrin and other granular eosinophilic material with spreading apart of histologic components occurred focally about blood vessels and was interpreted as interstitial degeneration. Occasional mononuclear cells, predominantly histiocytes and rarely lymphocytes, were present interstitially and perivascularly. The histiocytic aggregates, myocyte degeneration, and interstitial degeneration were not noted in patients with chronic inactive RHD. Because Aschoff nodules or histiocytic aggregates have historically been observed only in patients with RF, they were described as diagnostic of rheumatic myocarditis. Although myocytic or interstitial alterations occurred in the majority of the patients with definite rheumatic carditis and not in chronic RHD, these changes are known to exist in many other conditions and were not considered diagnostic.

The sensitivity of EMB (based on histiocytic aggregates) in patients with clinically certain carditis was only 30% and, therefore, no additional diagnostic information was obtained in the patients with clinical carditis by performing EMB. Low prevalence of Aschoff nodules in EMB specimens may reflect the actual sparse occurrence of these lesions or the inability of the biopsy to detect focal lesions. There seems to be a greater tendency for these lesions to be observed in more severe disease, because all patients demonstrating Aschoff nodules in the reported study had clinically overt CHF. This is also consistent with the higher prevalence of Aschoff nodules in autopsy material, which represents carditis severe enough to cause death.

EMBs were also performed in 23 patients who had preexisting RHD and developed a recurrence of rheumatic carditis.[66] The diagnosis of carditis was suspected because of a recent unexplained occurrence of CHF in 13 of the 23 patients who had at least 1 other major manifestation of RF. The clinical diagnosis of carditis was not considered certain because previous cardiac findings were not available and a documentation of change in clinical cardiac findings was not possible and none of the patients demonstrated pericarditis. The remaining 10 patients in this group had unexplained CHF, did not have the telltale major manifestations of RF, but did demonstrate minor manifestations of RF and a modest increase in antistreptococcal antibody titers. Previous cardiac findings were not known and demonstration of change in cardiac findings was not possible. Aschoff nodules were observed in EMB specimens from 40% of patients. In addition, interstitial fibrinoid change, occasional interstitial or perivascular mononuclear cells, and myocyte degenerative changes were seen in almost all patients.

The importance of unexplained CHF as an isolated manifestation of carditis, especially with recurrence of rheumatic activity, has been debated.[66,75,99] The revised Jones criteria[72] require the presence of a new murmur or an obvious increase in cardiac size for CHF to qualify as a major manifestation. These features are difficult to demonstrate, especially if previous cardiac status is not known. Biopsy provided confirmatory evidence of rheumatic myocarditis in two-fifths of patients. Less diagnostic histologic features (consistent with some form of myocardial injury) were observed in the majority of the remaining cases. This study suggested that a recent onset of unexplained CHF associated with underlying RHD indicated a high probability of rheumatic carditis in patients with raised ASO titers and minor manifestations of RF. Therefore, EMB does not appear necessary in this group. This assumption is in agreement with the recommendations of the American Heart Association,[73] which do not insist on the major manifestations in patients with preexisting RHD who present, in the recurrent attack, with several minor manifestations and evidence of recent streptococcal infection.

Radionuclide Imaging in Rheumatic Carditis

Radionuclide techniques are simple noninvasive modalities that are sensitive and specific for the evaluation of various disorders. Rheumatic myocarditis is characterized by the presence of myocardial inflammation with some evidence of damage to myocardial cells.[66] Whereas gallium-67 or radiolabeled leukocytes can provide a means for imaging myocardial inflammation, radiolabeled antimyosin antibody allows scintigraphic detection of myocardial cell damage.

Gallium-67 Scintigraphy—Inflammation is usually associated with increased capillary permeability and results in exudation of various macromolecules including transferrin. Gallium binds to transferrin and results in localization to the site of inflammation.[100] Gallium uptake in the heart has been reported in several disorders[101] such as pericarditis of viral,[101] bacterial,[102] tubercular,[103] or rheumatoid origin; myocarditis;[104] and bacterial endocarditis.[105] Calegaro et al.[106] prospectively studied 40 RF patients with gallium scans. The patients were divided into 2 groups; 21 patients had an initial episode of rheumatic carditis and 19 patients had no clinical and laboratory evidence of active disease. Of the 21 patients with active carditis, 18 demonstrated a positive gallium scan. All 19 quiescent patients had a negative scan. Therefore, sensitivity of the technique was 86%, specificity 100%, positive predictive value 100%, and negative predictive value 90%.

^{99m}Tc-labeled Leukocyte Imaging—A leukocyte labeled with a radioactive tracer behaves in the same manner as a nonlabeled leukocyte. It localizes to a site of infection under the influence of chemotactic factors, passes through the endothelial junctions, and gains access to inflammatory or infective foci.[107] There have been several reports of detection of endocarditis,[108] pericarditis,[109] and myocarditis[110] with leukocyte imaging. Kao et al.[110] used ^{99m}Tc-labeled white blood cells for the noninvasive detection of active rheumatic carditis in 10 patients with RF and in 15 with inactive RHD. Six of the 10 patients with RF had a positive scan; none of the 15 patients with inactive RHD demonstrated positive scans. The labeled leukocyte scan demonstrated a sensitivity of 60% and a specificity of 100% for the diagnosis of active carditis.

Antimyosin Antibody Imaging—Whereas gallium and leukocyte imaging reveal myocardial inflammation in rheumatic carditis, ^{111}In-labeled antimyosin antibody imaging provides evidence of myocardial damage. Its uptake is based on the loss of sarcolemmal integrity in damaged myocytes. A discrete and well-defined localization of antimyosin antibody in a coronary territory has been demonstrated in acute myocardial infarction,[111,112] whereas diffuse antimyosin uptake is seen in disorders such as myocarditis and cardiac allograft rejection.[113] Narula et al.[114] used ^{111}In-labeled antimyosin antibody to evaluate rheumatic carditis in 14 patients; 10 patients had rheumatic carditis based on clinical judgment, and the remaining 4 had either noncarditic manifestations of RF or chronic RHD. Eight of 10 patients thought to have rheumatic carditis had positive antimyosin scans. In most cases antimyosin uptake was modest at best, and intense uptake was seen only in the presence of associated pericarditis or CHF. All 4 patients with no clinical evidence of rheumatic carditis had a negative antimyosin scan. Although radionuclide imaging offers noninvasive evaluation of carditis, the experience is not adequate to allow application for the diagnosis of RF. In summary, gallium-67, leukocyte imaging, and antimyosin scintigraphy confirm the predominantly infiltrative, rather than degenerative, nature of rheumatic carditis.

SUGGESTED GUIDELINES FOR THE CLINICAL DIAGNOSIS OF CARDITIS

Although RF affects endocardial, myocardial, and pericardial layers to varying degrees, rheumatic carditis is almost always associated with a murmur of valvulitis (Table 21-3). Myocarditis or pericarditis (or both) is associated with valvulitis, and their isolated presence when not associated with a murmur should be labeled rheumatic in origin with great caution.

Valvulitis

Rheumatic carditis should be suspected in a patient who does not have a history of RHD and who develops a new apical systolic murmur or MR (with or without an apical mid-diastolic murmur) or basal diastolic murmur of AR (or both). The characteristics of murmurs were described in the revised Jones criteria.[72] The incorporation of the Doppler echocardiographic evidence of valvular regurgitation in the Jones criteria for the diagnosis of RF can be best considered based on epidemiologic burden of disease and socioeconomic status of various countries.[76] It is also mandatory to state that echocardiographic demonstration of valvular regurgitation must not be a prerequisite and that the diagnosis of rheumatic valvular incompetence should be considered after the best effort to exclude the regurgitation likely to be associated with a normal valve.

Echocardiography will have a role in developed countries that have widespread access to health care and have a low burden of RF, such as in the United States. In these countries, the patients almost always present during first attacks of RF and the advantages of routine echocardiographic study outweigh the small cost and workload imposed. Finding a normal heart or nonrheumatic cause of cardiac murmur by Doppler echocardiographic study saves

Table 21-3
Diagnosis of Acute Rheumatic Carditis*

Criteria	First attack	Recurrence

Valvulitis	New onset
	    Apical systolic murmur
	    Carey Coombs murmur
	    Aortic regurgitation murmur
		Change in murmur
		New-onset murmur

Myocarditis	Unexplained cardiomegaly Unexplained CHF/gallop sounds	Worsening cardiomegaly Worsening CHF
Pericarditis	Pericardial rub Unexplained pericardial effusion Pericardial effusion	Pericardial rub
Miscellaneous methods	Echocardiographic imaging[†] Nuclear imaging[‡] Morphologic evidence at operation Histologic evidence at biopsy or pathologic study	

CHF, congestive heart failure.
*Needs supportive evidence for the presence of acute rheumatic fever using the Jones criteria. In patients with known rheumatic heart disease, acute rheumatic fever can be diagnosed with minor criteria along with evidence for antecedent streptococcal infection.
[†]These would be considered soft criteria.
[‡]Significance of these methods is controversial.
Modified from Narula et al.[66] By permission of the American Heart Association.

prolonged prophylaxis in this population. On the other hand, it is expected that application of a Doppler echocardiographic study will confirm whether absence of an audible murmur is truly so and will protect patients with carditis from being misclassified owing to sub-optimal auscultation skills[83,85] and from inadequate secondary prophylaxis. With this strategy, overdiagnosis of subclinical carditis is bound to occur but is not likely to lead to prolonged prophylactic regimens because the duration of secondary prophylaxis can be optimized based on the persistence of valvular regurgitation on serial echocardiographic studies. Therefore, detecting subclinical carditis and even mislabeling a variable proportion of patients as having rheumatic carditis until their clinical situation is resolved would not seem to overtreat the RF patients.

In the developing countries in contrast to the developed nations, the incidence of RF and prevalence of RHD are high, access to medical care and echocardiography is limited, overcrowding and aggressive transmission of streptococcal infection deserve prolonged and frequent secondary prophylaxis, patients with a first attack of RF rarely seek medical attention, and most patients are likely to have established RHD at presentation with RF. Echocardiography is not likely to provide incremental diagnostic benefit in first episodes of RF because patients present late in the course of disease when the regurgitant murmurs are almost always likely to be audible. Similarly, echocardiographic study is not likely to support the diagnosis of subclinical carditis in patients with established RHD. The centers equipped with echo-Doppler facilities are not accessible to most of the population, and the cost and workload imposed on tertiary care centers with wider use of echocardiography in RF are likely to be enormous. Detecting NCEC may impose substantial cost on poor health budgets for requirements of longer prophylaxis. Because prophylaxis is initiated in RF patients regardless of the presence of carditis, an echocardiographic study can be performed at discontinuation of prophylaxis and the presence of RHD could constitute an indication for lifelong prophylaxis. Therefore, echocardiography during acute attack, even in the first episode, is not recommended for the diagnosis of RF in developing countries at present. The role of echocardiography in the diagnosis and management of established RHD remains unquestioned in any population.

Myocarditis

Myocarditis in the absence of valvulitis is not likely to be rheumatic in origin and is usually associated with an apical systolic or basal diastolic murmur. Tachycardia is an early sign of myocarditis, and its absence makes the diagnosis of myocarditis unlikely. If myocardial involvement from RF is severe, signs and symptoms of CHF may be present. Impairment in left ventricular systolic function does not occur in RF, and the signs and symptoms of CHF may result from significant left ventricular volume overload and severe valvular incompetence. Cardiomegaly is noted on radiography or echocardiography or both. Unexplained worsening of CHF in a suspected recurrence of RF indicates the presence of active rheumatic carditis if supported by adequate minor manifestations and supporting evidence of preceding streptococcal infection.

Pericarditis

Pericardial involvement in RF may result in distant heart sounds, a friction rub, and chest pain. At times the friction rub can mask the murmur of MR that might become evident only when the pericarditis subsides. The presence of pericardial effusion can be confirmed using echocardiography, and Doppler interrogation for MR may confirm the diagnosis of carditis in the context of RF. Large effusions and tamponade are rare. The electrocardiogram may show low-voltage QRS complexes and ST-T changes, and radiography may reveal an enlarged cardiac silhouette. Pericarditis in the absence of valvular involvement is unlikely to be of rheumatic origin. In the absence of a significant murmur, other causes of pericarditis should be sought, such as juvenile rheumatoid arthritis, other collagen vascular diseases, or infectious pericarditis.

DIAGNOSIS OF CARDITIC RECURRENCE

The original Jones criteria elaborated on the diagnosis of rheumatic recurrences and recommended that "minor manifestations of rheumatic fever in the absence of other causation are presumptive evidence of rheumatic fever (even initial) if the patient has rheumatic heart disease."[69] This implies that Jones did not believe that the criteria need necessarily be fulfilled for the diagnosis of a rheumatic recurrence.[73] However, the subsequent revisions of the Jones criteria by the American Heart Association did not confirm this intention until 1992, when application of the Jones criteria was limited to only the diagnosis of the primary RF episodes. The clinical diagnosis of rheumatic carditis in a recurrence has become a loosely diagnosed entity and is not likely to allow comparison of studies from different regions of the world.

The authors believe that the definite previous history of RF and RHD should be re-admitted as a major criterion for the diagnosis of a rheumatic recurrence. Individuals with a history of RF or RHD are at high risk for recurrent RF when infected with group A streptococci. One must have a high awareness for evaluation of any potential rheumatic complaint in these patients, especially with the evidence of preceding streptococcal infection. Therefore, a diagnosis of rheumatic recurrence may be made when a single major or several minor manifestations are present in a patient with a reliable history of RF or RHD and supporting evidence is present of a recent group A streptococcal infection. In addition, EMB study patients with suspected RF in the setting of preexisting RHD have demonstrated that acute unexplained worsening of CHF provides a presumptive diagnosis of carditis if it is supported by several minor manifestations and high ASO titers. A firm diagnosis of a rheumatic recurrence can be made only after exclusion of an intercurrent illness or complication of RHD, such as infective endocarditis which can mimic a rheumatic recurrence.[73]

MANAGEMENT OF RHEUMATIC CARDITIS

RISK OF DEVELOPMENT OF RHD IN RF

Risk stratification in RF has been the subject of many studies, and the following factors appear to influence the prognostication.

RF Recurrences

Many studies have shown that recurrences of RF contribute to increased cardiovascular mortality[115-117] and increased prevalence of residual heart disease.[56,64,91,93,97] RF recurrences may also be responsible for the aggressive nature of the disease in the tropics, with increased prevalence of heart disease,[53,115] particularly mitral stenosis.[118]

Carditis in Index RF Episode

One of the most important prognostic factors in RF is the detection of carditis in an acute episode of RF.[119] Patients with recurrences eventually develop greater cardiac damage not because cardiac damage occurred in later episodes but because patients with cardiac damage in the first attack were more prone to the first attack. This divides the RF population into 2 distinct subsets with and without initial cardiac involvement. Those with cardiac involvement in the first attack develop more severe and new cardiac damage with each subsequent attack, leading to severe RHD[91] regardless of the degree of carditis in the first episode. The patients who escape cardiac involvement in the initial attacks have fewer recurrences, and recurrences rarely involve the heart.[75,91,93-96,98,118,120,121]

Practice of Secondary Prophylaxis

Secondary prophylaxis prevents further recurrences, reduces new cardiac damage, and facilitates resolution of previous damage. In a widely quoted study of outcomes in RF,[95] a regurgitant lesion of the mitral valve disappeared in almost three-fourths of patients who received secondary prophylaxis. This relatively benign process was not observed in a small group of patients who were not receiving prophylaxis. The importance of secondary prophylaxis was further emphasized by evaluation of the incidence of residual heart disease at 5 years after the first RF attack in 2 groups of patients with good and poor prophylaxis. There was a significant difference in outcomes in patients with carditis during the initial attack, and the greatest difference was seen in patients with mild carditis. Prophylaxis did not seem to reduce the incidence of residual heart disease in the patients with severe carditis. On the other hand, the incidence of heart disease was minimal in the noncarditic group, regardless of prophylaxis.[92]

Prevalence of Streptococcal Infection in the Community

It has been tacitly believed that only certain streptococcal strains are rheumatogenic, even in patients not receiving prophylaxis.[121-123] Streptococci with large mucoid capsules and those with high M protein load are particularly virulent.[10] Whereas strains such as the M type 5, 18, 3, 6, 14, 19, and 24 have resulted in large epidemics, others such as M2, 4, 12, and 28 have not caused significant RF, even during epidemics of streptococcal sore throat.[10] Bacterial strains have shown unexplained spontaneous alterations in virulence over the years,[10,124,125] and such a change has been proposed to account for the resurgence of RF in the United States.[126] Similarly, streptococcal types common during previous epidemics are now being isolated less frequently, which may partially account for a decline in the prevalence of RHD.

Demographic Characteristics

The rate of RF recurrence is highest in the first year after an index attack and decreases in proportion with interval after the previous attack.[81,115,127,128] Similarly, the risk decreases with increasing age of the patient. The risk of recurrence remains small but significant even up to 20 years after an attack of RF,[115] and patients with more than 1 episode of RF have higher recurrence rates.[81,128,129]

TREATMENT OF THE ACUTE EPISODE OF RHEUMATIC CARDITIS

Medical management of RF has not changed since the mid-1950s and has not been shown to significantly alter the natural history of the disease. The treatment of an acute episode initially involves eradication of residual streptococcal infection by using an antibiotic regimen.[130] Anti-inflammatory agents such as aspirin have been used for controlling the arthritis, milder forms of carditis, and indices of systemic inflammation. Relatively high doses of aspirin are needed: up to 8 to 10 g/day (100 mg/kg per day) for 3 to 4 weeks. This period of treatment has been arbitrarily selected from the average duration of persistence of inflammation in the untreated patients from earlier studies.

Corticosteroids are used in moderate-to-severe forms of rheumatic carditis.[131] Because RF is considered to be an aberrant immune response to the cross-reactive streptococcal antigens, the anti-inflammatory and immunosuppressive effects of steroids make them a logical choice. Steroids rapidly resolve the toxic state, reduce inflammation,[57] and help early resolution of pericardial effusions.[53] It has been proposed that steroids may reduce the incidence of new murmurs[132] and help murmurs disappear faster,[133] and there is some evidence that steroids may be lifesaving in severe carditis.[134] Almost 135 reports, including 11 randomized trials, on the role of steroids have compared them to salicylates for the treatment of RF. None of the major trials were able to demonstrate superiority of steroids in modifying the natural history of RF or reducing the prevalence of residual heart disease. However, most investigators believed that steroids controlled acute symptoms faster[135,136] and helped to resolve mitral murmurs.[137] A meta-analysis of these studies has not demonstrated a significant difference in reducing residual RHD.[138] However, the studies analyzed were old, used varying methodology and entry criteria, allowed a significant number of patients to cross over to the steroid group, and did not have sufficient power in some cases.[136,138] Most importantly, these studies did not include a sufficient number of patients with severe carditis who are expected to benefit the most. Moreover, the results were influenced predominantly by a negative trial, and the meta-analysis had a large degree of uncertainty.

The authors believe that corticosteroids must be used in severe carditis. A short course of steroids (prednisone, 1-2 mg/kg per d) is used for 2 to 4 weeks. Prednisone should be tapered once the acute symptoms resolve, usually after the first 2 weeks. Although there are no definitive end points for discontinuing anti-inflammatory therapy, resolution of clinical symptoms and normalization of acute phase reactants usually guide the duration of therapy. Steroid taper is often covered with salicylates to prevent a relapse. If CHF continues to persist despite steroid therapy, surgical repair of mechanical lesions should be considered promptly.

SURGICAL INTERVENTION IN THE ACUTE EPISODE OF SEVERE RHEUMATIC CARDITIS

Surgical intervention during rheumatic activity has been considered contraindicated because some studies showed that operation in such patients is associated with increased mortality.[139,140] However, patients can be operated on in the acute stage of rheumatic carditis with gratifying results and valve repair or replacement in patients with severe CHF could be lifesaving. Operation quickly reverses the prolonged course of CHF and should be considered early in the course of refractory disease, especially because it is well recognized that CHF during an acute RF episode is due to severe MR. Essop et al.[65] reported 32 cases of mitral or mitral and aortic valve replacement during active carditis with no mortality. The operation was associated with a rapid improvement, including significant reduction in left ventricular dimensions. In another series with a 5-year follow-up in 254 patients, Skoularigis et al.[141] compared the outcomes of mitral valve repair in patients with chronic RHD and active RF. Acute and long-term mortality were about 2.6% and 15%; there was a high incidence of valve failure needing reoperation (27%). Thus, mitral valve repair or replacement should be undertaken only in an acute episode of rheumatic carditis when CHF is refractory despite optimum anti-inflammatory treatment.

STRATEGIES FOR THE PREVENTION OF RF

The rheumatic carditis remains an enigma and little is known about its pathogenesis. However, this has not precluded successful prophylaxis. Primary prophylaxis involves effective recognition and treatment of streptococcal sore throats to prevent the development of RF. Secondary prophylaxis is aimed at prevention of streptococcal sore throats in patients with previous episodes of RF to prevent recurrences of disease (Table 21-4).

Although streptococcal pharyngitis is the only precipitating cause of RF, primordial preventive efforts to eradicate streptococcal infections (as was done with the smallpox virus), are not feasible at present. It is unlikely that dramatic socioeconomic changes would occur in the near future in the Third World countries, and yet there is no certainty of its effectiveness given the resurgence of RF in the United States. Mass chemoprophylaxis for primordial or primary prevention has been feasible in some high-risk situations[6,135,142] such as naval recruitment centers. Universal application of such a strategy is excessively wasteful, cannot be applied on a long-term basis, and even has a poor efficacy unless carefully targeted.[21] Attempts have been made with some success to identify susceptible

Table 21-4
Prevention of Rheumatic Fever

Agent	Dose	Mode	Duration
Primary prevention (treatment of streptococcal tonsillopharyngitis)*			
Benzathine penicillin G		IM	Once
< 27 kg (60 lb)	0.6 million U		
> 27 kg (60 lb)	1.2 million U		
Penicillin V		PO	10 days
Children	250 mg bid/tid		
Adolescents and adults	500 mg bid/tid		
Erythromycin (maximum 1 g/d)		PO	10 days
(with penicillin allergy)			
Estolate	20-40 mg/kg per d		
Ethylsuccinate	40 mg/kg per d		
Secondary prevention			
Benzathine penicillin G[†]	1.2 million U	IM	Every 4 wk[‡]
Penicillin V[§]	250 mg bid	PO	Daily
Sulfadiazine[//]		PO	Daily
< 27 kg (60 lb)	500 mg		
> 27 kg (60 lb)	1,000 mg		
Erythromycin (with penicillin and sulfa allergy)	250 mg bid	PO	Daily

bid, 2 times a day; IM, intramuscular; PO, orally; tid, 3 times a day.
*Drugs not useful in primary prevention: sulfonamides, trimethoprim, tetracyclines, and chloramphenicol.
[†]Use drug at room temperature and with procaine penicillin to reduce pain.
[‡]Consider 3 weekly in high-risk situations including Third World countries.
[§]May interfere with oral contraception.
[//]Avoid in pregnancy. More effective than penicillin and better choice if tolerated.
(Based on recommendations modified from Dajani A, Taubert K, Ferrieri P, Peter G, Shulman S, and other Committee members and the Committee on Rheumatic Fever, Endocarditis, and Kawasaki Disease of the Council on Cardiovascular Disease in the Young, the American Heart Association. Treatment of acute streptococcal pharyngitis and prevention of rheumatic fever: a statement for health professionals. Pediatrics 1995;96:758-764. By permission of the American Academy of Pediatrics.)

individuals by using genetic markers.[34,35] The other possible strategy entails rapid identification of streptococcal infections in people who have pharyngitis. Characterization of clinically manifest pharyngitis is grossly inadequate because RF is often precipitated by subclinical streptococcal infections.[56,121] In addition, there are significant problems with the early detection of streptococcal sore throats for primary prevention such as delay in seeking medical help, delay in diagnosis, and differentiating carriers from active infection. It is therefore not possible for the physicians to intervene effectively at this stage until a vaccine is developed for prevention of streptococcal infection.

The most effective strategy is secondary prevention, which entails preventing recurrent RF episodes in patients with a prior history of RF. Secondary prophylaxis is associated with the most satisfying outcome,[119,143] and it has been shown to be effective. The population targeted is at a higher risk of cardiac damage and increased likelihood of recurrences. These subjects are more easily identified, form a smaller proportion of the population than that for primary prophylaxis, and are motivated to follow medical advice.[143] Strategies and protocols for secondary prophylaxis are available in various reviews on the subject (Tables 21-4 and 21-5).[119]

VACCINE FOR PRIMARY PREVENTION OF RF

Immunization is one of the most cost-effective means of preventing morbidity and mortality from infectious diseases. Routine immunization, particularly of children, has resulted in reported decreases of 90% or more in cases of measles, mumps, rubella, polio, tetanus, diphtheria, and pertussis. Vaccines also offer the opportunity not only to control but also to eradicate some diseases. The experience with smallpox has shown that the eradication of disease is a remarkably good economic and medical investment. Because of the biotechnology revolution, the development of a vaccine to prevent RF has made some headway. There are several different strategies currently being used to develop group A streptococcal vaccines, but the main focus has been based on the M protein.

M-PROTEIN VACCINES

One strategy is to incorporate common, protective M-protein epitopes into vaccines that would prevent colonization of mucosal surfaces and thus interrupt infection at the earliest steps. A second approach is to incorporate type-specific, M-protein epitopes into multivalent vaccines that are designed to evoke serum bactericidal antibodies and mucosal IgA. Complete characterization of the M-protein molecule has allowed the development of M-protein-derived vaccines. Whole M-protein vaccines are not a feasible approach because of the cross-reactivity between the M protein and host proteins. Opsonic antibodies directed against the N-terminus of the M protein are mostly responsible for serotypic immunity. Therefore, the approach has focused on M serotypes, which would provide coverage against a large number of group A streptococcal strains. Two approaches that have been pursued by researchers of M-protein-based vaccines include identifying and

Table 21-5
Duration of Secondary Rheumatic Fever Prophylaxis*

Category	Risk of recurrent streptococcal infections[†]		
	High	Not high	
		≤ 40 y	> 40 y[‡]
RHD	Lifelong	Till 40 y[‡]	None[‡]
Hx carditis and no RHD[§]	Till 40 y of age[‡]	Till 21 y of age[‡,//] or 10 y since last attack	None[¶]
RF and no carditis	Till 21 y of age[‡,//] or 10 y from last attack	Till 21 y of age[//,¶] or 5 y since last attack	None[¶]

Hx, history; RF, rheumatic fever; RHD, residual rheumatic heart disease of any severity.
*Each case is judged individually after considering the clinical situation and patient wishes. Patients from developing countries, with large RF burden, should be considered at high risk for recurrent streptococcal infections.
[†]Modify prophylaxis in epidemic situations, especially if virulent streptococci reemerge.
[‡]Should be at least 10 years since last attack and should not have history of multiple attacks.
[§]Use echo if possible to prove or disprove RHD.
[//]Whichever is longer in duration.
[¶]Should be at least 5 years since last attack and should not have history of multiple attacks.

combining multiple opsonic epitopes from the N-terminus and identifying vaccine candidates from the conserved region of the M protein.

Multivalent Group A Streptococcal Vaccines

Multivalent vaccines with protective epitopes without autoimmune epitopes have been constructed from the amino terminal of the M protein. However, it is unclear how many B-cell epitopes should be combined to produce an effective vaccine. It is tacitly believed that N-terminal epitopes from group A streptococci from endemic regions should be obtained to offer coverage for at least all strains of the organism within an endemic region. One group of investigators constructed a trivalent hybrid peptide against 3 separate M epitopes; rabbits immunized with this peptide were able to recognize all 3 serotypes.[144] The same group of investigators[145,146] constructed a recombinant, hybrid protein that contained amino-terminal fragments from up to 8 different M proteins that have each previously been shown to be opsonic and not host cross-reactive. The hybrid protein was able to raise a high titer in rabbits that reacts with each of the 8 native M proteins, and these antibodies opsonized 6 of the 8 representative serotypes of group A streptococci.

These encouraging studies should lay the foundation for the development of multivalent vaccines containing type-specific epitopes more accessible to the immune system and more defined in terms of purity.

CONSERVED DOMAIN VACCINES

Other investigators have used the highly conserved carboxy-terminal of the M protein to develop a broad-based vaccine. A collection of peptides from the carboxy-terminal region of the M protein is able to induce protection in mice, including prevention of pharyngeal colonization[147,148] and protection from death after mucosal challenge.[149] However, these epitopes occur in a region of the M protein known to induce host cross-reactive antibodies and T cells, making such a vaccine almost impossible to use in a clinical setting. Therefore, investigators have attempted to identify protective epitopes from the 'C' repeat region that are not host cross-reactive. One peptide known as p145 is recognized in more than 90% of individual sera. Minimal epitopes were then mapped from this peptide and using chimeric peptides, investigators were able to separate the minimal T- and B-cell epitopes within p145. This allowed the design of a vaccine that eliminates the potential of inducing harmful host activation of cross-reactive T cells.

Brandt et al.[150] reported a combined approach. They identified a minimum, helical, non-host-cross-reactive peptide from the conserved C-terminal half of the protein and displayed it within a non-M-protein peptide sequence designed to maintain helical folding, J14. Because this region of M protein was identified in only 70% of group A streptococci isolates, they obtained common N-terminal sequences found in communities with endemic group A streptococci. They then used 7 serotypic peptides with J14 by using a new technique that enabled the immunogen to display all the individual peptides pendant from an alkaline backbone. Their construct demonstrated excellent immunogenicity and protection in mice. Their results suggest that new generation multiepitope vaccines may provide a safe and effective way to prevent endemic streptococcal infection and subsequent morbidity.

NON-M-PROTEIN VACCINES

In addition to M protein, other antigens are being targeted for vaccine development and include C5a peptidase and cysteine protease. Such an approach should be able to induce nonserotype-specific immunity.

C5a Peptidase

C5a peptidase is a protease that inactivates complement-derived chemotaxin C5a and is coded by the gene *scpA*. The *scpA* gene has been found in more than 40 serotypes of group A streptococcal infection,[151] and antibodies to C5a peptidase are detectable in all adults.[152]

However, antibody concentrations peak between age 9 and 12 years, correlating with exposure to group A streptococci. Intranasal immunization of mice with purified C5a resulted in significantly reduced levels of colonization of group A streptococci on pharyngeal challenge with 5 different strains compared with unimmunized controls.[153,154] Therefore, a C5a peptidase vaccine could potentially protect against nearly all serotypes of group A streptococcal infection.

Cysteine Protease

Streptococcal cysteine protease is another potential vaccine that can induce non-type-specific immunity to group A streptococcal infection. Intraperitoneal administration of rabbit antistreptococcal cysteine protease IgG to mice has been shown to improve survival after challenge of highly virulent strains of group A streptococcal infection.[155] However, further studies are required to determine potential toxic effects of this vaccine.

Lipoteichoic Acid

Lipoteichoic acid is present on the surface of group A streptococci and plays a role in the adhesion to pharyngeal mucosa. Intranasal administration of lipoteichoic acid to mice blocks colonization and reduces mortality after intranasal challenge of group A streptococci.[156] Also group A streptococci pretreated with antilipoteichoic acid antibody are less virulent to mice. These data suggest that lipoteichoic acid is an important candidate as a vaccine to protect against group A streptococcal infection.

Hyaluronic Acid

Most strains of group A streptococci produce hyaluronic acid, and the gene for hyaluronic acid is present in all group A streptococcal strains.[157] The hyaluronic acid capsule influences M-protein-mediated adherence, and capsule expression generally promotes colonization of group A streptococci in the pharynx. Therefore, modulating the hyaluronic acid capsule can prevent pharyngeal colonization of group A streptococci.

VACCINE DELIVERY SYSTEMS

An important consideration in the development of vaccines is the mode of delivery. Development of vaccines against RF is focussed on the parenteral and the mucosal delivery of the vaccines.

Parenteral Delivery

Administration of adjuvant potentially enhances the efficacy of a vaccine and alum is one of the choices, although the magnitude of the antibody response happens to be suboptimal. Human-compatible adjuvants that induce strong antibody responses are being investigated.

Mucosal Delivery

It is generally believed that a mucosal vaccine is an optimal approach because the portal of entry of streptococcus is the nasopharynx. Fischetti[38] investigated the role of IgA in immunity to group A streptococcal infection. Mice were protected against intranasal group A streptococcal challenge after passive transfer of affinity-purified human IgA to M protein M6. Mice immunized intranasally with conserved epitopes of M protein conjugated to the B unit of cholera could induce detectable levels of M-protein-specific salivary IgA and serum IgG, and these mice showed significant reduction in colonization by group A streptococcus after challenge with either the M6 or M24 group A streptococci. IgA specific for p145 is capable of opsonizing group A streptococcus in vitro in the presence of complement.[158] Other successful oral vaccine strategies include use of genetically altered strains of *Salmonella*, *Escherichia coli* heated-labile toxin, and *Streptococcus gordonii* for delivery of recombinant M-protein antigens. If proven successful, the commensal delivery system would be ideal for developing countries. A live vector would be easy to administer and probably would not require additional doses. Also, since gram-positive bacteria are stable for long periods in the lyophilized state, a cold chain would not be required for *S gordonii*. *S gordonii* can persist for more than 2 years and is transmitted to other members of the family. This could be ideal for developing nations. However, it remains to be demonstrated whether the recombinant vaccine will induce a protective immune response in humans to the M-protein fragment expressed on its surface.

In summary, a streptococcal vaccine that evokes broad-spectrum immunity will have significant impact on populations living in areas of high endemicity with group A streptococci. The major problem with developing a vaccine for RF is the complexity of vaccine constructs. Epidemiologic data suggest that numerous serotypes of group A streptococci can induce RF. By using a limited number of serotypes and assuming 100% serotype specificity, the vaccines can at best prevent about three-fourths of the infections causing RF. Strain variation of M-protein structures means that the vaccines will be less efficacious. Another important determinant of serotype-specific M-protein vaccine efficacy is the proportion of strains within a population that is nontypeable. Although future studies in the laboratory should address issues related to strain variation of M proteins and the absolute number of serotypes within the nontypeable strains, ultimate determination of efficacy depends on the outcome of large-scale clinical trials. Clearly, epidemiologic data suggest that it may be necessary to reformulate vaccine constructs periodically to represent the most current serotypes prevalent at any given time, as is currently done for influenza vaccines. Finally, the most effective vaccine strategies may require the combination of M-protein vaccines with non-M-protein vaccines. Such vaccines may not prevent group A streptococcal infections but may have a significant impact on the devastating sequelae, particularly due to RF. Another important area is the ways in which the candidate vaccines can be delivered effectively. Development of an effective vaccine, therefore, is highly complicated but not outside the realm of possibility.

REFERENCES

1. WHO Study Group. Rheumatic fever and rheumatic heart disease. World Health Organ Tech Rep Ser 1988;764:1-58.

2. Massell BF, Narula J. Rheumatic fever and rheumatic carditis. In: Braunwald E, ed. Atlas of heart diseases. Volume 2: Cardiomyopathies, myocarditis, and pericardial disease. Edited by Abelmann WH). Philadelphia: Current Medicine, 1995:10.1-10.20.

3. English PC. Emergence of rheumatic fever in the nineteenth century. Milbank Q 1989;67 Suppl 1:33-49.

4. Bland EF. Rheumatic fever: the way it was. Circulation 1987;76:1190-1195.

5. Rammelkamp CH, Denny FW, Wannamaker LW. Studies on the epidemiology of rheumatic fever in the armed services. In: Thomas L, ed. Rheumatic fever. Minneapolis: University of Minnesota Press, 1952:72-89.

6. Arguedas A, Mohs E. Prevention of rheumatic fever in Costa Rica. J Pediatr 1992;121:569-572.

7. Ayoub EM, Barrett DJ, Maclaren NK, Krischer JP. Association of class II human histocompatibility leukocyte antigens with rheumatic fever. J Clin Invest 1986;77:2019-2026.

8. Bisno AL. The resurgence of acute rheumatic fever in the United States. Annu Rev Med 1990;41:319-329.

9. Veasy LG, Wiedmeier SE, Orsmond GS, Ruttenberg HD, Boucek MM, Roth SJ, Tait VF, Thompson JA, Daly JA, Kaplan EL, Hill HR. Resurgence of acute rheumatic fever in the intermountain area of the United States. N Engl J Med 1987;316:421-427.

10. Stollerman GH. Rheumatogenic group A streptococci and the return of rheumatic fever. Adv Intern Med 1990;35:1-25.

11. Newsholme A. The Milroy lectures on the natural history and affinities of rheumatic fever: a study in epidemiology. Lancet 1895;1:589-592.

12. Read FEM, Ciocco A, Taussig HB. Frequency of rheumatic manifestations among siblings, parents, uncles, aunts and grandparents of rheumatic and control patients. Am J Hyg 1938;27:719-737.

13. Pickles WN. Rheumatic family. Lancet 1943;2:241.

14. Schwentker FF. The epidemiology of rheumatic fever. In: Thomas L, ed. Rheumatic fever. Minneapolis: University of Minnesota Press, 1952:17-27.

15. Taranta A, Torosdag S, Metrakos JD, Jegier W, Uchida I. Rheumatic fever in monozygotic and dizygotic twins (abstract). Circulation 1959;20:778.

16. DiSciascio G, Taranta A. Rheumatic fever in children. Am Heart J 1980;99:635-658.

17. Paul JR. The epidemiology of rheumatic fever. 3rd ed. New York: American Heart Association, 1957:81-92.

18. Bisno AL. Landmark perspective: the rise and fall of rheumatic fever. JAMA 1985;254:538-541.

19. Pope RM. Rheumatic fever in the 1980s. Bull Rheum Dis 1989;38:1-8.

20. Markowitz M. The decline of rheumatic fever: role of medical intervention. Lewis W. Wannamaker Memorial Lecture. J Pediatr 1985;106:545-550.

21. Chun LT, Reddy DV, Yamamoto LG. Rheumatic fever in children and adolescents in Hawaii. Pediatrics 1987;79:549-552.

22. Wannamaker LW. Changes and changing concepts in the biology of group A streptococci and in the epidemiology of streptococcal infections. Rev Infect Dis 1979;1:967-975.

23. Sasazuki T, Kaneoka H, Nishimura Y, Kaneoka R, Hayama M, Ohkuni H. An HLA-linked immune suppression gene in man. J Exp Med 1980;152:297s-313s.

24. Guilherme L, Weidebach W, Kiss MH, Snitcowsky R, Kalil J. Association of human leukocyte class II antigens with rheumatic fever or rheumatic heart disease in a Brazilian population. Circulation 1991;83:1995-1998.

25. Hafez M, Chakravarti A, el-Shennawy F, el-Morsi Z, el-Sallab SH, Al-Tonbary Y. HLA antigens and acute rheumatic fever: evidence of a recessive susceptibility gene linked to HLA. Genet Epidemiol 1985;2:273-282.

26. Jhinghan B, Mehra NK, Reddy KS, Taneja V, Vaidya MC, Bhatia ML. HLA, blood groups and secretor status in patients with established rheumatic fever and rheumatic heart disease. Tissue Antigens 1986;27:172-178.

27. Anastasiou-Nana MI, Anderson JL, Carlquist JF, Nanas JN. HLA-DR typing and lymphocyte subset evaluation in rheumatic heart disease: a search for immune response factors. Am Heart J 1986;112:992-997.

28. Maharaj B, Hammond MG, Appadoo B, Leary WP, Pudifin DJ. HLA-A, B, DR, and DQ antigens in black patients with severe chronic rheumatic heart disease. Circulation 1987;76:259-261.

29. Taneja V, Mehra NK, Reddy KS, Narula J, Tandon R, Vaidya MC, Bhatia ML. HLA-DR/DQ antigens and reactivity to B cell alloantigen D8/17 in Indian patients with rheumatic heart disease. Circulation 1989;80:335-340.

30. Guilherme L, Weidebach W, Kiss MH, Snitcowsky R, Kalil J. Association of human leukocyte class II antigens with rheumatic fever or rheumatic heart disease in a Brazilian population. Circulation 1991;83:1995-1998.

31. Weidebach W, Goldberg AC, Chiarella JM, Guilherme L, Snitcowsky R, Pileggi F, Kalil J. HLA class II antigens in rheumatic fever. Analysis of the DR locus by restriction fragment-length poly- morphism and oligotyping. Hum Immunol 1994;40:253-258.

32. Rajapakse CN, Halim K, Al-Orainey I, Al-Nozha M, Al-Aska AK. A genetic marker for rheumatic heart disease. Br Heart J 1987;58:659-662.

33. Ozkan M, Carin M, Sonmez G, Senocak M, Ozdemir M, Yakut C. HLA antigens in Turkish race with rheumatic heart disease. Circulation 1993;87:1974-1978.

34. Khanna AK, Buskirk DR, Williams RC Jr, Gibofsky A, Crow MK, Menon A, Fotino M, Reid HM, Poon-King T, Rubinstein P, Zabriskie JB. Presence of a non-HLA B cell antigen in rheumatic fever patients and their families as defined by a monoclonal antibody. J Clin Invest 1989;83:1710-1716.

35. Patarroyo ME, Winchester RJ, Vejerano A, Gibofsky A, Chalem F, Zabriskie JB, Kunkel HG. Association of a B-cell alloantigen with susceptibility to rheumatic fever. Nature 1979;278:173-174.

36. Stollerman GH. The nature of rheumatogenic streptococci. Mt Sinai J Med 1996;63:144-158.

37. Martin DR, Single LA. Molecular epidemiology of group A streptococcus M type 1 infections. J Infect Dis 1993;167:1112-1117.

38. Fischetti VA. Streptococcal M protein: molecular design and biological behavior. Clin Microbiol Rev 1989;2:285-314.

39. Guilherme L, Cunha-Neto E, Coelho V, Snitcowsky R, Pomerantzeff PM, Assis RV, Pedra F, Neumann J, Goldberg A, Patarroyo ME, Pileggi F, Kalil J. Human heart-infiltrating T-cell clones from rheumatic heart disease patients recognize both streptococcal and cardiac proteins. Circulation 1995;92:415-420.

40. Ayoub EM, Dudding BA. Streptococcal group A carbohydrate antibody in rheumatic and non- rheumatic bacterial endocarditis. J Lab Clin Med 1970;76:322-332.

41. Ayoub EM. The search for host determinants of susceptibility to rheumatic fever: the missing link. T. Duckett Jones Memorial Lecture. Circulation 1984;69:197-201.

42. Baggenstoss AH, Titus JL. Rheumatic and collagen disorders of the heart. In: Gould SE, ed. Pathology of the heart and blood vessels. 3rd ed. Springfield, IL: Charles C Thomas, 1968:649-722.

43. Gross L, Ehrlich JC. Histologic studies on the Aschoff body. Am J Pathol 1930;6:621-623.

44. Gross L, Ehrlich JC. Studies on myocardial Aschoff body: descriptive classification of lesions. Am J Pathol 1934;10:467-488.

45. Gross L, Ehrlich JC. Studies on myocardial Aschoff body: life cycle, sites of predilection and relation to clinical course of rheumatic fever. Am J Pathol 1934;10:489-504.

46. Gross L, Friedberg CK. Lesions of the cardiac valve rings in rheumatic fever. Am J Pathol 1935;12:469-493.

47. Silver MD. Blood flow obstruction related to tricuspid, pulmonary, and mitral valves. In: Silver MD, ed. Cardiovascular pathology. 2nd ed. Vol. 2. New York: Churchill Livingstone, 1991:933-960.

48. Gulizia JM, Cunningham MW, McManus BM. Immunoreactivity of anti-streptococcal mono-clonal antibodies to human heart valves. Evidence for multiple cross-reactive epitopes. Am J Pathol 1991;138:285-301.

49. Gulizia JM, Engel PJ, McManus BM. Acute rheumatic carditis: diagnostic and therapeutic challenges in the era of heart transplantation. J Heart Lung Transplant 1993;12:372-380.

50. Marboe CC, Knowles DM II, Weiss MB, Fenoglio JJ Jr. Monoclonal antibody identification of mononuclear cells in endomyocardial biopsy specimens from a patient with rheumatic carditis. Hum Pathol 1985;16:332-338.

51. Kaplan MH. Streptococcal cross reactions with tissue antigens: cardiac myofibers, smooth muscle, and heart valve fibroblasts; significance for pathogenesis of rheumatic fever. In: Read SE, Zabriskie JB, eds. Streptococcal diseases and the immune response. New York: Academic Press, 1980:625-632.

52. Edwards BS, Edwards JE. Congestive heart failure in rheumatic carditis: valvular or myocardial origin? J Am Coll Cardiol 1993;22:830-831.

53. Feinstein AR, Spagnuolo M. The clinical patterns of acute rheumatic fever: a reappraisal. Medicine (Baltimore) 1962;41:279-305.

54. Majeed HA, Khan N, Dabbagh M, Najdi K, Khateeb N. Acute rheumatic fever during childhood in Kuwait: the mild nature of the initial attack. Ann Trop Paediatr 1981;1:13-20.

55. Sanyal SK, Thapar MK, Ahmed SH, Hooja V, Tewari P. The initial attack of acute rheumatic fever during childhood in North India; a prospective study of the clinical profile. Circulation 1974;49:7-12.

56. Feinstein AR, Spagnuolo M, Wood HF, Taranta A, Tursky E, Kleinberg E. Rheumatic fever in children and adolescents. A long-term epidemiologic study of subsequent prophylaxis, streptococcal infections, and clinical sequelae. VI. Clinical features of streptococcal infections and rheumatic recurrences. Ann Intern Med 1964;60 Suppl 5:68-86.

57. Massell BF, Fyler DC, Roy SB. The clinical picture of rheumatic fever: diagnosis, immediate prognosis, course, and therapeutic implications. Am J Cardiol 1958;1:436-449.

58. Kinare SG. Chronic valvular heart disease. Ann Indian Acad Med Sci 1972;8:48-51.

59. Vasan RS, Shrivastava S, Vijayakumar M, Narang R, Lister BC, Narula J. Echocardiographic evaluation of patients with acute rheumatic fever and rheumatic carditis. Circulation 1996;94:73-82.

60. Kinsley RH, Girdwood RW, Milner S. Surgical treatment during the acute phase of rheumatic carditis. Surg Annu 1981;13:299-323.

61. Marcus RH, Sareli P, Pocock WA, Meyer TE, Magalhaes MP, Grieve T, Antunes MJ, Barlow JB. Functional anatomy of severe mitral regurgitation in active rheumatic carditis. Am J Cardiol 1989;63:577-584.

62. de Moor MM, Lachman PI, Human DG. Rupture of tendinous chords during acute rheumatic carditis in young children. Int J Cardiol 1986;12:353-357.

63. Stollerman GH. Rheumatic carditis. Lancet 1995;346:390-392.

64. Feinstein AR, Wood HF, Spagnuolo M, Taranta A, Jonas S, Kleinberg E, Tursky E. Rheumatic fever in children and adolescents. A long-term epidemiologic study of subsequent prophylaxis, streptococcal infections, and clinical sequelae. VII. Cardiac changes and sequelae. Ann Intern Med 1964;60 Suppl 5:87-123.

65. Essop MR, Wisenbaugh T, Sareli P. Evidence against a myocardial factor as the cause of left ventricular dilation in active rheumatic carditis. J Am Coll Cardiol 1993;22:826-829.

66. Narula J, Chopra P, Talwar KK, Reddy KS, Vasan RS, Tandon R, Bhatia ML, Southern JF. Does endomyocardial biopsy aid in the diagnosis of active rheumatic carditis? Circulation 1993;88:2198-2205.

67. Tan AT, Mah PK, Chia BL. Cardiac tamponade in acute rheumatic carditis. Ann Rheum Dis 1983;42:699-701.

68. Przybojewski JZ. Rheumatic constrictive pericarditis. A case report and review of the literature. S Afr Med J 1981;59:682-686.

69. Jones TD. The diagnosis of rheumatic fever. JAMA 1944;126:481-484.

70. Rutstein DD, Bauer W, Dorfman A, Gross RE, Lichty JA, Taussig HB, Whittemore R. Jones criteria (modified) for guidance in the diagnosis of rheumatic fever. Report of the Committee on Standards and Criteria for Programs of Care. Circulation 1956;13:617-620.

71. Stollerman GH, Markowitz M, Taranta A, Wannamaker LW, Whittemore R. Jones criteria (revised) for guidance in the diagnosis of rheumatic fever. Report of the Adhoc Committee on Rheumatic Fever and Congenital Heart Disease of American Heart Association. Circulation 1965;32:664-668.

72. Shulman ST, Kaplan EL, Bisno AL, Millard HD, Amren DP, Houser H, Sanders WE Jr, Durack DT, Watanakunakorn C. Jones criteria (revised) for guidance in the diagnosis of rheumatic fever. Committee on Rheumatic Fever, Endocarditis and Kawasaki Disease of the American Heart Association. Circulation 1984;70:204A-208A.

73. Special Writing Group of the Committee on Rheumatic Fever, Endocarditis, and Kawasaki Disease of the Council on Cardiovascular Disease in the Young of the American Heart Association. Guidelines for the diagnosis of rheumatic fever. Jones criteria, 1992 update. JAMA 1992;268:2069-2073.

74. Okuni M. Problems in the clinical application of revised Jones diagnostic criteria for rheumatic fever. Jpn Heart J 1971;12:436-441.

75. Feinstein AR, Spagnuolo M. Mimetic features of rheumatic-fever recurrences. N Engl J Med 1960;262:533-540.

76. Narula J, Chandrasekhar Y, Rahimtoola S. Diagnosis of active rheumatic carditis. The echoes of change. Circulation 1999;100:1576-1581.

77. Veasy LG, Tani LY, Hill HR. Persistence of acute rheumatic fever in the intermountain area of the United States. J Pediatr 1994;124:9-16.

78. Folger GM Jr, Hajar R. Doppler echocardiographic findings of mitral and aortic valvular regurgitation in children manifesting only rheumatic arthritis. Am J Cardiol 1989;63:1278-1280.

79. Folger GM Jr, Hajar R, Robida A, Hajar HA. Occurrence of valvar heart disease in acute rheumatic fever without evident carditis: colour-flow Doppler identification. Br Heart J 1992;67:434-438.

80. Abernethy M, Bass N, Sharpe N, Grant C, Neutze J, Clarkson P, Greaves S, Lennon D, Snow S, Whalley G. Doppler echocardiography and the early diagnosis of carditis in acute rheumatic fever. Aust N Z J Med 1994;24:530-535.

81. Taranta A, Kleinberg E, Feinstein AR, Wood HF, Tursky E, Simpson R. Rheumatic fever in children

and adolescents: a long-term epidemiologic study of subsequent prophylaxis, streptococcal infections, and clinical sequelae. V. Relation of the rheumatic fever recurrence rate per streptococcal infection to pre-existing clinical features of the patients. Ann Intern Med 1964;60 Suppl 5:58-67.

82. Butterworth JS, Reppert EH. Auscultatory acumen in the general medical population. JAMA 1960;174:32-34.

83. Mangione S, Nieman LZ, Gracely E, Kaye D. The teaching and practice of cardiac auscultation during internal medicine and cardiology training. A nationwide survey. Ann Intern Med 1993;119:47-54.

84. Shaver JA. Cardiac auscultation: a cost-effective diagnostic skill. Curr Probl Cardiol 1995;20:441-530.

85. St. Clair EW, Oddone EZ, Waugh RA, Corey GR, Feussner JR. Assessing housestaff diagnostic skills using a cardiology patient simulator. Ann Intern Med 1992;117:751-756.

86. Wilson NJ, Neutze JM. Echocardiographic diagnosis of subclinical carditis in acute rheumatic fever. Int J Cardiol 1995;50:1-6.

87. Brand A, Dollberg S, Keren A. The prevalence of valvular regurgitation in children with structurally normal hearts: a color Doppler echocardiographic study. Am Heart J 1992;123:177-180.

88. Choong CY, Abascal VM, Weyman J, Levine RA, Gentile F, Thomas JD, Weyman AE. Prevalence of valvular regurgitation by Doppler echocardiography in patients with structurally normal hearts by two-dimensional echocardiography. Am Heart J 1989;117:636-642.

89. Berger M, Hecht SR, Van Tosh A, Lingam U. Pulsed and continuous wave Doppler echocardiographic assessment of valvular regurgitation in normal subjects. J Am Coll Cardiol 1989;13:1540-1545.

90. Sahn DJ, Maciel BC. Physiological valvular regurgitation. Doppler echocardiography and the potential for iatrogenic heart disease. Circulation 1988;78:1075-1077.

91. Feinstein AR, Stern EK. Clinical effects of recurrent attacks of acute rheumatic fever: a prospective epidemiologic study of 105 episodes. J Chronic Dis 1967;20:13-27.

92. Majeed HA, Yousof AM, Khuffash FA, Yusuf AR, Farwana S, Khan N. The natural history of acute rheumatic fever in Kuwait: a prospective six year follow-up report. J Chronic Dis 1986;39:361-369.

93. Majeed HA, Shaltout A, Yousof AM. Recurrences of acute rheumatic fever. A prospective study of 79 episodes. Am J Dis Child 1984;138:341-345.

94. Sanyal SK, Berry AM, Duggal S, Hooja V, Ghosh S. Sequelae of the initial attack of acute rheumatic fever in children from North India. A prospective 5-year follow-up study. Circulation 1982;65:375-379.

95. Tompkins DG, Boxerbaum B, Liebman J. Long-term prognosis of rheumatic fever patients receiving regular intramuscular benzathine penicillin. Circulation 1972;45:543-551.

96. United Kingdom and United States Joint Report on Rheumatic Heart Disease. The natural history of rheumatic fever and rheumatic heart disease. Ten-year report of a cooperative clinical trial of ACTH, cortisone, and aspirin. Circulation 1965;32:457-476.

97. Feinstein AR, Stern EK, Spagnuolo M. The prognosis of acute rheumatic fever. Am Heart J 1964;68:817-834.

98. Majeed HA, Batnager S, Yousof AM, Khuffash F, Yusuf AR. Acute rheumatic fever and the evolution of rheumatic heart disease: a prospective 12 year follow-up report. J Clin Epidemiol 1992;45:871-875.

99. Markowitz M. Evolution and critique of changes in the Jones criteria for the diagnosis of rheumatic fever. N Z Med J 1988;101:392-394.

100. Tsan MF. Mechanism of gallium-67 accumulation in inflammatory lesions. J Nucl Med 1985;26:88-92.

101. Taillefer R, Dionne D. Gallium-67 uptake by the heart. Semin Nucl Med 1983;13:176-177.

102. Shreiner DP, Krishnaswami V, Murphy JH. Unsuspected purulent pericarditis detected by gallium-67 scanning: a case report. Clin Nucl Med 1981;6:411-412.

103. Haase D, Marrie TJ, Martin R, Hayne O. Gallium scanning in tuberculous pericarditis. Clin Nucl Med 1981;6:275.

104. O'Connell JB, Robinson JA, Henkin RE, Gunnar RM. Gallium-67 citrate scanning for noninvasive detection of inflammation in pericardial diseases. Am J Cardiol 1980;46:879-884.

105. Wiseman J, Rouleau J, Rigo P, Strauss HW, Pitt B. Gallium-67 myocardial imaging for the detection of bacterial endocarditis. Radiology 1976;120:135-138.

106. Calegaro JU, de Carvalho AC, Campos ER, Medeiros M, Gomes Ed. [Gallium-67 in rheumatic fever: preliminary report.] Arq Bras Cardiol 1991;56:487-492.

107. Dewanjee MK. Cardiac and vascular imaging with labeled platelets and leukocytes. Semin Nucl Med 1984;14:154-187.

108. Oates E, Sarno RC. Detection of bacterial endocarditis with indium-111 labeled leukocytes. Clin Nucl Med 1988;13:691-693.

109. Greenberg ML, Niebulski HI, Uretsky BF, Salerni R, Klein HA, Forstate WJ, Starzl TE. Occult purulent pericarditis detected by indium-111 leukocyte imaging. Chest 1984;85:701-703.

110. Kao CH, Hsieh KS, Wang YL, Chen CW, Wang SJ, Yeh SH. ^{99}Tcm-HMPAO-labelled white blood cell scanning for the detection of carditis in the differentiation of rheumatic fever and inactive rheumatic heart disease in children. Nucl Med Commun 1992;13:478-481.

111. Khaw BA, Gold HR, Yasuda T, Leinbach RC, Kanke M, Fallon JT, Barlai-Kovach M, Strauss HW, Sheehan F, Haber E. Scintigraphic quantification of myocardial necrosis in patients after intravenous injection of myosin-specific antibody. Circulation 1986;74:501-508.

112. Khaw BA, Strauss HW, Carvalho A, Locke E, Gold HK, Haber E. Reply: concerning the labeling of DTPA-coupled proteins with Tc-99m (letter). J Nucl Med 1983;24:545.

113. Narula J, Reddy KS, Khaw B-A. Can indium-111 antimyosin scintigraphy complement the Jones criteria in the diagnosis of active rheumatic carditis? In: Khaw B-A, Narula J, Strauss HW, eds. Monoclonal antibodies in cardiovascular diseases. Philadelphia: Lea & Febiger, 1994:109-117.

114. Narula J, Malhotra A, Yasuda T, Talwar KK, Reddy KS, Chopra P, Southern JF, Vasan RS, Tandon R, Bhatia ML, Khaw BA, Strauss HW. Usefulness of antimyosin antibody imaging for the detection of active rheumatic myocarditis. Am J Cardiol 1999;84:946-950, A7.

115. Bland EF, Jones TD. Rheumatic fever and rheumatic heart disease: a twenty year report on 1000 patients followed since childhood. Circulation 1951;4:836-843.

116. Lue HC, Tseng WP, Lin GJ, Hsieh KH, Hsieh RP, Chiou JF. Clinical and epidemiological features of rheumatic fever and rheumatic heart disease in Taiwan and the Far East. Indian Heart J 1983;35:139-146.

117. Griffith GC, Taranta A. Should adults with rheumatic heart disease be kept on continuous penicillin prophylaxis? Am J Cardiol 1966;18:627-629.

118. Thomas GT. Five-year follow-up on patients with rheumatic fever treated by bed rest, steroids, or salicylate. Br Med J 1961;1:1635-1639.

119. Chandrashekhar Y. Secondary prevention of rheumatic fever: theory, practice, and analysis of available studies. In: Narula J, Virmani R, Reddy KS, Tandon R, eds. Rheumatic fever. Washington, DC: American Registry of Pathology, Armed Forces Institute of Pathology, 1999:399-442.

120. Findlay L. The rheumatic infection in childhood. London: E. Arnold, 1931.

121. Kuttner AG, Krumwiede E. Observations on effect of streptococcal upper respiratory infections on rheumatic children: 3-year study. J Clin Invest 1941;20:273-287.

122. Bisno AL, Pearce IA, Stollerman GH. Streptococcal infections that fail to cause recurrences of rheumatic fever. J Infect Dis 1977;136:278-285.

123. Saslaw MS, Streitfeld MM. Group A beta hemolytic streptococci and rheumatic fever in Miami, Florida. I. Bacteriologic observations from October 1954 through May 1955. Dis Chest 1959;35:175-193.

124. Kaplan EL, Johnson DR, Cleary PP. Group A streptococcal serotypes isolated from patients and sibling contacts during the resurgence of rheumatic fever in the United States in the mid-1980s. J Infect Dis 1989;159:101-103.

125. Schwartz B, Facklam RR, Breiman RF. Changing epidemiology of group A streptococcal infection in the USA. Lancet 1990;336:1167-1171.

126. Johnson DR, Stevens DL, Kaplan EL. Epidemiologic analysis of group A streptococcal serotypes associated with severe systemic infections, rheumatic fever, or uncomplicated pharyngitis. J Infect Dis 1992;166:374-382.

127. Spagnuolo M, Pasternack B, Taranta A. Risk of rheumatic-fever recurrences after streptococcal infections. Prospective study of clinical and social factors. N Engl J Med 1971;285:641-647.

128. Stollerman GH. Factors determining the attack rate of rheumatic fever. JAMA 1961;177:823-828.

129. Hansen AE. Rheumatic recrudescences: diagnosis and prevention. J Pediatr 1946;28:296-308.

130. Dajani A, Taubert K, Ferrieri P, Peter G, Shulman S. Treatment of acute streptococcal pharyngitis and prevention of rheumatic fever: a statement for health professionals. Committee on Rheumatic Fever, Endocarditis, and Kawasaki Disease of the Council on Cardiovascular Disease in the Young, the American Heart Association. Pediatrics 1995;96:758-764.

131. Hench PS, Slocumb CH, Barnes AR, Smith HL, Polley HF, Kendall EC. The effects of the adrenal cortical hormone 17-hydroxy-11-dehydrocorticosterone (compound E) on the acute phase of rheumatic fever: preliminary report. Proc Staff Meet Mayo Clin 1949;24:277-297.

132. Rothman PE. Treatment of rheumatic carditis. A critical evaluation. Clin Pediatr (Phila) 1965;4:619-625.

133. Markowitz M, Kuttner G. Treatment of acute rheumatic fever. Am J Dis Child 1962;104:313-320.

134. Amigo MC, Martinez-Lavin M, Reyes PA. Acute rheumatic fever. Rheum Dis Clin North Am 1993;19:333-350.

135. Combined Rheumatic Fever Study Group. A comparison of short-term, intensive prednisone and acetyl salicylic acid therapy in the treatment of acute rheumatic fever. N Engl J Med 1965;272:63-70.

136. Stolzer BL, Houser HB, Clark EJ. Therapeutic agents in rheumatic carditis: comparative effects of acetylsalicylic acid, corticotropin, and cortisone. Arch Intern Med 1955;95:677-688.

137. Dorfman A, Gross JI, Lorincz AE. The treatment of acute rheumatic fever. Pediatrics 1961;27:692-706.

138. Albert DA, Harel L, Karrison T. The treatment of rheumatic carditis: a review and meta-analysis. Medicine (Baltimore) 1995;74:1-12.

139. Duran CM, Gometza B, De Vol EB. Valve repair in rheumatic mitral disease. Circulation 1991;84 Suppl:III125-III132.

140. Lewis BS, Geft IL, Milo S, Gotsman MS. Echocardiography and valve replacement in the critically ill patient with acute rheumatic carditis. Ann Thorac Surg 1979;27:529-535.

141. Skoularigis J, Sinovich V, Joubert G, Sareli P. Evaluation of the long-term results of mitral valve repair in 254 young patients with rheumatic mitral regurgitation. Circulation 1994;90:II167-II174.

142. Schneider WF, Chapman S, Schulz VB, Krause RM, Lancefield RC. Prevention of streptococcal pharyngitis among military personnel and their civilian dependents by mass prophylaxis. N Engl J Med 1964;270:1205-1212.

143. Strasser T. Cost-effective control of rheumatic fever in the community. Health Policy 1985;5:159-164.

144. Beachey EH, Seyer JM, Dale JB. Protective immunogenicity and T lymphocyte specificity of a trivalent hybrid peptide containing NH2-terminal sequences of types 5, 6, and 24 M proteins synthesized in tandem. J Exp Med 1987;166:647-656.

145. Dale JB, Chiang EY, Lederer JW. Recombinant tetravalent group A streptococcal M protein vaccine. J Immunol 1993;151:2188-2194.

146. Dale JB, Simmons M, Chiang EC, Chiang EY. Recombinant, octavalent group A streptococcal M protein vaccine. Vaccine 1996;14:944-948.

147. Bessen D, Fischetti VA. Influence of intranasal immunization with synthetic peptides corresponding to conserved epitopes of M protein on mucosal colonization by group A streptococci. Infect Immun 1988;56:2666-2672.

148. Bessen D, Fischetti VA. Synthetic peptide vaccine against mucosal colonization by group A streptococci. I. Protection against a heterologous M serotype with shared C repeat region epitopes. J Immunol 1990;145:1251-1256.

149. Bronze MS, Courtney HS, Dale JB. Epitopes of group A streptococcal M protein that evoke cross-protective local immune responses. J Immunol 1992;148:888-893.

150. Brandt ER, Sriprakash KS, Hobb RI, Hayman WA, Zeng W, Batzloff MR, Jackson DC, Good MF. New multi-determinant strategy for a group A streptococcal vaccine designed for the Australian Aboriginal population. Nat Med 2000;6:455-459.

151. Chen CC, Cleary PP. Complete nucleotide sequence of the streptococcal C5a peptidase gene of *Streptococcus pyogenes*. J Biol Chem 1990;265:3161-3167.

152. O'Connor SP, Darip D, Fraley K, Nelson CM, Kaplan EL, Cleary PP. The human antibody response to streptococcal C5a peptidase. J Infect Dis 1991;163:109-116.

153. Ji Y, McLandsborough L, Kondagunta A, Cleary PP. C5a peptidase alters clearance and trafficking of group A streptococci by infected mice. Infect Immun 1996;64:503-510.

154. Ji Y, Carlson B, Kondagunta A, Cleary PP. Intranasal immunization with C5a peptidase prevents nasopharyngeal colonization of mice by the group A *Streptococcus*. Infect Immun 1997;65:2080-2087.

155. Kapur V, Maffei JT, Greer RS, Li LL, Adams GJ, Musser JM. Vaccination with streptococcal extracellular cysteine protease (interleukin-1 beta convertase) protects mice against challenge with heterologous group A streptococci. Microb Pathog 1994;16:443-450.

156. Dale JB, Baird RW, Courtney HS, Hasty DL, Bronze MS. Passive protection of mice against group A streptococcal pharyngeal infection by lipoteichoic acid. J Infect Dis 1994;169:319-323.

157. Schrager HM, Alberti S, Cywes C, Dougherty GJ, Wessels MR. Hyaluronic acid capsule modulates M protein-mediated adherence and acts as a ligand for attachment of group A *Streptococcus* to CD44 on human keratinocytes. J Clin Invest 1998;101:1708-1716.

158. Brandt ER, Good MF. Vaccine strategies to prevent rheumatic fever. Immunol Res 1999;19:89-103.

Myocarditis Associated With Human Immunodeficiency Virus Infection and Acquired Immunodeficiency Syndrome

Lyle J. Olson, M.D.

Acquired immunodeficiency syndrome (AIDS) has been recognized for more than 20 years, during which time it has become a worldwide pandemic. AIDS is caused by human immunodeficiency virus type I (HIV-1), one of the Lentivirinae subfamily of retroviruses. Initially, HIV-1 causes an indolent, chronic infection with a clinical latency of several years characterized by persistent viremia and poor humoral response.[1] The major targets of HIV-1 are CD4$^+$ T lymphocytes. The gradual depletion of this cell line culminates in the profound immunodeficiency characteristic of AIDS.[2] Infected individuals most often succumb to opportunistic infection or malignancy.

Individuals at highest risk for HIV infection include male homosexuals, intravenous drug users, and those who have intimate contact with HIV-infected individuals. Worldwide, an estimated 40 million people are infected with HIV-1 and another 10 million people have AIDS.[3] In the United States, more than 1 million people are HIV positive, of whom more than 440,000 have been diagnosed with AIDS.[4] Among men age 25 to 40 years in the United States, AIDS became the leading cause of death in 1992 and is also a leading cause of death in women.[3]

Clinically recognized cardiac complications of HIV-1 infection and AIDS are numerous (Table 22-1), although relatively infrequent compared to HIV-associated diseases of the lungs, brain, and gastrointestinal tract.[5,6] Congestive heart failure is the leading cause of death in pediatric patients with AIDS.[7] The cardiovascular complications of HIV infection and AIDS in adults may be increasing as survival is prolonged because of earlier detection and more effective therapy and supportive care.[8,9] The pericardium is the most common site of *clinically recognized* cardiovascular involvement associated with HIV-1 infection or AIDS in adults, whereas antemortem diagnosis of myocardial involvement is relatively uncommon.[10-13] By comparison, myocarditis is the most common cardiac *pathologic finding* at autopsy of HIV-infected patients; the prevalence is as high as 70%.[14-19] However, it is uncertain whether the myocarditis so frequently observed at autopsy is clinically relevant. In the majority of cases a specific etiologic factor cannot be identified, whereas in a smaller proportion of cases opportunistic pathogens are observed.

Table 22-1
Cardiac Lesions in Acquired Immunodeficiency Syndrome

Myocarditis
Pericarditis
Endocarditis
Dilated cardiomyopathy
Kaposi sarcoma
Malignant lymphoma
Arteriopathy
Myocardial infarction

Myocarditis associated with HIV-1 infection or AIDS is most often characterized as a focal, nonspecific lymphocytic process in the setting of left ventricular (LV) dysfunction. The entire spectrum of cardiovascular complications of AIDS and HIV infection is beyond the scope of this chapter, which is limited to nonspecific and infectious myocarditis associated with AIDS and HIV-1 infection.

PREVALENCE OF LV DYSFUNCTION IN HIV-1 INFECTION

LV dysfunction associated with AIDS is well recognized and led to the notion that direct myocardial infection by HIV may cause this disorder. However, clinically overt myocarditis associated with HIV infection or AIDS is probably an uncommon entity, and the link between myocarditis and LV dysfunction is not definitively proven.

The prevalence of LV dysfunction in HIV-infected patients is related to the stage of disease; patients with overt AIDS are more likely to have LV dysfunction than patients at earlier stages of HIV infection.[20] Echocardiographic studies performed at tertiary care centers have estimated that overt structural heart disease is present in as many as 10% to 40% of patients with AIDS or HIV infection.[10,21-23] Cardiac involvement is often subclinical as echocardiographic studies have demonstrated LV dysfunction in 41% of asymptomatic HIV-positive individuals.[10] However, in the primary care setting, AIDS cardiac complications are unusual. One autopsy series demonstrated no cardiac disease in 115 consecutive autopsies of patients who died of AIDS-related complications.[16]

The natural history of structural heart disease in HIV-infected individuals has been well described in a prospective and serial echocardiographic study of 952 *asymptomatic* patients with normal baseline LV function. The incidence of LV dysfunction was 1.5% per year, with a prevalence of 8% at 5 years.[20] This relatively low prevalence compared with previous reports suggests that structural heart disease is relatively uncommon and related to the stage of HIV disease. It seems likely that the relatively high frequency of LV dysfunction described in earlier reports was due to referral bias.

NONSPECIFIC MYOCARDITIS

Myocarditis identified at autopsy or on endomyocardial biopsy in HIV-infected patients is most often nonspecific and manifested as focal, inflammatory lymphocytic infiltrates without myocyte necrosis. Other reported histopathologic findings include lymphocytic infiltration with myocyte necrosis fulfilling the Dallas criteria or myocyte damage without associated cellular inflammatory infiltrate.[17,20] The autopsy finding of focal myocarditis in many patients who die of AIDS-related complications, but have no known premortem heart disease, suggests that focal lymphocytic infiltration may have no clinical significance. By comparison, diffuse lymphocytic myocarditis meeting the Dallas criteria appears rare.[17]

The prevalence of nonspecific myocarditis is related to the stage of HIV infection and the presence of structural heart disease. In one study of HIV-infected patients with a premortem diagnosis of *dilated cardiomyopathy*, histologic findings consistent with lymphocytic myocarditis by the Dallas criteria were identified in 63 of 76 patients (83%).[20] By comparison, in HIV-infected patients without LV dysfunction the prevalence of nonspecific lymphocytic myocarditis was relatively low.[20]

PATHOGENESIS

The first clinical report to suggest a relationship between nonspecific myocarditis and dilated cardiomyopathy in AIDS patients appeared in 1986;[24] 3 patients had clinical, echocardiographic, and pathologic findings of dilated cardiomyopathy and 2 of the patients had focal lymphocytic infiltration associated with myocyte necrosis. Subsequent reports suggested an association between focal nonspecific myocarditis at autopsy and clinical cardiomyopathy.[20,25] Numerous hypotheses have been suggested to account for the etiology of nonspecific myocarditis and cardiomyopathy observed in HIV-infected patients, including direct HIV-1 infection of myocardial cells or coinfection with other cardiotropic viruses,[26-30] cytokine cardiotoxicity,[31-33] postviral cardiac autoimmunity,[34,35] nutritional deficiencies,[36-39] and cardiotoxicity from illicit drugs[40-43] or pharmacologic agents.[28,44-49]

The histologic findings of a monoclonal or oligoclonal inflammatory cellular infiltrate suggest a viral or autoimmune cause for the myocarditis associated with HIV infection. Myocarditis is more likely in individuals with more profound immunosuppression because a CD4 count less than 400 cells/μL is more frequently observed in patients with dilated cardiomyopathy.[20] In this same series, inflammatory myocardial cellular infiltrates were predominantly CD3 lymphocytes in 12 patients and CD8 lymphocytes in 64 patients. A separate report[19] described 35 HIV-infected patients with global LV dysfunction who underwent endomyocardial biopsy in which active or borderline myocarditis was observed in 55% of patients. For those patients with biopsy-proven myocarditis, mean LV ejection fraction was 28% whereas for patients without myocarditis it was 48%. The cellular infiltrate was primarily composed of CD8 T lymphocytes.

Although it has been suspected that myocarditis and cardiomyopathy associated with HIV-1 infection may be caused by direct viral infection of myocytes, definite evidence for this is lacking. Difficulty in demonstration of a link among HIV-1 infection, myocarditis, and cardiomyopathy in AIDS is related, in part, to lack of a suitable in vivo model of the disease. Because of the limited host range of HIV-1 and the difficulty in handling nonhuman primates infected with simian immunodeficiency virus-1, little investigation has been reported of myocarditis or cardiomyopathy associated with AIDS in animal models.[50]

What is the potential for direct myocardial infection? HIV-1 invades T cells by attachment to a CD4 surface-membrane receptor. However, there are no CD4 receptors on myocyte surface membranes. It is possible that the virus gains access to myocytes by other mechanisms, although the evidence to support this concept is limited. It is also possible that injury to myocytes may facilitate entry of the HIV virion; Epstein-Barr virus (EBV) promotes entry of HIV into CD4 receptor negative cells, with subsequent replication.[51]

The presence of viral genomic material within the myocytes of HIV-infected patients with myocarditis and cardiomyopathy does not definitely establish viral infection as causal. Furthermore, the significance of the finding of viral transcripts within cells is uncertain because patients may or may not have LV dysfunction.[35] HIV-1 genomic material reportedly was detected within the genome of myocardial cells, although typically the findings have been sparse and may not have represented myocyte infection because the HIV nucleic acid sequence may actually have been located in endothelial cells or macrophages.[26,29,52,53] In one study, in 58 of 63 patients with AIDS, LV dysfunction, and biopsy-proven nonspecific lymphocytic myocarditis, a positive hybridization signal was observed but staining was weak and affected myocytes were generally not surrounded by inflammatory cells.[20]

In adults with AIDS-associated myocarditis, non-HIV viruses or viral genomic material identified in myocardial tissue has included cytomegalovirus (CMV), coxsackievirus group B, and Epstein-Barr virus.[20,54] In an autopsy study of 32 children who died with advanced HIV disease, including 23 with histologic evidence of myocarditis, viral sequences detected by polymerase chain reaction included adenovirus in 6, CMV in 3, and both adenovirus and CMV in 2. No other viruses were detected by polymerase chain reaction, including HIV.[55]

A high proportion of HIV-seropositive patients with LV dysfunction have evidence of latent infection of myocytes with CMV immediate-early genes.[54] Although observation of the intranuclear inclusions of active, lytic CMV infection is unusual, it has been suggested that latent viral infection may promote enhanced major histocompatibility complex expression, thereby provoking immune-mediated injury typical of animal models of myocarditis.[54]

Immune-mediated mechanisms other than direct myocardial viral infection may account for the cellular infiltrates and cardiomyopathy observed in AIDS patients. Herskowitz et al.[34] demonstrated circulating autoantibodies in 4 of 6 AIDS patients with cardiomyopathy, whereas AIDS patients without cardiomyopathy did not have these antibodies. In the patients with autoantibodies, antimyosin antibodies were identified. In these same individuals, no evidence of HIV-1 or other viruses was identified from myocardial biopsy specimens evaluated by in situ hybridization, lending support to an autoimmune mechanism of disease. A study by Gu et al.[56] used monoclonal antibodies to HIV core proteins that reacted with myocyte antigens in 38 of 42 AIDS patients (and 11 of 28 non-AIDS patients), suggesting antibodies occurring in AIDS patients may react with antigenic epitopes of myocytes, thereby promoting autoimmune-mediated heart muscle disease.

Multiple cytokines are suspected of having a role in the mediation of myocardial inflammation, myocyte necrosis, and ventricular dysfunction in myocarditis, although specifics are incompletely understood in human disease.[57] The mononuclear cells characteristic of lymphocytic myocarditis, including the focal nonspecific myocarditis of AIDS, are a likely source of cytokines that promote inflammation and maintenance of immune response, which may lead to impaired contractile function and fibrosis. Matsumori et al.[58] showed that patients with myocarditis have markedly increased concentrations of cytokines, including tumor necrosis factor-α and interleukin-1 and -6. In animal models of myocarditis, similar profiles of cytokine activation have been described and have been demonstrated directly in cardiac tissue.[59] Tumor necrosis factor-α has been demonstrated to be a negative inotrope[31] and is increased in patients with congestive heart failure,[60] AIDS,[61,62] and myocarditis.[58] HIV may cause myocyte injury by an "innocent bystander destruction" mechanism, as may occur in AIDS-associated encephalitis.[63] However, whether these mechanisms operate in the myocarditis and dilated cardiomyopathy of AIDS is unknown.

INFECTIOUS MYOCARDITIS

Opportunistic infections are a common complication of AIDS and the most frequent cause of morbidity and mortality. However, relatively few pathogens have been isolated from the myocardium of AIDS patients (Table 22-2). Myocardial involvement is usually associated with disseminated disease and multiple foci of infection. Typically, infectious organisms are identified in patients dying of noncardiac causes, and the findings of myocardial abnormalities are regarded as incidental. Opportunistic pathogens represent diverse causes of infectious disease, including bacteria, fungi, protozoa, and viruses.

PROTOZOAL

Toxoplasma gondii is the most frequently documented infectious cause of myocarditis associated with AIDS, and the heart is the second most common site of infection after the brain. Autopsy series have described *T gondii* myocarditis (myocardial toxoplasmosis) in 1% to 16% of patients dying of AIDS.[14,17,64] Evidence of myocardial toxoplasmosis includes trophozoites or pseudocysts in myocardial fibers. A minority of cases have associated myocarditis with focal areas of necrosis and lymphocytic infiltrates.[65] Antemortem diagnosis of toxoplasma myocarditis associated with LV dysfunction has been described, including successful treatment.[66,67]

Table 22-2
Opportunistic Myocardial Pathogens Associated With AIDS or HIV Infection

Bacterial
  Mycobacterium tuberculosis
  Mycobacterium avium complex

Fungal
  Cryptococcus neoformans
  Aspergillus fumigatus
  Candida albicans
  Histoplasma capsulatum
  Coccidioides immitis

Protozoal
  Toxoplasma gondii

Viral
  HIV
  Cytomegalovirus
  Herpes simplex
  Coxsackie B
  Epstein-Barr virus
  Adenovirus

AIDS, acquired immunodeficiency syndrome; HIV, human immunodeficiency virus.

BACTERIAL

Pericardial tuberculosis has been reported in association with AIDS, typically in the setting of widespread disease. However, myocardial tuberculosis appears rare.[5,68]

FUNGAL

Fungal myocarditis is an unusual complication of disseminated infection that is identified most often at autopsy. Various fungal organisms identified in the myocardium at autopsy with associated myocarditis have included *Aspergillus fumigatus*, *Candida albicans*, *Histoplasma capsulatum*, *Coccidioides immitis*, and *Cryptococcus neoformans*. Cardiac cryptococcus has been diagnosed in association with congestive heart failure and resolved after therapy with amphotericin B and flucytosine.[68-70]

VIRAL

Several viruses have been implicated in myocarditis associated with AIDS (Table 22-3). CMV is a common opportunistic pathogen in AIDS, but it is associated less frequently with

Table 22-3
Viruses Implicated in AIDS-associated Myocarditis

Cytomegalovirus
Coxsackie B
Human immunodeficiency virus
Epstein-Barr virus
Adenovirus

AIDS, acquired immunodeficiency syndrome.

myocarditis.[71] In an autopsy series of AIDS patients, CMV was identified histologically from various organ systems by the detection of inclusion bodies in 43 of 56 patients (77%); however, inclusion bodies with myocarditis were detected in only 4 of these cases.[72] When inclusion bodies are the criteria for the detection and diagnosis of solid organ involvement by CMV, the rate of infection is underestimated compared to in situ DNA hybridization techniques.[54,73]

Other viruses identified by culture or polymerase chain reaction within the myocardium of HIV-infected or AIDS patients, either at antemortem endomyocardial biopsy or from autopsy material, have included Epstein-Barr and coxsackie B virus in adults[20] and adenovirus in children.[55] These viruses may be present as either primary infection or as coinfection and can occur with or without associated myocarditis and with or without associated LV dysfunction.

DIFFERENTIAL DIAGNOSIS OF LV DYSFUNCTION IN AIDS

It is difficult to assess the clinical significance of viral infection of the myocardium in HIV-infected patients. AIDS or HIV-infected patients with myocarditis most often present with signs and symptoms of congestive heart failure or asymptomatic LV dysfunction. The diagnosis of dilated cardiomyopathy in this setting is best established by echocardiography. More specific diagnosis can be established by endomyocardial biopsy, as clinically indicated. However, in the vast majority of cases endomyocardial biopsy will not identify a specific cause that will modify therapy. In a minority of patients, biopsy may establish a treatable cause of myocarditis. Therefore, the clinician should consider the specifics of each case before making a recommendation regarding whether endomyocardial biopsy is necessary.

Aside from nonspecific or infectious myocarditis, the differential diagnosis of LV dysfunction in the AIDS patient includes drug toxicity from either abuse of illicit substances or iatrogenic disease from agents used in the therapy for AIDS. AIDS patients often take a great variety of prescription and nonprescription drugs and use illicit drugs.[74] Alcohol, cocaine, or heroin may contribute to LV dysfunction in many cases.[40,41,43,74-76] Pharmacotherapy is also potentially associated with LV dysfunction in AIDS patients. Therapeutic agents implicated as potential cardiac toxins include zidovudine,[28,77,78] interleukin-2,[79] and interferon alfa-2.[46,80]

If neoplastic infiltration is suspected as a cause of LV dysfunction, cardiac computed tomography or magnetic resonance imaging may be a useful adjunct to echocardiography for characterizing cardiac involvement. Neoplastic infiltration of the heart by Kaposi sarcoma is frequently seen at autopsy and usually associated with widespread disease in the terminal phases of AIDS.[81] Non-Hodgkin lymphoma is also observed in this setting and also associated with widespread disease.[82]

In addition to HIV-related cardiac conditions, differential diagnosis also includes non-HIV disease, because the latency of HIV disease may be long and patients are at risk for development of hypertensive heart disease, coronary artery disease, or other causes of LV dysfunction.

TREATMENT

The prognosis of HIV-infected and AIDS patients with dilated cardiomyopathy is generally poor. Patients with nonreversible LV dysfunction have a mean survival of only 101 days as a result of complications of heart failure or advanced AIDS.[83]

No clinical treatment trials of HIV-infected patients with myocarditis have been reported. Accordingly, treatment is supportive and directed at the underlying disorder, systemic infectious and neoplastic complications, and LV dysfunction.

Angiotensin-converting enzyme inhibitors, digitalis, diuretics, and beta-adrenergic receptor blockers are indicated in patients with stable classes II and III LV systolic dysfunction. Antiarrhythmic drugs and anticoagulation therapy are also used in the standard manner.

There is no role for immunosuppressive therapy in the treatment of the HIV-infected or AIDS patient with suspected or proven myocarditis because immunosuppression in nonimmunocompromised patients has not been shown to be efficacious for management.[84] Moreover, it seems imprudent to treat severely immunocompromised patients with augmented immunosuppression.

The role of antiretroviral therapy for treatment of dilated cardiomyopathy or myocarditis in HIV-infected patients is uncertain; it has not been demonstrated to be beneficial in a carefully designed study.[85] Moreover, some authors have described an association between the use of zidovudine and the development of heart failure.[28]

SUMMARY

Cardiac dysfunction should be considered in the differential diagnosis of any HIV-infected patient with dyspnea or cardiomegaly. In the setting of AIDS or HIV infection, the diagnosis of dilated cardiomyopathy is established by echocardiography. A significant proportion, perhaps exceeding 80%, of patients with dilated cardiomyopathy may have focal, nonspecific lymphocytic myocarditis.[20] Although viruses, in general, are well established as a cause of acute myocarditis, a causal role for viruses in the pathogenesis of dilated cardiomyopathy has not been demonstrated conclusively, including HIV infection. Moreover, it is uncertain whether the myocarditis frequently observed in AIDS patients with LV dysfunction is caused by *any* viral infection, including HIV.

A low CD4 count is an excellent predictor of the presence of LV dysfunction.[20] The risk of dilated cardiomyopathy may also be increased with a history of illicit drug use.[74,76]

Myocarditis due to HIV-1 myocyte infection does not seem to be the most likely cause of LV dysfunction in patients with AIDS. It is more likely that the cause of LV dysfunction and congestive heart failure in this setting is multifactorial, related to drug toxicity, non-HIV viral infection, poor nutrition, or cytokines.

REFERENCES

1. Letvin NL. Animal models for AIDS. Immunol Today 1990;11:322-326.
2. Fauci AS. The human immunodeficiency virus: infectivity and mechanisms of pathogenesis. Science 1988;239:617-622.
3. Centers for Disease Control. Update: mortality attributable to HIV infection among persons aged 25-44 years—United States, 1991 and 1992. MMWR Morb Mortal Wkly Rep 1993;42:869-872.
4. Ward J, Peterson L, Jaffe H. Current trends in the epidemiology of HIV/AIDS. In: Sande MA, Volberding PA, eds. The medical management of AIDS. 5th ed. Philadelphia: WB Saunders, 1997:3-13.
5. Miller-Catchpole R, Variakojis D, Anastasi J, Abrahams C. The Chicago AIDS autopsy study: opportunistic infections, neoplasms, and findings from selected organ systems with a comparison to national data. Chicago Associated Pathologists. Mod Pathol 1989;2:277-294.
6. Moskowitz L, Hensley GT, Chan JC, Adams K. Immediate causes of death in acquired immunodeficiency syndrome. Arch Pathol Lab Med 1985;109:735-738.
7. Johann-Liang R, Cervia JS, Noel GJ. Characteristics of human immunodeficiency virus-infected children at the time of death: an experience in the 1990s. Pediatr Infect Dis J 1997;16:1145-1150.
8. Hoover DR, Saah AJ, Bacellar H, Phair J, Detels R, Anderson R, Kaslow RA. Clinical manifestations of AIDS in the era of pneumocystis prophylaxis. Multicenter AIDS Cohort Study. N Engl J Med 1993;329:1922-1926.
9. Palella FJ Jr, Delaney KM, Moorman AC, Loveless MO, Fuhrer J, Satten GA, Aschman DJ, Holmberg SD. Declining morbidity and mortality among patients with advanced human immunodeficiency virus infection. HIV Outpatient Study Investigators. N Engl J Med 1998;338:853-860.

10. Corallo S, Mutinelli MR, Moroni M, Lazzarin A, Celano V, Repossini A, Baroldi G. Echocardiography detects myocardial damage in AIDS: prospective study in 102 patients. Eur Heart J 1988;9:887-892.

11. Akhras F, Dubrey S, Gazzard B, Noble MI. Emerging patterns of heart disease in HIV infected homosexual subjects with and without opportunistic infections; a prospective colour flow Doppler echocardiographic study. Eur Heart J 1994;15:68-75.

12. Hsia J, Ross AM. Pericardial effusion and pericardiocentesis in human immunodeficiency virus infection. Am J Cardiol 1994;74:94-96.

13. Heidenreich PA, Eisenberg MJ, Kee LL, Somelofski CA, Hollander H, Schiller NB, Cheitlin MD. Pericardial effusion in AIDS. Incidence and survival. Circulation 1995;92:3229-3234.

14. Baroldi G, Corallo S, Moroni M, Repossini A, Mutinelli MR, Lazzarin A, Antonacci CM, Cristina S, Negri C. Focal lymphocytic myocarditis in acquired immunodeficiency syndrome (AIDS): a correlative morphologic and clinical study in 26 consecutive fatal cases. J Am Coll Cardiol 1988;12:463-469.

15. Webb JG, Chan-Yan C, Kiess MC. Cardiac dysfunction associated with the acquired immuno-deficiency syndrome (AIDS). Clin Cardiol 1988;11:423-426.

16. Lewis W. AIDS: cardiac findings from 115 autopsies. Prog Cardiovasc Dis 1989;32:207-215.

17. Anderson DW, Virmani R, Reilly JM, O'Leary T, Cunnion RE, Robinowitz M, Macher AM, Punja U, Villaflor ST, Parrillo JE, Roberts WC. Prevalent myocarditis at necropsy in the acquired immunodeficiency syndrome. J Am Coll Cardiol 1988;11:792-799.

18. Magno J, Margaretten W, Cheitlin M. Myocardial involvement in acquired immunodeficiency syndrome: incidence in a large autopsy study (abstract). Circulation 1988;78 Suppl 2:II-459.

19. Herskowitz A, Willoughby SB, Beschorner WE, Neumann DA, Baughman KL. Myocarditis associated with severe left ventricular dysfunction in late stage HIV infection (abstract). Circulation 1992;86 Suppl 1:I-6.

20. Barbaro G, Di Lorenzo G, Grisorio B, Barbarini G. Incidence of dilated cardiomyopathy and detection of HIV in myocardial cells of HIV-positive patients. Gruppo Italiano per lo Studio Cardiologico dei Pazienti Affetti da AIDS. N Engl J Med 1998;339:1093-1099.

21. Blanchard DG, Hagenhoff C, Chow LC, McCann HA, Dittrich HC. Reversibility of cardiac abnormalities in human immunodeficiency virus (HIV)-infected individuals: a serial echocardio-graphic study. J Am Coll Cardiol 1991;17:1270-1276.

22. Herskowitz A, Vlahov D, Willoughby S, Chaisson RE, Schulman SP, Neumann DA, Baughman KL. Prevalence and incidence of left ventricular dysfunction in patients with human immunodeficiency virus infection. Am J Cardiol 1993;71:955-958.

23. De Castro S, d'Amati G, Gallo P, Cartoni D, Santopadre P, Vullo V, Cirelli A, Migliau G. Frequency of development of acute global left ventricular dysfunction in human immunodeficiency virus infection. J Am Coll Cardiol 1994;24:1018-1024.

24. Cohen IS, Anderson DW, Virmani R, Reen BM, Macher AM, Sennesh J, DiLorenzo P, Redfield RR. Congestive cardiomyopathy in association with the acquired immunodeficiency syndrome. N Engl J Med 1986;315:628-630.

25. Reilly JM, Cunnion RE, Anderson DW, O'Leary TJ, Simmons JT, Lane HC, Fauci AS, Roberts WC, Virmani R, Parrillo JE. Frequency of myocarditis, left ventricular dysfunction and ventricular tachycardia in the acquired immune deficiency syndrome. Am J Cardiol 1988;62:789-793.

26. Grody WW, Cheng L, Lewis W. Infection of the heart by the human immunodeficiency virus. Am J Cardiol 1990;66:203-206.

27. Wu AY, Forouhar F, Cartun RW, Berman MM, Shiue ST, Louie AT, Grunnet M. Identification of human immunodeficiency virus in the heart of a patient with acquired immunodeficiency syndrome. Mod Pathol 1990;3:625-630.

28. Herskowitz A, Willoughby SB, Baughman KL, Schulman SP, Bartlett JD. Cardiomyopathy associated with antiretroviral therapy in patients with HIV infection: a report of six cases. Ann Intern Med 1992;116:311-313.

29. Lipshultz SE, Fox CH, Perez-Atayde AR, Sanders SP, Colan SD, McIntosh K, Winter HS. Identification of human immunodeficiency virus-1 RNA and DNA in the heart of a child with cardiovascular abnormalities and congenital acquired immune deficiency syndrome. Am J Cardiol 1990;66:246-250.

30. Rodriguez ER, Nasim S, Hsia J, Sandin RL, Ferreira A, Hilliard BA, Ross AM, Garrett CT. Cardiac myocytes and dendritic cells harbor human immunodeficiency virus in infected patients with and without cardiac dysfunction: detection by multiplex, nested, polymerase chain reaction in individually microdissected cells from right ventricular endomyocardial biopsy tissue. Am J Cardiol 1991;68:1511-1520.

31. Suffredini AF, Fromm RE, Parker MM, Brenner M, Kovacs JA, Wesley RA, Parrillo JE. The cardio-vascular response of normal humans to the administration of endotoxin. N Engl J Med 1989;321:280-287.

32. Lahdevirta J, Maury CP, Teppo AM, Repo H. Elevated levels of circulating cachectin/tumor necrosis factor in patients with acquired immunodeficiency syndrome. Am J Med 1988;85:289-291.

33. Levine B, Kalman J, Mayer L, Fillit HM, Packer M. Elevated circulating levels of tumor necrosis factor in severe chronic heart failure. N Engl J Med 1990;323:236-241.

34. Herskowitz A, Ansari AA, Neumann DA, Beschorner WE, Oliveira M, Chaisson RE, Rose NR, Bartlett JG, Weiss JL, Baughman KL. Cardiomyopathy in acquired immunodeficiency syndrome: evidence for autoimmunity (abstract). Circulation 1989;80 Suppl 2:II-322.

35. Herskowitz A, Willoughby S, Wu TC, Beschorner WE, Neumann DA, Rose NR, Baughman KL, Ansari AA. Immunopathogenesis of HIV-1-associated cardiomyopathy. Clin Immunol Immunopathol 1993;68:234-241.

36. Schocken DD, Holloway JD, Powers PS. Weight loss and the heart: effects of anorexia nervosa and starvation. Arch Intern Med 1989;149:877-881.

37. Goldberg SJ, Comerci GD, Feldman L. Cardiac output and regional myocardial contraction in anorexia nervosa. J Adolesc Health Care 1988;9:15-21.

38. Dworkin BM, Rosenthal WS, Wormser GP, Weiss L. Selenium deficiency in the acquired immuno-deficiency syndrome. JPEN J Parenter Enteral Nutr 1986;10:405-407.

39. Dworkin BM, Antonecchia PP, Smith F, Weiss L, Davidian M, Rubin D, Rosenthal WS. Reduced cardiac selenium content in the acquired immunodeficiency syndrome. JPEN J Parenter Enteral Nutr 1989;13:644-647.

40. Tazelaar HD, Karch SB, Stephens BG, Billingham ME. Cocaine and the heart. Hum Pathol 1987;18:195-199.

41. Virmani R, Robinowitz M, Smialek JE, Smyth DF. Cardiovascular effects of cocaine: an autopsy study of 40 patients. Am Heart J 1988;115:1068-1076.

42. Wiener RS, Lockhart JT, Schwartz RG. Dilated cardiomyopathy and cocaine abuse. Report of two cases. Am J Med 1986;81:699-701.

43. Regan TJ. Alcohol and the cardiovascular system. JAMA 1990;264:377-381.

44. Dalakas MC, Illa I, Pezeshkpour GH, Laukaitis JP, Cohen B, Griffin JL. Mitochondrial myopathy caused by long-term zidovudine therapy. N Engl J Med 1990;322:1098-1105.

45. Lipshultz SE, Orav EJ, Sanders SP, Hale AR, McIntosh K, Colan SD. Cardiac structure and function in children with human immunodeficiency virus infection treated with zidovudine. N Engl J Med 1992;327:1260-1265.

46. Deyton LR, Walker RE, Kovacs JA, Herpin B, Parker M, Masur H, Fauci AS, Lane HC. Reversible cardiac dysfunction associated with interferon alfa therapy in AIDS patients with Kaposi's sarcoma.

N Engl J Med 1989;321:1246-1249.

47. Sonnenblick M, Rosenmann D, Rosin A. Reversible cardiomyopathy induced by interferon. BMJ 1990;300:1174-1175.

48. Stein KM, Haronian H, Mensah GA, Acosta A, Jacobs J, Kligfield P. Ventricular tachycardia and torsades de pointes complicating pentamidine therapy of *Pneumocystis carinii* pneumonia in the acquired immunodeficiency syndrome. Am J Cardiol 1990;66:888-889.

49. Brown DL, Sather S, Cheitlin MD. Reversible cardiac dysfunction associated with foscarnet therapy for cytomegalovirus esophagitis in an AIDS patient. Am Heart J 1993;125:1439-1441.

50. Lewis W. Cardiomyopathy in AIDS: a pathophysiological perspective. Prog Cardiovasc Dis 2000;43:151-170.

51. Goldblum N, Daefler S, Llana T, Ablashi D, Josephs S, Salahuddin Z. Susceptibility to HIV-1 infection of a human B-lymphoblastoid cell line, DG75, transfected with subgenomic DNA fragments of Epstein-Barr virus. Dev Biol Stand 1990;72:309-313.

52. Flomenbaum M, Soeiro R, Udem SA, Kress Y, Factor SM. Proliferative membranopathy and human immunodeficiency virus in AIDS hearts. J Acquir Immune Defic Syndr 1989;2:129-135.

53. Cenacchi G, Re MC, Furlini G, La Placa M, Binetti G, Rapezzi C, Alampi G, Magnani B. Human immunodeficiency virus type 1 antigen detection in endomyocardial biopsy: an immunomorphological study. Microbiologica 1990;13:145-149.

54. Wu TC, Pizzorno MC, Hayward GS, Willoughby S, Neumann DA, Rose NR, Ansari AA, Beschorner WE, Baughman KL, Herskowitz A. In situ detection of human cytomegalovirus immediate-early gene transcripts within cardiac myocytes of patients with HIV-associated cardiomyopathy. AIDS 1992;6:777-785.

55. Bowles NE, Kearney DL, Ni J, Perez-Atayde AR, Kline MW, Bricker JT, Ayres NA, Lipshultz SE, Shearer WT, Towbin JA. The detection of viral genomes by polymerase chain reaction in the myocardium of pediatric patients with advanced HIV disease. J Am Coll Cardiol 1999;34:857-865.

56. Gu J, Dische R, Anderson V, Zavallos E, Schloo B, Douglas K, Forte M, McGrath LB. Evidence for an autoimmune mechanism of the cardiac pathology in AIDS patients (abstract). Circulation 1992;86 Suppl 1:I-795.

57. Liu PP, Mason JW. Advances in the understanding of myocarditis. Circulation 2001;104:1076-1082.

58. Matsumori A, Yamada T, Suzuki H, Matoba Y, Sasayama S. Increased circulating cytokines in patients with myocarditis and cardiomyopathy. Br Heart J 1994;72:561-566.

59. Yamada T, Matsumori A, Sasayama S. Therapeutic effect of anti-tumor necrosis factor-alpha antibody on the murine model of viral myocarditis induced by encephalomyocarditis virus. Circulation 1994;89:846-851.

60. Sharma R, Coats AJ, Anker SD. The role of inflammatory mediators in chronic heart failure: cytokines, nitric oxide, and endothelin-1. Int J Cardiol 2000;72:175-186.

61. Odeh M. The role of tumour necrosis factor-alpha in acquired immunodeficiency syndrome. J Intern Med 1990;228:549-556.

62. Yamamoto N. The role of cytokines in the acquired immunodeficiency syndrome. Int J Clin Lab Res 1995;25:29-34.

63. Ho DD, Pomerantz RJ, Kaplan JC. Pathogenesis of infection with human immunodeficiency virus. N Engl J Med 1987;317:278-286.

64. Matturri L, Quattrone P, Varesi C, Rossi L. Cardiac toxoplasmosis in pathology of acquired immunodeficiency syndrome. Panminerva Med 1990;32:194-196.

65. Jautzke G, Sell M, Thalmann U, Janitschke K, Gottschalk J, Schurmann D, Ruf B. Extracerebral toxoplasmosis in AIDS. Histological and immunohistological findings based on 80 autopsy cases. Pathol Res Pract 1993;189:428-436.

66. Grange F, Kinney EL, Monsuez JJ, Rybojad M, Derouin F, Khuong MA, Janier M. Successful therapy for *Toxoplasma gondii* myocarditis in acquired immunodeficiency syndrome. Am Heart J 1990;120:443-444.

67. Albrecht H, Stellbrink HJ, Fenske S, Schafer H, Greten H. Successful treatment of *Toxoplasma gondii* myocarditis in an AIDS patient. Eur J Clin Microbiol Infect Dis 1994;13:500-504.

68. Kinney EL, Monsuez JJ, Kitzis M, Vittecoq D. Treatment of AIDS-associated heart disease. Angiology 1989;40:970-976.

69. Lewis W, Lipsick J, Cammarosano C. Cryptococcal myocarditis in acquired immune deficiency syndrome. Am J Cardiol 1985;55:1240.

70. Lafont A, Wolff M, Marche C, Clair B, Regnier B. Overwhelming myocarditis due to *Cryptococcus neoformans* in an AIDS patient. Lancet 1987;2:1145-1146.

71. Michaels AD, Lederman RJ, MacGregor JS, Cheitlin MD. Cardiovascular involvement in AIDS. Curr Probl Cardiol 1997;22:115-148.

72. Niedt GW, Schinella RA. Acquired immunodeficiency syndrome. Clinicopathologic study of 56 autopsies. Arch Pathol Lab Med 1985;109:727-734.

73. Myerson D, Hackman RC, Nelson JA, Ward DC, McDougall JK. Widespread presence of histologically occult cytomegalovirus. Hum Pathol 1984;15:430-439.

74. Brown J, King A, Francis CK. Cardiovascular effects of alcohol, cocaine, and acquired immune deficiency. Cardiovasc Clin 1991;21:341-376.

75. Peng SK, French WJ, Pelikan PC. Direct cocaine cardiotoxicity demonstrated by endomyocardial biopsy. Arch Pathol Lab Med 1989;113:842-845.

76. Soodini G, Morgan JP. Can cocaine abuse exacerbate the cardiac toxicity of human immunodeficiency virus? Clin Cardiol 2001;24:177-181.

77. Lewis W, Papoian T, Gonzalez B, Louie H, Kelly DP, Payne RM, Grody WW. Mitochondrial ultrastructural and molecular changes induced by zidovudine in rat hearts. Lab Invest 1991;65:228-236.

78. d'Amati G, Kwan W, Lewis W. Dilated cardiomyopathy in a zidovudine-treated AIDS patient. Cardiovasc Pathol 1992;1:317-320.

79. Samlowski WE, Ward JH, Craven CM, Freedman RA. Severe myocarditis following high-dose interleukin-2 administration. Arch Pathol Lab Med 1989;113:838-841.

80. Zimmerman S, Adkins D, Graham M, Petruska P, Bowers C, Vrahnos D, Spitzer G. Irreversible, severe congestive cardiomyopathy occurring in association with interferon alpha therapy. Cancer Biother 1994;9:291-299.

81. Silver MA, Macher AM, Reichert CM, Levens DL, Parrillo JE, Longo DL, Roberts WC. Cardiac involvement by Kaposi's sarcoma in acquired immune deficiency syndrome (AIDS). Am J Cardiol 1984;53:983-985.

82. Holladay AO, Siegel RJ, Schwartz DA. Cardiac malignant lymphoma in acquired immune deficiency syndrome. Cancer 1992;70:2203-2207.

83. Currie PF, Jacob AJ, Foreman AR, Elton RA, Brettle RP, Boon NA. Heart muscle disease related to HIV infection: prognostic implications. BMJ 1994;309:1605-1607.

84. Mason JW, O'Connell JB, Herskowitz A, Rose NR, McManus BM, Billingham ME, Moon TE. A clinical trial of immunosuppressive therapy for myocarditis. The Myocarditis Treatment Trial Investigators. N Engl J Med 1995;333:269-275.

85. Domanski MJ, Sloas MM, Follmann DA, Scalise PP III, Tucker EE, Egan D, Pizzo PA. Effect of zidovudine and didanosine treatment on heart function in children infected with human immunodeficiency virus. J Pediatr 1995;127:137-146.

Childhood Myocarditis and Dilated Cardiomyopathy

Neil E. Bowles, Ph.D., and Jeffrey A. Towbin, M.D.

Myocarditis, particularly in children, remains a major cause of morbidity and mortality worldwide.[1,2] Dilated cardiomyopathy (DCM) is the major reason for cardiac transplantation in the United States and Europe, with an annual incidence of 2 to 8 cases per 100,000 and an estimated prevalence of 36 per 100,000.[3] The idiopathic form of DCM accounts for approximately 50% of the patients undergoing transplantation. Each year in the United States more than 750,000 cases of heart failure are reported,[4] with approximately 250,000 deaths, and myocarditis or DCM probably accounts for 25% of these cases.[5] At present, the treatment of these conditions is limited to management of the symptoms or transplantation, and the cost is thought to be $3 billion to $4 billion annually. Therefore, understanding the basis for this disorder and developing preventive and disease-specific therapies would have a major impact on health care in the United States. In this review, we describe some of the progress toward understanding the etiologies of these disorders in children and clarification of the mechanisms of pathogenesis.

DIAGNOSIS OF VIRAL INFECTION

HISTORICAL PERSPECTIVES

Viral infections of the heart are important causes of morbidity and mortality in children and adults. A patient who has acute myocarditis, the best studied of these infections, typically presents with severe clinical manifestations, especially in the newborn period.[6] Idiopathic DCM appears to occur as a late sequela of acute or chronic viral myocarditis,[1,7-10] due to persistence of virus[7] or an autoimmune phenomenon due to previous exposure to the inciting virus.[11] The affected individual may require long-term medical therapy for congestive heart failure and, in many cases, heart transplantation may be required. In some cases, sudden cardiac death occurs,[8] particularly in athletes.[12]

Endomyocardial biopsy (EMB) and histopathologic study demonstrating cellular infiltrates (particularly lymphocytes), edema, myocyte necrosis, and myocardial scarring were developed to improve diagnostic capabilities, but results were inconsistent among pathologists. The so-called Dallas criteria,[13] described in 1987, were developed in an attempt to improve the high rate of diagnostic disagreement among pathologists by using uniform criteria. However, because of insensitivity[14] and possible risks involved in biopsies, particularly in small or critically ill children, many centers abandoned EMB as a diagnostic tool.

An initial association between virus infection and the development of myocardial disease was made several decades ago. Grist and Bell[15] presented comprehensive serologic data correlating enterovirus infection with myocarditis. However, the role of these viruses in

DCM was less well established and based mainly on the observation of high titers of neutralizing antibody in cases of sudden-onset disease.[16] This led to the proposal that DCM is a progression from an enteroviral myocarditis.

Enteroviruses, and particularly the coxsackievirus B (CVB) group, have a major positive tropism for skeletal and cardiac muscle. However, isolation of infectious virus from patients with heart muscle disease is rare.[17] For example, in a study of EMB samples from 70 patients with myocarditis or DCM, no enterovirus was isolated from or virus-specific antigens detected in any of these samples,[18] despite evidence of virus association from retrospective serologic study.

Detection of virus-specific IgM is more significant, in that it usually reflects recent or persisting infection. CVB-specific IgM was detected in nearly 40% of patients with myocarditis compared with none of the controls.[19] Such IgM responses have been shown to persist for up to 6 months.[20] CVB-specific IgM responses have also been reported in patients with end-stage DCM undergoing cardiac transplantation, with the IgM responses persisting for up to 19 months before transplantation.[21]

The concept of an enteroviral origin of heart muscle disease is reinforced by animal models of myocarditis and DCM. A cardiotropic strain of coxsackievirus B3 (CVB3) induces inflammatory heart muscle disease in mice. Infectious virus cannot be isolated from myocardium after the first 2 to 3 weeks,[22,23] although many of the animals progress to left ventricular disease reminiscent of DCM,[24,25] supporting the hypothesis that DCM can be a sequela of a viral myocarditis.

MOLECULAR DIAGNOSTIC TECHNIQUES

The failure to isolate virus or to detect viral antigens in patient EMB samples, despite the serologic demonstration of persistent infection, prompted the development of virus-specific molecular hybridization probes. These were designed to detect the presence of enteroviral RNA sequences in myocardial or other tissue samples. The studies by Bowles and coworkers[26,27] and by Kandolf et al.[28,29] led to the direct demonstration of persisting enteroviral infection of the myocardium in myocarditis patients and supported the hypothesis that DCM was caused by enteroviral persistence and is a late sequela of viral myocarditis. Polymerase chain reaction (PCR) has been used in the rapid detection of viral sequences in many tissues and body fluids, including the myocardium of patients with suspected myocarditis or DCM.[30-36] Evidence from our laboratory suggested that adenovirus often is found in hearts of affected children and could be an important cause of myocarditis and DCM.[37,38]

We (unpublished data) have studied more than 750 myocardial samples from patients with myocarditis or DCM (or both) by using PCR to detect a range of viruses, including the enteroviruses, adenoviruses, cytomegalovirus (CMV), herpes simplex virus, Epstein-Barr virus, parvovirus, influenza virus, and respiratory syncytial virus. The patients were divided into groups by age: neonates (age between 1 day and 1 month); infants (age between 1 month and 1 year); toddlers (age between 1 year and 5 years); children (age between 5 years and 13 years); adolescents (age between 13 years and 18 years); and adults (age greater than 18 years). More than 65% of the samples came from patients between the ages of 1 day and 13 years; more than 600 of the patients had a diagnosis of myocarditis, and the remainder had DCM. More than 200 samples from individuals with medical histories inconsistent with these criteria were included as unaffected, age-matched controls.

The overall prognosis of the patients with acute myocarditis was poor, with an overall mortality of more than 50%. Approximately 40% of the DCM patients underwent heart transplantation. The majority of patients with myocarditis had poor recovery of their cardiac function, while the remaining patients had mild recovery with persistence of depressed cardiac function or complete recovery or underwent transplantation.

Serologic findings consistent with viral infection were seen in 38% of patients studied, primarily enterovirus and CMV, from acute and convalescent titers. Only 7 patients had positive postmortem viral cultures from multiple organs, including the heart. Four of these patients had postmortem cultures positive for enterovirus from heart, brain, liver, and kidney, and 3 patients grew adenovirus from specimens of the lungs and heart. Two patients grew CMV from specimens of the heart and lungs (1 in a patient whose sample grew enterovirus, 1 in a patient whose sample grew adenovirus). One other child had adenoviral particles in the heart by electron microscopy but had negative viral cultures.

PCR amplified a viral product in approximately 40% of the samples obtained from patients with myocarditis compared with 1.5% of control samples. Of these positive myocarditis samples, adenovirus was detected in more than 50% (80% adenovirus type 2, 20% type 5; Fig. 23-1 and 23-2; see color plate 41) and enterovirus in 33%, whereas the remainder were mainly CMV but also included a few herpes simplex virus type 1, Epstein-Barr virus, parvovirus, influenza, and respiratory syncytial virus positives. Compared with the positive peripheral cultures obtained, 80% amplified viral genome, with 76% agreement in the results obtained by PCR. PCR analysis of blood drawn from 300 patients at the same time that tissue was obtained demonstrated only 3 of 300 blood samples analyzed by PCR amplified viral genome (CMV in 2, enterovirus in 1).

In the patients with DCM, 20% were positive for viral genome: adenovirus in 60% of the PCR-positive samples and enterovirus in the remaining 40%. None of the blood samples from these patients were PCR positive.

These data show that adenovirus is detected at least as often as the enteroviruses in the hearts of children and adult patients.[37-39] Further, no significant differences were observed among age groups with respect to the relative frequencies of detection of adenovirus and enterovirus.

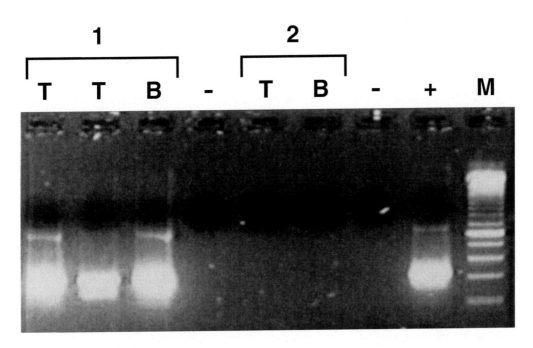

Fig. 23-1. The detection of adenovirus DNA by nested polymerase chain reaction in tracheal aspirate (*T*) and endomyocardial biopsy (*B*) samples in 2 patients: one positive for adenovirus type 5 (patient 1) and the other negative (patient 2). Lanes - are water controls and + is adenovirus type 2 positive control DNA. Lane M is a 100-bp DNA ladder (Life Technologies). The adenovirus identified in each of the samples from patient 1 was determined to be type 5 by DNA sequencing of the polymerase chain reaction product.

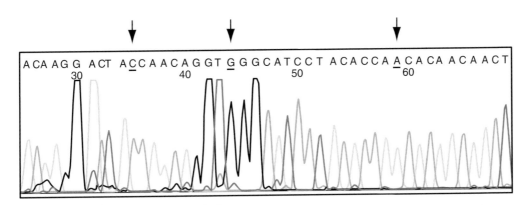

Fig. 23-2. DNA sequence analysis of an adenovirus-specific polymerase chain reaction product. The region shown is highly divergent between adenovirus serotypes, allowing rapid identification of the virus amplified—in this case adenovirus type 5. Analysis of the 3 nucleotides indicated is sufficient to differentiate all adenovirus serotypes sequenced to date. See color plate 41.

Different isolates of CVB3 vary in their cardiovirulence. Tu et al.[40] reported that a single nucleotide difference, at position 234 of the CVB3 genome, determined the phenotype of the virus. If this nucleotide was a cytidine, the virus was attenuated compared to another strain of CVB3 with uridine at this location. Subsequently it was reported that in natural isolates of CVB3, regardless of cardiovirulence, this position was invariably uridine, suggesting that other nucleotides are important in determining the viral phenotype.[41] By construction of chimeras from cardiovirulent and noncardiovirulent strains of CVB3, critical regions were identified within the 5′ untranslated region, including within stem-loop motifs associated with the internal ribosome entry site.[42] In addition, 2 amino acid changes within the VP2 and VP3 structural proteins had some additive effects on cardiovirulence. DNA sequencing of the genome of adenovirus variants detected by PCR could potentially distinguish between cardiovirulent and noncardiovirulent adenovirus subtypes, although the size of the adenoviral genome and the number of adenoviral types (more than 40 have been identified) may make such an analysis impractical and likely uninformative. To date, it appears that the group C adenoviruses are primarily associated with heart muscle disease.

HEART DISEASE IN CHILDREN INFECTED WITH HUMAN IMMUNODEFICIENCY VIRUS

Human immunodeficiency virus (HIV) infection is increasingly recognized as an important cause of heart disease, particularly myocarditis and DCM. However, the pathogenesis of the heart-muscle disease in the acquired immunodeficiency syndrome is unclear. CMV sequences have been detected in myocardial samples. For example, Wu et al.[43] reported a study of the role of CMV infection in the development of HIV-associated cardiomyopathy. Using probes derived from the CMV immediate-early and delayed-early genes, they analyzed by in situ hybridization EMB samples from 12 HIV-infected patients with global left ventricular hypokinesis demonstrated on 2-dimensional echocardiography and 8 autopsy cardiac samples from HIV-infected patients without cardiac disease during life. Of the 12 EMB specimens, 6 had hybridization for transcripts of the CMV immediate-early gene, consistent with nonpermissive or latent infection. Similar patterns were not found in any of the 8 autopsy control samples. All 6 patients presented with unexplained congestive heart failure and had biopsy samples with immunohistochemical evidence of increased myocardial major histocompatibility complex (MHC) class I expression, a finding typical of non-HIV myocarditis. None of the EMB samples had characteristic CMV inclusions and no specific hybridization was noted with the delayed-early gene probe, suggesting that no active viral DNA replication was present. Only 2 of the 6 patients with myocyte hybridization with the immediate-early probe had clinical evidence of solid organ infection with CMV at presentation with cardiovascular complaints.

The first comprehensive study of the etiologic basis of heart disease was reported by Barbaro et al.[44] They performed a prospective, long-term clinical and echocardiographic follow-up study of 952 asymptomatic HIV-positive patients to assess the incidence of DCM. All patients with a diagnosis of DCM underwent EMB for histologic, immuno-histologic, and virologic assessment. During a mean follow-up period of 60 months, an echocardiographic diagnosis of DCM was made in 76 patients (8%). The incidence of DCM was higher in patients with a CD4 count of less than 400 cells/µL and in those who received therapy with zidovudine. A histologic diagnosis of myocarditis was made in 63 of the patients with DCM (83%). Inflammatory infiltrates were predominantly composed of CD3 and CD8 lymphocytes, with staining for MHC class I antigens in 71% of the patients. In the myocytes of 58 patients, HIV nucleic acid sequences were detected by in situ hybridization, and active myocarditis was documented in 36 of the 58. Among these 36 patients, 6 were also infected with CVB (17%), 2 with CMV (6%), and 1 with Epstein-Barr virus (3%). They concluded that DCM might be related to a direct action of HIV on the myocardial tissue or to an autoimmune process induced by HIV, possibly in associa-tion with other cardiotropic viruses. Although these data indicate a similar origin for myocarditis and DCM in HIV-infected adults and non-HIV-infected adults, the frequency of detection of CMV was somewhat lower than in previous studies.[43]

In 1999 we[45] reported a similar study in 32 pediatric patients with advanced HIV disease. In 13 of the 32 samples (41%) from HIV-infected children, 1 or more virus types were detected. The virus identified most often was adenovirus (10 of 32 = 31%), followed by CMV (7 of 32 = 22%).

DNA sequence analysis of the adenoviruses amplified from the HIV-infected patient samples demonstrated only adenovirus type 5. This is in contrast to the apparent pre-dominance of adenovirus type 2 in non-HIV-infected children with myocarditis or DCM (see previous section). This difference may reflect a different spectrum of adenoviral sus-ceptibility in HIV-infected and non-HIV-infected children or a difference in viral pathogenesis in immunocompromised children. However, it does appear that the group C adenoviruses are identified most often in myocardial samples.

Active myocarditis was observed in 11 of the 32 HIV-infected patient myocardial samples (34%), and infiltrates borderline for myocarditis were observed in another 13 cases—a frequency of myocarditis considerably higher than in the study by Barbaro et al.[44] However, the pediatric patients studied were those with advanced, end-stage disease, whereas the patients studied by Barbaro and colleagues were initially asymptomatic. Our results may indicate that children with HIV are more prone to the development of myocarditis, perhaps because of a greater susceptibility to infection with cardiotropic viruses. Adenovirus was detected in 4 of the 11 samples with myocarditis, in 3 samples with borderline infiltrates, in 1 patient with infiltrates confined to the epicardium, and in 2 with no histologic evidence of inflammation. Of the 2 patients with adenovirus but no inflammation, 1 was reported to have died of congestive heart failure and the other of adenoviral pneumonia. Adenovirus was detected in 3 of the 6 patients with congestive heart failure; only 1 had myocardial infiltrates, and these were confined to the epicardium. Among the 3 patients with DCM, 1 was positive for adenovirus. Seven of the 18 patients (39%) with postmortem cardiomegaly were positive for adenovirus by PCR. Two patients were reported to have adenoviral pneumonia at the time of death; both patients were positive for adenoviral DNA by PCR, including 1 with disseminated infection and positive myocardial culture.

Interestingly, 6 of 10 patients positive for adenovirus had other organisms identified in the heart. All 6 had myocardial inflammation; however, only 1 had clinical cardiac symptoms. This contrasts sharply with the findings in 4 patients in whom adenovirus was the sole myocardial isolate; all 4 were symptomatic and only 2 of 4 had myocardial infiltrates. The frequency of postmortem cardiomegaly was similar in both groups of patients. These clinical and pathologic features in patients with PCR evidence of adenovirus support a pathogenic role for this virus in the development of heart disease in HIV-infected pediatric patients.

CMV was detected in 3 myocarditis samples and in 4 samples with borderline lymphocytic infiltrates. Extracardiac systemic infection with the virus was detected by culture or by histologic study (or both) in 6 of the 7 patients, considerably more often than detected in adult patients by Wu and colleagues.[43] Two patients had clinical cardiac symptoms, including 1 who had terminal acute congestive heart failure and myocardial infiltrates borderline for myocarditis. In the other, borderline myocarditis and disseminated systemic CMV infection were identified. Clinically, the heart was enlarged on chest radiograph and the patient was hypotensive. Another patient positive for CMV by myocardial culture and PCR was clinically asymptomatic but had myocarditis and mildly decreased left ventricular function assessed 1 week before death.

The relatively mild inflammatory infiltrates in most of the virus-positive samples could result from several things, including the fact that these HIV-infected patients were immunocompromised, precluding a significant cellular immune response against infected cells. Indeed, in 26 of 29 patients with CD4 lymphocyte counts available to permit Centers for Disease Control and Prevention classification, class C3 reflected severe immunosuppression. Additionally, we have observed in non-HIV-infected myocarditis patients that the level of inflammatory infiltration is less in adenovirus-infected samples than in, for example, enterovirus-infected samples.[37]

These data indicate that in HIV-infected children and adults, myocarditis and DCM can develop as a result of infection of the myocardium by the same viruses that infect non-immunocompromised individuals (ie, adenovirus, enteroviruses, and CMV).

ALTERNATIVE DIAGNOSTIC APPROACHES

Other important causes of morbidity and mortality in children are infectious disorders of the respiratory tract.[46] Rapid respiratory and metabolic deterioration may occur, requiring intubation and mechanical ventilation. Respiratory decompensation is often accompanied by cardiac dysfunction due to myocarditis.[10,47,48]

To determine whether the analysis of tracheal aspirate samples would be informative for the diagnosis of viral myocarditis, Akhtar et al.[49] analyzed tracheal aspirate samples and EMB samples from 10 patients presenting with myocarditis or DCM, with or without presumed pneumonia by PCR, for evidence of viral infection. Of the 7 patients with PCR-positive tracheal aspirate samples, 4 were also positive by aspirate culture (enterovirus). In all cases, PCR performed on EMB specimens identified the same virus as detected in the tracheal aspirate samples. In the case of the child diagnosed by tracheal aspirate PCR to have EBV, EMB PCR also identified this relatively uncommon cause of pneumonitis and myocarditis. Confirmation of this diagnosis was later provided by serologic test during convalescence. Another patient who presented clinically with myocarditis and pneumonitis was positive by PCR for adenovirus from 2 consecutive tracheal aspirate samples (Fig. 23-1) and also was positive by PCR for adenovirus from EMB samples. In another case of myocarditis with pneumonia, the PCR, in addition to amplifying the same agent as isolated by culture (enterovirus), also amplified the adenovirus genome. Adenovirus respiratory tract infections are common in children, and in this case it may have contributed to myocardial injury.

These results suggest that tracheal aspirate samples are a useful substrate for PCR analysis in intubated pediatric patients with suspected viral pneumonitis, with or without myocarditis. Tracheal aspirate sample PCR may provide a safer means than EMB to arrive at an etiologic diagnosis in viral myocarditis, especially when the right ventricular free wall and outflow tracts are pathologically thinned. However, these results should not be generalized to include, for example, any unselected patient with intubated respiratory disease or children with known cardiac dysfunction and recurrent cardiac decompensation. Confirmation of these findings is needed before changes in diagnostic methodology are embraced.

TRANSPLANT REJECTION AND MYOCARDITIS

Cardiac transplantation in children is a lifesaving procedure aimed at sustaining long-term, productive survival in recipients. The major short-term and long-term risks preventing extended survival include allograft rejection, coronary artery disease in the transplanted organ, and lymphoproliferative disease, but the underlying causes of these disorders are not completely understood. The diagnosis of allograft rejection relies on histopathologic criteria but these criteria are known to mimic myocarditis in patients who have not received a transplant.[50,51]

The association between viral genome in the myocardium and concomitant rejection is known. Schowengerdt et al.[50,51] reported results of the analysis by PCR of 40 patients who underwent serial right ventricular EMB for rejection surveillance after heart transplantation, with viruses identified in 41 samples from 21 patients. Viral genomes amplified included CMV in 16 samples, adenovirus in 14, enterovirus in 6, parvovirus in 3, and HSV in 2. In 13 of the 21 patients positive for viral genome, EMB histologic scores were consistent with multifocal moderate-to-severe rejection (Internal Society for Heart and Lung Transplantation scores of 3A or greater). However, the longer-term implications of the detection of virus by PCR are unclear.

Adenovirus infection in the transplanted lung is significantly associated with graft failure, histologic obliterative bronchiolitis, and death. Bridges et al.[52] reported that of 16 patients undergoing lung or heart-lung transplantation, virus was identified in the transplanted lung during follow-up on 26 occasions; adenovirus was identified most frequently (8 of 16 patients) and had the greatest impact on outcome. In 2 patients with early fulminant infection, adenovirus was also identified in the donor. Adenovirus was significantly associated with respiratory failure leading to death or graft loss and with the histologic diagnosis of obliterative bronchiolitis.

In a study of 45 explanted hearts from patients who underwent heart transplantation, enteroviral genome was detectable in only 1 of 27 patients with DCM and in 1 patient with lymphocytic myocarditis.[53] The enterovirus-positive DCM patient showed a higher index of severe rejection (> 3A) in the first 6 months, compared with the other patients tested; the enterovirus-positive myocarditis patient died of disease recurrence 2 months after transplantation.

These findings suggest that the identification of virus, and particularly adenovirus and enterovirus, is predictive of a poor prognosis in organ transplant recipients, further confirming the similarity between myocarditis and rejection. They also indicate a need for the development of a rapid viral diagnostic technique to determine the suitability of a donor organ for transplantation.

ANIMAL MODELS OF MYOCARDITIS/DCM

In many strains of mice, inoculation with CVB3 results in myocarditis.[10] The myocardium heals once infectious virus is cleared. However, in some strains of immunocompetent weanling mice, such as C3H/HeJ or A.SW, virus can be isolated from the myocardium during the first few days after inoculation. Histopathologic changes characteristic of myocarditis develop only after infectious virus is no longer present. In such models myocardial damage is biphasic. The initial acute phase involves virus replication and cell lysis, with immune clearance of virus, followed by a chronic phase that involves infiltration of the myocardium by inflammatory cells and the production of cardiac-specific auto-antibodies. A murine model of DCM, after infection with encephalomyocarditis virus, has been described.[54,55] About 3 months after the development of myocarditis, cardiac dilatation, myocardial fibrosis, and hypertrophy of myocardial fibers occur, in the absence of cellular infiltration or myocardial necrosis. Despite the fact that infectious virus cannot be isolated after the first few days, viral genomic RNA sequences were detected in some samples at 3 months. A similar model using CVB3 in Swiss ICR mice has been described.[56]

To date there have been no animal models of adenovirus-induced heart disease reported. However, the cotton rat (*Sigmodon hispidus*) is susceptible to infection by some strains of human adenovirus,[57] and it was reported that the intranasal inoculation of cotton rats with Ad5 resulted in the development of pneumonitis.[58] Cellular infiltration of the interstitial and intra-alveolar areas and the peribronchiolar and perivascular regions was seen, with moderate damage occurring to the bronchiolar epithelium. The histologic changes could be divided into 2 phases. The first, probably due to the action of cytokines, involved the infiltration of primarily monocytes, macrophages, and neutrophils, but rarely lymphocytes, into the alveoli, bronchial epithelium, and peribronchiolar regions. The second phase, probably a cytotoxic T-cell response to the virus, involved a predominantly lymphocytic infiltrate into the peribronchiolar and perivascular areas. The degree of histopathologic change depended on the initial adenovirus dose, with doses of greater than 10^8 plaque-forming units (pfu) resulting in severe damage to the type II alveolar cells.

We[59] have begun to develop a model of adenovirus-induced myocarditis in the cotton rat. Adenovirus type 5 (10^7 pfu) was administered to cotton rats by intranasal (IN), intra-peritoneal (IP), or intracardiac (IC) injection. The animals were killed (2 per group) after 4, 14, or 28 days. In addition, 2 IC injected animals were killed after 3 months.

Adenoviral DNA was detected in the lungs of all animals at days 4 and 14, except for 1 animal receiving virus by IP injection that was negative at day 14. At day 28, only the animals administered virus by the IN or IC route were positive (3-month IC animals were not tested). Adenoviral DNA was detected in the hearts of all animals inoculated by the IC route, even at 3 months postinjection (Figure 23-3). Adenoviral DNA was detected in the hearts of only IN and IP animals at day 4 and 1 IP injected animal at day 14.

Animals inoculated IN were considered normal, whereas animals inoculated IP had borderline myocarditis at day 4 and myocarditis at days 14 and 28 (Fig. 23-4; see color plate 42). Even at day 14 there was evidence of fibrosis and myocyte necrosis. Animals inoculated IC had epicarditis, with subepicardial myocarditis at day 4 and myocarditis at 14 days, 28 days, and 3 months.

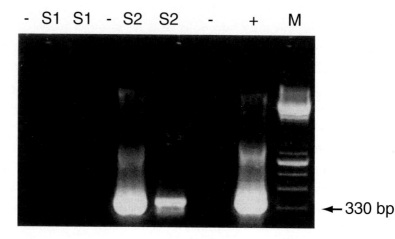

Fig. 23-3. The detection of adenoviral DNA by nested polymerase chain reaction in myocardial samples from 2 cotton rats injected with adenovirus, 3 months postinjection (lanes S2). Lanes S1 are myocardial samples from sham-infected animals. See Figure 23-1 for details.

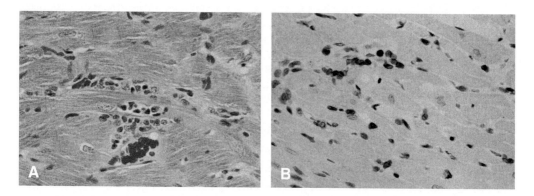

Fig. 23-4. Myocarditis in the cotton rat heart. *A*, Hematoxylin-eosin staining shows a discrete cluster of lymphocytes and macrophages adjacent to a degenerating myocyte. There is also focal loss of myocytes with early fibrous scarring. *B*, T-cell immunostain demonstrates a cluster of cells surrounding myocytes. (x132.) See color plate 42.

From these preliminary data, it appears that the IP and IC administration of adenovirus result in the development of myocarditis in the cotton rat. The myocarditis demonstrated in these animals is histologically mild, similar to adenovirus myocarditis in humans. Further, wild-type adenovirus is capable of persisting in the myocardium of cotton rats for at least 3 months.

PATHOGENESIS OF HEART FAILURE IN MYOCARDITIS AND DCM

VIRAL PERSISTENCE

Although the evidence is compelling that enteroviruses are capable of persisting in the myocardium of patients with myocarditis or DCM in the absence of virus-antigen expression or the formation of infectious virions, few reports relate to the specific nature of the mechanism. During a normal lytic infection, enteroviral RNA replication is mediated by the virus-encoded RNA-dependent RNA polymerase via a replication intermediate, comprising the positive-sense genomic strand and a negative-template strand. The positive-strand RNA is normally present in 100-fold excess over the negative strand as a result of asymmetric synthesis. However, in the myocardium of patients with myocarditis or DCM infected with enterovirus, approximately equimolar amounts of the positive and negative strands are synthesized.[60,61] It is possible that the synthesis of complementary RNA strands results in interference in translation of the genomic RNA because of the RNA-RNA hybridization: such double-stranded RNA is likely to be more stable than single-stranded RNA.

Most of the information relating to adenovirus latency or persistence has come from the study of infected tonsils or adenoids. Infectious virus can rarely be isolated directly from the tissue but is recovered after cultivation of the tissue[62] or from stimulated lymphocytes[63] in vitro. After propagation of tonsillar tissue in vitro, adenoviral DNA can be detected in high molecular weight DNA fractions, suggesting that the viral genome has been integrated into the host chromosomes.[64] Latent infection of lung by adenovirus can also cause chronic obstructive pulmonary disease,[65] with adenoviral DNA integrating in a linear fashion and subsequent rearrangement and amplification of the early regions, particularly E1A.[65] The E1A region has been implicated in the sensitization of the infected cells to destruction by cytokines[66] and in the induction of apoptosis.[67] This region could be an important component of the mechanism of inflammatory responses against chronically infected cells.

APOPTOSIS AND IMMUNE RESPONSE

Little is understood about the pathogenesis underlying the development of heart failure associated with myocarditis or DCM. Although the pathologic features of acute myocarditis are well documented, hearts from patients with DCM display relatively nonspecific histologic changes. These include widespread myocardial fibrosis and associated hypertrophy of surviving cardiomyocytes. Apoptosis of cardiomyocytes may be responsible for these changes.[68] In a small number of cases apoptotic cells were detected in myocardial tissue samples from patients with DCM by an in situ labeling protocol (TUNEL), including adenovirus-infected samples.[69,70]

Thus, it is possible that in adenovirus-infected cardiomyocytes the dissociated expression of E1A and E1B could result in the induction of apoptosis by overexpression of E1A, by underexpression of E1B, or by expression of mutated forms of the E1B gene products. Alternatively, other adenoviral gene products may influence the apoptotic pathway in, as yet, uncharacterized ways.

Another effect of the expression of E1A is to shut down the expression of α-myosin heavy chain by transcriptional repression.[71] The long-term effect of this on the myocardium could be to impair cardiac myocyte function, potentially leading to congestive heart failure.

The adenoviruses have strategies for modulating the immune response. Several adenoviral-encoded proteins are capable of interacting with host immune components.[67] These include proteins encoded by the E3 region that can protect cells from tumor necrosis factor (TNF)-mediated lysis[72] and down-regulation of MHC class I antigen expression.[73] The E1A proteins are capable of promoting the induction of apoptosis,[67] inhibiting interleukin (IL)-6 expression,[74] and interfering with IL-6 signal transduction pathways.[75] These functions of E1A may be particularly pertinent for explaining the myocardial abnormalities observed in DCM patients: IL-6 promotes lymphocyte activation, and this was reduced in the adenovirus-infected patient samples in the study by Pauschinger et al.[39]

The presence of mononuclear cell infiltrates within the heart is a characteristic of myocarditis. These mononuclear cells are a significant source of the cytokines IL-1β and TNF. Henke et al.[76] demonstrated the release of TNF-α and IL-1β by human monocytes exposed to CVB3. Both of these cytokines participate in leukocyte activation, which may promote a specific lymphocyte response during viral infection. However, these cytokines may also promote cardiac fibroblast activity.[77] Therefore, local secretion of cytokines in the myocardium may perpetuate the inflammatory process and lead to the fibrosis associated with cardiomyopathy and resultant deteriorating cardiac function. Evidence also implicates IL-1β and TNF-α as potential inhibitors of cardiac myocyte β-adrenergic responsiveness.[78] Further, TNF-α is capable of inducing apoptosis. Transgenic mice expressing TNF-α in the myocardium have been described.[79-81] Severe cardiac dysfunction indicated by biventricular dysfunction and depressed ejection fraction was evident in these transgenic mice, and the mice died prematurely. At necropsy globular dilated hearts were observed, and on histologic examination there was evidence of myocyte apoptosis and severe inflammatory infiltration of the walls of all chambers, indicative of an acute myocarditis. There was also significant ventricular fibrosis. These data support a role for TNF-α in the pathogenesis of myocarditis and idiopathic DCM. The prolonged expression of inflammatory cytokines and immunomodulators, such as TNF-α and IL-1β, has been reported in patients with chronic myocarditis or DCM.

Another possible effect of cytokine expression is the induction of inducible nitric oxide synthase. Increased expression of nitric oxide synthase has been proposed to account for some of the dilation associated with DCM[82] and has been demonstrated in a murine CVB3-induced myocarditis model.[83] In a study of a cardiac myosin-induced myocarditis model in mice, it was shown that nitric oxide synthase expression is induced in both macrophages and cardiomyocytes.[84] However, nitric oxide synthesis did not appear to be essential for the development of pathologic conditions because myocarditis developed in mice lacking interferon regulatory transcription factor-1, a transcription factor that controls expression of inducible nitric oxide synthase. Despite the failure to synthesize nitric oxide synthase in the myocardium, the prevalence and severity of disease in interferon regulatory transcription factor-1-deficient animals were similar to control animals. In addition, no difference was detected in animals lacking the interferon regulatory transcription factor-2 gene, a negative regulator of interferon regulatory transcription factor-1-induced transcription.

CYTOSKELETON DYSFUNCTION IN DCM: THE COMMON FINAL PATHWAY HYPOTHESIS

In addition to the acquired form of DCM, inherited forms of the disease are described frequently. During the past several years, clues have emerged to the underlying cause of familial DCM, and the underlying basis for other inherited cardiovascular diseases.[85,86] For instance, the basis for familial hypertrophic cardiomyopathy, a primary heart muscle disease in which ventricular wall thickening (hypertrophy) and diastolic dysfunction occur, has been demonstrated to be mutations in genes encoding sarcomeric proteins such as β-myosin heavy chain, α-tropomyosin, cardiac troponin T, cardiac troponin I, myosin-binding protein-C, cardiac actin, and the essential and regulatory myosin light chains.[87] In addition, the inherited long QT syndromes have been shown to be due to mutations in genes encoding ion channels, such as the potassium channel genes *KVLQT1*, *KCNE1*, *KCNE2*, and *HERG* and the cardiac sodium channel gene *SCN5A*.[88] Because of the consistent protein classes mutated in phenotypically similar patients (ie, sarcomeric proteins in familial hypertrophic cardiomyopathy; ion channels in long QT syndromes), we hypothesized that a common final pathway is disturbed in individual cardiovascular disorders and that similar protein types would also be mutated in DCM.[85,86]

Currently, only 5 genes have been identified and characterized in cases of familial DCM. In Barth syndrome, the gene *G4.5*, which encodes a novel protein family called taffazins, is mutated.[89] Although well characterized at the molecular level, the function of the encoded protein is not known. In contrast, dystrophin is the gene responsible for X-linked DCM and is well defined.[90-92] This gene, which also causes Duchenne and Becker muscular dystrophy when mutated, encodes a large (427 kDa) cytoskeletal protein that resides at the inner face of the sarcolemma (Fig. 23-5; see color plate 43),[93] colocalizing with β-spectrin and vinculin. Dystrophin protein is thought to assume a rod-shaped structure with an actin-binding domain at the amino terminus. The carboxy-terminal domain is associated with a large transmembrane glycoprotein complex, the dystrophin-associated glycoprotein complex, which is thought to mechanically stabilize the plasma membrane of muscle cells (Fig. 23-5). This complex is formed by the dystroglycan subcomplex (α-dystroglycan and β-dystroglycan), sarcoglycan subcomplex (α-, β-, γ-, and δ-sarcoglycan), caveolin-3, neuronal nitric oxide synthase, syntrophin, α-dystrobrevin, and sarcospan and serves as a link among cytoplasmic actin, the membrane, and the extracellular matrix of muscle (Fig. 23-5). Mutations in dystrophin or dystrophin-associated glycoprotein complex subcomplexes result in a wide spectrum of skeletal myopathy or cardiomyopathy (or both) in humans and animal models such as the mouse or hamster.[94-102]

The third mutant gene thus far identified, *cardiac actin*, has been identified as the gene responsible for 15q14-linked autosomal dominant familial DCM.[103] It has also been shown to cause familial hypertrophic cardiomyopathy.[104] This mutant gene appears to cause a DCM phenotype when mutated near the dystrophin-binding domain, whereas mutations that result in disruption of the protein at its interaction with the sarcomere result in familial hypertrophic cardiomyopathy. The actin-dystrophin link, when disrupted, dissociates the actin cytoskeleton from the muscle membrane and extracellular matrix, leading to cellular degeneration and necrosis and a DCM phenotype. Disruption of the sarcomere instead leads to familial hypertrophic cardiomyopathy.

The other 2 genes identified in familial DCM include *desmin* (2q35)[105] and *lamin A/C* (1p1-1q21),[106] both of which are thought to cause abnormalities of structural support when mutated. Desmin is a component of the intermediate filaments while lamin A/C makes up part of the inner nuclear envelope (Fig. 23-5). Interestingly, these genes are associated with skeletal myopathy and, in some cases, with conduction system disease.[107-109] We[85,86] hypothesized that DCM is a disease of the cytoarchitecture—the cytoskeleton and dystrophin-associated glycoprotein complex in particular.

Other supportive data for this hypothesis exist. Maeda et al.[110] identified absence of the metavinculin transcript in the cardiac tissue from a patient with idiopathic DCM and confirmed the metavinculin abnormality by immunoblot, which demonstrated the absence of metavinculin protein in the heart. Metavinculin has a role in attaching the sarcomere to the cardiomyocyte membrane by complexing with nonsarcomeric actin microfilaments complexed with other cytoskeletal proteins (talin, α-actinin, vinculin), which are linked to cadherin or to the integrin receptor. Arber et al.[94] showed that deficiency of muscle LIM protein in a mouse model results in DCM, heart failure, and disruption of cardiac myocyte cytoskeletal architecture. Muscle LIM protein is a structural protein that appears to link the actin cytoskeleton to the contractile apparatus and, although no mutations have been identified in humans, fits well with the Common Final Pathway hypothesis for DCM.

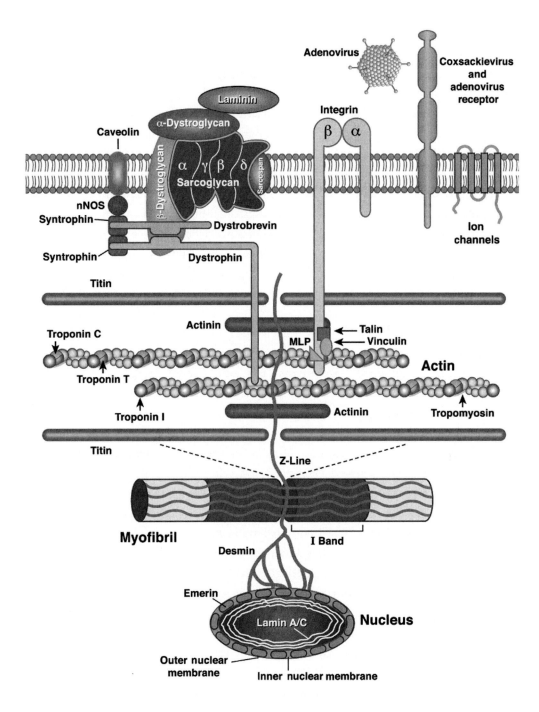

Fig. 23-5. Schematic representation of the cytoarchitecture of the cardiomyocyte, including components of the cytoskeleton, intermediate filaments, nuclear envelope, and dystrophin-associated glycoprotein complex. *MLP*, muscle LIM protein; *nNOS*, neuronal nitric oxide synthase. See color plate 43.

It is possible that vinculin, which maps to the 10q21-q23 region, and caveolin-3, which maps to 3p25, could be responsible for the familial DCM linked to these regions of the human genome.[111,112]

Badorff et al.[113] reported that the CVB3-encoded 2A protease cleaves dystrophin in cultured myocytes and in infected mouse hearts. This leads to disruption of dystrophin and the dystrophin-associated glycoprotein complex. Thus, it appears likely that one of the effects of the infection of the heart by the enteroviruses is the disruption of the sarcolemma. In addition, both TNF-α and IL-1β activate the GTPase Cdc42.[114,115] Constitutively active forms of this protein induce actin polymerization.[115,116] Thus, continuous stimulation of this signaling pathway could affect the integrity of the cytoskeleton. Whether viruses act directly on the cytoarchitecture or indirectly through inflammatory mediators, it appears that the Common Final Pathway hypothesis may be relevant to the pathogenesis of acquired and inherited forms of DCM in children and adults.

NOVEL THERAPEUTICS

Conventional treatments for myocarditis include bed rest, diuretics, digitalis, angiotensin-converting enzyme inhibitors, β-adrenergic blockade, and antiarrhythmic medication. Because of the idea that myocarditis involves, at least in part, autoreactive immunologic damage, trials of immunosuppressive agents have been undertaken. The results have varied. For example, in one multicenter myocarditis trial, patients were studied during the acute phase of disease and no difference was observed between patients receiving immunosuppressive or conventional therapy.[117] However, studies in patients with chronic myocarditis suggest that immunosuppression may be efficacious in these patients,[118] with significant improvement in ejection fraction and New York Heart Association classification.

Intravenous administration of immunoglobulin has been used for the treatment of autoimmune diseases,[119-121] including Kawasaki disease. Trials of intravenously administered immunoglobulin in acute myocarditis patients suggested that this treatment may improve left ventricular function, with patients experiencing better survival during the first year than the control group.[122] Further, in the CVB3-induced myocarditis model in the mouse, intravenously administered immunoglobulin therapy during the acute phase resulted in reduced inflammation and improved survival.[120] The successful treatment was reported of a patient with adenovirus-induced myocarditis with high-dose intravenously administered immunoglobulin.[123] However, a randomized trial of intravenously administered immunoglobulin for DCM in adults failed to demonstrate benefit.[124]

The observation that some patients succumb to idiopathic DCM, long after the healing of myocarditis, but with evidence that viral sequences persist in the myocardium, suggests that other approaches may be beneficial for the treatment of this condition. Most antiviral therapies (eg, ganciclovir or zidovudine) rely on viral replication to be effective. In chronic myocarditis or idiopathic DCM, it is not obvious that viral replication is occurring or directly responsible for the pathogenic changes.

The possible role of CVB-encoded protease in the development of a pathologic cardiac condition by cleavage of dystrophin raises the possibility of an alternative approach to treating viral heart disease. Virus-specific protease inhibitors have been widely used for the treatment of HIV infection with considerable efficacy.[125,126] Enterovirus-specific protease inhibitors have been described, including one for poliovirus 2A and one for rhinovirus 3C.[127,128]

The identification of specific agents as causes of these conditions suggests that approaches directed toward the protection of humans from these viruses would be beneficial. The highly efficacious poliovirus vaccines[129] that have almost eliminated poliomyelitis suggest that the development of coxsackievirus B-specific vaccines is possible.[130] Support for such an approach comes from studies of endocardial fibroelastosis (EFE).

EFE is characterized by a diffuse thickening of the left ventricular endocardium. This results from proliferation of fibrous and elastic tissue and leads to decreased compliance and impaired diastolic function. Most patients have a dilated left ventricular chamber (dilated form), although some display ventricular hypoplasia. EFE usually occurs in infants and young children, who present with signs of congestive heart failure, and most cases are of unknown etiology. In the past, the incidence of EFE in the United States was relatively high—approximately 1 per 5,000 live births. In recent decades, however, the incidence has declined significantly for unknown reasons.

It was suggested that idiopathic cases of EFE result from increased endocardial mural tension produced by the left ventricular dilatation due to myocarditis.[131] Hutchins and Vie[131] studied 64 children with either myocarditis or primary EFE; of these, 5 had myocarditis only, 18 had idiopathic EFE, and the remaining 41 had evidence of both myocarditis and EFE. With longer survival, the severity of myocarditis decreased but was replaced by an increase in EFE. By 4 months, no patient had histologic evidence of myocarditis, which is reminiscent of the association between myocarditis and DCM.

The link between viral myocarditis and EFE, therefore, supported a role for chronic viral infection in the etiology of EFE.[131] However, as with myocarditis, there was little direct evidence for viral infection of the myocardium of patients with EFE by classical virologic techniques. Fruhling et al.[132] reported that a significant proportion of myocardial samples from EFE patients was culture-positive for coxsackievirus B. It also was proposed that EFE might develop in a particular subset of patients with viral myocarditis—those with mumps virus-induced disease. A link between mumps virus infection and EFE was established by positive skin reactivity tests.[133] In 1 case, the mother had a mumps infection during the first trimester of pregnancy, whereas 2 other patients were exposed to mumps. It was suggested that intrauterine infection with the mumps virus may be involved in some cases of EFE.

It was first suggested in 1918 that myocarditis was a rare complication of mumps virus infection.[134] In 1984 a link was established among mumps, myocarditis, and subsequent cardiomyopathy.[135]

Ni et al.[136] identified mumps RNA by reverse transcription PCR in more than 70% of EFE samples, whereas 28% amplified adenovirus. These data support an etiologic role for viral infection in EFE and the hypothesis that EFE is a sequela of a viral myocarditis, particularly due to mumps virus. None of the samples obtained after 1980 were positive for mumps virus. Thus, it is possible that the remaining cases of EFE are caused by a different etiologic agent, such as adenovirus.

A mumps virus origin for EFE may also explain the dramatic decline in incidence in the last few decades. Since the introduction of the mumps vaccine, the prevalence of epidemic parotitis has decreased significantly.[137] Therefore, unlike the pattern of infection of the enteroviruses, which show periodic peaks in infection rates, the decline in incidence of EFE seems to reflect the decreased prevalence of mumps virus in the population. These data support the efficacy of a virus-specific vaccination (eg, adenovirus group C and CVB) in the prevention of an acquired form of heart disease.

Adenovirus-specific vaccines are already available for some serotypes, and the vaccine is provided for military personnel in the United States. However, this vaccine does not protect against the group C adenoviruses most commonly associated with heart disease. No data are available on the difference in the frequency of myocarditis in these individuals versus the general population.

THE COMMON COXSACKIEVIRUS B-ADENOVIRUS RECEPTOR

It has remained something of a conundrum why 2 such divergent virus families as the human adenoviruses and coxackievirus B cause these diseases. The description of the common human coxsackievirus B-adenovirus receptor (CAR) offers at least a partial explanation.[138-140]

CAR is a 46-kDa transmembrane glycoprotein with 2 extracellular immunoglobulin-like domains. Transfection of nonpermissive cells with a cDNA clone encoding this receptor allows both coxsackievirus B and adenovirus (through the fiber protein) attachment and infection.[138] In humans, this protein is expressed highly in the heart, pancreas, testes, and prostate and to some degree in many other tissues.[140] The human *CAR* gene consisting of 7 exons is encoded at 21q11.2,[141] and pseudogenes are located on chromosomes 15, 18, and 21.

It has been postulated that the physiologic function of CAR is as a cellular adhesion molecule, which in the developing brain is important in neural network formation.[142] However, the broad spectrum of tissues encoding this protein suggests that its function is more general in cell-to-cell contact and cardiomyocyte adhesion.

CAR is not limited to humans and mice. Ito et al.[143] reported that it is strongly expressed in the myocardium of newborn rats. Although in adult rats myocardial expression is reduced, in a rat model of myocarditis induced by immunization with cardiac myosin, CAR expression is enhanced during the active phase due to induction by inflammatory mediators. It is unknown whether such a phenomenon occurs in humans, but the increased expression of CAR should be considered as a host factor in the pathogenesis of viral myocarditis and DCM.

Adenovirus uses a second receptor for cell entry, the vitronectin receptor (α_5 integrin and β_3 integrin). Although the interactions of CAR with components of the cytoskeleton are not yet identified, the vitronectin receptor interacts with vinculin and actin[144,145] (Fig. 23-5). Whether disturbances in these interactions contribute to the susceptibility or pathogenesis of myocarditis or DCM is under investigation.

ACKNOWLEDGMENTS

Neil E. Bowles, Ph.D., is supported by a grant from the American Heart Association, Texas Affiliate, and by the Abercrombie Cardiology Fund of Texas Children's Hospital. Jeffrey A. Towbin, M.D., is supported by the Texas Children's Hospital Foundation Chair in Pediatric Cardiovascular Research and by grants from the National Heart, Lung and Blood Institute.

REFERENCES

1. Dec GW, Fuster V. Idiopathic dilated cardiomyopathy. N Engl J Med 1994;331:1564-1575.
2. Keeling PJ, Gang Y, Smith G, Seo H, Bent SE, Murday V, Caforio AL, McKenna WJ. Familial dilated cardiomyopathy in the United Kingdom. Br Heart J 1995;73:417-421.
3. Manolio TA, Baughman KL, Rodeheffer R, Pearson TA, Bristow JD, Michels VV, Abelmann WH, Harlan WR. Prevalence and etiology of idiopathic dilated cardiomyopathy (summary of a National Heart, Lung, and Blood Institute workshop). Am J Cardiol 1992;69:1458-1466.
4. O'Connell JB, Bristow MR. Economic impact of heart failure in the United States: time for a different approach. J Heart Lung Transplant 1994;13:S107-S112.
5. Sole MJ, Liu P. Viral myocarditis: a paradigm for understanding the pathogenesis and treatment of dilated cardiomyopathy. J Am Coll Cardiol 1993;22 Suppl A:99A-105A.
6. Rosenberg HS, McNamara DG. Acute myocarditis in infancy and childhood. Prog Cardiovasc Dis 1964;7:179-197.

7. Chow LH, Beisel KW, McManus BM. Enteroviral infection of mice with severe combined immuno-deficiency. Evidence for direct viral pathogenesis of myocardial injury. Lab Invest 1992;66:24-31.

8. Noren GR, Staley NA, Bandt CM, Kaplan EL. Occurrence of myocarditis in sudden death in children. J Forensic Sci 1977;22:188-196.

9. O'Connell JB. The role of myocarditis in end-stage dilated cardiomyopathy. Tex Heart Inst J 1987;14:268-275.

10. Woodruff JF. Viral myocarditis. A review. Am J Pathol 1980;101:425-484.

11. Huber SA. Autoimmunity in myocarditis: relevance of animal models. Clin Immunol Immunopathol 1997;83:93-102.

12. Maron BJ. Sudden death in young athletes. Lessons from the Hank Gathers affair. N Engl J Med 1993;329:55-57.

13. Aretz HT, Billingham ME, Edwards WD, Factor SM, Fallon JT, Fenoglio JJ Jr, Olsen EG, Schoen FJ. Myocarditis. A histopathologic definition and classification. Am J Cardiovasc Pathol 1987;1:3-14.

14. Chow LH, Radio SJ, Sears TD, McManus BM. Insensitivity of right ventricular endomyocardial biopsy in the diagnosis of myocarditis. J Am Coll Cardiol 1989;14:915-920.

15. Grist NR, Bell EJ. A six-year study of coxsackievirus B infections in heart disease. J Hyg (Lond) 1974;73:165-172.

16. Goodwin JF. Myocarditis as a possible cause of cardiomyopathy. In: Just H, Schuster H-P, eds. Myocarditis, cardiomyopathy: selected problems of pathogenesis and clinic. Berlin: Springer-Verlag, 1983:7-11.

17. Grist NR, Bell EJ, Assaad F. Enteroviruses in human disease. Prog Med Virol 1978;24:114-157.

18. Morgan-Capner P, Richardson PJ, McSorley C, Daley K, Pattison JR. Virus investigations in heart muscle disease. In: Bolte H-D, ed. Viral heart disease. Berlin: Springer-Verlag, 1984:95-115.

19. El-Hagrassy MM, Banatvala JE, Coltart DJ. Coxsackie-B-virus-specific IgM responses in patients with cardiac and other diseases. Lancet 1980;2:1160-1162.

20. McCartney RA, Banatvala JE, Bell EJ. Routine use of μ-antibody-capture ELISA for the serological diagnosis of Coxsackie B virus infections. J Med Virol 1986;19:205-212.

21. Muir P, Nicholson F, Tilzey AJ, Signy M, English TA, Banatvala JE. Chronic relapsing pericarditis and dilated cardiomyopathy: serological evidence of persistent enterovirus infection. Lancet 1989;1:804-807.

22. Huber SA, Lodge PA. Coxsackievirus B-3 myocarditis in Balb/c mice. Evidence for autoimmunity to myocyte antigens. Am J Pathol 1984;116:21-29.

23. Huber SA, Lodge PA. Coxsackievirus B-3 myocarditis. Identification of different pathogenic mechanisms in DBA/2 and Balb/c mice. Am J Pathol 1986;122:284-291.

24. Andreoletti L, Hober D, Becquart P, Belaich S, Copin MC, Lambert V, Wattre P. Experimental CVB3-induced chronic myocarditis in two murine strains: evidence of interrelationships between virus replication and myocardial damage in persistent cardiac infection. J Med Virol 1997;52:206-214.

25. Neumann DA, Lane JR, Allen GS, Herskowitz A, Rose NR. Viral myocarditis leading to cardiomyopathy: do cytokines contribute to pathogenesis? Clin Immunol Immunopathol 1993;68:181-190.

26. Bowles NE, Richardson PJ, Olsen EG, Archard LC. Detection of Coxsackie-B-virus-specific RNA sequences in myocardial biopsy samples from patients with myocarditis and dilated cardiomyopathy. Lancet 1986;1:1120-1123.

27. Bowles NE, Rose ML, Taylor P, Banner NR, Morgan-Capner P, Cunningham L, Archard LC, Yacoub MH. End-stage dilated cardiomyopathy. Persistence of enterovirus RNA in myocardium at cardiac transplantation and lack of immune response. Circulation 1989;80:1128-1136.

28. Kandolf R, Ameis D, Kirschner P, Canu A, Hofschneider PH. In situ detection of enteroviral

genomes in myocardial cells by nucleic acid hybridization: an approach to the diagnosis of viral heart disease. Proc Natl Acad Sci U S A 1987;84:6272-6276.

29. Kandolf R, Klingel K, Mertsching H, Canu A, Hohenadl C, Zell R, Reimann BY, Heim A, McManus BM, Foulis AK, Schultheiss H-P, Erdmann E, Riecker G. Molecular studies on enteroviral heart disease: patterns of acute and persistent infections. Eur Heart J 1991;12 Suppl D:49-55.

30. Chapman NM, Tracy S, Gauntt CJ, Fortmueller U. Molecular detection and identification of enteroviruses using enzymatic amplification and nucleic acid hybridization. J Clin Microbiol 1990;28:843-850.

31. Grasso M, Arbustini E, Silini E, Diegoli M, Percivalle E, Ratti G, Bramerio M, Gavazzi A, Vigano M, Milanesi G. Search for Coxsackievirus B3 RNA in idiopathic dilated cardiomyopathy using gene amplification by polymerase chain reaction. Am J Cardiol 1992;69:658-664.

32. Jin O, Sole MJ, Butany JW, Chia WK, McLaughlin PR, Liu P, Liew CC. Detection of enterovirus RNA in myocardial biopsies from patients with myocarditis and cardiomyopathy using gene amplification by polymerase chain reaction. Circulation 1990;82:8-16.

33. Muir P, Nicholson F, Jhetam M, Neogi S, Banatvala JE. Rapid diagnosis of enterovirus infection by magnetic bead extraction and polymerase chain reaction detection of enterovirus RNA in clinical specimens. J Clin Microbiol 1993;31:31-38.

34. Redline RW, Genest DR, Tycko B. Detection of enteroviral infection in paraffin-embedded tissue by the RNA polymerase chain reaction technique. Am J Clin Pathol 1991;96:568-571.

35. Weiss LM, Liu XF, Chang KL, Billingham ME. Detection of enteroviral RNA in idiopathic dilated cardiomyopathy and other human cardiac tissues. J Clin Invest 1992;90:156-159.

36. Weiss LM, Movahed LA, Billingham ME, Cleary ML. Detection of Coxsackievirus B3 RNA in myocardial tissues by the polymerase chain reaction. Am J Pathol 1991;138:497-503.

37. Griffin LD, Kearney D, Ni J, Jaffe R, Fricker FJ, Webber S, Demmler G, Gelb BD, Towbin JA. Analysis of formalin-fixed and frozen myocardial autopsy samples for viral genome in childhood myocarditis and dilated cardiomyopathy with endocardial fibroelastosis using polymerase chain reaction (PCR). Cardiovasc Pathol 1995;4:3-11.

38. Martin AB, Webber S, Fricker FJ, Jaffe R, Demmler G, Kearney D, Zhang YH, Bodurtha J, Gelb B, Ni J, Bricker JT, Towbin JA. Acute myocarditis. Rapid diagnosis by PCR in children. Circulation 1994;90:330-339.

39. Pauschinger M, Bowles NE, Fuentes-Garcia FJ, Pham V, Kuhl U, Schwimmbeck PL, Schultheiss HP, Towbin JA. Detection of adenoviral genome in the myocardium of adult patients with idiopathic left ventricular dysfunction. Circulation 1999;99:1348-1354.

40. Tu Z, Chapman NM, Hufnagel G, Tracy S, Romero JR, Barry WH, Zhao L, Currey K, Shapiro B. The cardiovirulent phenotype of coxsackievirus B3 is determined at a single site in the genomic 5' nontranslated region. J Virol 1995;69:4607-4618.

41. Chapman NM, Romero JR, Pallansch MA, Tracy S. Sites other than nucleotide 234 determine cardiovirulence in natural isolates of coxsackievirus B3. J Med Virol 1997;52:258-261.

42. Lee C, Maull E, Chapman N, Tracy S, Gauntt C. Genomic regions of coxsackievirus B3 associated with cardiovirulence. J Med Virol 1997;52:341-347.

43. Wu TC, Pizzorno MC, Hayward GS, Willoughby S, Neumann DA, Rose NR, Ansari AA, Beschorner WE, Baughman KL, Herskowitz A. In situ detection of human cytomegalovirus immediate-early gene transcripts within cardiac myocytes of patients with HIV-associated cardiomyopathy. AIDS 1992;6:777-785.

44. Barbaro G, Di Lorenzo G, Grisorio B, Barbarini G. Incidence of dilated cardiomyopathy and detection of HIV in myocardial cells of HIV-positive patients. Gruppo Italiano per lo Studio Cardiologico dei Pazienti Affetti de AIDS. N Engl J Med 1998;339:1093-1099.

45. Bowles NE, Kearney DL, Ni J, Perez-Atayde AR, Kline MW, Bricker JT, Ayres NA, Lipshultz SE, Shearer WT, Towbin JA. The detection of viral genomes by polymerase chain reaction in the myocardium of pediatric patients with advanced HIV disease. J Am Coll Cardiol 1999;34:857-865.

46. Greenberg SB. Viral pneumonia. Infect Dis Clin North Am 1991;5:603-621.

47. Gardiner AJ, Short D. Four faces of acute myopericarditis. Br Heart J 1973;35:433-442.

48. Henson D, Mufson MA. Myocarditis and pneumonitis with type 21 adenovirus infection. Association with fatal myocarditis and pneumonitis. Am J Dis Child 1971;121:334-336.

49. Akhtar N, Ni J, Stromberg D, Rosenthal GL, Bowles NE, Towbin JA. Tracheal aspirate as a substrate for polymerase chain reaction detection of viral genome in childhood pneumonia and myocarditis. Circulation 1999;99:2011-2018.

50. Schowengerdt KO, Ni J, Denfield SW, Gajarski RJ, Bowles NE, Rosenthal G, Kearney DL, Price JK, Rogers BB, Schauer GM, Chinnock RE, Towbin JA. Association of parvovirus B19 genome in children with myocarditis and cardiac allograft rejection: diagnosis using the polymerase chain reaction. Circulation 1997;96:3549-3554.

51. Schowengerdt KO, Ni J, Denfield SW, Gajarski RJ, Radovancevic B, Frazier HO, Demmler GJ, Kearney D, Bricker JT, Towbin JA. Diagnosis, surveillance, and epidemiologic evaluation of viral infections in pediatric cardiac transplant recipients with the use of the polymerase chain reaction. J Heart Lung Transplant 1996;15:111-123.

52. Bridges ND, Spray TL, Collins MH, Bowles NE, Towbin JA. Adenovirus infection in the lung results in graft failure after lung transplantation. J Thorac Cardiovasc Surg 1998;116:617-623.

53. Calabrese F, Valente M, Thiene G, Angelini A, Testolin L, Biasolo MA, Soteriou B, Livi U, Palu G. Enteroviral genome in native hearts may influence outcome of patients who undergo cardiac transplantation. Diagn Mol Pathol 1999;8:39-46.

54. Kyu B, Matsumori A, Sato Y, Okada I, Chapman NM, Tracy S. Cardiac persistence of cardioviral RNA detected by polymerase chain reaction in a murine model of dilated cardiomyopathy. Circulation 1992;86:522-530.

55. Matsumori A, Kawai C. An animal model of congestive (dilated) cardiomyopathy: dilatation and hypertrophy of the heart in the chronic stage in DBA/2 mice with myocarditis caused by encephalomyocarditis virus. Circulation 1982;66:355-360.

56. Reyes MP, Ho KL, Smith F, Lerner AM. A mouse model of dilated-type cardiomyopathy due to coxsackievirus B3. J Infect Dis 1981;144:232-236.

57. Pacini DL, Dubovi EJ, Clyde WA Jr. A new animal model for human respiratory tract disease due to adenovirus. J Infect Dis 1984;150:92-97.

58. Prince GA, Porter DD, Jenson AB, Horswood RL, Chanock RM, Ginsberg HS. Pathogenesis of adenovirus type 5 pneumonia in cotton rats (Sigmodon hispidus). J Virol 1993;67:101-111.

59. Bowles NE, Kearney DL, Gilbert B, Jacobs TN, Moore-Poveda D, Wyde PR, Towbin JA. An animal model of adenovirus-induced myocarditis. Pediatr Res 1999;45 no. 4:20a.

60. Cunningham L, Bowles NE, Lane RJ, Dubowitz V, Archard LC. Persistence of enteroviral RNA in chronic fatigue syndrome is associated with the abnormal production of equal amounts of positive and negative strands of enteroviral RNA. J Gen Virol 1990;71:1399-1402.

61. Why HJ, Archard LC, Richardson PJ. Dilated cardiomyopathy—new insights into the pathogenesis. Postgrad Med J 1994;70 Suppl 1:S2-S7.

62. Evans AS. Latent adenovirus infections of the human respiratory tract. Am J Hyg 1958;67:256-266.

63. Lambriex M, Van der Veen J. Comparison of replication of adenovirus type 2 and type 4 in human lymphocyte cultures. Infect Immun 1976;14:618-622.

64. Green M, Wold WS, Mackey JK, Rigden P. Analysis of human tonsil and cancer DNAs and RNAs for DNA sequences of group C (serotypes 1, 2, 5, and 6) human adenoviruses. Proc Natl Acad Sci U S A 1979;76:6606-6610.

65. Matsuse T, Hayashi S, Kuwano K, Keunecke H, Jefferies WA, Hogg JC. Latent adenoviral infection in the pathogenesis of chronic airways obstruction. Am Rev Respir Dis 1992;146:177-184.

66. Duerksen-Hughes P, Wold WS, Gooding LR. Adenovirus E1A renders infected cells sensitive to cytolysis by tumor necrosis factor. J Immunol 1989;143:4193-4200.

67. White E. Regulation of apoptosis by the transforming genes of the DNA tumor virus adenovirus. Proc Soc Exp Biol Med 1993;204:30-39.

68. James TN. Normal and abnormal consequences of apoptosis in the human heart. From postnatal morphogenesis to paroxysmal arrhythmias. Circulation 1994;90:556-573.

69. Bowles NE, Kearney D, Ni J, Towbin JA. Association of adenovirus infection with apoptosis in the pathogenesis of myocarditis and dilated cardiomyopathy. Pediatr Res 1997;41:19a.

70. Narula J, Haider N, Virmani R, DiSalvo TG, Kolodgie FD, Hajjar RJ, Schmidt U, Semigran MJ, Dec GW, Khaw BA. Apoptosis in myocytes in end-stage heart failure. N Engl J Med 1996;335:1182-1189.

71. Bishopric NH, Zeng GQ, Sato B, Webster KA. Adenovirus E1A inhibits cardiac myocyte-specific gene expression through its amino terminus. J Biol Chem 1997;272:20584-20594.

72. Gooding LR, Elmore LW, Tollefson AE, Brady HA, Wold WS. A 14,700 MW protein from the E3 region of adenovirus inhibits cytolysis by tumor necrosis factor. Cell 1988;53:341-346.

73. Burgert HG, Maryanski JL, Kvist S. "E3/19K" protein of adenovirus type 2 inhibits lysis of cytolytic T lymphocytes by blocking cell-surface expression of histocompatibility class I antigens. Proc Natl Acad Sci U S A 1987;84:1356-1360.

74. Janaswami PM, Kalvakolanu DV, Zhang Y, Sen GC. Transcriptional repression of interleukin-6 gene by adenoviral E1A proteins. J Biol Chem 1992;267:24886-24891.

75. Takeda T, Nakajima K, Kojima H, Hirano T. E1A repression of IL-6-induced gene activation by blocking the assembly of IL-6 response element binding complexes. J Immunol 1994;153:4573-4582.

76. Henke A, Mohr C, Sprenger H, Graebner C, Stelzner A, Nain M, Gemsa D. Coxsackievirus B3-induced production of tumor necrosis factor-alpha, IL-1 beta, and IL-6 in human monocytes. J Immunol 1992;148:2270-2277.

77. Postlethwaite AE, Kang AH. Induction of fibroblast proliferation by human mononuclear leukocyte-derived proteins. Arthritis Rheum 1983;26:22-27.

78. Gulick T, Chung MK, Pieper SJ, Lange LG, Schreiner GF. Interleukin 1 and tumor necrosis factor inhibit cardiac myocyte beta-adrenergic responsiveness. Proc Natl Acad Sci U S A 1989;86:6753-6757.

79. Bryant D, Becker L, Richardson J, Shelton J, Franco F, Peshock R, Thompson M, Giroir B. Cardiac failure in transgenic mice with myocardial expression of tumor necrosis factor-alpha. Circulation 1998;97:1375-1381.

80. Kubota T, McTiernan CF, Frye CS, Demetris AJ, Feldman AM. Cardiac-specific overexpression of tumor necrosis factor-alpha causes lethal myocarditis in transgenic mice. J Card Fail 1997;3:117-124.

81. Kubota T, McTiernan CF, Frye CS, Slawson SE, Lemster BH, Koretsky AP, Demetris AJ, Feldman AM. Dilated cardiomyopathy in transgenic mice with cardiac-specific overexpression of tumor necrosis factor-alpha. Circ Res 1997;81:627-635.

82. de Belder AJ, Radomski MW, Why HJ, Richardson PJ, Martin JF. Myocardial calcium-independent nitric oxide synthase activity is present in dilated cardiomyopathy, myocarditis, and postpartum cardiomyopathy but not in ischaemic or valvar heart disease. Br Heart J 1995;74:426-430.

83. Mikami S, Kawashima S, Kanazawa K, Hirata K, Katayama Y, Hotta H, Hayashi Y, Ito H, Yokoyama M. Expression of nitric oxide synthase in a murine model of viral myocarditis induced by coxsackievirus B3. Biochem Biophys Res Commun 1996;220:983-989.

84. Bachmaier K, Neu N, Pummerer C, Duncan GS, Mak TW, Matsuyama T, Penninger JM. iNOS expression and nitrotyrosine formation in the myocardium in response to inflammation is controlled by the interferon regulatory transcription factor 1. Circulation 1997;96:585-591.

85. Bowles NE, Bowles KR, Towbin JA. The "final common pathway" hypothesis and inherited cardiovascular disease. The role of cytoskeletal proteins in dilated cardiomyopathy. Herz 2000;25:168-175.

86. Towbin JA, Bowles KR, Bowles NE. Etiologies of cardiomyopathy and heart failure. Nat Med 1999;5:266-267.

87. Bonne G, Carrier L, Richard P, Hainque B, Schwartz K. Familial hypertrophic cardiomyopathy: from mutations to functional defects. Circ Res 1998;83:580-593.

88. Wang Q, Bowles NE, Towbin JA. The molecular basis of long QT syndrome and prospects for therapy. Mol Med Today 1998;4:382-388.

89. Bione S, D'Adamo P, Maestrini E, Gedeon AK, Bolhuis PA, Toniolo D. A novel X-linked gene, G4.5. is responsible for Barth syndrome. Nat Genet 1996;12:385-389.

90. Muntoni F, Cau M, Ganau A, Congiu R, Arvedi G, Mateddu A, Marrosu MG, Cianchetti C, Realdi G, Cao A, Melis MA. Brief report: deletion of the dystrophin muscle-promoter region associated with X-linked dilated cardiomyopathy. N Engl J Med 1993;329:921-925.

91. Muntoni F, Wilson L, Marrosu G, Marrosu MG, Cianchetti C, Mestroni L, Ganau A, Dubowitz V, Sewry C. A mutation in the dystrophin gene selectively affecting dystrophin expression in the heart. J Clin Invest 1995;96:693-699.

92. Ortiz-Lopez R, Li H, Su J, Goytia V, Towbin JA. Evidence for a dystrophin missense mutation as a cause of X-linked dilated cardiomyopathy. Circulation 1997;95:2434-2440.

93. Hoffman EP, Brown RH Jr, Kunkel LM. Dystrophin: the protein product of the Duchenne muscular dystrophy locus. Cell 1987;51:919-928.

94. Arber S, Hunter JJ, Ross J Jr, Hongo M, Sansig G, Borg J, Perriard JC, Chien KR, Caroni P. MLP-deficient mice exhibit a disruption of cardiac cytoarchitectural organization, dilated cardiomyopathy, and heart failure. Cell 1997;88:393-403.

95. Bies RD, Maeda M, Roberds SL, Holder E, Bohlmeyer T, Young JB, Campbell KP. A 5' dystrophin duplication mutation causes membrane deficiency of alpha-dystroglycan in a family with X-linked cardiomyopathy. J Mol Cell Cardiol 1997;29:3175-3188.

96. Maeda M, Holder E, Lowes B, Valent S, Bies RD. Dilated cardiomyopathy associated with deficiency of the cytoskeletal protein metavinculin. Circulation 1997;95:17-20.

97. Nigro G, Politano L, Nigro V, Petretta VR, Comi LI. Mutation of dystrophin gene and cardiomyopathy. Neuromuscul Disord 1994;4:371-379.

98. Nigro V, de Sa Moreira E, Piluso G, Vainzof M, Belsito A, Politano L, Puca AA, Passos-Bueno MR, Zatz M. Autosomal recessive limb-girdle muscular dystrophy, LGMD2F, is caused by a mutation in the delta-sarcoglycan gene. Nat Genet 1996;14:195-198.

99. Nigro V, Okazaki Y, Belsito A, Piluso G, Matsuda Y, Politano L, Nigro G, Ventura C, Abbondanza C, Molinari AM, Acampora D, Nishimura M, Hayashizaki Y, Puca GA. Identification of the Syrian hamster cardiomyopathy gene. Hum Mol Genet 1997;6:601-607.

100. Sakamoto A, Abe M, Masaki T. Delineation of genomic deletion in cardiomyopathic hamster. FEBS Lett 1999;447:124-128.

101. Sakamoto A, Ono K, Abe M, Jasmin G, Eki T, Murakami Y, Masaki T, Toyo-oka T, Hanaoka F. Both hypertrophic and dilated cardiomyopathies are caused by mutation of the same gene, delta-sarcoglycan, in hamster: an animal model of disrupted dystrophin-associated glycoprotein complex. Proc Natl Acad Sci U S A 1997;94:13873-13878.

102. Towbin JA, Hejtmancik JF, Brink P, Gelb B, Zhu XM, Chamberlain JS, McCabe ER, Swift M. X-linked dilated cardiomyopathy. Molecular genetic evidence of linkage to the Duchenne muscular dystrophy (dystrophin) gene at the Xp21 locus. Circulation 1993;87:1854-1865.

103. Olson TM, Michels VV, Thibodeau SN, Tai YS, Keating MT. Actin mutations in dilated cardiomyopathy, a heritable form of heart failure. Science 1998;280:750-752.

104. Mogensen J, Klausen IC, Pedersen AK, Egeblad H, Bross P, Kruse TA, Gregersen N, Hansen PS, Baandrup U, Borglum AD. Alpha-cardiac actin is a novel disease gene in familial hypertrophic cardiomyopathy. J Clin Invest 1999;103:R39-R43.

105. Li D, Tapscoft T, Gonzalez O, Burch PE, Quinones MA, Zoghbi WA, Hill R, Bachinski LL, Mann DL, Roberts R. Desmin mutation responsible for idiopathic dilated cardiomyopathy. Circulation 1999;100:461-464.

106. Fatkin D, MacRae C, Sasaki T, Wolff MR, Porcu M, Frenneaux M, Atherton J, Vidaillet HJ Jr, Spudich S, De Girolami U, Seidman JG, Seidman C, Muntoni F, Muehle G, Johnson W, McDonough B. Missense mutations in the rod domain of the lamin A/C gene as causes of dilated cardiomyopathy and conduction-system disease. N Engl J Med 1999;341:1715-1724.

107. Bonne G, Di Barletta MR, Varnous S, Becane HM, Hammouda EH, Merlini L, Muntoni F, Greenberg CR, Gary F, Urtizberea JA, Duboc D, Fardeau M, Toniolo D, Schwartz K. Mutations in the gene encoding lamin A/C cause autosomal dominant Emery-Dreifuss muscular dystrophy. Nat Genet 1999;21:285-288.

108. Muchir A, Bonne G, van der Kooi AJ, van Meegen M, Baas F, Bolhuis PA, de Visser M, Schwartz K. Identification of mutations in the gene encoding lamins A/C in autosomal dominant limb girdle muscular dystrophy with atrioventricular conduction disturbances (LGMD1B). Hum Mol Genet 2000;9:1453-1459.

109. Raffaele Di Barletta M, Ricci E, Galluzzi G, Tonali P, Mora M, Morandi L, Romorini A, Voit T, Orstavik KH, Merlini L, Trevisan C, Biancalana V, Housmanowa-Petrusewicz I, Bione S, Ricotti R, Schwartz K, Bonne G, Toniolo D. Different mutations in the LMNA gene cause autosomal dominant and autosomal recessive Emery-Dreifuss muscular dystrophy. Am J Hum Genet 2000;66:1407-1412.

110. Maeda M, Nakao S, Miyazato H, Setoguchi M, Arima S, Higuchi I, Osame M, Taira A, Nomoto K, Toda H, Tahara M, Atsuchi Y, Tanaka H. Cardiac dystrophin abnormalities in Becker muscular dystrophy assessed by endomyocardial biopsy. Am Heart J 1995;129:702-707.

111. Bowles KR, Gajarski R, Porter P, Goytia V, Bachinski L, Roberts R, Pignateli R, Towbin JA. Gene mapping of familial autosomal dominant dilated cardiomyopathy to chromosome 10q21-23. J Clin Invest 1996;98:1355-1360.

112. Olson TM, Keating MT. Mapping a cardiomyopathy locus to chromosome 3p22-p25. J Clin Invest 1996;97:528-532.

113. Badorff C, Lee GH, Lamphear BJ, Martone ME, Campbell KP, Rhoads RE, Knowlton KU. Enteroviral protease 2A cleaves dystrophin: evidence of cytoskeletal disruption in an acquired cardiomyopathy. Nat Med 1999;5:320-326.

114. Puls A, Eliopoulos AG, Nobes CD, Bridges T, Young LS, Hall A. Activation of the small GTPase Cdc42 by the inflammatory cytokines TNF (alpha) and IL-1, and by the Epstein-Barr virus transforming protein LMP1. J Cell Sci 1999;112:2983-2992.

115. Wojciak-Stothard B, Entwistle A, Garg R, Ridley AJ. Regulation of TNF-alpha-induced reorganization of the actin cytoskeleton and cell-cell junctions by Rho, Rac, and Cdc42 in human endothelial cells. J Cell Physiol 1998;176:150-165.

116. Binks M, Jones GE, Brickell PM, Kinnon C, Katz DR, Thrasher AJ. Intrinsic dendritic cell abnormalities in Wiskott-Aldrich syndrome. Eur J Immunol 1998;28:3259-3267.

117. Mason JW, O'Connell JB, Herskowitz A, Rose NR, McManus BM, Billingham ME, Moon TE. A clinical trial of immunosuppressive therapy for myocarditis. The Myocarditis Treatment Trial Investigators. N Engl J Med 1995;333:269-275.

118. Maisch B, Schonian U, Hengstenberg C, Herzum M, Hufnagel G, Bethge C, Bittinger A, Neumann K. Immunosuppressive treatment in autoreactive myocarditis—results from a controlled trial. Postgrad Med J 1994;70 Suppl 1:S29-S34.

119. Bozkurt B, Villaneuva FS, Holubkov R, Tokarczyk T, Alvarez RJ Jr, MacGowan GA, Murali S, Rosenblum WD, Feldman AM, McNamara DM. Intravenous immune globulin in the therapy of peripartum cardiomyopathy. J Am Coll Cardiol 1999;34:177-180.

120. Takada H, Kishimoto C, Hiraoka Y. Therapy with immunoglobulin suppresses myocarditis in a murine coxsackievirus B3 model. Antiviral and anti-inflammatory effects. Circulation 1995;92:1604-1611.

121. Takeda Y, Yasuda S, Miyazaki S, Daikoku S, Nakatani S, Nonogi H. High-dose immunoglobulin G therapy for fulminant myocarditis. Jpn Circ J 1998;62:871-872.

122. Drucker NA, Colan SD, Lewis AB, Beiser AS, Wessel DL, Takahashi M, Baker AL, Perez-Atayde AR, Newburger JW. Gamma-globulin treatment of acute myocarditis in the pediatric population. Circulation 1994;89:252-257.

123. Briassoulis G, Papadopoulos G, Zavras N, Pailopoulos V, Hatzis T, Thanopoulos V. Cardiac troponin 1 in fulminant adenovirus myocarditis treated with a 24-hour infusion of high-dose intravenous immunoglobulin. Pediatr Cardiol 2000;21:391-394.

124. McNamara DM, Holubkov R, Starling RC, Dec GW, Loh E, Torre-Amione G, Gass A, Janosko K, Tokarczyk T, Kessler P, Mann DL, Feldman AM. Controlled trial of intravenous immune globulin in recent-onset dilated cardiomyopathy. Circulation 2001;103:2254-2259.

125. Hellen CU, Wimmer E. Viral proteases as targets for chemotherapeutic intervention. Curr Opin Biotechnol 1992;3:643-649.

126. Tomasselli AG, Heinrikson RL. Targeting the HIV-protease in AIDS therapy: a current clinical perspective. Biochim Biophys Acta 2000;1477:189-214.

127. Molla A, Hellen CU, Wimmer E. Inhibition of proteolytic activity of poliovirus and rhinovirus 2A proteinases by elastase-specific inhibitors. J Virol 1993;67:4688-4695.

128. Patick AK, Binford SL, Brothers MA, Jackson RL, Ford CE, Diem MD, Maldonado F, Dragovich PS, Zhou R, Prins TJ, Fuhrman SA, Meador JW, Zalman LS, Matthews DA, Worland ST. In vitro antiviral activity of AG7088, a potent inhibitor of human rhinovirus 3C protease. Antimicrob Agents Chemother 1999;43:2444-2450.

129. Melnick JL. Current status of poliovirus infections. Clin Microbiol Rev 1996;9:293-300.

130. Hofling K, Tracy S, Chapman N, Kim KS, Smith Leser J. Expression of an antigenic adenovirus epitope in a group B coxsackievirus. J Virol 2000;74:4570-4578.

131. Hutchins GM, Vie SA. The progression of interstitial myocarditis to idiopathic endocardial fibro-elastosis. Am J Pathol 1972;66:483-496.

132. Fruhling L, Korn R, Lavillaureix J, Surjus A, Fossereau S. Chronic fibroelastic myoendocarditis of the newborn and the infant (fibroelastosis). New morphological, etiological and pathogenic data. Relation to certain cardiac abnormalities. [French.] Ann Anat Path (Paris) 1962;7:227-303.

133. Noren GR, Adams P Jr, Anderson RC. Positive skin reactivity to mumps virus antigen in endo-cardial fibroelastosis. J Pediatr 1963;62:604-606.

134. Pujol M. Oreillons et myocardite. Arch Med Pharm Mil Par 1918;69:527-538.

135. Baandrup U, Mortensen SA. Fatal mumps myocarditis. Acta Med Scand 1984;216:331-333.

136. Ni J, Bowles NE, Kim YH, Demmler G, Kearney D, Bricker JT, Towbin JA. Viral infection of the myocardium in endocardial fibroelastosis. Molecular evidence for the role of mumps virus as an etiologic agent. Circulation 1997;95:133-139.

137. van Loon FPL, Holmes SJ, Sirotkin BI, Williams WW, Cochi SL, Hadler SC, Lindegren ML. Mumps surveillance—United States, 1988-1993. MMWR CDC Surveill Summ 1995;44 no. SS-3:1-14.

138. Bergelson JM, Cunningham JA, Droguett G, Kurt-Jones EA, Krithivas A, Hong JS, Horwitz MS, Crowell RL, Finberg RW. Isolation of a common receptor for Coxsackie B viruses and adenoviruses 2 and 5. Science 1997;275:1320-1323.

139. Carson SD, Chapman NN, Tracy SM. Purification of the putative coxsackievirus B receptor from HeLa cells. Biochem Biophys Res Commun 1997;233:325-328.

140. Tomko RP, Xu R, Philipson L. HCAR and MCAR: the human and mouse cellular receptors for subgroup C adenoviruses and group B coxsackieviruses. Proc Natl Acad Sci U S A 1997;94:3352-3356.

141. Bowles KR, Gibson J, Wu J, Shaffer LG, Towbin JA, Bowles NE. Genomic organization and chromosomal localization of the human Coxsackievirus B-adenovirus receptor gene. Hum Genet 1999; 105:354-359.

142. Honda T, Saitoh H, Masuko M, Katagiri-Abe T, Tominaga K, Kozakai I, Kobayashi K, Kumanishi T, Watanabe YG, Odani S, Kuwano R. The coxsackievirus-adenovirus receptor protein as a cell adhesion molecule in the developing mouse brain. Brain Res Mol Brain Res 2000;77:19-28.

143. Ito M, Kodama M, Masuko M, Yamaura M, Fuse K, Uesugi Y, Hirono S, Okura Y, Kato K, Hotta Y, Honda T, Kuwano R, Aizawa Y. Expression of coxsackievirus and adenovirus receptor in hearts of rats with experimental autoimmune myocarditis. Circ Res 2000;86:275-280.

144. Anderson DH, Johnson LV, Hageman GS. Vitronectin receptor expression and distribution at the photoreceptor-retinal pigment epithelial interface. J Comp Neurol 1995;360:1-16.

145. Conforti G, Calza M, Beltran-Nunez A. Alpha v beta 5 integrin is localized at focal contacts by HT-1080 fibrosarcoma cells and human skin fibroblasts attached to vitronectin. Cell Adhes Commun 1994;1:279-293.

Peripartum Cardiomyopathy

Joseph G. Murphy, M.D.

INTRODUCTION

Peripartum cardiomyopathy (PPCM) is an enigmatic disease about which our knowledge is primarily descriptive, with little real understanding of the pathophysiology of the condition. It is a rare cause of often fulminant heart failure that suddenly strikes previously healthy female patients either during the last trimester of pregnancy or during the immediate peripartum period. It is unusual in several regards: first, we know little about the nature of the myocardial insult; second, it may remit spontaneously after delivery, with apparent complete resolution of ventricular dysfunction as judged on echocardiography; and finally, patients remain at increased risk for a recurrence with subsequent pregnancies even if ventricular function appears to recover normally.

New-onset heart failure presenting during late pregnancy or after childbirth has been recognized at least since the 1700s. Gouley et al.[1] in the 1930s are generally credited with providing the first detailed description of new-onset heart failure in late pregnancy and linking the clinical findings to dilated cardiomyopathy. An important diagnostic point is that PPCM occurs, by definition, only in women without preexisting heart disease. There are many patients with preexisting ventricular dysfunction of a known specific etiology (eg, ischemic, alcoholic, congenital valvular heart disease) or an undetermined etiology (eg, preexisting dilated cardiomyopathy) who experience new-onset heart failure during pregnancy who are specifically excluded by this definition of PPCM. PPCM is relatively rare but has high reported mortality rates of between 10% and 50% in a population of young women in whom the expected mortality would otherwise be less than 0.1% per annum. An unusual feature of PPCM is the variability of prognosis. This spans the gambit of death within hours or days of presentation due to fulminant heart failure, gradual recovery with residual left ventricular dysfunction, to complete recovery with no sequelae evident either clinically or echocardiographically. Even when left ventricular function returns to normal by standard echocardiographic criteria, exercise tolerance may remain abnormal and the condition may reappear with subsequent pregnancies.

In April 1997, the National Heart, Lung, and Blood Institute (NHLBI) and the Office of Rare Diseases of the National Institutes of Health (NIH) convened a Workshop on Peripartum Cardiomyopathy.[2] The objectives for the workshop on PPCM were to "(1) summarize existing information on PPCM, specifically its definition, epidemiology, cause, clinical characteristics, treatment, and prognosis; (2) review diagnostic criteria and discuss means of differentiating early symptoms of heart failure from normal physiological changes associated with pregnancy, such as tachypnea and fatigue during the third trimester of pregnancy; (3) develop recommendations for future research on PPCM; and (4) discuss educational measures to increase awareness of PPCM and thus facilitate prompt diagnosis." This workshop produced a written report that standardized the definition of PPCM and provided a framework for management and future research into the condition.

DEFINITION OF PERIPARTUM CARDIOMYOPATHY

The NHLBI/NIH workshop defined PPCM on the basis of 4 criteria adapted from earlier work by Demakis et al.[3] These criteria are summarized in Table 24-1. In contrast to an earlier definition of PPCM, the workshop adopted an interval from 1 month before delivery to 5 months postpartum as the allowable time for the onset of new ventricular dysfunction. Exacerbation of a preexisting dilated cardiomyopathy as a result of the hemodynamic stress of pregnancy (primarily increased cardiac output and blood volume) or new heart failure presenting during the early month of pregnancy was specifically excluded from this definition of PPCM. Many previous case reports of PPCM included patients presenting with unexplained heart failure early in pregnancy and probably also those with underlying dilated cardiomyopathy unmasked by the hemodynamic or hormonal stress of pregnancy. PPCM as defined by the NHLBI/NIH workshop panel includes only patients without a history of recognizable heart disease and without another explanation for the cardiomyopathy. This definition of PPCM while epidemiologically strong is scientifically nonrigorous because it is not based on true disease causation. Patients presenting with heart failure before the last month of pregnancy may have pregnancy-induced cardiomyopathy/heart failure but are excluded on semantic grounds by this definition of PPCM. Also, the duration of pregnancy varies among patients such that the last month of pregnancy for an individual patient may in fact not be the 9th month of actual pregnancy. In summary, the definition of PPCM adopted by the NHLBI/NIH workshop provides consistency but is less than scientifically rigorous. When the underlying pathogenesis of PPCM is better understood, it is hoped that the diagnostic criteria will be reformulated accordingly.

Table 24-1
Definition of Peripartum Cardiomyopathy

Classic
 Development of cardiac failure in the last month of pregnancy
  or within 5 months of delivery
 Absence of an identifiable cause for the cardiac failure
 Absence of recognizable heart disease prior to the last
  month of pregnancy

Additional
 Left ventricular systolic dysfunction demonstrated by classic
  echocardiographic criteria, such as depressed shortening
  fraction or ejection fraction

From Pearson et al.[2] By permission of the American Medical Association.

INCIDENCE AND RISK FACTORS
FOR PERIPARTUM CARDIOMYOPATHY

The true incidence of PPCM is not known. This is because most PPCM series are reported from tertiary referral hospitals and by their nature contain significant referral bias. To date, no population-based estimate of the occurrence of left ventricular dysfunction in pregnant women has been reported. The best reported incidence rates for PPCM range between 1 per 1,500 and 1 per 15,000 live births; the currently accepted best estimate of incidence in the United States is approximately 1 per 3,000 live births. From the 1999 birth rate of 14.5 live births per 1,000 population in the United States, this translates into about 1,500 new cases of PPCM each year in the United States.[4] A variant of PPCM occurs in northern Nigeria that may be related to the local tribal custom of ingesting large quantities of salt during pregnancy.

Several risk factors for PPCM have been identified but without any apparent unifying causation. These risk factors include multiple pregnancies, advanced maternal age, twin or triplet pregnancy, preeclampsia and gestational hypertension, and African American race. It is unclear whether race represents an independent risk factor or whether it is the interaction of race with hypertension that increases the risk of PPCM.

Rural Haiti appears to have a high incidence of PPCM—possible incidence rates of 1:300 to 1:400 live births (Personal observation and communications from Hospital Albert Schweitzer, Deschapelle, Artibomte Valley, Haiti). The average per capita annual wage is about $300 in the rural areas. Infant mortality exceeds 10%, the prevalence of human immunodeficiency virus in the general population is between 3% and 6%, and the average life expectancy is approximately 49 years. Most rural patients are anemic as a result of hookworm disease, and many also carry sickle cell trait or have sickle cell disease. The incidence of tuberculosis is among the highest on earth. Multiple possible etiologies exist to explain the high incidence of PPCM, including deficiency of trace elements such as selenium.

IS PERIPARTUM CARDIOMYOPATHY A DISTINCT DISEASE?

There is much confusion in the scientific literature over whether PPCM is truly an independent entity. Much of this problem is due to a multiplicity of definitions of PPCM used by various authors. The consensus definition of PPCM promulgated by the NHLBI/NIH workshop would have excluded many previous case reports of patients with underlying idiopathic cardiomyopathy that have been published as PPCM cases in the world literature. The NHLBI/NIH workshop on PPCM considered PPCM a distinct disease entity rather than an exacerbation of a clinically silent underlying cardiomyopathy with heart failure precipitated by the hemodynamic stresses of pregnancy. Two factors led to this assertion:

the reported incidence of PPCM is much higher than the observed incidence of dilated cardiomyopathy in women of child-bearing age and the high frequency of histologic myocarditis in some PPCM studies. This would not be expected in a patient population presenting with decompensation of preexisting heart disease due to acute hemodynamic stress.

Reliable community-based epidemiologic data comparing the incidence of dilated cardiomyopathy in pregnant women with that of age-matched nonpregnant women have not been reported. Many pathologic mechanisms have been proposed to explain PPCM, including viral myocarditis, an abnormal cellular immunologic response to pregnancy, left ventricular dysfunction due to fluid overload, an abnormal inflammatory mediator response by cytokines, and prolonged tocolysis. In addition, the role of family history and genetic factors in PPCM is unknown. Approximately 10% of patients with idiopathic cardiomyopathy have a family history of dilated cardiomyopathy and there have been a few reports of familial PPCM,[5-7] raising the possibility that some cases of PPCM are actually familial dilated cardiomyopathy unmasked by pregnancy.

IS MYOCARDITIS THE CAUSE OF PERIPARTUM CARDIOMYOPATHY?

Viral myocarditis, either as a primary infection or as a recrudescence of a previous subclinical infection due to the relative immunologic suppression characteristic of pregnancy, is a possible etiologic factor in PPCM. In 1982, Melvin and colleagues[8] first reported myocarditis diagnosed by endomyocardial biopsy in 3 consecutive patients with PPCM. The incidence of myocarditis in subsequent authors' series has varied widely.

Rizeq et al.[9] from Stanford reviewed their experience with endomyocardial biopsies in PPCM. In this study, a retrospective review was performed of endomyocardial biopsy specimens from 34 patients with PPCM. There was a low incidence of active myocarditis (8.8%, 3 of 34 patients), comparable to that found in an age- and sex-matched control population of patients with dilated cardiomyopathy undergoing cardiac transplantation (9.1%, 2 of 22 patients).

The strongest support for myocarditis as the predominant cause of PPCM comes from the Johns Hopkins experience as reported by Midei et al.[10] This group was clinically aggressive in their performance of endomyocardial biopsies on patients with symptoms of congestive heart failure and suspected PPCM at presentation. Histologically, patients with borderline myocarditis as well as those with active myocarditis were classified as having myocarditis in this series.

The high incidence of histologic myocarditis (76% of patients) has not been confirmed by reports on endomyocardial biopsy in suspected PPCM from other authors. Several reasons have been advanced for this discordance, including the higher proportion of inner-city African American patients included in the Hopkins study and the liberal criteria of including patients with borderline histologic myocarditis in the final myocarditis tally. Other studies of endomyocardial biopsy in PPCM have been criticized because of the delay between patient presentation and endomyocardial biopsy. The issue of avoidance of fluoroscopy needed during endomyocardial biopsy in pregnant women may delay or cancel endomyocardial biopsy in some PPCM patients. It is postulated that the altered immune state characteristic of pregnancy may allow unchecked viral replication and thus a greater likelihood of histologic myocarditis in the setting of PPCM.

Studies in pregnant mice demonstrated enhanced susceptibility to viral myocarditis due to coxsackieviruses and echoviruses.[11,12] No published studies to date have reported the prevalence of viral genome studied by polymerase chain reaction in endomyocardial biopsy specimens from patients with PPCM. Felker et al.,[13] in a follow-up study from Johns Hopkins, reported the long-term prognosis in their population of patients with PPCM. In this study, the prevalence of myocarditis on endomyocardial biopsy and the clinical variables associated with poor outcome were analyzed in 42 women with PPCM over a 15-year period. All patients underwent endomyocardial biopsy and right-sided heart catheterization. Three patients (7%) died and 3 patients (7%) underwent heart transplantation during a median follow-up of 8.6 years. Endomyocardial biopsy demonstrated a high prevalence of active myocarditis (62%), but the presence or absence of active myocarditis was not associated with a poorer long-term survival. The authors concluded that in patients with PPCM, 1) long-term survival is better than has been reported, 2) the prevalence of myocarditis was high, and 3) decreased left ventricular stroke work index was associated with worse clinical outcomes.

O'Connell et al.[14] reported on 14 patients with PPCM; 29% had histologic evidence of active myocarditis on endomyocardial biopsy compared with 9% of patients who had idiopathic dilated cardiomyopathy. A review of endomyocardial biopsy specimens obtained over 20 years at Mayo Clinic in patients with PPCM found no significant evidence that myocarditis, as judged by the Dallas criteria, was the cause of PPCM.[15] Why is there such a large discrepancy among series in the incidence of histologic active myocarditis in patients with PPCM? There are several explanations. Variations in histologic interpretation, the timing of endomyocardial biopsy, and sampling error may be responsible for the discrepancies in some reported results.[16] Myocarditis currently as defined by the Dallas criteria is interstitial and perivascular lymphomononuclear invasion in the presence of myocyte necrosis with or without fibrosis. Other sources of variability are likely the result of the inclusion of patients in some series outside the accepted period of PPCM, the difficulties in establishing the diagnosis of myocarditis by endomyocardial biopsy,[16,17] the inclusion of patients who have borderline myocarditis in some series, the possible geographic variability of patient populations affected, and the variable interval between clinical presentation and the endomyocardial biopsy. The pathogenesis of viral myocarditis may be linked to development of cellular immunity to myocardial antigens.[18] The use of electron micrography and molecular biologic techniques should permit us to move beyond purely histologic criteria for the diagnosis of myocarditis to identification of viral particles in myocardium. The hypothesis is that if viral genetic products are present in the myocardium, the immune system may have been improperly directed against otherwise immune-tolerated cardiac tissue proteins, leading to inflammation, cytokine activation, and eventually ventricular dysfunction.

PREGNANCY AND THE ALTERED IMMUNE RESPONSE

It is well documented that there are significant changes in immune function during normal pregnancy. Many immunologically based diseases improve or deteriorate dramatically during pregnancy. Specific examples include the disease flares that frequently characterize ulcerative colitis, rheumatoid arthritis, and multiple sclerosis in pregnant patients. Thus, many researchers have suggested that the cause of PPCM lies in a similar immunologic disturbance. It has been postulated that the maternal immune system forms antibodies to the myometrium, placenta, or fetus that cross-react with myocardial antigens. Some patients with PPCM develop antibodies to smooth muscle and actin. However, there is little direct evidence for an autoimmune etiology of PPCM.

A novel speculation on the causation of PPCM is the migration into the maternal myocardium of fetal stem cells, which provoke maternal autoantibodies that induce an autoimmune myocarditis. This theory postulates that fetal cells cross the placental fetomaternal vascular barrier and migrate into the maternal circulation. Many of these cells are antigenic and are destroyed rapidly by the maternal immune system, but it is possible that some fetal cells may survive in the maternal circulation because of weak immunogenicity or the maternal immunosuppressed state. These cells then populate the maternal myocardium for a time. After delivery maternal immunocompetence improves, leading to an antigenic response to the fetal cells. There are several arguments against this theory: analogous diseases of other organs that would also be expected to be populated by fetal cells (eg, lungs, liver) do not occur in the peripartum period. Fetal ventricular function almost always remains normal despite severe maternal left ventricular dysfunction.

PPCM may be associated with high titers of autoantibodies against select cardiac tissue proteins[2] (Table 24-2). However, antimyocardial antibodies and other autoantibodies are a frequent incidental finding in pregnant women without clinical evidence of PPCM.

Table 24-2
Serum Values of Antibodies to Cardiac Muscle Proteins in Patients With Peripartum Cardiomyopathy and Idiopathic Dilated Cardiomyopathy*

Patient group	Antibody titers[†]		
	< 1:20	1:20-1:160	> 1:160
ANT			
Idiopathic CM	16/56 (28)	29/56 (52)	11/56 (20)
Peripartum CM	1/10 (10)	1/10 (10)	8/10 (80)
BCKD			
Idiopathic CM	30/56 (53)	21/56 (38)	5/56 (9)
Peripartum CM	0/10 (0)	2/10 (20)	8/10 (80)
Myosin			
Idiopathic CM	18/56 (32)	27/56 (48)	11/56 (20)
Peripartum CM	1/10 (10)	1/10 (10)	8/10 (80)

ANT, adenine nucleotide translocator; BCKD, branched chain α-keto acid dehydrogenase; CM, cardiomyopathy. Data presented as no./total (%) of patients in each group.
*A. Ansari, M.D., unpublished data, 1997.
[†]Reciprocal of the highest dilation of serum samples showing reactivity arbitrarily divided into those with low (< 1:20), medium (1:20-1:160), and high (> 1:160) titers.
From Pearson et al.[2] By permission of the American Medical Association.

HEMODYNAMIC CHANGES IN NORMAL PREGNANCY

Normal pregnancy is associated with major hemodynamic changes that progress throughout pregnancy. In brief, blood volume (preload) and cardiac output increase while afterload decreases. Geva et al.[19] reported a 10% increase in left ventricular end-diastolic volume, a 45% increase in cardiac output, and a 26% decrease in end-systolic wall stress (a measure of myocardial afterload). In addition, Geva et al.[19] reported a reversible decrease in left ventricular systolic function in the 2nd and 3rd trimesters that persisted into the early postpartum period but returned to baseline shortly thereafter. Could PPCM, in part, be due to an exaggeration of this "normal" decrease in systolic function?

Russo et al.[20] reported on an animal study that tested the hypothesis of whether PPCM was associated with chronic β-mimetic tocolytic therapy. On gestational day 20 (normal term, 31 days), Alza miniosmotic pumps were implanted in the subcutaneous tissue of pregnant New Zealand white rabbits. Each pump was filled with terbutaline (20 μg/μL,

$n = 7$) or saline solution ($n = 7$) that was infused continuously for 7 days. The rabbits were killed on the 28th gestational day. Maternal hearts were placed on a Langendorff (isolated) perfusion apparatus for assessment of cardiac function. At a constant perfusion pressure and heart rate, left ventricular diastolic pressure varied while left ventricular developed pressure and left ventricular ± rate of pressure rise (index values of left ventricular contractility and relaxation) were measured. Hearts taken from terbutaline-treated rabbits exhibited arrhythmias and mechanical alternans in 5 of 7 cases versus 1 of 7 in the saline solution group. At a preload of 0 mm Hg, both left ventricular developed pressure (88.0 vs. 48.4 mm Hg, $P < 0.001$) and left ventricular rate of pressure rise (1,406 vs. 653 mm Hg/s, $P < 0.001$) were less in terbutaline-treated rabbits. At a preload of 10 mm Hg, left ventricular developed pressure (104.4 vs. 56.7 mm Hg, $P < 0.01$) and rate of pressure rise (1,424 vs. 694 mm Hg/s, $P < 0.001$) were also significantly less in terbutaline-treated rabbits. Left ventricular relaxation was impaired at all preloads. The authors concluded that chronic administration of terbutaline during late pregnancy in an animal model significantly depressed global maternal cardiac function.

Hibbard[21] reported a case-control study of whether long-term β-mimetic therapy of at least 9 days for preterm contractions was associated with subsequent development of PPCM. The controls for the 15 cardiomyopathic patients were chosen by a computer-generated random patient selection. Medical records were retrospectively reviewed to determine exposure to terbutaline. Although 4 of the PPCM patients (26.7%) had received long-term terbutaline therapy, only 3 of 60 controls (5.0%) had. When confounding variables including smoking and maternal age were analyzed, terbutaline therapy remained significantly associated with the development of PPCM (odds ratio, 6.91; CI, 1.30-36.85) ($P = 0.02$).

Sliwa et al.[22] evaluated the relationship of outcome in 29 patients with PPCM to circulating plasma concentrations of cytokines and Fas receptors (an apoptosis-signaling receptor). Tumor necrosis factor-α, interleukin-6, and Fas/APO-1 values were significantly increased in the study patients compared with 20 healthy volunteers. sFas/APO-1 levels were significantly higher in the 8 patients who died than in survivors. In 34% of the patients, left ventricular function almost completely returned to normal, and overall the mean ejection fraction improved from 27 ± 10% to 43 ± 16% ($P = 0.00003$). This study differed from previous studies of PPCM in that all patients were treated with diuretics, digoxin, enalapril, and carvedilol. The authors concluded that inflammatory cytokine values were significantly increased in patients with PPCM in spite of treatment with angiotensin-converting enzyme inhibitors and β-adrenergic receptor blockers.

Cenac et al.[23] investigated nutritional and trace element status and plasma concentrations of albumin, prealbumin (transthyretin), retinol binding protein, copper, selenium, and zinc in 35 African women (Republic of Niger) with peripartum cardiac failure due to PPCM. The results were compared with those for a control group of African women living under the same conditions but without peripartum cardiac failure. Plasma albumin and prealbumin were lower in patients with PPCM than they were in controls. For retinol binding protein, the difference was not statistically significant. The plasma concentrations of selenium and zinc were also lower in patients than they were in controls. The authors suggested that nutritional deficiencies might play a role in the pathophysiology of PPCM.

De Belder et al.[24] determined the activity of the calcium-dependent constitutive nitric oxide synthase (cNOS) and calcium-independent inducible NOS (iNOS) in endomyocardial biopsy samples from patients with cardiomyopathy from different causes, including PPCM (n = 3), noninflammatory dilated cardiomyopathy (n = 6), and inflammatory cardiomyopathy (n = 5). Myocardial tissue from patients with dilated cardiomyopathy, inflammatory cardiomyopathy, and PPCM showed considerable iNOS activity and little or no cNOS activity. In contrast, myocardial tissue from patients with dilated or nondilated hearts of ischemic or valvular etiology showed cNOS and little, if any, iNOS activity. Plasma tumor necrosis factor-α was detectable only in patients with inflammatory dilated cardiomyopathy. The authors concluded that generation of nitric oxide by iNOS accounts for some of the dilatation and impaired contractility associated with inflammatory and noninflammatory dilated cardiomyopathy and PPCM.

CLINICAL PRESENTATION OF PATIENTS WITH PPCM

The clinical presentation of patients with PPCM is similar to that of patients with dilated cardiomyopathies and heart failure. The diagnostic dilemma is that some of the early symptoms of PPCM may mimic features of normal pregnancy such as increasing dyspnea on exercise, fatigue, and peripheral edema. Many pregnant women with no left ventricular dysfunction also have dyspnea on exertion and peripheral edema. Less common symptoms are chest and abdominal pain, palpitations, hemoptysis, or neurologic deficits due to cardioembolic phenomena. Physical examination at the time of diagnosis may show jugular venous distension, resting tachycardia, hypotension, ventricular gallop rhythm, mitral regurgitation murmur, hepatosplenomegaly, ascites, and peripheral edema. The presentation is similar in patients presenting before and after delivery. Most patients present in New York Heart Association class III or IV heart failure. Patients may also present with palpitation without clinical evidence of heart failure. Patients with lesser degrees of left ventricular dysfunction may be largely asymptomatic and without clinical features of heart failure. Some of the patients may be diagnosed because of an intercurrent echocardiogram for other reasons (eg, murmur). Routine ancillary studies include electrocardiogram, chest radiograph, and echocardiography. The electrocardiogram usually shows nonspecific changes, including left ventricular hypertrophy or ST-T wave changes. The electrocardiogram may also be normal. The chest radiograph may show cardiomegaly with left ventricular enlargement, pulmonary edema, and bilateral pleural effusions. Echocardiography is the standard for diagnosing PPCM and for determining the severity of left ventricular dysfunction. Echocardiographic changes include increased left ventricular end-diastolic dimensions and decreased ejection fraction. Left atrial enlargement and mitral regurgitation are also commonly seen.

Cardiac catheterization may be considered in selected patients for evaluation of cardiac function and endomyocardial biopsy. If PPCM is severe, cardiac catheterization usually shows increased left and right filling pressures, decreased cardiac output, and pulmonary hypertension. It is usually possible to avoid catheterization in most affected postpartum patients. The role of endomyocardial biopsy is controversial. Although some authors recommend biopsy for all symptomatic PPCM patients, others recommend a conservative approach. Midei and associates[10] recommended that endomyocardial biopsy be undertaken in patients without resolution of PPCM symptoms within 1 week of presentation. Endomyocardial biopsy has a high false-negative rate because of the focal nature of the infiltrate, and results may depend on the timing of biopsy. Because PPCM has no characteristic histologic features, we do not know the false-negative rate. Furthermore, the demonstration of myocarditis on biopsy is unlikely to change individual patient treatment. Both immunosuppressive and steroid therapy have been used in patients with active myocarditis but are of unproven or no benefit.

Coronary angiography is rarely indicated in patients with PPCM except for those few young female patients with risk factors for coronary artery disease, including long-standing diabetes mellitus with complications, prior mediastinal irradiation for Hodgkin disease, or possibly heavy cigarette smoking. Immunologic studies, such as immunofluorescence staining of endomyocardial biopsy specimens, viral genome studies, and sarcolemma antibody detection in maternal and cord blood may also be considered on an individual basis.

DIAGNOSIS AND INVESTIGATION OF PERIPARTUM CARDIOMYOPATHY

The early diagnosis of PPCM is a challenge because most women in the last month of a normal pregnancy experience some dyspnea, fatigue, and pedal edema, symptoms identical to those of early congestive heart failure. Many cases of less severe PPCM probably go unrecognized, leading to an underestimation of disease incidence. Added symptoms and signs that raise the suspicion of PPCM include paroxysmal nocturnal dyspnea, orthopnea, severe cough, increased jugular venous pressure, loud S_3 new murmurs consistent with tricuspid and mitral valve regurgitation, and pulmonary rales. There are no specific clinical criteria for differentiating subtle symptoms of early heart failure from normal late pregnancy, so it is important that a high degree of suspicion be maintained to identify the cases of PPCM. The current standard for the diagnosis of PPCM rests on the echocardiographic identification of new left ventricular systolic dysfunction during the peripartum period. The diagnosis of PPCM also requires exclusion of other causes of cardiomyopathy. PPCM is confirmed by standard echocardiographic assessment of left ventricular systolic dysfunction and size and left ventricular systolic and diastolic diameters and ejection fraction. Strong consideration should be given to screening family members of PPCM patients because PPCM may be the forme fruste of a genetic predisposition to cardiomyopathy.

MANAGEMENT OF PERIPARTUM CARDIOMYOPATHY

Management of PPCM depends critically on whether the baby is delivered or not at the time of diagnosis. There are no clinical trials that specifically address the treatment of patients with PPCM. In brief, the treatment of the mother is similar to treatment of a patient who has conventional heart failure, with several important exceptions. Standard heart failure therapy, including diuretics, vasodilators, and sometimes digoxin, should be started as dictated by the clinical situation.

Angiotensin-converting enzyme inhibitors are contraindicated during pregnancy because of teratogenicity and possible adverse effects on placental blood flow, but they should be considered a mainstay of treatment for PPCM after delivery. Safe alternatives during pregnancy include hydralazine and nitrates. Many calcium channel blockers have negative inotropic properties and are contraindicated.

Second-generation β-receptor antagonists have beneficial effects in patients who have congestive heart failure and dilated cardiomyopathy. Clinical trials demonstrated safety, clinical benefit, and a mortality reduction in dilated cardiomyopathy. These drugs, although not contraindicated in pregnancy, have not been tested for use in PPCM. A reasonable approach is the use of β-receptor antagonists in the postpartum period in patients who continue to have symptoms and echocardiographic evidence of left ventricular compromise despite more than 2 weeks of standard heart failure management.[2]

Patients with severe heart failure require hospitalization and aggressive hemodynamic support, including, if needed, intravenous inotropic agents and invasive monitoring. Immunosuppressive therapy should be considered in patients with myocarditis documented by endomyocardial biopsy who fail to improve with 2 weeks of standard heart failure therapy. The landmark Myocarditis Treatment Trial did not demonstrate a benefit for immunosuppressive therapy in patients with biopsy-proven lymphocytic myocarditis, but it did not specifically evaluate patients with PPCM.[25] Pregnancy or PPCM was a specific exclusion criterion for the Myocarditis Treatment Trial. In contrast, Bozkurt et al.[26] reported that patients with PPCM treated with intravenous immunoglobulin had a greater improvement in ejection fraction during early follow-up than patients treated conventionally. In this retrospective study, the clinical outcomes of 6 women with PPCM treated with intravenous immunoglobulin (2 g/kg) were compared with those of 11 recent historical control subjects. All women in the study had class II-IV heart failure and a left ventricular ejection fraction < 40%. The 2 groups did not differ in terms of baseline left ventricular ejection fraction, left ventricular end-diastolic diameter, months to presentation, age, or multiparity. The improvement in left ventricular ejection fraction in patients treated with immunoglobulin was significantly greater than in the conventionally treated group (increase of 26 ± 8 ejection fraction units vs. 13 ± 13, $P = 0.042$).

HEART TRANSPLANT IN PERIPARTUM CARDIOMYOPATHY

Patients with PPCM who fail maximal medical management should be considered candidates for cardiac transplantation. In a study by Keogh et al.[27] of 10 PPCM patients who underwent heart transplantation, survival was similar to age-matched women undergoing heart transplantation for other reasons, but they noted a higher rate ($P = 0.05$) of biopsy-proven early rejection. PPCM patients had severe persistent episodes of rejection (40% of these rejection episodes required cytolytic therapy).

Aravot et al.[28] published their experience in 6 consecutive cases of PPCM treated by heart transplantation in which there were 2 postoperative deaths attributable to infection and rejection. Rickenbacher et al.[29] reported a 25% mortality rate during the first 6 months post-transplantation for their patients with PPCM. Aziz et al.[30] reported a good short-term outcome following cardiac transplantation in 3 patients after PPCM.

Johnson et al.[31] reported the overall experience from a large multi-institutional database of 3,244 adult heart transplant recipients. They compared the outcome of 40 women who underwent transplantation for PPCM with that of 200 women of childbearing age who underwent transplantation for other indications. Also, the outcome of 543 women with a history of pregnancy was compared with that of 101 nulliparous women and 2,562 men. The authors concluded that the long-term outcome of patients with a history of PPCM was similar to that of women of childbearing age who underwent transplantation for other reasons. Parous women had a significantly shorter time to first rejection ($P < 0.0001$) and a greater cumulative rejection than nulliparous women or men. By multivariable analysis, the risk factors for cumulative rejection at 1 year were a history of pregnancy ($P < 0.0001$), younger recipient age ($P < 0.0001$), induction therapy ($P < 0.0001$), and number of human leukocyte antigen-DR mismatches ($P = 0.007$). The authors concluded that previous pregnancy and not female sex per se was associated with an increased frequency of rejection after heart transplantation.

WHAT IS THE RISK OF ADDITIONAL PREGNANCIES IN PATIENTS WITH PERIPARTUM CARDIOMYOPATHY?

Future pregnancies in patients with PPCM are at increased risk of precipitating recurrent heart failure or progressive left ventricular dysfunction. Patients who have had PPCM, even if asymptomatic, are at increased risk for recurrence compared with baseline risk.

Elkayam et al.[32] reported the outcome of additional pregnancies in 44 women who had a history of PPCM and subsequently had a total of 60 pregnancies (Fig. 24-1). These patients were grouped into those in whom left ventricular function had returned to normal by echocardiographic criteria (28 patients) (group 1) and those with persistent left ventricular dysfunction (16 patients) (group 2). Both groups had a new reduction in the mean (± SD) left ventricular ejection fraction: from 56 ± 7% to 49 ± 10% in group 1 ($P = 0.002$) and from 36 ± 9% to 32 ± 11% in group 2 ($P = 0.08$). New symptoms of heart failure occurred during pregnancies in 21% of group 1 and 44% of group 2. The mortality rate was 0% in group 1 and 19% in group 2 ($P = 0.06$) (Table 24-3). The frequency of premature delivery was higher in group 2 (37%) than in group 1 (11%), as was that of therapeutic abortions (25% vs. 4%). The authors concluded that subsequent pregnancy in women with a history of PPCM is associated with a significant decrease in left ventricular function that can result

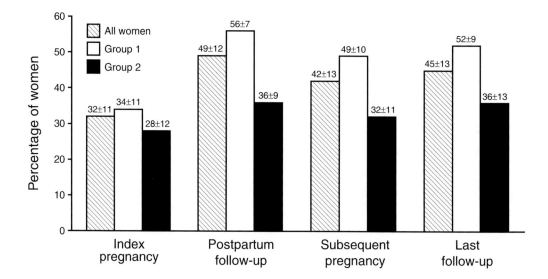

Fig. 24-1. Mean (±SD) left ventricular ejection fraction in 44 women at the time of the diagnosis of peripartum cardiomyopathy (index pregnancy), at postpartum follow-up, during the first subsequent pregnancy, and at the last follow-up a mean of 72 months after the first subsequent pregnancy. Group 1 included all the women with a left ventricular ejection fraction of 50% or higher before subsequent pregnancies, and group 2 included all those with a left ventricular ejection fraction of less than 50% before subsequent pregnancies. For group 1, $P < 0.001$ for the comparison between postpartum follow-up and the index pregnancy, $P = 0.002$ for the comparison between subsequent pregnancy and postpartum follow-up, and $P = 0.06$ for the comparison between last follow-up and subsequent pregnancy. For group 2, $P = 0.05$ for the comparison between postpartum follow-up and the index pregnancy, and $P = 0.08$ for the comparison between subsequent pregnancy and postpartum follow-up. (From Elkayam et al.[32] By permission of the Massachusetts Medical Society.)

in clinical heart failure or death and that a return of normal ventricular indices is not protective against a poor outcome at a subsequent pregnancy.

Patients with PPCM and residual left ventricular dysfunction have a significant risk of death if they become pregnant again. It remains unclear how to distinguish patients with recovered left ventricular function into those who can safely undergo subsequent pregnancy and those who cannot. In Demakis and associates' series,[3] 8 of 21 patients with return to normal heart size had subsequent pregnancies and only 2 experienced temporary recurrence of heart failure. Of the 13 patients with persistent cardiomegaly, 6 had subsequent pregnancies. Three of those 6 patients died. Ostrzega and Elkayam[33] examined 63 women diagnosed with PPCM who had 67 subsequent pregnancies. The maternal mortality was 2% in the patients with a history of PPCM who had recovery of left ventricular function compared with an 8% mortality among the patients with persistent left ventricular dysfunction.

Albanesi Filho and da Silva[34] prospectively studied 34 patients with the diagnosis of PPCM (mean age, 26 years). At first diagnosis, 5 were New York Heart Association functional class II for heart failure, 1 in functional class III, and 28 in functional class IV. After standard heart failure treatment, patients were advised to avoid further pregnancies.

Table 24-3
Incidence of Maternal Complications During the First Subsequent Pregnancy in Women Who Had Had Peripartum Cardiomyopathy*

Group	Women, no.	Symptoms of heart failure	> 20% Decrease in LVEF	Decreased LVEF at follow-up	Death
		Women, no. (%)			
All women	44				
Group 1	28	6 (21)	6 (21)	4 (14)	0
Group 2	16	7 (44)	4 (25)	5 (31)	3 (19)[†]
Women who did not have abortions	35				
Group 1	23	6 (26)	4 (17)	2 (9)	0
Group 2	12	6 (50)	4 (33)	5 (42)	3 (25)[‡]

*Group 1 consisted of women with recovered left ventricular function, defined as a left ventricular ejection fraction (LVEF) of 50% or higher, before the subsequent pregnancy; group 2 consisted of women with persistent left ventricular dysfunction (an LVEF of less than 50%).

[†]$P = 0.06$ for the comparison with group 1.

[‡]$P = 0.05$ for the comparison with group 1.

From Elkayam et al.[32] By permission of the Massachusetts Medical Society.

There were 12 (35.3%) subsequent pregnancies in patients aged 19 to 44 years (mean, 32 years), divided into 2 groups: group 1 had 6 patients whose heart size had returned to normal and group 2 had 6 patients with persistent cardiomegaly. Group 1 had initially mild clinical manifestations (3 patients were in functional class II, 1 in functional class III, and 2 in functional class IV) and complete recovery of cardiac function (functional class I). A new pregnancy was tolerated well in 5 (83.3%); 1 patient presented with preeclampsia and progressed to functional class II. Five patients are in functional class I and 1 is in functional class II. Group 2 patients had more severe heart failure at the onset of PPCM (1 in functional class II and 5 in functional class IV). During follow-up, 4 patients were in functional class I and 2 were in functional class II. A new pregnancy was tolerated well in all of them but the eldest, who had had 2 pregnancies and had a progressive worsening of clinical status. She died 8 years after the last pregnancy and 13 years after the diagnosis of PPCM. The remaining 5 patients are still alive, 3 in functional class I and 2 in functional class II, with worsening of functional class in 1. Subsequent pregnancies occurred between 3 and 7 years after the diagnosis of PPCM. The authors concluded that subsequent pregnancies are tolerated well after PPCM but not devoid of risk. A minimum interval of 3 years after the recovery of cardiac function seems to be optimal before subsequent pregnancies.

The long-term prognosis in PPCM varies and depends primarily on the extent to which left ventricular size and function return to normal. If the ejection fraction remains depressed 6 months after delivery, this is considered a poor prognostic indicator. In a study by Demakis et al.,[3] approximately half of the 27 women studied had persistent left ventricular dysfunction. This group had a high cardiac mortality (85% over 5 years) compared with the group in whom cardiac size returned to normal, who experienced no cardiac deaths in the same period. A further study by Sutton et al.[35] corroborated these results: 7 of 14 patients had a dramatic improvement in left ventricular ejection fraction soon after delivery, but 6 of the 7 patients in whom ventricular function remained abnormal died. Survivors had a higher mean ejection fraction (23% vs. 11%) and smaller mean left ventricular cavity size (5.8 vs. 6.9 cm) at presentation. Historically, PPCM has also been associated with multiparity.

Patients who have had a single episode of PPCM are at increased risk of a recurrence of heart failure compared with baseline risk. Patients whose left ventricular size or function does not return to normal are at high risk for recurrent PPCM with further pregnancies and should avoid subsequent pregnancy. Patients in whom ventricular function returns to normal echocardiographically pose a dilemma. In the study reported by Demakis et al.,[3] 8 of 14 patients in whom heart size returned to normal after a single episode of PPCM had subsequent pregnancies, and 2 patients developed clinical heart failure. Sutton et al.[35] reported no heart failure in 4 women whose heart size returned to normal after PPCM in a prior pregnancy. There is considerable interest in methods of identifying patients in whom left ventricular size and function have returned to normal, but who remain at risk of future heart failure.

Contractile reserve, the ability of the left ventricle to augment ventricular function in response to inotropes, usually dobutamine, has been studied in PPCM patients by Lampert et al.[36] (Fig. 24-2 and 24-3). Other authors also documented recurrent heart failure even if left ventricular size and function apparently return to normal.[37]

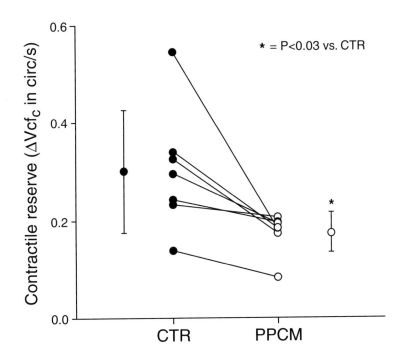

Fig. 24-2. Contractile reserve among recovered patients with peripartum cardiomyopathy and controls (*CTR*). Contractile reserve was defined as vertical deviation (change in rate-corrected velocity of circumferential fiber shortening in circulation per second) between baseline contractility line and dobutamine-induced shift in data point. Contractile reserve (*Delta Vcf*c) values are depicted for study patients (*open circles*) and respective controls (*closed circles*), each matched for age, race, and parity (*lines*). Contractile reserve was significantly lower in patients with a history of peripartum cardiomyopathy and recovered left ventricular function than in controls (*P* < 0.03). *PPCM*, peripartum cardiomyopathy with recovered left ventricular function. (From Lampert et al.[36] By permission of Mosby-Year Book.)

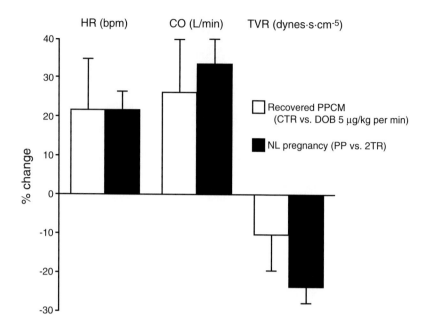

Fig. 24-3. Comparison of hemodynamic changes induced by dobutamine (*DOB*) in patients with recovered peripartum cardiomyopathy (*PPCM*) and in normal pregnancy (*CTR*). These results depict percent change in heart rate (*HR*), cardiac output (*CO*), and total vascular resistance (*TVR*) in 7 patients with recovered peripartum cardiomyopathy after infusion of dobutamine (5 µg/kg per min) (*white bars*) and 15 normal pregnant women (*black bars*). In latter group, percent change corresponds to those of second trimester (*2TR*) compared with 8 weeks post partum (*PP*). Results are expressed as mean ± SEM. (From Lampert et al.[36] By permission of Mosby-Year Book.)

REFERENCES

1. Gouley BA, McMillan TM, Bellet S. Idiopathic myocardial degeneration associated with pregnancy and especially puerperium. Am J Med Sci 1937;194:185-199.

2. Pearson GD, Veille J-C, Rahimtoola S, Hsia J, Oakley CM, Hosenpud JD, Ansari A, Baughman KL. Peripartum cardiomyopathy: National Heart, Lung, and Blood Institute and Office of Rare Diseases (National Institutes of Health) Workshop Recommendations and Review. JAMA 2000;283:1183-1188.

3. Demakis JG, Rahimtoola SH, Sutton GC, Meadows WR, Szanto PB, Tobin JR, Gunnar RM. Natural course of peripartum cardiomyopathy. Circulation 1971;44:1053-1061.

4. Ventura SJ, Peters KD, Martin JA, Maurer JD. Births and deaths: United States, 1996. Mon Vital Stat Rep 1997;46 Suppl 2:1-40.

5. Pierce JA, Price BO, Joyce JW. Familial occurrence of postpartal heart failure. Arch Intern Med 1963;111:651-655.

6. Massad LS, Reiss CK, Mutch DG, Haskel EJ. Familial peripartum cardiomyopathy after molar pregnancy. Obstet Gynecol 1993;81:886-888.

7. Pearl W. Familial occurrence of peripartum cardiomyopathy. Am Heart J 1995;129:421-422.

8. Melvin KR, Richardson PJ, Olsen EG, Daly K, Jackson G. Peripartum cardiomyopathy due to myocarditis. N Engl J Med 1982;307:731-734.

9. Rizeq MN, Rickenbacher PR, Fowler MB, Billingham ME. Incidence of myocarditis in peripartum cardiomyopathy. Am J Cardiol 1994;74:474-477.

10. Midei MG, DeMent SH, Feldman AM, Hutchins GM, Baughman KL. Peripartum myocarditis and cardiomyopathy. Circulation 1990;81:922-928.

11. Farber PA, Glasgow LA. Viral myocarditis during pregnancy: encephalomyocarditis virus infection in mice. Am Heart J 1970;80:96-102.

12. Lyden DC, Huber SA. Aggravation of coxsackievirus, group B, type 3-induced myocarditis and increase in cellular immunity to myocyte antigens in pregnant Balb/c mice and animals treated with progesterone. Cell Immunol 1984;87:462-472.

13. Felker GM, Jaeger CJ, Klodas E, Thiemann DR, Hare JM, Hruban RH, Kasper EK, Baughman KL. Myocarditis and long-term survival in peripartum cardiomyopathy. Am Heart J 2000;140:785-791.

14. O'Connell JB, Costanzo-Nordin MR, Subramanian R, Robinson JA, Wallis DE, Scanlon PJ, Gunnar RM. Peripartum cardiomyopathy: clinical, hemodynamic, histologic and prognostic characteristics. J Am Coll Cardiol 1986;8:52-56.

15. Davis MD, Murphy JG, Olson LJ, Warnes CA, Edwards WD, Rodeheffer RJ, Gersh BJ. Natural history and endomyocardial biopsy findings in peripartum cardiomyopathy (abstract). Circulation 1992;86 Suppl 1:I-439.

16. Chow LH, Radio SJ, Sears TD, McManus BM. Insensitivity of right ventricular endomyocardial biopsy in the diagnosis of myocarditis. J Am Coll Cardiol 1989;14:915-920.

17. Hauck AJ, Kearney DL, Edwards WD. Evaluation of postmortem endomyocardial biopsy specimens from 38 patients with lymphocytic myocarditis: implications for role of sampling error. Mayo Clin Proc 1989;64:1235-1245.

18. Lange LG, Schreiner GF. Immune mechanisms of cardiac disease. N Engl J Med 1994;330:1129-1135.

19. Geva T, Mauer MB, Striker L, Kirshon B, Pivarnik JM. Effects of physiologic load of pregnancy on left ventricular contractility and remodeling. Am Heart J 1997;133:53-59.

20. Russo LR, Besinger RE, Tomich PG, Thomas JX Jr. Effect of chronic tocolytic therapy on maternal ventricular function in pregnant rabbits. Am J Obstet Gynecol 1996;175:847-852.

21. Hibbard JU. Chronic terbutaline therapy and peripartum cardiomyopathy: a case-control study. Hypertens Pregnancy 1996;15:183-191.

22. Sliwa K, Skudicky D, Bergemann A, Candy G, Puren A, Sareli P. Peripartum cardiomyopathy: analysis of clinical outcome, left ventricular function, plasma levels of cytokines and Fas/APO-1. J Am Coll Cardiol 2000;35:701-705.

23. Cenac A, Simonoff M, Djibo A. Nutritional status and plasma trace elements in peripartum cardiomyopathy. A comparative study in Niger. J Cardiovasc Risk 1996;3:483-487.

24. de Belder AJ, Radomski MW, Why HJ, Richardson PJ, Martin JF. Myocardial calcium-independent nitric oxide synthase activity is present in dilated cardiomyopathy, myocarditis, and postpartum cardiomyopathy but not in ischaemic or valvar heart disease. Br Heart J 1995;74:426-430.

25. Mason JW, O'Connell JB, Herskowitz A, Rose NR, McManus BM, Billingham ME, Moon TE. A clinical trial of immunosuppressive therapy for myocarditis. The Myocarditis Treatment Trial Investigators. N Engl J Med 1995;333:269-275.

26. Bozkurt B, Villanueva FS, Holubkov R, Tokarczyk T, Alvarez RJ Jr, MacGowan GA, Murali S, Rosenblum WD, Feldman AM, McNamara DM. Intravenous immune globulin in the therapy of peripartum cardiomyopathy. J Am Coll Cardiol 1999;34:177-180.

27. Keogh A, Macdonald P, Spratt P, Marshman D, Larbalestier R, Kaan A. Outcome in peripartum cardiomyopathy after heart transplantation. J Heart Lung Transplant 1994;13:202-207.

28. Aravot DJ, Banner NR, Dhalla N, Fitzgerald M, Khaghani A, Radley-Smith R, Yacoub MH. Heart transplantation for peripartum cardiomyopathy. Lancet 1987;2:1024.

29. Rickenbacher PR, Rizeq MN, Hunt SA, Billingham ME, Fowler MB. Long-term outcome after heart transplantation for peripartum cardiomyopathy. Am Heart J 1994;127:1318-1323.

30. Aziz TM, Burgess MI, Acladious NN, Campbell CS, Rahman AN, Yonan N, Deiraniya AK. Heart transplantation for peripartum cardiomyopathy: a report of three cases and a literature review. Cardiovasc Surg 1999;7:565-567.

31. Johnson MR, Naftel DC, Hobbs RE, Kobashigawa JA, Pitts DE, Levine TB, Tolman D, Bhat G, Kirklin JK, Bourge RC. The incremental risk of female sex in heart transplantation: a multi-institutional study of peripartum cardiomyopathy and pregnancy. Cardiac Transplant Research Database Group. J Heart Lung Transplant 1997;16:801-812.

32. Elkayam U, Tummala PP, Rao K, Akhter MW, Karaalp IS, Wani OR, Hameed A, Gviazda I, Shotan A. Maternal and fetal outcomes of subsequent pregnancies in women with peripartum cardiomyopathy. N Engl J Med 2001;344:1567-1571.

33. Ostrzega E, Elkayam U. Risk of subsequent pregnancy in women with a history of peripartum cardiomyopathy: results of a survey (abstract). Circulation 1995;92 Suppl 1:I-333.

34. Albanesi Filho FM, da Silva TT. Natural course of subsequent pregnancy after peripartum cardiomyopathy. Arq Bras Cardiol 1999;73:47-57.

35. Sutton MS, Cole P, Plappert M, Saltzman D, Goldhaber S. Effects of subsequent pregnancy on left ventricular function in peripartum cardiomyopathy. Am Heart J 1991;121:1776-1778.

36. Lampert MB, Weinert L, Hibbard J, Korcarz C, Lindheimer M, Lang RM. Contractile reserve in patients with peripartum cardiomyopathy and recovered left ventricular function. Am J Obstet Gynecol 1997;176:189-195.

37. Ceci O, Berardesca C, Caradonna F, Corsano P, Guglielmi R, Nappi L. Recurrent peripartum cardiomyopathy. Eur J Obstet Gynecol Reprod Biol 1998;76:29-30.

Index